Current Trends, Innovations and Issues in Nursing Practice and Education

Current Trends, Innovations and Issues in Nursing Practice and Education

Guest Editors

Antonio Martinez-Sabater
Elena Chover-Sierra
Carles Saus-Ortega

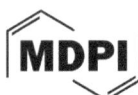

Basel • Beijing • Wuhan • Barcelona • Belgrade • Novi Sad • Cluj • Manchester

Guest Editors

Antonio Martinez-Sabater	Elena Chover-Sierra	Carles Saus-Ortega
Nursing Department	Nursing Department	Nursing Department
University of Valencia	University of Valencia	University of Valencia
Valencia	Valencia	Valencia
Spain	Spain	Spain

Editorial Office
MDPI AG
Grosspeteranlage 5
4052 Basel, Switzerland

This is a reprint of the Special Issue, published open access by the journal *Nursing Reports* (ISSN 2039-4403), freely accessible at: https://www.mdpi.com/journal/nursrep/special_issues/O80F4L4FRB.

For citation purposes, cite each article independently as indicated on the article page online and as indicated below:

Lastname, A.A.; Lastname, B.B. Article Title. *Journal Name* **Year**, *Volume Number*, Page Range.

ISBN 978-3-7258-3996-4 (Hbk)
ISBN 978-3-7258-3995-7 (PDF)
https://doi.org/10.3390/books978-3-7258-3995-7

© 2025 by the authors. Articles in this book are Open Access and distributed under the Creative Commons Attribution (CC BY) license. The book as a whole is distributed by MDPI under the terms and conditions of the Creative Commons Attribution-NonCommercial-NoDerivs (CC BY-NC-ND) license (https://creativecommons.org/licenses/by-nc-nd/4.0/).

Contents

About the Editors ix

Preface xi

Laura A. Robinson, Pamela R. Short and Andrew D. Frugé
Sleep Quality and Interoception Are Associated with Generalized Anxiety in Baccalaureate Nursing Students: A Cross-Sectional Study
Reprinted from: *Nurs. Rep.* **2024**, *15*, 90, https://doi.org/10.3390/nursrep14020090 1

Héctor González-de la Torre, María-Naira Hernández-De Luis, Sergio Mies-Padilla, Rafaela Camacho-Bejarano, José Verdú-Soriano and Claudio-Alberto Rodríguez-Suárez
Effectiveness of "Escape Room" Educational Technology in Nurses' Education: A Systematic Review
Reprinted from: *Nurs. Rep.* **2024**, *14*, 91, https://doi.org/10.3390/nursrep14020091 10

Anne White, Mary Beth Maguire, Austin Brown and Diane Keen
Impact of Artificial Intelligence on Nursing Students' Attitudes toward Older Adults: A Pre/Post-Study
Reprinted from: *Nurs. Rep.* **2024**, *14*, 85, https://doi.org/10.3390/nursrep14020085 29

Berit Sandberg
Effects of Arts-Based Pedagogy on Competence Development in Nursing: A Critical Systematic Review
Reprinted from: *Nurs. Rep.* **2024**, *14*, 83, https://doi.org/10.3390/nursrep14020083 36

L. Iván Mayor-Silva, Alfonso Meneses-Monroy, Leyre Rodriguez-Leal and Guillermo Moreno
An Exploration of Resilience and Positive Affect among Undergraduate Nursing Students: A Longitudinal Observational Study
Reprinted from: *Nurs. Rep.* **2024**, *14*, 67, https://doi.org/10.3390/nursrep14020067 66

Ingrid Rachel Strand, Unni Knutstad, Anton Havnes and Mette Sagbakken
Addressing a Critical Voice in Clinical Practice: Experiences of Nursing Students, Teachers, and Supervisors—A Qualitative Study
Reprinted from: *Nurs. Rep.* **2024**, *14*, 61, https://doi.org/10.3390/nursrep14020061 78

Lydia Pfeifer, Sophia Fries, Alexander Stirner, Lisa Nagel, Christian Cohnen, Leona Aschentrup, et al.
Positive Aspects and Potential Drawbacks of Implementing Digital Teaching/Learning Scenarios in Health Professions Using Nursing Education as an Example: A Research Report from Germany
Reprinted from: *Nurs. Rep.* **2024**, *14*, 36, https://doi.org/10.3390/nursrep14010036 91

Leodoro J. Labrague
Umbrella Review: Stress Levels, Sources of Stress, and Coping Mechanisms among Student Nurses
Reprinted from: *Nurs. Rep.* **2024**, *14*, 28, https://doi.org/10.3390/nursrep14010028 105

L. S. Hlahla, C. Ngoatle, M. N. Kgatla and E. M. Mathapo-Thobakgale
Challenges Faced by University of Limpopo Learner Nurses during Psychiatry Clinical Exposure: A Qualitative Study
Reprinted from: *Nurs. Rep.* **2024**, *14*, 14, https://doi.org/10.3390/nursrep14010014 119

Guillermo Moreno, Alfonso Meneses-Monroy, Samir Mohamedi-Abdelkader, Felice Curcio, Raquel Domínguez-Capilla, Carmen Martínez-Rincón, et al.
Virtual Active Learning to Maximize Knowledge Acquisition in Nursing Students: A Comparative Study
Reprinted from: Nurs. Rep. 2024, 14, 11, https://doi.org/10.3390/nursrep14010011 129

Irene Tárrega-Piquer, María Jesús Valero-Chillerón, Víctor Manuel González-Chordá, Irene Llagostera-Reverter, Águeda Cervera-Gasch, Laura Andreu-Pejo, et al.
Nomophobia and Its Relationship with Social Anxiety and Procrastination in Nursing Students: An Observational Study
Reprinted from: Nurs. Rep. 2023, 13, 140, https://doi.org/10.3390/nursrep13040140 141

Hanan A. Alkorashy and Hanan A. Alotaibi
Locus of Control and Self-Directed Learning Readiness of Nursing Students during the COVID-19 Pandemic: A Cross-Sectional Study from Saudi Arabia
Reprinted from: Nurs. Rep. 2023, 13, 137, https://doi.org/10.3390/nursrep13040137 152

Laura Parra-Anguita, María Dolores López-Franco, Juan Miguel Martínez-Galiano, Manuel González-Cabrera, Sara Moreno-Cámara and Nani Granero-Moya
Evaluation of the Use of Project-Based Learning in the Nursing Degree
Reprinted from: Nurs. Rep. 2023, 13, 136, https://doi.org/10.3390/nursrep13040136 165

José Carlos López-García, Azucena González-Sanz, Elena Sutil-Rodríguez, Carlos Saus-Ortega, Regina Ruiz de Viñaspre-Hernádez, Raúl Juárez-Vela, et al.
Analysis of the Attitudes towards Sexuality in People with Intellectual Disabilities: A Cross-Sectional Study
Reprinted from: Nurs. Rep. 2023, 13, 134, https://doi.org/10.3390/nursrep13040134 175

Teresa Sufrate-Sorzano, Marco Di Nitto, María Elena Garrote-Cámara, Fidel Molina-Luque, José Ignacio Recio-Rodríguez, Pilar Asión-Polo, et al.
Media Exposure of Suicidal Behaviour: An Umbrella Review
Reprinted from: Nurs. Rep. 2023, 13, 125, https://doi.org/10.3390/nursrep13040125 186

Lisa A. Babkair, Razan A. Safhi, Raghad Balshram, Rahaf Safhei, Atheer Almahamdy, et al.
Nursing Care for Stroke Patients: Current Practice and Future Needs
Reprinted from: Nurs. Rep. 2023, 13, 106, https://doi.org/10.3390/nursrep13030106 200

Makoto Tsukuda, Atsuko Fukuda, Junko Shogaki and Ikuko Miyawaki
Validity and Reliability of a Short Form of the Questionnaire for the Reflective Practice of Nursing Involving Invasive Mechanical Ventilation: A Cross-Sectional Study
Reprinted from: Nurs. Rep. 2023, 13, 101, https://doi.org/10.3390/nursrep13030101 215

Florence M. F. Wong and David C. N. Wong
A Modified Guideline for High-Fidelity Patient Simulation to Improve Student Satisfaction and Self-Confidence in Learning: A Mixed Study
Reprinted from: Nurs. Rep. 2023, 13, 90, https://doi.org/10.3390/nursrep13030090 230

Yoonhee Seok, Yoomi Cho, Nayoung Kim and Eunyoung E. Suh
Degree of Alarm Fatigue and Mental Workload of Hospital Nurses in Intensive Care Units
Reprinted from: Nurs. Rep. 2023, 13, 83, https://doi.org/10.3390/nursrep13030083 240

Sofia de Sá, Ana Baião, Helena Marques, Maria do Céu Marques, Maria José Reis, Sandra Dias and Marta Catarino
The Influence of Smartphones on Adolescent Sleep: A Systematic Literature Review
Reprinted from: Nurs. Rep. 2023, 13, 54, https://doi.org/10.3390/nursrep13020054 250

Lars Kyte, Ingrid Lindaas, Hellen Dahl, Irene Valaker, Ole T. Kleiven and Solveig Sægrov
Nursing Students' Preferences for Learning Medical and Bioscience Subjects: A Qualitative Study
Reprinted from: *Nurs. Rep.* **2023**, *13*, 55, https://doi.org/10.3390/nursrep13020055 260

Makoto Tsukuda, Yoshiyasu Ito, Shota Kakazu, Katsuko Sakamoto and Junko Honda
Development and Validity of the Japanese Version of the Questionnaire on Factors That Influence Family Engagement in Acute Care Settings
Reprinted from: *Nurs. Rep.* **2023**, *13*, 53, https://doi.org/10.3390/nursrep13020053 272

Ramoipei J. Phage, Boitumelo J. Molato and Molekodi J. Matsipane
Challenges Regarding Transition from Case-Based Learning to Problem-Based Learning: A Qualitative Study with Student Nurses
Reprinted from: *Nurs. Rep.* **2023**, *13*, 36, https://doi.org/10.3390/nursrep13010036 283

Júlio Belo Fernandes, Josefa Domingos, John Dean, Sónia Fernandes, Rogério Ferreira, Cristina Lavareda Baixinho
Nurses' Motivations, Barriers, and Facilitators to Engage in a Peer Review Process: A Qualitative Study Protocol
Reprinted from: *Nurs. Rep.* **2023**, *13*, 29, https://doi.org/10.3390/nursrep13010029 298

Stefano Bambi, Eustachio Parente, Yari Bardacci, Samuele Baldassini Rodriguez, Carolina Forciniti, Lorenzo Ballerini, et al.
The Effectiveness of NIV and CPAP Training on the Job in COVID-19 Acute Care Wards: A Nurses' Self-Assessment of Skills
Reprinted from: *Nurs. Rep.* **2023**, *13*, 2, https://doi.org/10.3390/nursrep13010002 306

Karolina Krupa-Kotara, Mateusz Grajek, Agata Wypych-Ślusarska, Sandra Martynus-Depta, Klaudia Oleksiuk, Joanna Głogowska-Ligus, et al.
Properties of Polyunsaturated Fatty Acids in Primary and Secondary Prevention of Cardiovascular Diseases in the View of Patients (Silesia, Poland)
Reprinted from: *Nurs. Rep.* **2022**, *12*, 94, https://doi.org/10.3390/nursrep12040094 318

About the Editors

Antonio Martinez-Sabater

Professor Martinez-Sabater is a nurse and professor in the Department of Nursing at the University of Valencia. He combines teaching with care at the University Clinical Hospital of Valencia and his tenure as Dean of the Faculty of Nursing and Podiatry at the University of Valencia.

Elena Chover-Sierra

Dr. Elena Chover is a nurse and professor at the University of Valencia, combining her teaching work with her care work at the General University Hospital of Valencia. She has extensive research experience.

Carles Saus-Ortega

Professor Saus-Ortega is a nurse, midwife, and professor at the University of Valencia. She combines her teaching with her leadership as director of the La Fe School of Nursing and is a member of the GRIECE research group.

Preface

Nursing practice and education are undergoing a profound transformation, driven by technological advances and social and healthcare changes. This Special Issue of *Nursing Reports*, entitled "Current Trends, Innovations and Issues in Nursing Practice and Education" and edited by Drs. Antonio Martínez-Sabater, Elena Chover-Sierra, and Carles Saus-Ortega, brings together contributions that address the need to adapt the training of healthcare professionals from the undergraduate level, integrating knowledge, skills, and attitudes aimed at improving patient safety and quality of care.

The main objective is to explore and disseminate studies that analyze trends, challenges, and innovations that are shaping contemporary nursing. The scope includes theoretical and empirical research focused on undergraduate training, clinical practice, professional competencies, applied technology, and adaptation to changing contexts such as the COVID-19 pandemic.

The motivation for this publication arises from the urgency of updating pedagogical and professional models based on solid evidence. The pandemic acted as a catalyst for multiple changes, revealing both strengths and areas for improvement in nursing education and practice.

This issue presents works by authors from different countries, addressing diverse approaches: from care plans as a learning strategy to the use of simulation, gamification, health literacy, and the impact of the pandemic on clinical training.

We deeply thank the authors, reviewers, and the *Nursing Reports* editorial team for their commitment to quality and innovation. We also extend our appreciation to the institutions, students, and professionals who made this compendium possible.

Nursing is at a pivotal moment in which the ability to innovate and adapt will be essential to facing the challenges of the future. This Special Issue seeks to be not only a compilation of research but also an invitation to action, collaboration, and commitment to ethical and evidence-based practice.

Antonio Martinez-Sabater, Elena Chover-Sierra, and Carles Saus-Ortega
Guest Editors

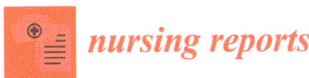

Communication

Sleep Quality and Interoception Are Associated with Generalized Anxiety in Baccalaureate Nursing Students: A Cross-Sectional Study

Laura A. Robinson [1,2], Pamela R. Short [2] and Andrew D. Frugé [2,*]

1. Department of Nutritional Science, Auburn University, Auburn, AL 36849, USA
2. College of Nursing, Auburn University, Auburn, AL 36849, USA
* Correspondence: fruge@auburn.edu

Abstract: Baccalaureate nursing students are at increased risk for anxiety and related mood disorders. We conducted a cross-sectional study to explore the relationships among anxiety symptoms measured by the Generalized Anxiety Disorder (GAD-7) questionnaire and lifestyle behaviors including habitual diet, sleep quality (Pittsburg Sleep Quality Index [PSQI]), and physical activity. Descriptive statistics were obtained for sample characteristics, and Pearson correlations and backward stepwise linear regression explored relationships between the GAD-7 scores, the Multidimensional Assessment of Interoceptive Awareness, version 2 (MAIA-2) subscales, and other variables. Sixty-eight students completed the survey, with 38% having moderate-to-severe anxiety. On average, respondents had moderate diet quality (Healthy Eating Index median 60/100 [range 51–75]), had high sleep quality (PSQI median 7/21 [range 4–10]), and were highly active, with a median of 43 (range 24–78) weekly metabolic equivalent (MET) hours. Sixty-seven out of 68 respondents indicated a willingness to change lifestyle behaviors; the most prevalent time-related factors were school and social commitments, with stress and financial constraints being reported among half or more of respondents. Regression analysis determined that PSQI ($\beta = 0.446$) and the MAIA-2 Not-Worrying subscale ($\beta = -0.366$) were significant ($p < 0.001$ for both) predictors of anxiety severity. These results indicate that mindfulness and sleep hygiene may be the most actionable foci for interventions to reduce anxiety in baccalaureate nursing students. This study was not registered as a clinical trial.

Keywords: nursing students; sleep quality; diet quality; anxiety; physical activity; interoception

1. Introduction

Anxiety disorders rank among the top ten leading causes of disability in adolescents and young adults, impacting approximately 301 million people globally [1,2]. Concurrently, psychological distress among American college students has reached unprecedented levels [3], with 61% of students reporting anxiety and depression as primary reasons for seeking counseling [4]. Amid a myriad of stress-inducing factors, eight in ten students report experiencing extreme stress regarding their uncertain future [3,5]. Baccalaureate nursing programs pose unique challenges as students must navigate rigorous and fast-paced coursework while consistently demonstrating robust critical thinking skills and effective time management [6]. The most prominent stressors for nursing students include academic demands, fear of making mistakes with patients or when handling technical equipment, relationships within the clinical environment, and the responsibilities associated with patient and family care [7,8]. The integration of theoretical knowledge and clinical practice in nursing education not only makes the process challenging and stressful but also leads to heightened anxiety, with studies indicating that over 30% of nursing students experience high levels of anxiety [9].

Several factors that predict academic stress and achievement are associated with life satisfaction, psychological well-being, one's relationship with happiness, and one's locus of control [10]. One study found that 66.5% of surveyed nursing students had experienced varying levels of anxiety crises, with 48.8% of these students choosing not to seek assistance for mitigation of their anxiety or stress [11]. Academic stress has been linked to health concerns such as physical exhaustion, sleeping disorders, irritability, negative thoughts, and heightened nervousness [12]. Additionally, increased stress levels have been observed to contribute to the consumption of unhealthy foods while simultaneously reducing the intake of healthy options [13]. College students experiencing higher stress levels demonstrated a greater tendency to dine out, indulge in sugary snacks, and skip meals, ultimately leading to overeating [14,15]. One study involving 523 students revealed that nearly 83% experienced moderate-to-high levels of stress, while over 80% exhibited low-to-medium levels of self-regulation in their eating habits [15]. Emotional eating and overeating have been linked to increased stress, depression, and increased body mass index (BMI) [16]. In contrast, regular physical activity and increased sleep have a positive influence on stress markers in adults [17,18].

Given the greater demands and potential stressors of nursing school and increased awareness of anxiety in undergraduate students, we sought to assess anxiety symptoms, diet quality, physical activity, sleep quality, and interoceptive awareness among undergraduate nursing students. Additionally, we aimed to explore the relationships among these factors to determine predictors of increased anxiety. We hypothesized that the majority of nursing students would report experiencing mild-to-moderate anxiety levels and exhibit lower interoceptive awareness.

2. Materials and Methods

2.1. Participants

A convenience sample was obtained after exempt Institutional Review Board (IRB) approval was provided by the Auburn University IRB. Students in the second and third semester of the baccalaureate nursing program were approached during the first week of their respective semesters. An email with an information letter and survey link was provided on 18 August 2023, and the Qualtrics survey was open a total of ten days, with additional reminders sent on days three and seven. Surveys were completed anonymously; however, students could opt in to a draw for one of 25 10USD gift cards via a separate

2.2. Measures

2.2.1. Generalized Anxiety

The seven-item generalized anxiety disorder screener (GAD-7) was used to assess anxiety symptom severity [19]. Each item is rated on a four-point Likert scale (0–3), with total scores ranging from 0 to 21, where higher scores indicate greater severity of anxiety. The GAD-7 has shown good reliability and construct validity with a Cronbach alpha ranging from $\alpha = 0.88$ to $\alpha = 0.93$ [19,20].

2.2.2. Interoceptive Awareness

Interoceptive awareness was assessed using the Multidimensional Assessment of Interoceptive Awareness, version 2 (MAIA-2). The MAIA-2 consists of a 37-item questionnaire measuring across eight subscales: (i) Noticing, which assesses awareness of various body sensations; (ii) Not-Distracting, which evaluates the tendency to avoid ignoring sensations of pain or discomfort; (iii) Not-Worrying, related to avoiding emotional distress in response to pain; (iv) Attention Regulation, concerning the control and maintenance of attention to body sensations; (v) Emotional Awareness, which links body sensations to emotional states; (vi) Self-Regulation, involving the management of psychological distress through body awareness; (vii) Body Listening, which focuses on gaining insights by listening to the body; and (viii) Trusting, the perception of the body as safe and reliable. The MAIA-2 employs a 6-point Likert scale (0–5) for scoring, with average scores for each subscale indicating the level of interoceptive awareness, where higher scores represent greater awareness.

The subscales exhibit Cronbach's alpha values ranging from 0.64 to 0.83, indicating their reliability [21].

2.2.3. Sleep Quality

Sleep quality was assessed using the Pittsburg Sleep Quality Index. The 19-item self-report questionnaire measures seven components of sleep: subjective sleep quality, sleep latency, sleep duration, habitual sleep efficiency, sleep disturbances, use of sleeping medication, and daytime dysfunction. A score above 5 on this scale effectively distinguishes between good and poor sleepers. The Global Sleep Quality scale, with a reported Cronbach's alpha of 0.83, demonstrates its reliability [22].

2.2.4. Physical Activity

The modified 5-item physical activity questionnaire (PAQ-M) assesses the number of hours spent weekly in physical activity across light, moderate, and vigorous activities as well as in resistance training. The PAQ-M has test–retest reliability with an intraclass correlation of 0.87 [23]. Times spent in each domain were multiplied by an average metabolic equivalent (MET) to estimate total MET hours per week of physical activity [24].

2.2.5. Diet Quality

Seven questions were used to assess habitual diet over the previous thirty days using the Global Assessment Tool 2.0 and Health Eating Score-5 (HES-5) [25]. A Cronbach test determined that HES-5 yielded an internal consistency reliability coefficient of 0.81 [26]. The short Healthy Eating Index (s-HEI) scoring criteria were used to scale responses to the Dietary Guidelines for Americans HEI, resulting in a relative diet quality score out of 100 [27].

2.2.6. Perceived Health and Willingness to Change

Perceived health was assessed with the first question from the RAND Short-Form 12-Item Health Survey [28], and four questions asked whether a change in health behaviors was currently a priority, the timing of willingness to change, and barriers to change [29]. In the general US population, the RAND Short-Form 12-Item Health Survey demonstrated reliability with test–retest correlations of 0.89 for the 12-item Physical Component Summary and 0.76 for the 12-item Mental Component Summary [28].

2.2.7. Demographics and Anthropometrics

Demographic variables were obtained using standard US census methods. Current height was reported in feet and inches, and current weight was reported in pounds. BMI was calculated and reported in kg/m^2.

2.3. Statistical Analysis

Statistical analyses were conducted in SPSS Version 29.0 (IBM Corp, Armonk, NY, USA). Descriptive statistics were obtained for sample characteristics, and Pearson correlations explored relationships between independent variables and GAD-7 scores and MAIA-2 subscales. Backward stepwise linear regression with GAD-7 score as the dependent variable was used to determine the predictive value of highly correlated factors.

3. Results

Of 180 potential second- and third-semester students, 68 (37.7%) completed the survey. Demographics characteristics were mostly representative of the nursing student population with regard to gender, race, and ethnicity (Table 1). Physical activity levels were skewed, ranging from 24 to 48 MET hours/week. Diet quality was moderate overall, ranging from 51 to 75 out of a possible 100 points. Sleep quality was concentrated on the low (better) end, ranging from 4 to 10 out of 21 points. Finally, most students had normal-weight BMI. According to GAD-7 scores, roughly 60% of respondents had minimal or mild anxiety, with 25% having moderate and 15% having severe anxiety. No students self-reported poor health, while slightly more than half of students reported very good or excellent health.

Table 1. Characteristics of baccalaureate nursing student participants.

	N (%)
Female gender	64 (94.1%)
White race	66 (97.1%)
Hispanic ethnicity	2 (2.9%)
Age; median (range)	21 (19–26)
Earned associate degree	2 (2.9%)
Prior military service	2 (2.9%)
Lifestyle factors	
MET hours/week; median (range)	43 (24–78)
Diet Quality (HEI Score); median (range)	60 (51–75)
Sleep Score (PSQI Global Score); median (range)	7 (4–10)
BMI; mean (SD)	23.2 (3.8)
GAD-7	
Minimal anxiety	25 (36.8%)
Mild anxiety	16 (23.5%)
Moderate anxiety	17 (25%)
Severe anxiety	10 (14.7%)
General health status	
Fair or good	31 (45.6%)
Very good or excellent	37 (54.4%)
Willing to change	67 (98.5%)
Barriers to change; median (range)	4 (1–8)

Sixty-seven out of 68 students reported they were willing to change their health behaviors, providing one to eight specific barriers, with four as the median. The most prevalent time-related factors were school and social commitments, with stress and financial constraints rounding out the other top choices reported by at least half of the students (Figure 1).

What barriers do you believe may hinder improvements in any of these health behaviors (diet, sleep, exercise, and/or stress reduction)?

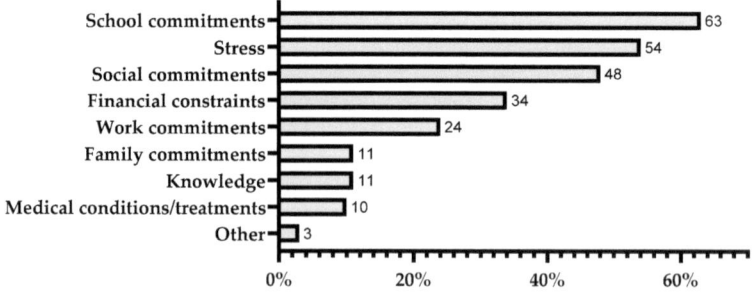

Figure 1. Self-reported perceived barriers to changing health behaviors in baccalaureate nursing students (n = 68).

Backward stepwise regression, with GAD-7 scores as the dependent variable, reduced five highly correlated independent variables to three, omitting barriers to change and the MAIA-2 Trusting subscale in the final model. Sleep quality (β = 0.446) and the MAIA-2 Not-Worrying subscale (β = -0.366) were the remaining significant ($p < 0.001$ for both) predictors of anxiety severity (Table 2).

Table 2. Backward stepwise regression of variables predicting anxiety severity in baccalaureate nursing students ($n = 68$).

Model	Dependent Variable: GAD-7	Beta	t	Sig.
	(Constant)		3.135	0.003
	Sleep quality (PSQI)	0.413	4.296	<0.001
	Perceived health	−0.159	−1.715	0.091
	Number of barriers to behavior change	0.128	1.450	0.152
	MAIA Not-Worrying	−0.361	−3.868	<0.001
	MAIA Trusting	−0.045	−0.477	0.635
2	(Constant)		3.295	<0.001
	Sleep quality (PSQI)	0.425	4.602	<0.001
	Perceived health	−0.173	−1.954	0.055
	Number of barriers to behavior change	0.133	1.526	0.132
	MAIA Not-Worrying	−0.357	−3.865	<0.001
3	(Constant)		4.679	<0.001
	Sleep quality (PSQI)	0.446	4.823	<0.001
	Perceived health	−0.168	−1.887	0.064
	MAIA Not-Worrying	−0.366	−3.93	<0.001

Correlations between GAD-7 score and MAIA-2 subscales are displayed in Figure 2. Anxiety symptom severity was most strongly associated with the Not-Worrying subscale ($r = -0.547$, $p < 0.001$), followed by the Trusting ($r = -0.262$, $p = 0.031$), Self-Regulation ($r = -0.256$, $p = 0.035$), and Attention Regulation ($r = -0.218$, $p = 0.075$) subscales.

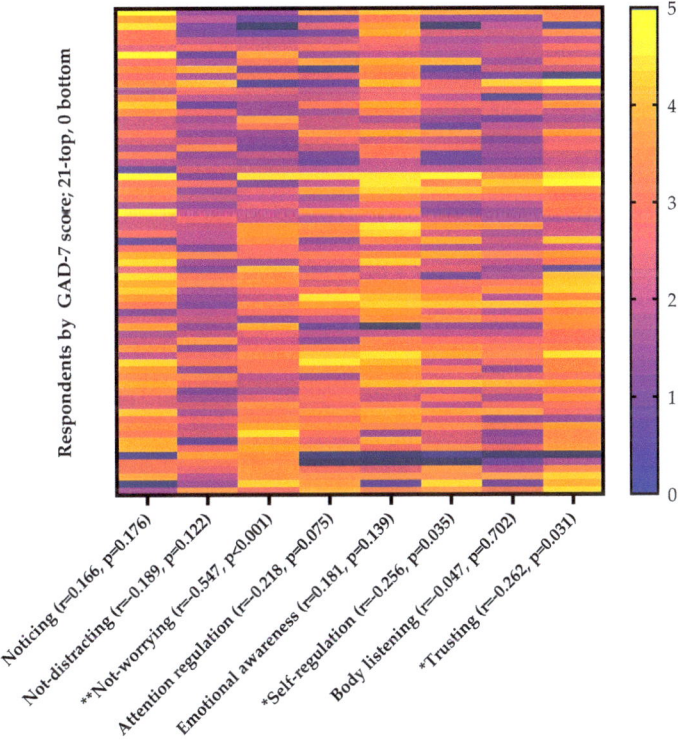

Figure 2. Heatmap of MAIA-2 subscales ordered by the respondents' GAD-7 score. Rows represent individual respondents' subscale scores, with respondents ($n = 68$) listed by decreasing GAD-7 scores from top to bottom. * $p < 0.05$; ** $p < 0.005$.

4. Discussion

In our study of baccalaureate nursing students, we found that respondents generally reported moderate diet quality and high sleep quality and maintained high levels of physical activity. However, GAD-7 testing showed that 40% of students experienced moderate-to-severe anxiety. Notably, sleep quality and the Not-Worrying subscale of the MAIA-2 questionnaire emerged as significant predictors of anxiety severity. Our analysis revealed that various MAIA-2 subscales, particularly Not-Worrying, Trusting, Self-Regulation, and Attention Regulation, exhibited the strongest correlations with anxiety symptom severity. Importantly, 99% of respondents reported that they were willing to change their health behaviors for the better.

Given that a majority of respondents self-reported minimal or mild anxiety levels along with moderate-to-high diet quality, physical activity, and sleep quality, our findings are consistent with previous research exploring the connections between health behaviors and mental health [6,17,18]. A systematic review conducted by Saha and colleagues [30] highlights the relationship between diet and symptoms of anxiety and depression in college students. Among the 21 studies reviewed, including four interventional studies, the majority demonstrated positive associations between a healthy diet and improved mental health during college. In a similar vein, a series of pilot studies investigated the impact of regular physical activity on mental health and well-being, as well as the health benefits of short-term aerobic exercise, in university students. These studies revealed a negative correlation between regular exercise and self-reported anxiety, depression, and perceived psychosomatic stress. Additionally, cardiovascular fitness was inversely associated with self-reported anxiety, depression, and stress related to uncertainty [31]. A cross-sectional study in Indian college students observed significant inverse relationships between moderate and high physical activity levels and anxiety and depression scores, while sleep quality was positively associated with anxiety and depression [32]. Furthermore, in a moderation mediation analysis conducted on higher education students from seven countries, it was found that perceived stress and anxiety were negatively associated with sleep quality, but this relationship was weakened by increased psychological resilience [33]. Collectively, these findings highlight the effects of lifestyle behaviors on reducing anxiety levels in college students.

Interoceptive awareness, as defined by Price and Hooven [34], refers to the capacity to recognize internal bodily sensations, encompassing heart rate, respiration, hunger, satiety, temperature, pain, and emotional sensations. Several studies have investigated the relationships between anxiety and interoception in this population. Our study found that the Not-Worrying, Trusting, and Self-Regulation subscales from the MAIA-2 displayed strong negative correlations with anxiety levels among nursing students. Other studies of college students have revealed that higher interoceptive scores are associated with increased feelings of self-efficacy in learning, improved self-regulation of attention, enhanced academic performance, and higher grade point averages [35,36]. Interoceptive awareness also serves as an effective measure for assessing the outcomes of stress and relaxation training in practicing nurses. One study found that Self-Regulation score was negatively correlated with and predictive of anxiety in both hospital nurses and university students, while nurses specifically exhibited higher anxiety levels and lower mean Body Listening scores compared to university students [37]. Similar to our findings, Kabir et al. found that MAIA-2 subscales Noticing, Not-Distracting, Not-Worrying, Emotional Awareness, Self-Regulation, and Trusting negatively predicted anxiety in both groups.

Despite the fact that most participants self-reported having very good or excellent health, a significant majority of them expressed a willingness to change their health behaviors. Participants identified school and social commitments, stress, and financial constraints as the most relevant perceived barriers to making changes in their health behaviors. While certain barriers may be non-modifiable (e.g., financial constraints and medical conditions), addressing stress and time management offers potential solutions to these challenges. In one trial, progressive muscle relaxation exercises performed for 45 min 5 days per week for two weeks, along with an additional 10–15 min training session performed every day at home, reduced anxiety among nursing students [38]. Similarly, a study conducted by Almarcha and colleagues found that participants involved in an exercise regime experienced increased mental health and interoceptive awareness scores. Interoceptive scores increased further for those who were able to co-design their exercise regime [39]. Finally, in a study assessing the impact of a time management training program on time management and anxiety among nursing undergraduate students, significant improvements were reported. Students paid more attention to the value of time, engaged in more time management behaviors, and increased their time efficacy [40].

Recent research offers strong evidence for the efficacy of targeted interventions in reducing stress and anxiety among nursing students and healthcare providers. For example, a systematic review identified 18 studies highlighting cognitive behavioral therapy (CBT) and mindfulness-based stress reduction (MBSR) as particularly effective in alleviating stress, anxiety, and depression among undergraduate nursing students [41]. Additionally, a specialized two-phase intervention program incorporating CBT and progressive muscle relaxation demonstrated significant reductions in stress and anxiety levels among nursing students after just the first three-month phase, enhancing their ability to manage clinical demands more effectively [42]. Moreover, Heeter and colleagues found that engaging in 10–12 min of yoga and meditation via smartphone apps over six weeks significantly enhanced participants' perceived ability to focus on body sensations and emotions. Such technology-assisted meditation programs have also been shown to enhance interoceptive awareness and reduce compassion fatigue and burnout among healthcare providers [43]. Building on these findings, future interventions could integrate cognitive behavioral strategies, reinforced peer support, and innovative technology-assisted mindfulness practices to comprehensively address the mental health needs and enhance the overall well-being of nursing students.

This study possesses noteworthy limitations that impact the generalizability of our findings. First, we acknowledge the subjective nature of our data, which is inherent in survey research. While we used validated assessments of dietary, physical activity, and sleep habits, recall bias is highly probable. Second, the sample was predominantly composed of white females. This lack of diversity makes it challenging to extrapolate the study's findings to a broader population, though it is representative of most baccalaureate nursing programs in the United States. Additionally, the administration of the survey exclusively in a southeastern United States university further limits its applicability to the national student population or associate degree nursing programs.

5. Conclusions

These results suggest that anxiety is highly prevalent among undergraduate nursing students, and mindfulness and sleep hygiene may be ideal behaviors to modify for anxiety reduction. Baccalaureate nursing programs are encouraged to assess and intervene to promote programmatic and long-term professional success for its current and future nursing students.

Author Contributions: Conceptualization, methodology, data curation, writing—review and editing, L.A.R., P.R.S. and A.D.F.; writing—original draft preparation, L.A.R.; visualization, A.D.F. All authors have read and agreed to the published version of the manuscript.

Funding: This research received no external funding.

Institutional Review Board Statement: The study was conducted in accordance with the Declaration of Helsinki and approved by the Auburn University Institutional Review Board (protocol code 23-389 EX 2308, approved 23 August 2023).

Informed Consent Statement: Informed consent was obtained from all subjects involved in the study.

Data Availability Statement: Data are available upon reasonable request to the corresponding author.

Public Involvement Statement: No public involvement in any aspect of this research.

Guidelines and Standards Statement: This manuscript was drafted against the STROBE guidelines for cross-sectional studies.

Conflicts of Interest: The authors declare no conflicts of interest.

References

1. Anxiety Disorders. 2023. Available online: https://www.who.int/news-room/fact-sheets/detail/anxiety-disorders (accessed on 10 January 2024).
2. Vos, T.; Allen, C.; Arora, M.; Barber, R.M.; Bhutta, Z.A.; Brown, A.; Carter, A.; Casey, D.C.; Charlson, F.J.; Chen, A.Z.; et al. Global, regional, and national incidence, prevalence, and years lived with disability for 310 diseases and injuries, 1990–2015: A systematic analysis for the Global Burden of Disease Study 2015. *Lancet* **2016**, *388*, 1545–1602. [CrossRef] [PubMed]
3. American Psychological Association. Stress in America™ 2023 A National Mental Health Crisis. 2023. Available online: https://www.apa.org/news/press/releases/stress/2023/november-2023-topline-data.pdf (accessed on 10 January 2024).
4. Center for Collegiate Mental Health. Center for Collegiate Mental Health 2022 Annual Report. 2023. Available online: https://ccmh.psu.edu/assets/docs/2022%20Annual%20Report.pdf (accessed on 10 January 2024).
5. Barbayannis, G.; Bandari, M.; Zheng, X.; Baquerizo, H.; Pecor, K.W.; Ming, X. Academic stress and mental well-being in college students: Correlations, affected groups, and COVID-19. *Front. Psychol.* **2022**, *13*, 886344. [CrossRef] [PubMed]
6. Kris-Etherton, P.M.; Petersen, K.S.; Hibbeln, J.R.; Hurley, D.; Kolick, V.; Peoples, S.; Rodriguez, N.; Woodward-Lopez, G. Nutrition and behavioral health disorders: Depression and anxiety. *Nutr. Rev.* **2021**, *79*, 247–260. [CrossRef] [PubMed]
7. Alzayyat, A.; Al-Gamal, E. A review of the literature regarding stress among nursing students during their clinical education. *Int. Nurs. Rev.* **2014**, *61*, 406–415. [CrossRef] [PubMed]
8. Pulido-Martos, M.; Augusto-Landa, J.M.; Lopez-Zafra, E. Sources of stress in nursing students: A systematic review of quantitative studies. *Int. Nurs. Rev.* **2012**, *59*, 15–25. [CrossRef]
9. Ahmed, F.A.; Alrashidi, N.; Mohamed, R.A.; Asiri, A.; Al Ali, A.; Aly, K.H.; Nouh, W.G.; Demerdash, N.A.; Marzouk, S.A.; Omar, A.M.; et al. Satisfaction and anxiety level during clinical training among nursing students. *BMC Nurs.* **2023**, *22*, 187. [CrossRef] [PubMed]
10. Karaman, M.A.; Lerma, E.; Vela, J.C.; Watson, J.C. Predictors of academic stress among college students. *J. Coll. Couns.* **2019**, *22*, 41–55. [CrossRef]
11. Martínez-Vázquez, S.; Martínez-Galiano, J.M.; Peinado-Molina, R.A.; Hernández-Martínez, A. Magnitude of general anxiety disorder among nursing students and its associated factors. *Health Sci. Rep.* **2023**, *6*, e1405. [CrossRef] [PubMed]
12. Casuso-Holgado, M.J.; Moreno-Morales, N.; Labajos-Manzanares, M.T.; Montero-Bancalero, F.J. The association between perceived health symptoms and academic stress in Spanish higher education students. *Eur. J. Educ. Psychol.* **2019**, *12*, 109–123. [CrossRef]
13. Hill, D.; Conner, M.; Clancy, F.; Moss, R.; Wilding, S.; Bristow, M.; O'connor, D.B. Stress and eating behaviours in healthy adults: A systematic review and meta-analysis. *Health Psychol. Rev.* **2022**, *16*, 280–304. [CrossRef]
14. Choi, J. Impact of stress levels on eating behaviors among college students. *Nutrients* **2020**, *12*, 1241. [CrossRef]
15. Ling, J.; Zahry, N.R. Relationships among perceived stress, emotional eating, and dietary intake in college students: Eating self-regulation as a mediator. *Appetite* **2021**, *163*, 105215. [CrossRef] [PubMed]
16. Bartschi, J.G.; Greenwood, L.-M. Food addiction as a mediator between depressive symptom severity and body mass index. *Appetite* **2023**, *190*, 107008. [CrossRef]
17. Lipert, A.; Kozłowski, R.; Timler, D.; Marczak, M.; Musiał, K.; Rasmus, P.; Kamecka, K.; Jegier, A. Physical Activity as a Predictor of the Level of Stress and Quality of Sleep during COVID-19 Lockdown. *Int. J. Environ. Res. Public Health* **2021**, *18*, 5811. [CrossRef]
18. Ye, J.; Jia, X.; Zhang, J.; Guo, K. Effect of physical exercise on sleep quality of college students: Chain intermediary effect of mindfulness and ruminative thinking. *Front. Psychol.* **2022**, *13*, 987537. [CrossRef]
19. Spitzer, R.L.; Kroenke, K.; Williams, J.B.; Löwe, B. A brief measure for assessing generalized anxiety disorder: The GAD-7. *Arch. Intern. Med.* **2006**, *166*, 1092–1097. [CrossRef] [PubMed]
20. Johnson, S.U.; Ulvenes, P.G.; Øktedalen, T.; Hoffart, A. Psychometric properties of the general anxiety disorder 7-item (GAD-7) scale in a heterogeneous psychiatric sample. *Front. Psychol.* **2019**, *10*, 449461. [CrossRef]
21. Mehling, W.E.; Acree, M.; Stewart, A.; Silas, J.; Jones, A. The multidimensional assessment of interoceptive awareness, version 2 (MAIA-2). *PLoS ONE* **2018**, *13*, e0208034. [CrossRef]
22. Buysse, D.J.; Reynolds, C.F., III; Monk, T.H.; Berman, S.R.; Kupfer, D.J. The Pittsburgh Sleep Quality Index: A new instrument for psychiatric practice and research. *Psychiatry Res.* **1989**, *28*, 193–213. [CrossRef]
23. Rubenstein, J.H.; Morgenstern, H.; Kellenberg, J.; Kalish, T.; Donovan, J.; Inadomi, J.; McConnell, D.; Stojanovska, J.; Schoenfeld, P. Validation of a new physical activity questionnaire for a sedentary population. *Dig. Dis. Sci.* **2011**, *56*, 2678–2687. [CrossRef]
24. Jetté, M.; Sidney, K.; Blümchen, G. Metabolic equivalents (METS) in exercise testing, exercise prescription, and evaluation of functional capacity. *Clin. Cardiol.* **1990**, *13*, 555–565. [CrossRef] [PubMed]
25. Shingleton, J.; Buttrey, S.; Orendorff, F.; Wright, E. *Global Assessment Tool (GAT) Trend Analysis*; Army TRADOC Analysis Center: Austin, TX, USA, 2016.

26. Purvis, D.L.; Lentino, C.V.; Jackson, T.K.; Murphy, K.J.; Deuster, P.A. Nutrition as a component of the performance triad: How healthy eating behaviors contribute to soldier performance and military readiness. *US Army Med. Dep. J.* **2013**. Available online: https://pubmed.ncbi.nlm.nih.gov/24146244/ (accessed on 10 January 2024).
27. Colby, S.; Zhou, W.; Allison, C.; Mathews, A.E.; Olfert, M.D.; Morrell, J.S.; Byrd-Bredbenner, C.; Greene, G.; Brown, O.; Kattelmann, K.; et al. Development and validation of the short healthy eating index survey with a college population to assess dietary quality and intake. *Nutrients* **2020**, *12*, 2611. [CrossRef] [PubMed]
28. Ware, J., Jr.; Kosinski, M.; Keller, S.D. A 12-Item Short-Form Health Survey: Construction of scales and preliminary tests of reliability and validity. *Med. Care* **1996**, *34*, 220–233. [CrossRef] [PubMed]
29. Allison, K.R.; Dwyer, J.J.M.; Makin, S. Perceived Barriers to Physical Activity among High School Students. *Prev. Med.* **1999**, *28*, 608–615. [CrossRef] [PubMed]
30. Saha, S.; Okafor, H.; Biediger-Friedman, L.; Behnke, A. Association between diet and symptoms of anxiety and depression in college students: A systematic review. *J. Am. Coll. Health* **2023**, *71*, 1270–1280. [CrossRef]
31. Huberty, J.; Green, J.; Glissmann, C.; Larkey, L.; Puzia, M.; Lee, C. Efficacy of the mindfulness meditation mobile app "calm" to reduce stress among college students: Randomized controlled trial. *JMIR mHealth uHealth* **2019**, *7*, e14273. [CrossRef] [PubMed]
32. Ghrouz, A.K.; Noohu, M.M.; Manzar, D.; Spence, D.W.; BaHammam, A.S.; Pandi-Perumal, S.R. Physical activity and sleep quality in relation to mental health among college students. *Sleep Breath.* **2019**, *23*, 627–634. [CrossRef] [PubMed]
33. Du, C.; Zan, M.C.H.; Cho, M.J.; Fenton, J.I.; Hsiao, P.Y.; Hsiao, R.; Keaver, L.; Lai, C.-C.; Lee, H.; Ludy, M.-J.; et al. Increased resilience weakens the relationship between perceived stress and anxiety on sleep quality: A moderated mediation analysis of higher education students from 7 countries. *Clocks Sleep* **2020**, *2*, 334–353. [CrossRef] [PubMed]
34. Price, C.J.; Hooven, C. Interoceptive Awareness Skills for Emotion Regulation: Theory and Approach of Mindful Awareness in Body-Oriented Therapy (MABT). *Front. Psychol.* **2018**, *9*, 798. [CrossRef]
35. Fagioli, S.; Pallini, S.; Mastandrea, S.; Barcaccia, B. Effectiveness of a Brief Online Mindfulness-Based Intervention for University Students. *Mindfulness* **2023**, *14*, 1234–1245. [CrossRef]
36. McMahon, S. *Mindful Success: A Correlational Study on Mindfulness, Interoceptive Awareness, Thought Suppression, Perceived Stress, and Academic Success*; California Institute of Integral Studies: San Francisco, CA, USA, 2021.
37. Kabir, R.S. Interoceptive attention tendencies predict trait anxiety in undergraduate students and hospital nurses participating in stress management programs. *Bull. Grad. Sch. Educ. Hiroshima Univ.* **2019**, *68*, 111–120.
38. Toqan, D.; Ayed, A.; Khalaf, I.A. Effect of progressive muscle relaxation exercise on anxiety among nursing students prior to critical care clinical training. *J. Public Health Res.* **2023**, *12*, 22799036231181668. [CrossRef] [PubMed]
39. Almarcha, M.; González, I.; Balagué, N.; Javierre, C. Prescribing or co-designing exercise in healthy adults? Effects on mental health and interoceptive awareness. *Front. Behav. Neurosci.* **2022**, *16*, 944193. [CrossRef] [PubMed]
40. Zhang, F.; Liu, J.; An, M.; Gu, H. The effect of time management training on time management and anxiety among nursing undergraduates. *Psychol. Health Med.* **2021**, *26*, 1073–1078. [CrossRef] [PubMed]
41. Aloufi, M.A.; Jarden, R.J.; Gerdtz, M.F.; Kapp, S. Reducing stress, anxiety and depression in undergraduate nursing students: Systematic review. *Nurse Educ. Today* **2021**, *102*, 104877. [CrossRef] [PubMed]
42. Ortega, R.H.; Pascual, J.L.G.; Araque, A.M.F. Impact of an intervention program with reinforcement on nursing students' stress and anxiety levels in their clinical practices. *Nurse Educ. Pract.* **2021**, *55*, 103179. [CrossRef]
43. Heeter, C.; Lehto, R.; Allbritton, M.; Day, T.; Wiseman, M. Effects of a Technology-Assisted Meditation Program on Healthcare Providers' Interoceptive Awareness, Compassion Fatigue, and Burnout. *J. Hosp. Palliat. Nurs.* **2017**, *19*, 314–322. [CrossRef]

Disclaimer/Publisher's Note: The statements, opinions and data contained in all publications are solely those of the individual author(s) and contributor(s) and not of MDPI and/or the editor(s). MDPI and/or the editor(s) disclaim responsibility for any injury to people or property resulting from any ideas, methods, instructions or products referred to in the content.

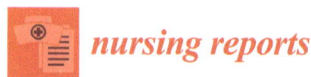

Systematic Review

Effectiveness of "Escape Room" Educational Technology in Nurses' Education: A Systematic Review

Héctor González-de la Torre [1,2,*], María-Naira Hernández-De Luis [3], Sergio Mies-Padilla [4], Rafaela Camacho-Bejarano [5], José Verdú-Soriano [6] and Claudio-Alberto Rodríguez-Suárez [1,2,*]

1. Research Support Unit, Insular Maternal and Child University Hospital Complex, Canary Health Service, 35016 Las Palmas de Gran Canaria, Spain
2. Nursing Department, Faculty of Healthcare Science, Universidad de Las Palmas de Gran Canaria (ULPGC), 35016 Las Palmas de Gran Canaria, Spain
3. Las Remudas Primary Health Care Centre, Canary Health Service, 35213 Las Palmas de Gran Canaria, Spain; mherluif@gobiernodecanarias.org
4. Department of Obstetrics and Gynaecology, Insular Maternal and Child University Hospital Complex, Canary Health Service, 35016 Las Palmas de Gran Canaria, Spain; sergio.mies101@alu.ulpgc.es
5. Department of Nursing, University of Huelva, 21007 Huelva, Spain; rafaela.camacho@denf.uhu.es
6. Department of Community Nursing, Preventive Medicine, Public Health and History of Science, Faculty of Health Sciences, University of Alicante (UA), 03690 Alicante, Spain; pepe.verdu@ua.es
* Correspondence: hector.gonzalez@ulpgc.es (H.G.-d.l.T.); claudioalberto.rodriguez@ulpgc.es (C.-A.R.-S.)

Abstract: Escape room games are educational gamification technologies that consist of introducing a team of players into a physical or digital space in search of clues to answer puzzles, riddles or enigmas and solve a mystery or problem. This study aims to determine the effectiveness of escape room games on the training of nursing students in an international context. A systematic review was carried out in MEDLINE, WOS, SCOPUS, CINAHL and LILACS databases using the MeSH terms "Education, Nursing" and "Educational Technology", and the free term "Escape room", combined with Boolean operators AND/OR. Intervention studies in Spanish, English and Portuguese were included, without limitation for the year of publication. Selection and critical appraisal were conducted by two independent reviewers. A total of $n = 13$ interventional studies were included ($n = 2$ Randomized Clinical Trials and $n = 11$ quasi-experimental design). Escape rooms are a recent and growing educational methodology, increasingly used in academia and in the training of nurses and nursing students. However, it is necessary to expand their use and the quality of the studies in a greater number of contexts. Furthermore, it is necessary to homogenize and standardize validated instruments to evaluate the effectiveness of escape rooms in the nursing education area.

Keywords: education; nursing; educational technology; gamification; systematic review

1. Introduction

The use of educational technologies aims to facilitate and improve learning through the creation, use and management of appropriate technological processes and resources [1]. These educational technologies should facilitate collaboration among students, stimulate student problem solving and seek an "authentic approach", improving their motivation and engagement [1,2]. This is why the search for more effective educational technologies has aroused great interest in the educational community [3,4]. This is especially applicable in the case of the education of health sciences students in general and nursing students in particular [1,4].

One of the educational technologies that has piqued the most interest in recent years has been gamification [4,5]. Although there is no uniform definition regarding this term [5], we can say that gamification includes the use of various game elements in the academic setting with the aim of improving the academic learning performance and motivation of students [5,6]. These game elements should be interpreted widely, as they can include

Citation: González-de la Torre, H.; Hernández-De Luis, M.-N.; Mies-Padilla, S.; Camacho-Bejarano, R.; Verdú-Soriano, J.; Rodríguez-Suárez, C.-A. Effectiveness of "Escape Room" Educational Technology in Nurses' Education: A Systematic Review. *Nurs. Rep.* **2024**, *14*, 1193–1211. https://doi.org/10.3390/nursrep14020091

Academic Editors: Antonio Martínez-Sabater, Elena Chover-Sierra and Carles Saus-Ortega

Received: 13 March 2024
Revised: 3 May 2024
Accepted: 9 May 2024
Published: 13 May 2024

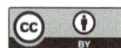

Copyright: © 2024 by the authors. Licensee MDPI, Basel, Switzerland. This article is an open access article distributed under the terms and conditions of the Creative Commons Attribution (CC BY) license (https://creativecommons.org/licenses/by/4.0/).

different techniques and methods [1,5,6], but always with the main purpose of using them to achieve a didactic and educational objective that should be clear and well defined [5]. Therefore, the main purpose should never be entertainment, but to improve students' learning of a specific subject or area, as well as to help in the acquisition of certain clinical-practical skills or competencies [5,7].

One of the educational techniques that have been included in gamification is the so-called "escape rooms" (ERs) [4,8]. ER games consist of introducing a team of players in a physical or digital space in search of clues to complete puzzles, riddles or enigmas, with the aim of solving a mystery or a problem. ER games have the aim of acquiring professional skills in a complementary way to other teaching methods [8,9]. ER games have been used in recent years in the field of health sciences education, including nursing studies, whether undergraduate or graduate [4,8,10].

Recently, Reinkemeyer et al. have examined the use of ER games in nursing, concluding that they are effective in improving nurses' knowledge on different topics [10]. According to these authors, the ER games were organized around four main narrative themes: group dynamics, training, theoretical aspects and identified barriers. However, this study did not perform statistical data extraction reporting on the effectiveness of ER games and did not undertake a joint analysis of the results. Thus, this review included only studies published in English. A new systematic review of this topic in other international contexts was proposed with the aim of evaluating the effectiveness of ER games in the specific training of nursing students based on the following review question: what is the effectiveness of the use of ER games as an educational technology for training nursing students at international context? Therefore, the aim of this review was to determine the effectiveness of ER games on the education of nursing students in the international context.

2. Materials and Methods

Design: A systematic review was carried out according to the methodology of the Joanna Briggs Institute (JBI) [11]. The report of the results followed the Preferred Reporting Items for Systematic Review and Meta-Analysis (PRISMA) Statement criteria [12]. The review protocol has been registered in PROSPERO under number CRD4202222374207. As this review is on the effectiveness of an intervention, the research question has been shaped using the following structure: Population (P), Intervention (I), Comparison (C) and Outcomes (O) [13], with P being undergraduate nursing students, I being ER games with physical or digital approaches, C being other gamification games or traditional educational techniques, and O being knowledge, satisfaction and attitudes with the training received.

Sources of information: The first step was to identify previous publications on the topic of interest through various searches in PROSPERO and Google Scholar® databases that could answer the search question. After this initial check, searches were conducted in December 2023 in the following Health Sciences databases: MEDLINE (PubMed), MEDLINE (OVID), SCI Expanded (Web of Science), SCOPUS (SCOPUS-Elsevier) and CINAHL (EbscoHOST).

Search strategies: The DeCS/MeSH descriptors "Education, Nursing" and "Educational Technology" were used, as well as the free term "Escape room" using Boolean operators AND/OR. Where appropriate, methodological filters were applied. The searches were piloted in PubMed. The search process was developed by one of the researchers (C.-A.R.-S.) and verified by a second researcher (H.G.-d.l.T) using the PRISMA-S for searching extension [14]. All references were exported to Mendeley Reference Manager Online® for screening. Table 1 shows the search strategies performed in each of the databases.

Inclusion criteria: Studies published up to December 2023 in Spanish, English or Portuguese that have addressed the use of ER games in the context of undergraduate education in nursing students were included. Only experimental intervention studies were included: randomized clinical trials (RCTs) and quasi-experimental studies (pre-post designs with or without a control group). No time limit was set for the year of publication.

Table 1. Search strategies in each of the databases.

Database	Date	Search Strategies
Medline (PubMed)	29 December 2023	("education, nursing"[MeSH Terms] OR "Nursing Education"[All Fields] OR ("education"[All Fields] AND "nursing"[All Fields]) OR "Nursing Education"[All Fields] OR ("educations"[All Fields] AND "nursing"[All Fields])) OR "Nursing Educations"[All Fields]) AND ("Gamification"[MeSH Terms] OR "escape room"[All Fields])
Medline (Ovid)	29 December 2023	Gamification.mp. "escape room".m_titl. 1 or 2 Education, Nursing.mp. 3 and 4
CINHAL (EbscoHOST)	29 December 2023	S1 TX gamification S2 TX "escape room" OR TX "scape room" OR TX "escape rooms" S3 TX "escape room" OR TX "scape room" OR TX "escape rooms") AND (S1 OR S2) S4 TX "nursing education" OR TX "education, nursing" S5(TX "nursing education" OR TX "education, nursing") AND (S3 AND S4)
Scopus (Scopus-Elsevier)	29 December 2023	(ALL ("escape room" OR "escape rooms" OR "scape room") OR INDEXTERMS (gamification)) AND (INDEXTERMS ("education, nursing" OR "nursing education"))
SCI Expanded (Web of Science)	29 December 2023	((TS = ("gamification")) OR TS = ("escape room" OR "scape room" OR "escape rooms")) AND TS = ("education, nursing" OR "nursing education")

Exclusion criteria: Studies conducted on graduate nurses, and other gamification games or traditional educational techniques were excluded. Other review studies (systematic, exploratory or narrative), studies with quantitative observational, analytical and descriptive designs, case studies and qualitative designs with any methodology were excluded. Publications that did not correspond to research studies (such as editorials and letters to the editor) were also excluded. Gray literature was not included.

Selection and classification of studies: After performing the searches, duplicate records were eliminated and screened by title and abstract. The full-text documents of the selected records were then retrieved to assess their eligibility according to inclusion and exclusion criteria. Screening was performed by peer review (H.G.-d.l.T. and S.M.-P.) and, in case of discrepancies, a third researcher decided (C.-A.R.-S.).

Definition of the study variables: Bibliometric variables on the affiliation of studies, as well as variables on the statistical results of the studies have been extracted. The main research outcome corresponded to the knowledge, and secondary outcomes were satisfaction and attitudes with the training research. However, knowledge, satisfaction and attitudes have been extracted from all studies, regardless of whether they were primary or secondary results. Additionally, other primary or secondary outcomes not included that have been reported in the different studies have also been extracted.

Evaluation and data extraction: Studies identified as potentially eligible for inclusion were distributed for peer review by two investigators (J.V.-S. and R.C.-B.) and discrepancies were resolved by a third researcher (M.-N.H.-D.L.). To assess the quality of the studies, the JBI critical appraisal tools appropriate to each research design were used, establishing as a criterion of good quality a score of more than 50% with respect to the items included in each tool (for RCT-13 items, a score ≥ 7 was considered good quality and for quasi-experimental studies—9 items, a score ≥ 5). Finally, the following information was extracted from the studies: country and year, design, main/secondary outcomes, instrument used to measure the effectiveness of ER games, characteristics of the ER games (type, setting and duration of the ER games sessions, size and composition of the groups) and the population in which it was performed. For continuous quantitative variables, statistical data on mean scores and standard deviations were extracted, and for qualitative variables, percentages and frequencies were extracted. The p-values were also extracted to test the hypothesis contrasts and the effect sizes when they were calculated. Data extraction was carried out independently by two researchers (H.G.-d.l.T. and S.M.-P.) and discrepancies were resolved by a third researcher (C.-A.R.-S.).

3. Results

The number of records retrieved was $n = 439$; after eliminating duplicates ($n = 160$) and gray literature ($n = 28$), $n = 251$ records were screened by title and abstract. Of these, $n = 215$ records were excluded because they did not meet the inclusion criteria, while $n = 36$ records met the criteria for full-text evaluation. After the critical appraisal process, $n = 13$ studies were included in the review, as shown in the flow diagram in Figure 1.

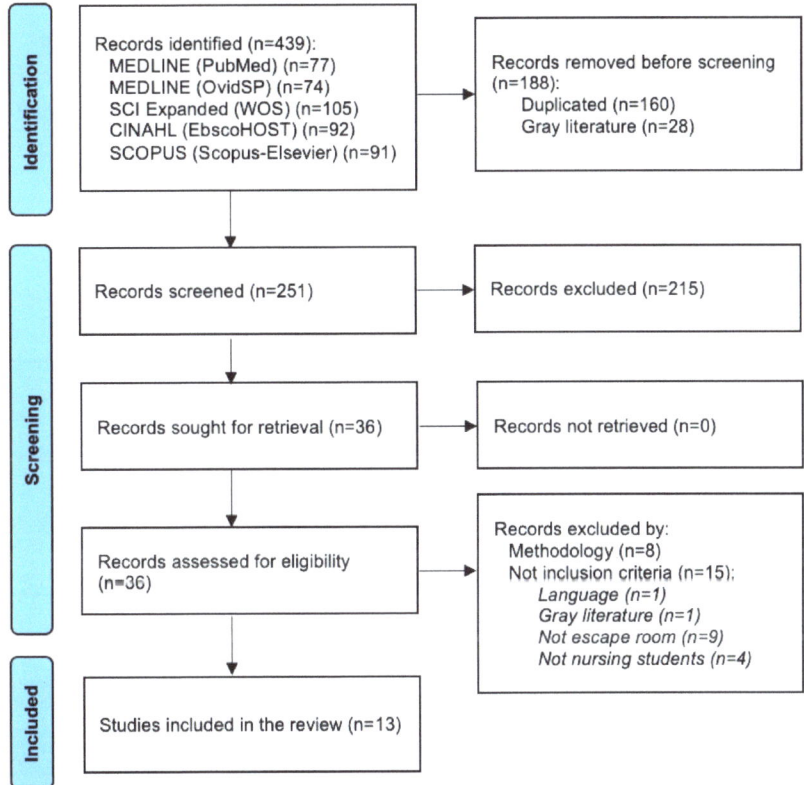

Figure 1. Flow diagram.

In the full-text critical appraisal process, $n = 8$ studies were excluded for not meeting the minimum methodological quality and $n = 15$ were excluded for not meeting the inclusion criteria (Table S1). The critical appraisal process of the included studies is shown in Supplementary Table S2.

Regarding the methodological design of the studies, RCTs ($n = 2$) and quasi-experimental studies ($n = 11$) were included. The quasi-experimental studies consisted of different designs such as pre- and post-experimental with control group ($n = 4$), pre- and post-experimental ($n = 6$) and quasi-experimental with control group ($n = 1$).

Table 2 shows the year and country of publication, design, themes and learning topics, aim and main/secondary outcomes and the conclusions for each study.

Table 2. Characteristics of the included studies.

Author (Year) Country	Design	Themes and Learning Topics	Aim and Main/Secondary Outcomes	Conclusions
Chen et al. (2023) China [15]	Quasi experimental pre-post with CG [1]	Gerontological Nursing (Safe Medication Care for the Elderly people)	To determine the effects of an intervention educational activity based on an ER [2] on nursing students' learning attitude and the game flow experience after they had received nursing classroom teaching on safe medication use in older adults *Main outcomes*: learnings attitudes and experience of game	During the teaching process of the Gerontological Nursing course, an ER added at the end of classroom teaching can improve nursing students' learning attitude and also help them to have a good game
Schmuhl et al. (2023) USA [16]	Quasi experimental pre-post	Interprofessional Collaboration and Opioid Use Disorder	To determine the impact of an innovative interprofessional educational activity on healthcare professional students' learning. The educational activity targeted student knowledge of opioid use disorder and perceptions of working with an interprofessional team while caring for patients with opioid use disorder *Main outcomes*: attitudes about interprofessional collaboration *Secondary outcomes*: perceptions about opioid use disorder	An interprofessional educational experience including both an asynchronous course and virtual synchronous ER can increase participant knowledge around opioid use disorder and may improve student perceptions of working with an interprofessional team and caring for patients with opioid use disorder
Yang et al. (2023) Taiwan [17]	Quasi experimental with CG	Maternity care	To identify the efficiency of ER activities in terms of enhancing nursing students' retention of maternity-related knowledge and their overall learning performance *Main outcomes*: knowledge about maternity care *Secondary outcomes*: students' confidence and critical thinking	Maternity ER emerged as an online game-based approach that effectively stimulated nursing students and can serve as a practical resource for engaging in maternity care learning
Hursman et al. (2022) USA [18]	Quasi experimental pre-post	Interprofessional Colaboration	To enhance interprofessional students' perceptions of their ability to communicate effectively and respectfully, work together to complete a task and to develop knowledge of the unique roles of members of the healthcare team *Main outcomes*: improvement in teamwork (effective communication) *Secondary outcomes*: perceptions and attitudes about gaming	This activity lays the groundwork for collaborative telehealth nursing that students will be exposed to in their future career. Results show the activity helped to build collaboration among team members, including those not in the same physical space. It also showed that virtual ER can be an effective activity to increase interprofessional teamwork perceptions in the online classroom environment and could prove to be useful in other online interprofessional settings
Millsaps et al. (2022) USA [19]	Quasi experimental pre-post	Neurological disorders with a focus on stroke	To promote engagement in undergraduate nursing coursework Main outcomes: knowledge about Stroke	ER experiences can be utilized in the preparation of associate degree nursing education to engage students while also ensuring that students meet key learning objectives

Table 2. Cont.

Author (Year) Country	Design	Themes and Learning Topics	Aim and Main/Secondary Outcomes	Conclusions
Molina-Torres et al. (2022) Spain [20]	Quasi experimental pre-post with CG	Anatomy	To evaluate the effectiveness of the ER for anatomy-related knowledge retention in nursing and the perceived value of the game. Main outcomes: knowledge about Anatomy. Secondary outcomes: satisfaction about gaming	According to the findings, the "Anatomy ER" is a game-based approach that motivates students and constitutes a down-to-earth resource for anatomy learning in healthcare students
Rodríguez-Ferrer et al. (2022) Spain [21]	RCT [3]	Stigma again Severe Mental Illness	To examine the effect of the Without Memories ER on nursing students' stigma against Severe Mental Illness. Main outcomes: modification of stigmatizing attitudes towards severe mental illness	The Without Memories ER can be used as an effective tool to educate and raise awareness about stigmatizing attitudes toward Severe Mental Illness in university students studying health care
Wettergreen et al. (2022) USA [22]	Quasi experimental pre-post	Interprofessional education and the opioid crisis	To evaluate the use of an interprofessional ER activity to increase clinical knowledge related to the opioid crisis. The secondary objective was to evaluate change in attitudes toward interprofessional collaboration. Main outcomes: knowledge related to the opioid crisis. Secondary outcomes: attitudes toward interprofessional collaboration	The use of an interprofessional ER as an educational method was effective in increasing some aspects of opioid crisis related knowledge and enhancing attitudes toward interprofessional collaboration. The educational model is applicable to various topics and inter-professional groups
Fusco et al. (2022) USA [23]	RCT	Interprofessional Collaboration Sepsis management and post-operative precautions (hip arthroplasty)	To extend our understanding of ER pedagogical design by investigating the impact of escape room puzzle content on changes in student immediate recall knowledge and demonstration of interprofessional skills during a subsequent interprofessional simulation. Main outcomes: knowledge of interprofessional collaboration about sepsis. Secondary outcomes: interprofessional collaborative skills during simulation	ER can be an innovative pedagogical tool that can positively impact immediate recall knowledge and interprofessional collaborative skills of health professions students
Foltz-Ramos et al. (2021) USA [24]	Quasi experimental pre-post with CG	Interprofessional Collaboration	To create and test the use of an interprofessional ER, as a method to improve teamwork, prior to interprofessional simulation. Main outcomes: improvement of students' performance in simulation. Secondary outcomes: attitudes toward interprofessional collaboration	ER can, in a brief period of time, improve teamwork and consequently performance during simulation. Findings support the use of ER in interprofessional education curriculum as a method to promote teamwork

Table 2. Cont.

Author (Year) Country	Design	Themes and Learning Topics	Aim and Main/Secondary Outcomes	Conclusions
Moore & Campbell (2021) Australia [25]	Quasi experimental pre-post	Interprofessional practice knowledge and competencies	To investigate the utility of an ER coupled with a debriefing workshop as an effective and engaging interprofessional learning activity. To evaluate the impact of the ER on participant knowledge about inter-professional practice and teamwork. To evaluate the impact of the ER through participant reflection on their personal contributions to the team. *Main outcomes*: knowledge about interprofessional practice and teamwork and improvement in interprofessional learning activity	The ER intervention added value to the placement curriculum and proved flexible for a heterogeneous student cohort
Gutiérrez-Puertas et al. (2020) Spain [26]	Quasi experimental with CG	Gameful experience Clinical skills	To understand the gameful experience and satisfaction of nursing students in the evaluation of their clinical skills using an ER. *Main outcomes*: satisfaction of clinical skills *Secondary outcomes*: experience of game	ER are a useful tool for the evaluation of nursing students compared with using the objective structured clinical evaluation
Morrel & Eukel (2020) USA [27]	Quasi experimental pre-post	Cardiovascular critical care	To evaluate the impact of a cardiovascular ER on student knowledge, as well as to understand student perceptions of the educational innovation. *Main outcomes*: knowledge about cardiovascular critical care. *Secondary outcomes*: perceptions about gaming	The cardiovascular ER increased student knowledge and was positively received by students. The educational innovation encouraged student engagement in learning, content application, peer communication, and nursing practice skills

[1] CG: Control group; [2] ER: Escape Room games; [3] RCT: Randomized Controlled Trial.

The thematic areas covered by studies were very disparate: gerontology, interprofessional collaboration, maternity care, neurological disorders, anatomy, severe mental illness interprofessional education or interprofessional practice, clinical skills and cardiovascular critical care. Four studies addressed the subject of interprofessional collaboration, although from different perspectives (effective communication and teamwork, interprofessional management of opioid use disorder, improve teamwork and sepsis management, and post-operative precautions).

Regarding the design of the ER games, the educational activities were also heterogeneous in different studies, with physical settings ($n = 8$), virtual/online settings ($n = 3$) or mixed (physical and virtual) settings ($n = 2$).

The clinical results of the studies are shown in Table 3.

Table 3. Clinical results of the included studies.

Author (Year)	Instruments	Type of ER Game (Setting) and Time Session (in Minutes)	Size Team (Nursing for Team)	Study Population/Sample (IG [1]/CG [2])	Lost Case (CG/IG)	Pre Mean (SD [3]) (IG/CG)	Post Mean (SD) (IG/CG)	p-Value	Size Effect	Other
Chen et al. (2023) [15]	- LAS [4]: 23 items, four subscales: learning interest, learning experience, learning habit, and professional recognition. Total range 23–92. Higher scores indicate better learning attitude. - GFEQ [5]: 19 items, 5 subscales: sense of control, telepresence, distorted sense of time, enjoyable feelings, and being unconscious of irrelevant surroundings. Total range 19–95. Higher scores indicate better game flow experience	Physical ER [6] (Geriatric nursing training room) (40)	6–8 (6–8)	84 Nursing students IG = 41 (6 group) CG = 33	None	- LAS: IG = 60.93 (2.33) CG = 61.51 (2.32) - CFEQ: IG = 63.27 (2.48)	- LAS: IG = 73.17 (1.67) CG = 61.63 (2.66) - CFEQ: IG = 81.29 (2.49)	- LAS: $p < 0.001$ t-test - GFEQ: $p < 0.001$ t-test	- LAS: Cohen's d 5.196 (post-test score) - GFEQ: Cohen's d 5.253	- LAS (total score 45) for the ER 43.83 (4.49)
Schmuhl et al. (2023) [16]	- ATHCT [7] (14 item). Likert (1 = strongly disagree, 2 = disagree, 3 = agree, 4 = strongly agree) - Survey to assess perceptions towards caring for patients with Opioid Use Disorder (11 item) Likert scale (1 = strongly disagree, 2 = disagree, 3 = agree, 4 = strongly agree)	Synchronous virtual ER hosted via zoom breakout rooms (30) Physical ER (simulated emergency room) (90)	Not reported (Team interprofessional)	402 health professional students (216 Nursing students) No CG	None	- ATHCT: Performed for 14 items but NP [8] for total score. - Opioid Use Disorder: Performed for 11 items but NP for total score	- ATHCT: Performed for 14 items but NP for total score. - Opioid Use Disorder: Performed for 11 items but NP for total score	- ATHCT: $p < 0.05$ t-test - Opioid Use Disorder: $p < 0.05$ (7 items) t-test	NC [9]	Following ER, students strongly agreed that their intentions were to change and work collaborative on interprofessional teams

Table 3. Cont.

Author (Year)	Instruments	Type of ER Game (Setting) and Time Session (in Minutes)	Size Team (Nursing for Team)	Study Population/Sample (IG [1]/CG [2])	Lost Case (CG/IG)	Pre Mean (SD [3]) (IG/CG)	Post Mean (SD) (IG/CG)	p-Value	Size Effect	Other
Yang et al. (2023) [17]	- Knowledge test of maternity care: 10 items (maximum score 100 points) - Problem-solving scale: 5 items 5-points Likert scale - Critical thinking questionnaire: 6 items to assess students' critical thinking abilities, knowledge and confidence	Online game-based ER (50)	6–7 (6–7)	42 Nursing students IG = 21 (Online game-based ER) CG = 21 (online learning without ER)	None	NP	- Knowledge: IG = 30.36 CG = 12.64 - Problem-solving: IG = 28.33 CG = 14.67 - Critical thinking: IG = 31.76 CG = 11.24	- Knowledge: $p < 0.001$ (Mann Whitney U) - Problem-solving: $p < 0.001$ (Mann Whitney U) - Critical thinking: $p < 0.001$ (Mann Whitney U)	NC	
Hursman et al. (2022) [18]	Questionnaire Pre-Post: - Pre-survey 8-item of core competencies for interprofessional collaborative practice - Post-survey 26-item same items more 17 items to evaluate the effectiveness, usefulness of the activity and attitudes toward gaming	Online ER (60)	5–7 (1–2)	176 heath science students (95 Nursing students) No CG	None	NP for 6 items	NP for 6 items	6 items ($p < 0.001$)	NC	
Millsaps et al. (2022) [19]	- 5 questions of knowledge about Stroke	Prequiz (10) Pre-briefing (25) Physical ER (30) Debriefing (25)	4 (4)	Undergraduate ASN [10] students (24 students) (12 morning session, and 12 afternoon session) No CG	None	Knowledge: 2.9 (1.06) Median: 3	Knowledge: 3.8 (0.66) Median: 4	$p = 0.001$ for median (Wilcoxon)	NC	Not indicated punctuation system

Table 3. Cont.

Author (Year)	Instruments	Type of ER Game (Setting) and Time Session (in Minutes)	Size Team (Nursing for Team)	Study Population/Sample IG[1]/CG[2]	Lost Case (CG/IG)	Pre Mean (SD[3]) (IG/CG)	Post Mean (SD) (IG/CG)	p-Value	Size Effect	Other
Molina-Torres et al. (2022) [20]	- 10 questions of Knowledge about Anatomy (0–10 points)	Physical ER (University classroom) (15)	4 (4)	248 Nursing students IG = 128 CG = 120	None	NP	Knowledge: IG = 8.94 (0.96) CG = 7.70 (1.25)	Post p = 0.001 (Student's t)	NC	Also measured IG satisfaction using Satisfaction Questionnaire [11] (26 questions 1 to 5; higher score higher satisfaction)
Rodríguez-Ferrer et al. (2022) [21]	- Attributional Questionnaire (14-point Likert 1–9; higher score greater number of stigmatizing attitudes toward people with severe mental illness) - Motivation Questionnaire for Cooperative Playful Learning Strategies (Likert scale 1–7)	Web-based ER (60)	4 (4)	316 nursing students randomized IG = 204 (ER no memories) CG = 112 (ER locked In)	IG = 7 CG = 3 Final sample n = 306 IG = 197 CG = 109	Higher scores greater stigma: IG = 47.57 (16.7) CG = 49.56 (16.03)	Higher scores greater stigma expressed: IG = 30.83 (14.79) CG = 49.55 (16.02)	Post p < 0.001 (ANOVA)	0.258	
Wettergreen et al. (2022) [22]	- SPICE-R [12] Instrument (multiple response and true/false). Likert scale 1–5 points (higher score greater agreement with the statement)	Pre-brief (10) Virtual and Physical ER (60) Debrief (20)	5 (not reported)	80 Heath science students (7 Nursing students) No CG	10 lost	SPICE-R Higher score greater agreement Mean: 4.48	SPICE-R Higher score greater agreement Mean: 4.64	Knowledge: post (p < 0.05) (McNemar's Exact Test)	NC	Pre Knowledge: [13] 62.92% Post Knowledge: 74.30%

Table 3. Cont.

Author (Year)	Instruments	Type of ER Game (Setting) and Time Session (in Minutes)	Size Team (Nursing for Team)	Study Population/Sample (IG [1]/CG [2])	Lost Case (CG/IG)	Pre Mean (SD [3]) (IG/CG)	Post Mean (SD) (IG/CG)	p-Value	Size Effect	Other
Fusco et al. (2022) [23]	- ISVS-21 [14] - OIPC [15] tool: First 10 items: Adequacy of team to a common vision of the situation. Remaining 10 items: Team's ability to develop a common action plan. For each item, rated a 3-point Likert (1 = inadequate, 2 = more-less adequate, 3 = adequate)	Physical ER (School of Nursing Simulation Center) (30)	4 (2)	233 Nursing and pharmacy students (118 Nursing students) IG = 120 (Simulation) CG = 113 (ER+ simulation)	None	- ISVS-21: IG = 5.3 (0.92) CG = 5.2 (1.0) - OIPC: NP	- ISVS-21: IG = 6.0 (0.72) CG = 5.9 (0.8) - OIPC: Median (IQR [16]) IG: Items 1–10: 27 (26–28) IG: Items 11–20: 27 (26–28) Total 55 (53–56) CG: Items 1–10: 26 (24–28) CG: Item 11–20: 27 (25–28) Total 53 (49–56)	- ISVS-21: Mean (SD) * IG = 0.72 (0.81) CG = 0.64 (1.0) - OIPC: Items 1–10 $p < 0.001$ Item 11–20 $p < 0.001$ Total $p < 0.001$	Cohen's d: IG = 0.89 CG = 0.61	

Table 3. Cont.

Author (Year)	Instruments	Type of ER Game (Setting) and Time Session (in Minutes)	Size Team (Nursing for Team)	Study Population/Sample (IG[1]/CG[2])	Lost Case (CG/IG)	Pre Mean (SD[3]) (IG/CG)	Post Mean (SD) (IG/CG)	p-Value	Size Effect	Other
Foltz-Ramos et al. (2021) [24]	- Knowledge Test (10 items multiple choice test) - ISVS-21: 21 items 7-point Likert scale. Items scores are added together and divided by 21 to calculate overall score	Physical ER (Simulation scenario in a Simulation center) (30)	5 (2)	Senior nursing, third-year pharmacy, and second-year physical therapy students IG = 133 (Nursing: 54) ER acute management of sepsis CG = 129 (Nursing: 55) ER general acute care	None	- Knowledge #1: IG = 6.8 (1.9) CG = 6.7 (1.6) - ISVS-21: IG = 5.1 (0.92) CG = 5.2 (0.97)	- Knowledge #2: IG = 7.7 (1.6) CG = 7.3 (1.7) - ISVS-21: IG = 6.0 (0.77) CG = 6.0 (0.82)	- Knowledge #3: p = 0.06 - ISVS-21: p = 0.70	NC	Three knowledge measures #1, #2, #3
Moore and Campbell (2021) [25]	- Sharif and Nahas' Questionnaire Adaptation - Knowledge questionnaire: 6 items about knowledge (1 = low–5 = excellent)	Welcome and formal consent (5) Physical ER (55) Comfort break and health care plan development, educational session and evaluation (90)	6 (at least one nursing student)	50 health science students (8 Nursing students) No CG	None	NP	NP	Knowledge difference of pre-post means for 6 questions values p < 0.001	NC	

Table 3. Cont.

Author (Year)	Instruments	Type of ER Game (Setting) and Time Session (in Minutes)	Size Team (Nursing for Team)	Study Population/Sample (IG[1]/CG[2])	Lost Case (CG/IG)	Pre Mean (SD[3]) (IG/CG)	Post Mean (SD) (IG/CG)	p-Value	Size Effect	Other
Gutiérrez-Puertas et al. (2020) [26]	- GAMEX [17]: 7 questions Likert scale (1 = never–5 = always) - Scale for level of satisfaction: scores between 13–52, higher scores indicate higher satisfaction - Practical examination of clinical skill: 10 questions (0, 0.25, 0.5, or 1 point)	Physical ER (30)	5 (5)	237 Nursing students IG = 117 (ER) CG = 120 (OSCE [18])	None	NP	Examination of clinical skills IG = 9.59 (0.36) CG = 7.46 (1.36)	p < 0.05 (Mann Whitney U)	NC	Results of GAMEX 6 dimensions Mean (SD): - Enjoyment 27.60 (3.02) (range 6–30) - Absorption 22.74 (4.88) (range 6–30) - Creative thinking 15.55 (3.23) (range 4–20) - Activation 16.09 (2.98) (range 4–20) - Absence of negative effects 4.66 (2.32) (range 3–15) - Dominance 13.52 (3.12) (range 4–20)
Morrel and Eukel (2020) [27]	Knowledge questionnaire: - Pre: 10 questions - Post: Same question + perception scale (11 item)	Physical ER (60)	4 (4)	31 Nursing students No CG	2 lost	NP	NP	p < 0.05	NC	

[1] IC: Intervention Group; [2] CG: Control Group; [3] SD: Standard Deviation; [4] LAS: Learning Attitude Scale; [5] GFEQ: Game Flow Experience Questionnaire; [6] ER: Escape Room games; [7] ATCHT: Attitudes Toward Health Care Teams; [8] NP: Not Performed; [9] NC: Not calculated; [10] ASN: Associate of science in nursing; [11] Gomez-Urquiza, J.L., Gomez-Salgado, J., Albendin-Garcia, L., Correa-Rodriguez, M., Gonzalez-Jimenez, E., Cañadas-De la Fuente, G.A., 2019. The impact on nursing students' opinions and motivation of using a "Nursing escape room" as a teaching game: a descriptive study. Nurse Educ. Today 72, 73–76; [12] SPICE-R: Student Perceptions of Interprofessional Clinical Education-Revised (SPICE-R: 10 questions. The authors did not analyze an overall score but performed a question-by-question analysis. The scores for the 10 questions were summed and divided by 10; [13] The average percentage of knowledge has been calculated for the 5 areas (epidemiology, alternatives to opioids, prescription drug monitoring program. Signs of overdose, opioid overdose reversal); [14] ISVS-21: Interprofessional Socialization and Valuing Scale; [15] OIPC: Observed Interprofessional Collaboration; [16] IQR: Interquartile Range; [17] GAMEX: Gameful Experience Scale; [18] OSCE: objective structured clinical examination; * Mean difference with statistically significant results.

4. Discussion

As a result of the quick development and diffusion of gamification, an increasing number of studies and reviews are being published each year examining this educational methodology in healthcare workers [28,29]. Gamification is associated with positive perceptual, cognitive, behavioral, affective, and motivational effects and outcomes [29,30], as well as having the potential to offer learners the opportunity to engage in active learning, solve clinical problems, and acquire experience in a risk-free environment without the need to involve patients [30].

Within gamification, ER games have been rapidly growing in recent years [8,10,31]. In addition to the effects previously pointed out, this learning system constitutes a method able to decrease the generation gap that sometimes exists between students and teachers [27], being an example of educational technology that can help to overcome the dissonance between traditional methodologies and the needs of more innovative educational methodologies demanded by the new generations of students [32], all with a very acceptable economic cost [33,34]. This implies that systems capable of collecting the perceptions and experiences of the participants should always be included in the design of the ER games since in this way key information can be obtained to identify aspects that can be improved [8]. Therefore, debriefing is a necessary element to be included in ER games [8,35], with some authors going so far as to state that in healthcare simulation, "debriefing is just as or even more important than the simulation" [36]. Some of the studies included in this review included various debriefing systems for this purpose [19,22,25], although without uniformity regarding the method used for this purpose. Some authors such as Eukel and Morrell [8] and Eukel et al. [33] recommend using a survey of their design.

Similarly, it is also desirable to assess participant satisfaction with the activity [8,36]. However, many of the studies included in this review did not evaluate it or did so only superficially [22]. Only Gutiérrez-Puertas et al. used a validated tool, the Gameful Experience Scale (GAMEX), although the aim of their work was directly to understand the gameful experience and satisfaction of nursing students in the evaluation of their clinical skills [26]. The GAMEX is an instrument developed by Eppman et al. [37] that measures the gameful experience and is composed of 27 items divided into 6 dimensions: Enjoyment, Absorption, Creative thinking, Activation, Absence of negative affect and Dominance. The responses are answered on a Likert-type scale, with values from 1 (never) to 5 (always), and a total score can be calculated or by dimensions. A higher score indicates a more positive experience regarding the gaming experience. The results reported by the study of Gutiérrez-Puertas et al. indicate acceptable satisfaction for the ER games experience in their case [38], like other studies included in this review that reported high degrees of satisfaction [39].

Although GAMEX is not a specific instrument for ER games, we consider it advisable to use this tool to evaluate the students' experience with respect to ER games, since in addition to being able to measure the participants' satisfaction with the activity in an objective way, it allows us to compare this educational technology against other types of gamification [40]. One dimension of this scale even allows the detection of the presence of eventual negative effects in the gamification activity. Elevated anxiety levels have been reported in nursing students related to clinical laboratory practicums and simulations [41,42]. Although more research addressing how ER games affect students' anxiety levels is needed [43], in the design of ER games it is always imperative to guarantee a sense of safety among participants [38].

The present study was designed to answer the guiding question of this review and was initially aimed at conducting a meta-analysis to evaluate the effectiveness of ER games as an educational technology specifically in nursing. As such, only studies of experimental design were exclusively included, unlike the recent review by Quek et al., which included studies of all types of designs [4]. However, the high clinical heterogeneity found did not allow a meta-analysis to be performed, being one of the main limitations of this review, although this aspect is not new and has already been pointed out. The Cochrane review on the effectiveness of gamification educational activities in health sciences personnel conducted by Akl et al. cannot perform this meta-analysis either due to the lack of methodologically robust studies [30]. Quek et al. were also unable to perform a meta-analysis, despite including studies with all types of healthcare students in their review [4]. Therefore, the most important aspect to highlight as a result of this review is the lack of uniformity and the enormous heterogeneity that exists between the various studies that have been carried out with ER games in nursing. This situation affects all the elements, from the study designs to the thematic areas, to the tools or instruments used in the evaluation of their effectiveness, but especially to the measure's outcomes of the studies. Even in those cases where a similar main outcome variable was assessed (e.g., measure of knowledge), the disparity of the topics and themes discouraged the performance of meta-analysis. This aspect should be considered in future studies carried out with ER games; as far as possible, researchers should try to standardize the interventions to be able to carry out more global evaluations of this educational technology.

A particularly relevant aspect concerns the study designs. All the studies included in our review are quasi-experimental, except for two RCTs by Rodriguez-Ferrer et al. [21] and Fusco et al. [23]. Regarding the quasi-experimental studies, only five studies had a control group [15,17,20,24,26]. Therefore, a priority aspect that emerges from our results is the need to conduct RCTs that provide more solid evidence of the effectiveness of ER games as an educational technology. This is extensible both to ER games aimed at nursing students and other health sciences students [4,31].

The data extracted from the included studies and reported on were sectioned by a population of nursing students versus pharmacy, physical therapy or health science students. In contrast to some of the previously mentioned reviews [4,30,31], this review focused exclusively on nursing students. However, studies of ER games in graduated nurses were not included, so the usefulness of ER games in the continuing education of already graduated nurses still needs to be explored in future studies. In addition, in some cases, nursing students were integrated into groups where there were students from other disciplines or areas [16,18,22–25].

Interprofessional collaboration and education is precisely one of the thematic areas where the use of ER games has been most explored [4,16,43,44]. Four studies (Hursman et al. [18], Wettergreen et al. [22], Fusco et al. [23], Foltz-Ramos et al. [24]) focused on this topic. Gamification is often used to encourage team building in businesses [3,7,44], so it is logical to also use this new tool for interdisciplinary team building in healthcare professionals, especially in areas that require close professional cooperation [44,45]. ER games can provide work teams with several benefits, in addition to the inherent effect of clinical simulation itself, as communication skills among the professionals that make up the teams are especially improved [22,45–47].

Although these aspects are undoubtedly important and are sufficient reason to implement ER games in educational programs, we should not forget that the central objective of any educational technology or methodology is the transmission of knowledge. Most of the studies included in the review were primarily motivated by the need to improve participants' knowledge of a specific subject area, either in a single group (with a before and after measurement) or by comparing two groups. All studies found statistically significant differences with respect to these improvements, which indicates ER games is useful for increasing participants' level of knowledge, something that has been previously pointed out in the literature [4,7,31,48]. However, we would like to call attention to several aspects that we consider important. On the one hand, none of the included studies used a validated instrument for the measurement and evaluation of knowledge; they always used ad hoc questionnaires, which provided little information on the psychometric properties or reliability of the instrument. This is one reason that has contributed to impeding the performance of a meta-analysis. Future studies should try to improve the choice of measurement instruments used to assess knowledge of the specific area, prioritizing the use, as far as possible, of validated instruments. On the other hand, in the academic context, it is known that after a certain period of time, knowledge can be decreased in students. Except for the study by Fusco et al. [23], no study performed several measurements in a post-intervention time interval to ensure or, at least, provide information on the permanence and integration of the acquired knowledge. More post-intervention measurements should be introduced in new studies to mitigate this problem.

In most of the studies, we have found similarities with respect to the number of team members, as well as the duration of the ER games, with groups composed of 4 to 7 participants predominating, similar to what is reported in the literature on ER games [4,10,48]. Eukel and Morrell recommend a team size of a maximum of 4 to 5 students to encourage active participation from all members [8]. Regarding the duration of ER games, most studies conducted ER games that did not exceed 60 min, with a minimum duration of 30 min (except in the case of the study by Molina et al. [20], whose duration was 15 min), similar to studies of ER games conducted in other health professionals [4,48].

Finally, it should be noted that studies have only been identified from 5 countries (USA, Australia, Spain, China and Taiwan), which suggests that this educational technology is not yet well implemented in many countries. This could be because in these countries, the universities have enough autonomy to implement new educational technologies. Further research is needed to investigate the factors that encourage the implementation of new educational technologies in certain contexts-countries as opposed to others.

Limitations

This review has some limitations. The most important is the one mentioned above, referring to the impossibility of being able to perform a meta-analysis, which is the appropriate methodological design to test the effectiveness of an intervention, in this case, the use of ER games in the training of nursing students. Also, the lack of methodologically robust studies available limits this study and its results. In addition to this aspect, we must recognize that an undetermined number of studies may have been left out of the review due to inadequate indexing, as there is sometimes confusion with the term's gamification, serious games and the like [5,7]. In fact, the lack of standardization and of a clear and unambiguous definition for ER games may influence the exclusion of studies where, according to the authors, ER games were used, either virtually or physically. Finally, some studies evaluated ER games in a set of participants that included nursing students, but not exclusively, which cannot ensure the effectiveness of the educational methodology in this particular population.

5. Conclusions

ER games are a recent and growing educational methodology, increasingly used in academia and in the training of nursing students. However, in many countries, this educational technology is not yet implemented. It is therefore necessary to expand its use and the quality of studies in a greater number of contexts and countries. In addition, it is necessary to homogenize and standardize validated instruments to evaluate the effectiveness and real impact of ER games in the area of nursing education. Finally, the usefulness of this type of technology in educational modalities other than the traditional one should be investigated. For example, digital ER games could be a useful technology to achieve student motivation in online educational programs.

Supplementary Materials: The following supporting information can be downloaded at https://www.mdpi.com/article/10.3390/nursrep14020091/s1, Table S1: Excluded studies from the review, Table S2: Critical appraisal process of the included studies.

Author Contributions: Conceptualization, H.G.-d.l.T. and C.-A.R.-S.; methodology, H.G.-d.l.T., M.-N.H.-D.L., S.M.-P., R.C.-B., J.V.-S. and C.-A.R.-S.; validation, H.G.-d.l.T., M.-N.H.-D.L., S.M.-P., R.C.-B., J.V.-S. and C.-A.R.-S.; resources, H.G.-d.l.T. and C.-A.R.-S.; writing—original draft preparation, H.G.-d.l.T. and C.-A.R.-S.; writing—review and editing, M.-N.H.-D.L., S.M.-P., R.C.-B. and J.V.-S.;

project administration, H.G.-d.l.T. and C.-A.R.-S.; funding acquisition, H.G.-d.l.T., M.-N.H.-D.L. and C.-A.R.-S. All authors have read and agreed to the published version of the manuscript.

Funding: This research received no external funding.

Institutional Review Board Statement: Not applicable.

Informed Consent Statement: Not applicable.

Data Availability Statement: No new data were created.

Public Involvement Statement: No public involvement in any aspect of this research.

Guidelines and Standards Statement: This manuscript was drafted against the Reporting follows the Preferred Reporting Items for Systematic reviews and Meta-Analyses (PRISMA) statement [12].

Use of Artificial Intelligence: AI or AI-assisted tools were not used in drafting any aspect of this manuscript.

Conflicts of Interest: The authors declare no conflicts of interest.

References

1. Kowitlawakul, Y.; Tan, J.J.M.; Suebnukarn, S.; Nguyen, H.D.; Poo, D.C.C.; Chai, J.; Wang, W.; Devi, K. Utilizing educational technology in enhancing undergraduate nursing students' engagement and motivation: A scoping review. *J. Prof. Nurs.* **2022**, *42*, 262–275. [CrossRef] [PubMed]
2. Jose, M.M.; Dufrene, C. Educational competencies and technologies for disaster preparedness in undergraduate nursing education: An integrative review. *Nurse Educ. Today* **2014**, *34*, 543–551. [CrossRef] [PubMed]
3. Dahalan, F.; Alias, N.; Shaharom, M.S.N. Gamification and Game Based Learning for Vocational Education and Training: A Systematic Literature Review. *Educ. Inf. Technol.* **2023**, *29*, 1279–1317. [CrossRef] [PubMed]
4. Quek, L.H.; Tan, A.J.Q.; Sim, M.J.J.; Ignacio, J.; Harder, N.; Lamb, A.; Chua, W.L.; Lau, S.T.; Liaw, S.Y. Educational escape rooms for healthcare students: A systematic review. *Nurse Educ. Today* **2024**, *132*, 106004. [CrossRef] [PubMed]
5. van Gaalen, A.E.J.; Brouwer, J.; Schönrock-Adema, J.; Bouwkamp-Timmer, T.; Jaarsma, A.D.C.; Georgiadis, J.R. Gamification of health professions education: A systematic review. *Adv. Health Sci. Educ. Theory Pract.* **2021**, *26*, 683–711. [CrossRef]
6. Li, Q.; Yin, X.; Yin, W.; Dong, X.; Li, Q. Evaluation of gamification techniques in learning abilities for higher school students using FAHP and EDAS methods. *Soft Comput.* **2023**, 1–19. [CrossRef]
7. Gorbanev, I.; Agudelo-Londoño, S.; González, R.A.; Cortes, A.; Pomares, A.; Delgadillo, V.; Yepes, F.J.; Muñoz, Ó. A systematic review of serious games in medical education: Quality of evidence and pedagogical strategy. *Med. Educ. Online* **2018**, *23*, 1438718. [CrossRef] [PubMed]
8. Eukel, H.; Morrell, B. Ensuring Educational Escape-Room Success: The Process of Designing, Piloting, Evaluating, Redesigning, and Re-Evaluating Educational Escape Rooms. *Simul. Gaming* **2021**, *52*, 18–23. [CrossRef]
9. Antón-Solanas, I.; Rodríguez-Roca, B.; Urcola-Pardo, F.; Anguas-Gracia, A.; Satústegui-Dordá, P.J.; Echániz-Serrano, E.; Subirón-Valera, A.B. An evaluation of undergraduate student nurses' gameful experience whilst playing a digital escape room as part of a FIRST year module: A cross-sectional study. *Nurse Educ. Today* **2022**, *118*, 105527. [CrossRef] [PubMed]
10. Reinkemeyer, E.A.; Chrisman, M.; Patel, S.E. Escape rooms in nursing education: An integrative review of their use, outcomes, and barriers to implementation. *Nurse Educ. Today* **2022**, *119*, 105571. [CrossRef] [PubMed]
11. Aromataris, E.; Munn, Z. (Eds.) *JBI Manual for Evidence Synthesis*; JBI: Adelaide, Australia, 2020. Available online: https://synthesismanual.jbi.global (accessed on 17 January 2024).
12. Page, M.J.; McKenzie, J.E.; Bossuyt, P.M.; Boutron, I.; Hoffmann, T.C.; Mulrow, C.D.; Shamseer, L.; Tetzlaff, J.M.; Akl, E.A.; Brennan, S.E.; et al. The PRISMA 2020 statement: An updated guideline for reporting systematic reviews. *BMJ* **2021**, *372*, 71. [CrossRef]
13. Munn, Z.; Stern, C.; Aromataris, E.; Lockwood, C.; Jordan, Z. What kind of systematic review should I conduct? A proposed typology and guidance for systematic reviewers in the medical and health sciences. *BMC Med. Res. Methodol.* **2018**, *18*, 5. [CrossRef]
14. Rethlefsen, M.L.; Kirtley, S.; Waffenschmidt, S.; Ayala, A.P.; Moher, D.; Page, M.J.; Koffel, J.B.; PRISMA-S Group. PRISMA-S: An extension to the PRISMA Statement for Reporting Literature Searches in Systematic Reviews. *Syst. Rev.* **2021**, *10*, 39. [CrossRef]
15. Chen, D.; Liu, F.; Zhu, C.; Tai, C.; Zhang, Y.; Wang, X. The effect of an escape room game on college nursing students' learning attitude and game flow experiences in teaching safe medication care for the elderly: An intervention educational study. *BMC Med. Educ.* **2023**, *23*, 945. [CrossRef]
16. Schmuhl, K.K.; Nagel, S.; Tamburro, R.; Jewell, T.M.; Gilbert, E.; Gonzalez, A.; Sullivan, D.L.; Sprague, J.E. Better together: Utilizing an interprofessional course and escape room to educate healthcare students about opioid use disorder. *BMC Med. Educ.* **2023**, *23*, 917. [CrossRef]
17. Yang, C.L.; Chang, C.Y.; Jen, H.J. Facilitating undergraduate students' problem-solving and critical thinking competence via online escape room learning. *Nurse Educ. Pract.* **2023**, *73*, 103828. [CrossRef]

18. Hursman, A.; Richter, L.M.; Frenzel, J.; Viets Nice, J.; Monson, E. An online escape room used to support the growth of teamwork in health professions students. *J. Interprof. Educ. Pract.* **2022**, *29*, 100545. [CrossRef]
19. Millsaps, E.R.; Swihart, A.K.; Lemar, H.B. Time is brain: Utilizing escape rooms as an alternative educational assignment in undergraduate nursing education. *Teach. Learn. Nurs.* **2022**, *17*, 323–327. [CrossRef]
20. Molina-Torres, G.; Cardona, D.; Requena, M.; Rodriguez-Arrastia, M.; Roman, P.; Ropero-Padilla, C. The impact of using an "anatomy escape room" on nursing students: A comparative study. *Nurse Educ. Today* **2022**, *109*, 105205. [CrossRef]
21. Rodriguez-Ferrer, J.M.; Manzano-León, A.; Cangas, A.J.; Aguilar-Parra, J.M. A Web-Based Escape Room to Raise Awareness About Severe Mental Illness Among University Students: Randomized Controlled Trial. *JMIR Serious Games* **2022**, *10*, e34222. [CrossRef]
22. Wettergreen, S.A.; Stewart, M.P.; Huntsberry, A.M. Evaluation of an escape room approach to interprofessional education and the opioid crisis. *Curr. Pharm. Teach. Learn.* **2022**, *14*, 387–392. [CrossRef]
23. Fusco, N.M.; Foltz-Ramos, K.; Ohtake, P.J. An Interprofessional Escape Room Experience to Improve Knowledge and Collaboration among Health Professions Students. *Am. J. Pharm. Educ.* **2022**, *86*, ajpe8823. [CrossRef] [PubMed]
24. Foltz-Ramos, K.; Fusco, N.M.; Paige, J.B. Saving patient x: A quasi-experimental study of teamwork and performance in simulation following an interprofessional escape room. *J. Interprof. Care* **2021**, 1–8. [CrossRef]
25. Moore, L.; Campbell, N. Effectiveness of an escape room for undergraduate interprofessional learning: A mixed methods single group pre-post evaluation. *BMC Med. Educ.* **2021**, *21*, 220. [CrossRef]
26. Gutiérrez-Puertas, L.; Márquez-Hernández, V.V.; Román-López, P.; Rodríguez-Arrastia, M.J.; Ropero-Padilla, C.; Molina-Torres, G. Escape Rooms as a Clinical Evaluation Method for Nursing Students. *Clin. Simul. Nurs.* **2020**, *49*, 73–80. [CrossRef]
27. Morrell, B.L.M.; Eukel, H.N. Escape the Generational Gap: A Cardiovascular Escape Room for Nursing Education. *J. Nurs. Educ.* **2020**, *59*, 111–115. [CrossRef]
28. Katonai, Z.; Gupta, R.; Heuss, S.; Fehr, T.; Ebneter, M.; Maier, T.; Meier, T.; Bux, D.; Thackaberry, J.; Schneeberger, A.R. Serious Games and Gamification: Health Care Workers' Experience, Attitudes, and Knowledge. *Acad. Psychiatry* **2023**, *47*, 169–173. [CrossRef]
29. Gentry, S.V.; Gauthier, A.; L'Estrade Ehrstrom, B.; Wortley, D.; Lilienthal, A.; Tudor Car, L.; Dauwels-Okutsu, S.; Nikolaou, C.K.; Zary, N.; Campbell, J.; et al. Serious Gaming and Gamification Education in Health Professions: Systematic Review. *J. Med. Internet Res.* **2019**, *21*, e12994. [CrossRef]
30. Akl, E.A.; Kairouz, V.F.; Sackett, K.M.; Erdley, W.S.; Mustafa, R.A.; Fiander, M.; Gabriel, C.; Schünemann, H. Educational games for health professionals. *Cochrane Database Syst. Rev.* **2013**, *31*, CD006411. [CrossRef]
31. Hintze, T.D.; Samuel, N.; Braaten, B. A Systematic Review of Escape Room Gaming in Pharmacy Education. *Am. J. Pharm. Educ.* **2023**, *87*, 100048. [CrossRef]
32. Chicca, J.; Shellenbarger, T. Connecting with Generation Z: Approaches in nursing education. *Teach. Learn. Nurs.* **2018**, *13*, 180–184. [CrossRef]
33. Eukel, H.; Frenzel, J.; Frazier, K.; Miller, M. Unlocking Student Engagement: Creation, Adaptation, and Application of an Educational Escape Room across Three Pharmacy Campuses. *Simul. Gaming* **2020**, *51*, 167–179. [CrossRef]
34. Gómez-Urquiza, J.L.; Gómez-Salgado, J.; Albendín-García, L.; Correa-Rodríguez, M.; González-Jiménez, E.; Cañadas-De la Fuente, G.A. The impact on nursing students' opinions and motivation of using a "nursing escape room" as a teaching game: A descriptive study. *Nurse Educ. Today* **2019**, *72*, 73–76. [CrossRef] [PubMed]
35. Shah, A.S.; Pitt, M.; Norton, L. ESCAPE the Boring Lecture: Tips and Tricks on Building Puzzles for Medical Education Escape Rooms. *J. Med. Educ. Curric. Dev.* **2023**, *10*, 23821205231211200. [CrossRef] [PubMed]
36. Fanning, R.M.; Gaba, D.M. The role of debriefing in simulation-based learning. *Simul. Healthc.* **2007**, *2*, 115–125. [CrossRef]
37. Eppmann, R.; Bekk, M.; Klein, K. Gameful Experience in Gamification: Construction and Validation of a Gameful Experience Scale [GAMEX]. *J. Interact. Mark.* **2018**, *43*, 98–115. [CrossRef]
38. Gutiérrez-Puertas, L.; García-Viola, A.; Márquez-Hernández, V.V.; Garrido-Molina, J.M.; Granados-Gámez, G.; Aguilera-Manrique, G. Guess it (SVUAL): An app designed to help nursing students acquire and retain knowledge about basic and advanced life support techniques. *Nurse Educ. Pract.* **2021**, *50*, 102961. [CrossRef]
39. Kachaturoff, M.; Caboral-Stevens, M.; Gee, M.; Lan, V.M. Effects of peer-mentoring on stress and anxiety levels of undergraduate nursing students: An integrative review. *J. Prof. Nurs.* **2020**, *36*, 223–228. [CrossRef]
40. Najjar, R.H.; Lyman, B.; Miehl, N. Nursing students' experiences with high-fidelity simulation. *Int. J. Nurs. Educ. Scholarsh.* **2015**, *12*, 27–35. [CrossRef] [PubMed]
41. Reed, J.M.; Ferdig, R.E. Gaming and anxiety in the nursing simulation lab: A pilot study of an escape room. *J. Prof. Nurs.* **2021**, *37*, 298–305. [CrossRef]
42. Hudson, A.; Franklin, K.; Edwards, T.R.; Slivinski, A. Escaping the Silos: Utilization of a Pediatric Trauma Escape Room to Promote Interprofessional Education and Collaboration. *J. Trauma Nurs.* **2023**, *30*, 364–370. [CrossRef]
43. Fusco, N.M.; Foltz-Ramos, K.; Zhao, Y.; Ohtake, P.J. Virtual escape room paired with simulation improves health professions students' readiness to function in interprofessional teams. *Curr. Pharm. Teach. Learn.* **2023**, *15*, 311–318. [CrossRef]
44. Abensur Vuillaume, L.; Laudren, G.; Bosio, A.; Thévenot, P.; Pelaccia, T.; Chauvin, A. A Didactic Escape Game for Emergency Medicine Aimed at Learning to Work as a Team and Making Diagnoses: Methodology for Game Development. *JMIR Serious Games* **2021**, *9*, e27291. [CrossRef]

45. Guckian, J.; Eveson, L.; May, H. The great escape? The rise of the escape room in medical education. *Future Healthc. J.* **2020**, *7*, 112–115. [CrossRef]
46. Dams, V.; Burger, S.; Crawford, K.; Setter, R. Can You Escape? Creating an Escape Room to Facilitate Active Learning. *J. Nurses Prof. Dev.* **2018**, *34*, E1–E5. [CrossRef]
47. Friedrich, C.; Teaford, H.; Taubenheim, A.; Boland, P.; Sick, B. Escaping the professional silo: An escape room implemented in an interprofessional education curriculum. *J. Interprof. Care* **2019**, *33*, 573–575. [CrossRef] [PubMed]
48. Veldkamp, A.; van de Grint, L.; Knippels, M.-C.P.J.; van Joolingen, W.R. Escape Education: A Systematic Review on Escape Rooms in Education. *Educ. Res. Rev.* **2020**, *31*, 100364. [CrossRef]

Disclaimer/Publisher's Note: The statements, opinions and data contained in all publications are solely those of the individual author(s) and contributor(s) and not of MDPI and/or the editor(s). MDPI and/or the editor(s) disclaim responsibility for any injury to people or property resulting from any ideas, methods, instructions or products referred to in the content.

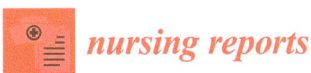

Communication

Impact of Artificial Intelligence on Nursing Students' Attitudes toward Older Adults: A Pre/Post-Study

Anne White [1,*], Mary Beth Maguire [1], Austin Brown [2] and Diane Keen [1]

1. Wellstar School of Nursing, Kennesaw State University, Kennesaw, GA 30144, USA; mbm2332@gmail.com (M.B.M.); dkeen2@kennesaw.edu (D.K.)
2. School of Data Science and Analytics, Kennesaw State University, Kennesaw, GA 30144, USA; abrow708@kennesaw.edu
* Correspondence: awhite@kennesaw.edu

Abstract: As the global population ages, nurses with a positive attitude toward caring for older adults is crucial. However, studies indicate that nursing students often exhibit negative attitudes toward older adults. This study aimed to determine if a three-phased educational intervention significantly improved nursing students' attitudes toward older adults. A pre/post-test study design was used to measure the change in nursing students' attitudes toward older adults, as measured by the UCLA Geriatrics Attitudes Survey, after participating in an Artificial Intelligence in Education learning event ($n = 151$). Results indicate that post-intervention scores (M = 35.07, SD = 5.34) increased from pre-intervention scores (M = 34.50, SD = 4.86). This difference was statistically significant at the 0.10 significance level (t = 1.88, $p = 0.06$). Incorporating artificial intelligence technology in a learning event is an effective educational strategy due to its convenience, repetition, and measurable learning outcomes. Improved attitudes toward older adults are foundational for delivering competent care to a rapidly growing aging population. This study was prospectively registered with the university's Institutional Review Board (IRB) on 30 July 2021 with the registration number IRB-FY22-3.

Keywords: artificial intelligence; simulation training; aging; geriatrics; attitudes survey

Citation: White, A.; Maguire, M.B.; Brown, A.; Keen, D. Impact of Artificial Intelligence on Nursing Students' Attitudes toward Older Adults: A Pre/Post-Study. *Nurs. Rep.* 2024, 14, 1129–1135. https://doi.org/10.3390/nursrep14020085

Academic Editor: Richard Gray

Received: 25 February 2024
Revised: 24 April 2024
Accepted: 26 April 2024
Published: 29 April 2024

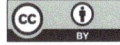

Copyright: © 2024 by the authors. Licensee MDPI, Basel, Switzerland. This article is an open access article distributed under the terms and conditions of the Creative Commons Attribution (CC BY) license (https://creativecommons.org/licenses/by/4.0/).

1. Introduction

As the global population ages, the demand for competent healthcare professionals with a positive attitude toward caring for older adults becomes increasingly crucial. Nurses hold a critical role in providing high-quality care to this vulnerable population. However, studies have indicated that nursing students often exhibit negative attitudes toward older adults, which can significantly impact their future practice of caring for older adults [1,2].

Recent reports have highlighted the need to improve the quality of geriatric care healthcare professionals provide, specifically emphasizing nursing education [3]. It has been observed that nursing students often harbor ageist attitudes, negative stereotypes, and limited knowledge about the unique healthcare needs of older adults [4]. These attitudes can hinder effective communication, compassionate care, and the overall well-being of older adults [5,6]. Consequently, efforts to address these attitudes and promote positive perceptions of senior care are essential in preparing a skilled nursing workforce to meet the demands of our aging population.

Ageism, defined as prejudice or discrimination against individuals based on age, remains a prevalent issue in healthcare settings, including nursing education [7]. Negative stereotypes and attitudes toward older adults can undermine the quality of care provided to this vulnerable population. A study by Allen et al. found that nursing students often held ageist beliefs, perceiving older adults as less capable, less deserving of care, and having limited potential for recovery [8]. Such attitudes can impact patient outcomes and the overall healthcare experience for older adults [9]. Therefore, addressing ageism within nursing education is imperative to develop a compassionate and person-centered approach to senior care.

Attitudes of healthcare professionals, particularly nurses, greatly influence the quality of care delivered to older adults. Positive attitudes toward aging and geriatric care are associated with better patient outcomes, increased patient satisfaction, and improved interprofessional collaboration [5]. Conversely, negative attitudes and stereotypes can result in suboptimal care, inadequate communication, and decreased patient well-being [4]. A systematic review by Burns et al. revealed that nursing students who often exhibited negative attitudes toward older adults were linked to insufficient exposure to geriatric nursing and a limited understanding of the aging process [10]. Thus, fostering positive attitudes among nursing students is essential to improve the overall quality of care for older adults and address the existing attitude-related barriers to effective geriatric nursing practice.

Educational interventions have shown promise in positively influencing nursing students' attitudes toward caring for older adults. Several authors have used geriatric simulation exercises and reflective discussions to expose healthcare professions to older adults. The intervention significantly improved empathy toward aging and increased confidence in providing geriatric care [11,12]. An integrative review by Magan et al. found that past experiences with older adults and gerontology-focused teaching strategies effectively diminished ageist stereotypes and fostered positive attitudes and perceptions of older adults [12]. Similarly, a systematic review by Shirey et al. demonstrated the efficacy of educational interventions in improving nursing students' knowledge, skills, and attitudes related to geriatric nursing [13].

The literature is replete with evidence regarding the impact of nurses' attitudes when caring for older adults. Contemporary nursing education may influence students' attitudes by incorporating innovative technology. An emerging pedagogy type involves Artificial Intelligence in Education (AIED) [14]. Artificial intelligence is the use of computers and machines to mimic the problem-solving skills of the human mind [15]. Therefore, this study aimed to determine if a three-phased AIED intervention significantly improved nursing students' attitudes toward older adults.

2. Materials and Methods

2.1. Theoretical Framework

The Experiential Learning Theory was the theoretical framework to support this study. Kolb described it as a four-stage learning cycle: concrete experience (CE), reflective observation (RO), active experimentation (AE), and abstract conceptualization (AC). The CE is described as the experience, whereas the RO is the purposeful reflection after the experience. The AE represents the implementation of the learning, and the AC is learning from experience [16]. A key aspect of Kolb's theory is that learning is not a linear process but a continuous cycle. Learners may revisit stages multiple times to refine their understanding and develop their skills.

2.2. Design

The researchers used a pre/post-test study design to measure the change in attitudes toward older adults among students enrolled in a senior-level community health nursing course in a baccalaureate program in the southeastern United States.

2.3. Sample Demographics

The population of interest is students enrolled in a senior-level community health nursing course in a baccalaureate program in the Southeastern United States. Since all students enrolled in the course were required to participate in the intervention as part of their course requirements, this implies that the sampling technique is non-probabilistic, the sample size relative to the population size is nearly 100%, and that attrition will not have a substantial role in the study. Further, since the sample size is almost the same as the size of the target population, the study is as maximally powered as is feasible since further participant recruitment was not possible. Thus, traditional power analysis techniques were deemed irrelevant for the present study. The sample demographics included the gender and age of the students enrolled in the community health class.

2.4. Inclusion and Exclusion Criteria

The inclusion criteria were all students enrolled in the community health nursing course. Exclusion criteria were incomplete datasets.

2.5. Instrument

The UCLA Geriatric Attitude Scale (GAS) was used to measure nursing students' attitudes before and after the educational intervention [17]. The GAS is a widely used instrument that assesses attitudes toward aging and older adults, providing valuable insights into respondents' prevailing attitudes and beliefs [17]. The instrument contains five positively and nine negatively worded statements rated on a scale from 1 (strongly disagree) to 5 (strongly agree), with higher scores indicating more positive attitudes toward aging. The internal reliability for the instrument was Cronbach's alpha = 0.76 [10]. An alpha between 0.7 and 0.9 is considered acceptable.

2.6. Statistical Methods

Because the study aimed to determine if the AIED changed nursing student attitudes toward older adults, a paired means sample test was deemed appropriate. Traditionally, a paired means sample t-test is used in such cases. Still, as is well-known, the validity of this test depends upon the assumption of normality being reasonably met. Before performing the paired means sample t-test, both a visual and a testing method of evaluating normality were employed, with the former being a Quantile–Quantile plot and the latter being the classical Shapiro–Wilk test of normality. In addition to the p-value of the inferential test used, the effect size was also reported to contextualize the results better.

2.7. Intervention

The community health nursing course utilized a three-phased approach to the AIED event (Table 1). The learning activities focused on Millie Larsen, a National League for Nursing (NLN) Advanced Care for Seniors (ACES) unfolding case [18]. The case study was introduced in the class and served as the foundation for complimenting activities related to older adult care.

Table 1. Instructional teaching methods.

Phase One: Pre-AIED Event Activities
1. Pre-class readings
2. Ninety-minute interactive classroom session
3. Pre-simulation medical record review
4. Pre-simulation knowledge survey
Phase Two: AIED Event Activities
1. AI-driven virtual non-immersive simulator experience
2. Completion of OASIS form
3. Create report email to multidisciplinary team
Phase Three: Post-AIED Activities
1. Guided reflection/debrief
2. NLN Simulation Design Scale

Phase One included assigned pre-class readings, 90-min classroom instruction, a review of the simulated patient's medical record, and a 22-item pre-simulation knowledge survey regarding the information reviewed to validate the completion of the Phase One activity. Phase Two comprised an AI-driven, virtual, non-immersive simulation experience of Millie Larson in her home [19]. The AI-driven virtual simulation replicated a patient interview using advanced artificial intelligence and natural language processing technology. Faculty members programmed the simulator prompts to ensure accurate responses to inquiries and adherence to the desired learning outcomes. Students interacted with the virtual simulator on their personal computers. Leveraging their computer's microphone, learners engaged in dialogue with the virtual patient. Each student was equipped with an individual account granting unrestricted access, free of charge, due to an in-kind grant. The virtual nature of the technology allowed for repeated practice sessions at their convenience to complete an abbreviated Outcome and Assessment Information Set Start of Care (OASIS SOC) [20]. Also, students drafted an email to a simulated multidisciplinary team describing the findings of the simulated patient encounter. Phase Three included completing an online reflection and debrief related to the simulated encounter and completing the NLN Simulation Design Scale instrument [21]. Due to the asynchronous nature of the learning event, students were given one week to complete the activities.

2.8. Ethical Aspects

The university's Institutional Review Board (IRB) deemed the study exempt from review. Participants were informed that completing the learning activity was a course requirement. Additionally, all study-related data were de-identified and stored on password-protected computers.

3. Results

3.1. Sociodemographic of Sample

A total of 160 students enrolled in the course (N = 160), and only those who completed all data were included in the study (n = 151), or 94% of the population. Table 2 represents a summary of the demographic data. Most of the sample identified as female (90%) and were between 18 and 24 years old (59; 39%).

Table 2. Demographics.

Category	Frequency	Percentage
	n = 151	
	Gender	
Male	15	10%
Female	136	90%
	Age Range	
18–24	74	49%
25–34	59	39%
35–44	11	7%
45–54	6	4%
55–64	1	1%
65+	0	0%
Mean	27.7	
Median	25	
Standard Deviation	7.5	

3.2. Instrument Reliability

The instrument's internal reliability was Cronbach's alpha = 0.76 for the pre-intervention scores and 0.78 for the post-intervention scores.

3.3. Mean Differences of Scores

Because the study aimed to determine if the AIED changed nursing student attitudes toward older adults, a paired sample t-test was used to compare the pre- and post-experience scores. Of note, only students with pre- and post-experience scores were included in the analysis (n = 151). Results indicate that post-intervention scores (M = 35.07,

SD = 5.34) increased from pre-intervention scores (M = 34.50, SD = 4.86). This modest improvement (d = 0.15) was statistically significant at the 0.10 significance level (t = 1.88, p = 0.06). An item-by-item analysis is given in Table 3. To note, all statistical analyses were performed in the statistical software package R version 4.3.2.

Table 3. Item analysis pre- and post-intervention.

Question	Pre-Intervention Mean (SD)	Post-Intervention Mean (SD)
Most old people are pleasant to be with	3.95 (0.90)	4.26 (0.76)
The federal government should reallocate money from Medicare to research on AIDS or pediatric diseases	3.45 (1.13)	3.52 (1.20)
If I have the choice, I would rather see younger patients than elderly ones	2.65 (1.23)	2.72 (1.14)
It is society's responsibility to provide care for its elderly persons	4.15 (0.86)	4.29 (0.80)
Medicare for old people uses up too much human and material resources	4.21 (0.97)	4.29 (0.87)
As people grow older, they become less organized and more confused	3.06 (1.12)	3.45 (1.07)
Elderly patients tend to be more appreciative of the medical care I provide than are younger patients	3.28 (0.97)	3.38 (0.96)
Taking a medical history from elderly patients is frequently an ordeal	3.53 (0.99)	3.50 (1.14)
I tend to pay more attention and have more sympathy towards my elderly patients than my younger patients	2.86 (0.97)	2.97 (0.92)
Old people in general do not contribute much to society	4.47 (0.76)	4.50 (0.67)
Treatment of chronically ill old patients is hopeless	4.55 (0.69)	4.60 (0.66)
Old persons don't contribute their fair share towards paying for their health care	4.25 (0.84)	4.33 (0.85)
In general, old people act too slow for modern society	4.27 (0.88)	4.26 (0.93)
It is interesting listening to old people's accounts of their past experiences	4.71 (0.58)	4.68 (0.61)

4. Discussion

This study aimed to add to the existing literature by assessing the influence of an AIED event on nursing students' feelings around ageism and attitudes toward caring for older adults. The findings reveal a significant increase in attitude scores after the AIED event. The results of this study support previous studies that identified education and intergenerational contact as effective interventions to combat ageism, thus improving attitudes toward older adults [6,9,10,22]. The outcomes propose that employing a multi-phased approach with a virtually simulated experience might overcome ageism in healthcare among baccalaureate nursing students.

The AIED event allowed undergraduate nursing students to experience a realistic encounter with an older adult, raising students' awareness of their attitudes toward the geriatric population. This study's results are like those of other studies that used simulation as an educational intervention to positively influence nursing students' attitudes toward caring for older adults [11,12]. This study underscores the efficacy of the AIED event in challenging negative attitudes and promoting more positive perceptions of older adults among future nursing workforces.

Nurses need to be at the forefront of evolving simulation pedagogy to help progress technologies in a manner sensitive to inclusivity and matters related to vulnerable groups like the elderly. The use of an AIED event differs from prior studies that used traditional simulation methods to increase students' attitudes toward working with older adults [23]. The computer-based virtual simulation of Millie Larson in her home permitted students to interact with the scenario at their convenience, regardless of location or time of day, if they had an internet connection. Evidence suggests there may be inherent bias in AI-driven technologies because they are built upon current evidence [24]. It is essential to explore the algorithms of the virtual simulation to ensure the virtual patient is evolving through machine learning that is sensitive to matters related to diversity, equity, and inclusion.

5. Limitations

There are several limitations related to this study. First, a single-site research design was utilized. Each school of nursing is unique. Thus, future studies should evaluate the effectiveness of this AIED event at other organizations. Second, the study employed a single AIED at one point in the nursing curriculum. It would be essential to explore the effectiveness of AIED at several time points across a curriculum. Repeated exposure to the simulated learning event may reveal how attitudes in older adults are or are not retained. Third, Wilson et al. concluded in their critical review of quantitative measures of attitudes toward older adults that all instruments used to date have inherent weaknesses [25]. A reliable and valid instrument to quantify attitudes toward older people has yet to be developed [26]. Magan et al. also identified the need for a current, nursing-specific measure of attitudes toward older people [9]. Finally, future studies should explore translating these findings to the knowledge of older adults in actual clinical encounters.

6. Conclusions

In summary, ageism within healthcare and nursing education poses a significant barrier to effective geriatric care. Addressing negative attitudes and stereotypes is crucial for fostering a compassionate and person-centered approach to caring for older adults. This research aims to contribute to the existing literature by evaluating the impact of an educational intervention on nursing students' attitudes toward caring for older adults, as measured by the GAS. By exploring the effectiveness of the intervention, this study provides evidence to inform future educational strategies and enhance the quality of care for older adults.

Author Contributions: Conceptualization, A.W. and M.B.M.; methodology, A.W., M.B.M. and A.B.; software, A.B.; validation, A.W., M.B.M. and A.B.; formal analysis, A.B.; investigation, A.W., M.B.M. and D.K.; resources, A.W., M.B.M. and D.K.; data curation, A.B.; writing—original draft preparation, A.W., M.B.M., A.B. and D.K.; writing—review and editing, A.W., M.B.M., A.B. and D.K.; supervision, A.W. and M.B.M.; project administration, A.W. and M.B.M. All authors have read and agreed to the published version of the manuscript.

Funding: This research received no funding.

Institutional Review Board Statement: The study was conducted in accordance with the Declaration of Helsinki and approved by the Institutional Review Board of Kennesaw State University (IRB-FY22-3 on 30 July 2021.

Informed Consent Statement: Informed consent was obtained from all subjects involved in the study.

Data Availability Statement: The data presented in this study are available on request from the corresponding author.

Public Involvement Statement: No public involvement in any aspect of this research.

Guidelines and Standards Statement: This manuscript was drafted against the SQUIRE-ED (Standards for Quality Improvement Reporting Excellence in Education: Publication Guidelines for Educational Improvement) for quantitative research.

Use of Artificial Intelligence: AI or AI-assisted tools were not used in drafting any aspect of this manuscript.

Conflicts of Interest: The authors declare no conflicts of interest.

References

1. Gipson, C.S.; Delello, J.A.; McWhorter, R.R. Engaging nursing students and older adults through service-learning. *Work. Older People* **2021**, *25*, 84–93. [CrossRef]
2. Venables, H.; Wells, Y.; Fetherstonhaugh, D.; Wallace, H. Factors associated with nursing students' attitudes toward older people: A scoping review. *Gerontol. Geriatr. Educ.* **2023**, *44*, 131–150. [CrossRef] [PubMed]

3. World Health Organization (WHO). Aging and Health. 2022. Available online: https://www.who.int/news-room/fact-sheets/detail/ageing-and-health (accessed on 26 April 2024).
4. Attafuah, P.Y.A.; Amertil, N.; Sarfo, J.O.; Deegbe, D.A.; Nyonator, D.; Amponsah-Boama, C.; Abuosi, A.A. "I decided to attend to him because it's my duty": Student Nurses perception and attitude towards care of older adults. *BMC Med. Educ.* **2022**, *22*, 23. [CrossRef]
5. Jang, I.; Oh, D.; Kim, Y.K. Factors associated with nursing students' willingness to care for older adults in Korea and the United States. *Int. J. Nurs. Sci.* **2019**, *6*, 426–431. [CrossRef] [PubMed]
6. Rababa, M.; Hammouri, A.M.; Al-Rawashdeh, S. Association of nurses' characteristics and level of knowledge with ageist attitudes toward older adults: A systematic review. *Work. Older People* **2021**, *25*, 21–38. [CrossRef]
7. São José, J.M.S.; Amado, C.A.F.; Ilinca, S.; Buttigieg, S.C.; Taghizadeh Larsson, A. Ageism in Health Care: A Systematic Review of Operational Definitions and Inductive Conceptualizations. *Gerontologist* **2019**, *59*, e98–e108. [CrossRef] [PubMed]
8. Allen, J.; Hutchinson, A.M.; Brown, R.; Livingston, P.M. Quality care outcomes following transitional care interventions for older people from hospital to home: A systematic review. *BMC Health Serv. Res.* **2014**, *14*, 346. [CrossRef]
9. Magan, K.C.; Ricci, S.; Hathaway, E. Factors influencing baccalaureate nursing students' attitudes toward older adults: An integrative review. *J. Prof. Nurs.* **2023**, *47*, 1–8. [CrossRef] [PubMed]
10. Burnes, D.; Sheppard, C.; Henderson, C.R.; Wassel, M.; Cope, R.; Barber, C.; Pillemer, K. Interventions to Reduce Ageism Against Older Adults: A Systematic Review and Meta-Analysis. *Am. J. Public Health* **2019**, *109*, e1–e9. [CrossRef] [PubMed]
11. Kaulback, M.; Barker, N.; Yocom, D. Experiencing Empathy through a Polypharmacy Simulation Experience in Baccalaureate Nursing Education. *Clin. Simul. Nurs.* **2021**, *59*, 94–97. [CrossRef]
12. Prete, D.; Tamburri, L.; Rolston, N.; Sturgill, M.; Bridgeman, M. Using simulation to introduce students and healthcare professionals to losses experienced by older adults: A pre-post analysis. *BMC Med. Educ.* **2024**, *24*, 96. [CrossRef]
13. Shirey, M.R.; Williams, E.S.; Artman, K.M. Systematic review of educational interventions to enhance geriatric nursing knowledge, attitudes, and skills. *Geriatr. Nurs.* **2021**, *42*, 1071–1080. [CrossRef]
14. IBM. Artificial Intelligence 2023. Available online: https://www.ibm.com/topics/artificial-intelligence (accessed on 25 February 2024).
15. Randhawa, G.K.; Jackson, M. The role of artificial intelligence in learning and professional development for health professionals. *Healthc. Manag. Forum.* **2019**, *33*. [CrossRef]
16. Kolb, D.A. *Experiential Learning: Experience as the Source of Learning and Development*; Prentice-Hall: Upper Saddle River, NJ, USA, 1984.
17. Reuben, D.B.; Lee, M.; Davis, J.W., Jr.; Eslami, M.S.; Osterweil, D.G.; Melchiore, S.; Weintraub, N.T. Development and validation of a geriatrics attitudes scale for primary care residents. *J. Am. Geriatr. Soc.* **1998**, *46*, 1425–1430. [CrossRef] [PubMed]
18. Reese, C. Advancing Care Excellence for Seniors: Millie Larson. National League for Nursing. 2022. Available online: https://www.nln.org/education/teaching-resources/professional-development-programsteaching-resourcesace-all/ace-s/unfolding-cases/millie-larsen-a22fc65c-7836-6c70-9642-ff00005f0421 (accessed on 25 February 2024).
19. PCS. Spark Intelligent Digital Patients. 2023. Available online: https://www.pcs.ai/ (accessed on 23 February 2024).
20. Centers for Medicare & Medicaid Services (CMS) U.S. Department of Health & Human Services. Outcome and Assessment Information Set OASIS-D Guidance Manual. 2019. Available online: https://www.hhs.gov/guidance/document/outcome-and-assessment-information-set-oasis-d-guidance-manualoasis-d-guidance-manual (accessed on 23 February 2024).
21. National League for Nursing. Simulation Design Scale: Student Version. 2005. Available online: https://www.nln.org/docs/default-source/uploadedfiles/professional-development-programs/nln-instrument-simulation-design-scale.pdf?sfvrsn=56f5d60d_0programs/nln-instrument-simulation-design-scale.pdf?sfvrsn=56f5d60d_0 (accessed on 23 February 2024).
22. Shropshire, M.; Hovey, S.; Ford, C.; Cecilia Wendler, M. Older adults "Have so Much to Teach Us": A qualitative study of BSN student perceptions when anticipating clinical in the nursing home. *Int. J. Older People Nurs.* **2022**, *17*, e12438. [CrossRef] [PubMed]
23. Von Gerich, H.; Moen, H.; Block, L.J.; Chu, C.H.; Haley, D.; Hobensack, M.; Michalowski, M.; Mitchell, J.; Nibber, R.; Olalia, M.A.; et al. Artificial intelligence-based technologies in nursing: A scoping literature review of the evidence. *Int. J. Nurs. Stud.* **2021**, *127*. Available online: https://www.sciencedirect.com/science/article/pii/S0020748921002984 (accessed on 25 February 2024). [CrossRef] [PubMed]
24. Larkin, Z. AI Bias-What Is it and How to Avoid it. 2022. Available online: https://levity.ai/blog/ai-bias-how-to-avoid (accessed on 25 February 2024).
25. Wilson MA, G.; Kurrle, S.; Wilson, I. Medical student attitudes towards older people: A critical review of quantitative measures. *BMC Res. Notes* **2018**, *11*, 71. [CrossRef]
26. Stewart, T.J.; Roberts, E.; Eleazer, P.; Boland, R.; Wieland, D. Reliability and Validity Issues for Two Common Measures of Medical Students' Attitudes toward Older Adults. *Educ. Gerontol.* **2006**, *32*, 409–421. [CrossRef]

Disclaimer/Publisher's Note: The statements, opinions and data contained in all publications are solely those of the individual author(s) and contributor(s) and not of MDPI and/or the editor(s). MDPI and/or the editor(s) disclaim responsibility for any injury to people or property resulting from any ideas, methods, instructions or products referred to in the content.

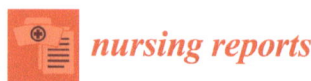

Review

Effects of Arts-Based Pedagogy on Competence Development in Nursing: A Critical Systematic Review

Berit Sandberg

HTW Business School, University of Applied Sciences Berlin, 10318 Berlin, Germany; berit.sandberg@htw-berlin.de

Abstract: The integration of arts-based methods into nursing education is a topic of growing interest in nursing practice. While there is an emerging body of research on this subject, evidence on competence development remains vague, largely due to methodological weaknesses. The purpose of this review is to evaluate the effectiveness of arts-based pedagogy in nursing, specifically in terms of students' changes in knowledge, skills, and attitudes. It explores which arts-based approaches to nursing education qualify as evidence-based practice in terms of nursing competence. A systematic critical review of research on arts-based pedagogy in nursing was conducted, identifying 43 relevant studies. These studies were assessed for methodological quality based on the CEC Standards for evidence-based practice, and 13 high-quality comparative studies representing a variety of arts-based approaches were selected. Creative drama was identified as the only evidence-based practice in the field, positively affecting empathy. The findings highlight a research gap in nursing education and emphasize the need for measurement and appraisal tools suitable for the peculiarities of arts-based pedagogy.

Keywords: arts-based learning; arts-based pedagogy; arts-based teaching; competence development; evidence-based practice; nursing education

Citation: Sandberg, B. Effects of Arts-Based Pedagogy on Competence Development in Nursing: A Critical Systematic Review. *Nurs. Rep.* **2024**, *14*, 1089–1118. https://doi.org/10.3390/nursrep14020083

Academic Editors: Antonio Martínez-Sabater, Elena Chover-Sierra and Carles Saus-Ortega

Received: 1 March 2024
Revised: 22 April 2024
Accepted: 23 April 2024
Published: 27 April 2024

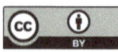

Copyright: © 2024 by the author. Licensee MDPI, Basel, Switzerland. This article is an open access article distributed under the terms and conditions of the Creative Commons Attribution (CC BY) license (https://creativecommons.org/licenses/by/4.0/).

1. Introduction

Nursing has been described as both an art and a science since Florence Nightingale's influential work, 'The Art of Nursing', was published in 1859 [1]. The artistic aspect of nursing has been a topic of discussion in the field of education for many years [2–6]. Scholars have complemented this concept by integrating liberal arts into nursing education [7–10]. This concept has been supported by professional associations [11] and global policy recommendations [12].

The inclusion of arts and humanities in the training of healthcare professionals aims to enhance learners' competencies in clinical and personal skills [12]. In nursing education, the arts and humanities help learners comprehend and appreciate human experiences. Some argue that knowledge of aesthetics can improve nurses' imaginative abilities and provide a more holistic understanding of themselves, human nature, and the caregiving process [13–16].

The integration of arts-based methods into nursing education has gained interest due to the growing recognition of the importance of a holistic approach to nursing [17,18]. This development aligns with the demand for competency-based education within curricula [12,19] and learner-centered approaches in the classroom, such as experiential learning [20].

In the sense of teaching *through the arts*, arts-based methods are a subfield of aesthetic teaching or aesthetic learning alongside teaching *about* and *in the arts* [15,21,22]. However, there is no appropriate term for using the arts as a didactic element. Common terms used in the literature include "arts-based learning" [23], "arts-based teaching" [24], "arts-based education" [25], and "arts-based pedagogy" [26,27]. These hyphenated terms highlight the interdisciplinary nature of arts-based teaching and learning, while also distinguishing it from artistic education and art pedagogy [28].

Arts-based pedagogy is a creative strategy that uses an art form to facilitate learning about another subject matter ([23], p. 53). This approach goes beyond decorative or entertaining elements in the classroom, such as background music (e.g., [29]). Learners engage with artistic works, perform them, or create their own. In this process, engagement with at least one art form, such as visual and performing arts, music, or literature, can aid in the acquisition of knowledge or skills in non-art subject areas [21,23,26]. Arts-based pedagogy facilitates experiential learning by considering sensory experience and aesthetic reflection as independent sources of knowledge and cognition [15,21].

Integrating arts and creative approaches into nursing education encourages students to explore beyond the traditional scientific and technical aspects of nursing and to engage with the emotional, social, and cultural aspects of the nursing profession. Arts-based approaches can increase learners' involvement, motivation, and attention by drawing from their experiences and creating an emotional connection to difficult topics [26,27,30,31]. This pedagogy complements training that primarily focuses on cognitive and psychomotor learning goals by addressing the affective level of learning [23,26,32].

Nursing practice requires a complex set of competencies, including clinical skills, interpersonal abilities, and humanistic practice [33]. Arts-based pedagogy has been used to address many of these competencies. Researchers suggest that arts-based nursing education can assist future nurses in developing a professional identity. The arts are believed to enhance critical thinking, diagnostic skills, and communication abilities. Enhancing empathy toward clients contributes to improved patient care quality and patient-centered nursing [30,34–39]. Additionally, arts-based approaches have been recognized to strengthen nursing students' resilience and help them cope with the high stress levels associated with the nursing profession [40,41].

Conceptual papers and empirical research generally present a positive view of arts-based nursing education and its effects, as reflected in relevant reviews. They either cover the entire field [27,32,42–44] or explore the integration of different genres within nursing education, such as the visual arts [31,45,46], drama [47,48], poetry [49–51], storytelling [52], and film (cinenurducation) [53,54].

However, many studies exploring the impact of art-based pedagogy in nursing education lack methodological quality and rigor. Most studies are qualitative and do not define what makes an intervention successful. It is suggested that qualitative studies may overestimate learning effects, while the actual development of competence may be lower than what a positive evaluation of arts-based learning experiences suggests [55]. In the case of quantitative research on arts-based pedagogy in nursing education, uncontrolled studies with limited internal validity are prevalent [56]. Outcome measures in many cases are not robust because they rely on participants' self-assessment [43,57].

A rigorous evaluation of arts-based nursing education is necessary to determine its impact on learners' knowledge acquisition, skill development, and attitudinal changes. Previous reviews have not systematically addressed this issue. Quantitative intervention studies are crucial in educational impact research because they allow for statistical verification of the causality between intervention and effect. They are an essential element of evidence-based practice (EBP), where the effectiveness of an intervention is the determining factor [58]. A practice is considered evidence-based if it is "supported by a sufficient number of research studies that (a) are of high methodological quality, (b) use appropriate research designs that allow for assessment of effectiveness, and (c) demonstrate meaningful effect sizes" ([59], p. 495).

This systematic review aims to determine if arts-based nursing education meets the criteria for evidence-based practice (EBP). It examines the extent to which rigorous research has been conducted on arts-based pedagogy in nursing, with attention to research design, methodological quality, and effect size [60–62]. As a critical review, this study explores the quality and credibility of quantitative research on arts-based nursing education. It aims to uncover potential methodological flaws or bias, make recommendations for future research, and inform practice in the field [63,64]. The paper takes a systematic approach to explore the impact of arts-based interventions on competence development as reflected in quantitative research. What are the reported effects on knowledge, skills, and attitudes resulting from art-based interventions? Is there scientifically robust research demonstrating their effectiveness [64]? The purpose of this review is to assess the effectiveness of art-based pedagogies in nursing and to support the concept of evidence-based nursing education [65].

2. Materials and Methods

This review follows the methodological approach for conducting systematic reviews as outlined by Kitchenham and Charters [66]. The approach includes the following stages: study selection, identification of research, quality assessment, data extraction, and data synthesis. The protocol for this systematic review was registered on INPLASY (INPLASY202440071).

2.1. Inclusion Criteria

2.1.1. Phenomena of Interest

As research on nursing education is the context of this study, the review encompasses all forms of training and development for nursing professionals, including secondary education in nursing degree programs and professional development. Secondary education in nursing degree programs as well as professional development are considered. The review also includes studies in which the participants were not exclusively nursing students or professionals.

This review focuses on arts-based pedagogy in nursing education. It includes studies in which learners receive works of visual art (painting, sculpture, graphics, photography, performance and media art, etc.), performing arts (theater, dance), music, film, or poetry. It also includes studies in which learners themselves create artifacts or actively engage in creative expressions such as theater, dance, narrative storytelling, etc. [67]. The review excludes methods that are not considered arts-based, such as photovoice, concept mapping, reflective writing, and standardized patient simulation using drama students. It considers interventions where the arts are integrated into regular nursing education, but not interventions limited to an examination context or self-contained art classes. Articles discussing the art of nursing, arts-based care methods, arts-based interventions in hospitals, or arts-based research methods in a nursing context are excluded.

2.1.2. Outcomes

This review examines competence development, defined as the process of enhancing knowledge, skills, and attitudes required to effectively perform tasks [68], with a focus on generic competency domains in nursing, such as professional attitude, clinical care, communication, and collaboration [33]. Only research that pertains to these domains is included, while studies that solely focus on learning experience and learner satisfaction, as well as research on learning and examination stress, are excluded.

2.1.3. Types of Studies

The review includes quantitative studies that enable the determination of causality between intervention and effect. It encompasses comparative studies with experimental or quasi-experimental designs, as well as non-experimental studies with a one-group pretest-posttest design [69]. Mixed-methods studies are included if they contain a relevant quantitative sub-study.

2.2. Literature Search and Screening

A systematic search for primary research studies was conducted in electronic databases relevant to nursing science, healthcare, and education. The databases searched were CINAHL, ERIC, Medline, PsycInfo, Scopus, and Web of Science. The Boolean phrase (nursing AND education OR nursing AND students) AND (art OR arts OR painting OR sculpture OR drawing OR music OR dance OR drama OR poetry OR photo* OR movie*) was applied to titles and abstracts. The full search strategy is displayed in Table S1. The database search was limited to articles with available abstracts and was supplemented by a manual backward search in relevant reviews [70].

To ensure the quality of the research, only peer-reviewed journal articles in English language published between January 1999 and December 2023, including electronic advance publications, were considered. This approach is in line with the growing body of relevant research since the mid-1990s [32]. Dissertations, book chapters, and other articles that might not have undergone independent review were excluded.

The database and manual searches together yielded an initial 2612 potentially relevant articles. Subsequently, titles and abstracts were screened against the inclusion criteria, resulting in 95 articles in total for full-text screening. After the screening process, 43 articles remained for evaluation. Search outcomes are displayed in Figure 1, using standard PRISMA flow diagram [71]. Screening was conducted by the author and a second reviewer using a review software, the Joanna Briggs Institute System for the Unified Management, Assessment, and Review of Information (JBI SUMARI) [72]. The concordance for title and abstract screening was initially established at a rate of 99.5% (12 conflicts). In the event that a conflict could not be resolved through discussion, the reviewers included the relevant studies for further examination [70,73]. The full-text screening yielded a 100% match.

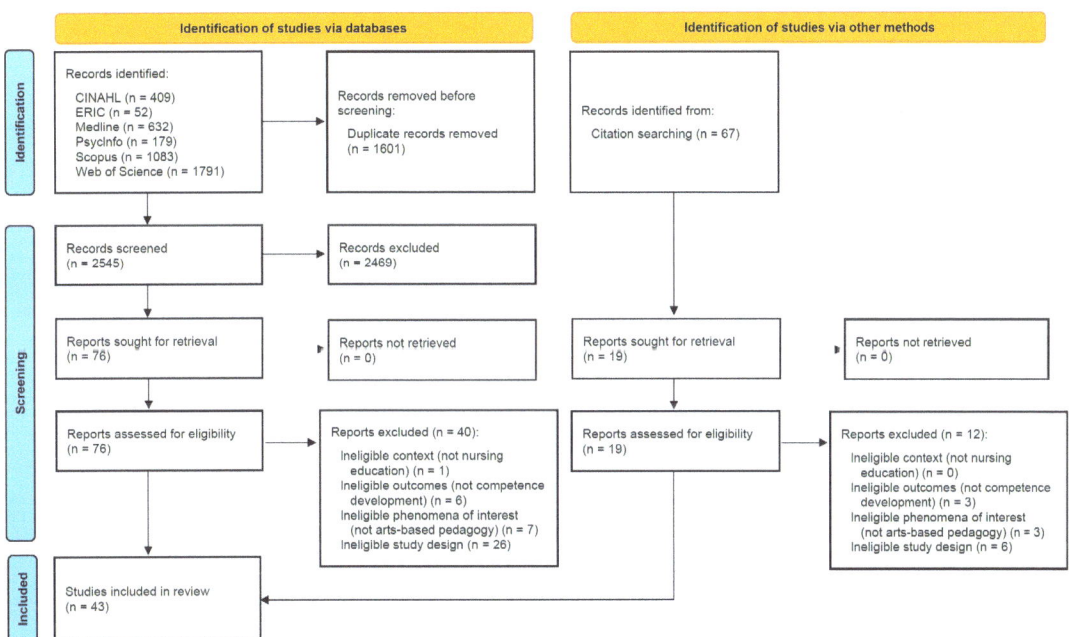

Figure 1. PRISMA flow diagram for literature search and selection.

2.3. Quality Assessment

The Council for Exceptional Children (CEC) Standards for Evidence-Based Practices in Special Education [74] is the selected assessment tool for this review. Evidence assessment tools developed for health research are not entirely applicable to evaluate articles in education research [75]. The CEC Standards were chosen because they are specifically designed for pedagogical intervention studies and allow for a more rigorous appraisal than other approaches in education research [76–78].

The CEC Standards encompass important research on comparative studies and single-case research in the field, as presented by Gersten and colleagues [79], Horner and colleagues [80], and Lane and colleagues [81], as well as the criteria established by the What

Works Clearinghouse (WWC) [82]. The CEC Standards are a common assessment tool in educational research. They are not exclusive to the field of special education [77], but they have also been used for systematic reviews in adult and higher education (e.g., [83–87]).

The CEC Standards guide the identification of evidence-based practices (EBPs) using 28 quality indicators (QIs) for the methodological soundness of group comparison studies and single-subject studies. The QIs cover eight areas: Context and Setting, Participants, Intervention Agents, Description of Practice, Implementation Fidelity, Internal Validity, Outcome Measures/Dependent Variables, and Data Analysis (Table 1). A study is considered sound if it meets all QIs in full. The CEC Standards also provide a grid for classifying the evidence base of practices based on high-quality research [82].

Table 1. CEC quality indicators. Source: [74].

Quality Indicator		Description	
1.	Context and setting	1.1	Describes critical features of the context or setting (school or classroom)
2.	Participants	2.1	Describes participants' demographics
		2.2	Describes disability or risk status and method for determining status
3.	Intervention agents	3.1	Describes role of the intervention agent, and background when relevant to review
		3.2	Describes agents' training or qualifications
4.	Description of practice	4.1	Describes detailed intervention procedures and agents' actions or cites accessible sources for that information
		4.2	Describes, when relevant, study materials described or cites accessible source
5.	Implementation fidelity	5.1	Assesses and reports implementation fidelity related to adherence with direct, reliable measures
		5.2	Assesses and reports implementation fidelity related to dosage or exposure with direct, reliable measures
		5.3	Assesses and reports implementation fidelity (adherence/dosage) throughout intervention and by unit of analysis
6.	Internal validity	6.1	Researcher controls and systematically manipulates independent variable
		6.2	Describes baseline or control conditions
		6.3	During baseline or control conditions, participants have no/extremely limited access to intervention
		6.4	Random assignment of groups
		6.8	Attrition is low across groups
		6.9	Attrition differential is low between groups or is controlled for
7.	Outcome measures/ dependent variables	7.1	Outcomes are socially important
		7.2	Defines and describes measurement of dependent variables
		7.3	Reports effects of intervention on all measures
		7.5	Provides evidence of adequate internal reliability
		7.6	Provides evidence of adequate validity
8.	Data analysis	8.1	Techniques are appropriate for detecting change in performance
		8.3	Reports appropriate effect size statistic(s) or provides data to calculate the effect size

Quality criteria sets must be adapted to the context and scope of the systematic review [58]. For this review, QIs 2.2 and 5.3 of the CEC Standards were excluded because they refer to requirements in special education and do not fit arts-based pedagogy. QIs 6.6 and 8.2 were also excluded because they apply to single-subject studies only. QIs 6.4, 6.8, and 6.9 are only applicable to group comparison studies.

The CEC standards should only be applied to experimental studies that meet the criteria for EBP [74]. However, this review includes non-experimental studies to identify methodological challenges and promising approaches in arts-based pedagogy. To assess the methodological quality of non-experimental studies, the CEC checklist was slightly modified. QI 6.5, originally intended for single-subject studies, is considered to be met if the study used a pretest-posttest-follow-up design, because such a design provides information about the long-term impact, stability, and causal effects of the intervention, which enhances validity [88].

The author and a second reviewer independently assessed all studies for methodological quality using extensive guidelines for interpreting the QIs [79–82]. The scoring was recorded in a quality indicator matrix that followed the CEC Standards [89]. Inter-rater agreement was calculated within the matrix at the indicator level to demonstrate the reliability of quality appraisal. The interrater-agreement percentage was initially 98.9% on average for all articles. Any discrepancies were discussed and resolved by the reviewers through mutual agreement [70]. The assessment results are presented for both comparative and non-experimental studies in Appendix A in Tables A1 and A2, respectively.

The CEC Standards require that all relevant QIs for the research design be met for a study to qualify as methodologically sound [74,82]. However, this benchmark has been criticized for being overly rigorous [81,90]. This review is based on a moderate understanding of evidence because, in educational research, it is appropriate to consider knowledge that does not correspond to the gold standard of evidence-based argumentation [91]. The scoring method suggested by Lane and colleagues [81] is followed, and QIs are weighed and given partial credit if met. A 80% cut-off point is applied to comparative studies. Studies that achieve 80% of QIs, equivalent to a score of 6.4, qualify as potential EBPs. Non-experimental studies, which represent a lower level of evidence than comparative studies [92], must meet the modified CEC Standards by 90%, equivalent to a score of 7.2.

2.4. Data Extraction

Data were extracted using summary tables for all comparative (Appendix A, Table A3) and non-experimental studies (Appendix A, Table A4). A concise summary is presented in Table 2. For mixed-methods studies, data extraction was limited to the characteristics of the quantitative sub-studies. The extraction was performed by the second reviewer and verified for accuracy in full by the author. The variables used for summarization were as follows: (a) intervention type, (b) study design, (c) participant characteristics and sample size, (d) data collection, (e) outcome measurements, and (f) key findings.

All studies were assessed for the certainty of evidence and categorized as having positive, mixed, neutral, or negative effects. The following criteria were established a priori [74,82]. Due to the heterogeneous nature of interventions and study designs, effect sizes were not taken into account. Studies are classified as having positive effects if statistically significant increases are demonstrated for all dependent variables. Studies are classified as yielding mixed effects if there are statistically significant increases in some dependent variables but not in others. Effects are classified as neutral if the intervention did not result in a statistically significant improvement in any of the dependent variables. If competencies deteriorate, the effect is termed negative.

Table 2. Summary of studies.

Author	Intervention	Study Design	Sample	Outcome	PE	No. of QIs Met Abs.	Wt.
Basit et al. (2023) [93] Turkey	Drama	Exp.	n = 49	Altruism Empathy	•	6	7.67
Briggs and Abell (2012) [94] USA	Movies	Exp.	n = 49	Empathy	•	6	7.33
Chen and Walsh (2009) [95] Taiwan	Visual art	Quasi-exp.	n = 194	Self-transcendence Attitudes toward elders		5	7.00
Dickens et al. (2018) [96] UK	Movies	Non-exp. (MMD)	n = 66	Attitudes toward people with PBD Knowledge about people with PBD		4	6.33
Dingwall et al. (2017) [97] UK	Drama	Non-exp. (MMD)	n = 63	Attitudes toward older people		2	4.17
Eaton and Donaldson (2016) [98] USA	Drama	Non-exp.	n = 12	Attitudes toward older adults	•	5	7.00
Emory et al. (2021) [99] USA	Music	Non-exp. (MMD)	n = 18	Attitudes toward older adults		3	5.83
Gazarian et al. (2014) [100] USA	Digital storytelling	Non-exp.	n = 36	Patient advocacy		3	5.00
Grossman et al. (2014) [101] USA	Visual art	Non-exp.	n = 19	Mindfulness Observational skills	•	3	5.33
Guo et al. (2021) [102] China	Visual art	Exp.	n = 99	Observational skills Diagnostic skills		7	7.50
HadaviBavili and İlçioğlu (2024) [103] Turkey	Visual art	Exp.	n = 181	Attitudes and self-efficacy toward anatomy courses		4	5.50
Hançer Tok and Cerit (2021) [104] Turkey	Drama	Exp.	n = 40	Attitudes toward caring for dying patients	•	8	8.00
Honan Pellico et al. (2012) [105] USA	Music	Exp.	n = 78	Auditory skills	•	6	7.33
Honan Pellico et al. (2014) [106] USA	Visual art Music	Non-exp.	n = 23	Perceptual aptitude skill (auditory and visual)		3	5.67
Honan et al. (2016) [107] USA	Visual art Music	Non-exp.	n = 39	Perceptual aptitude skill (auditory and visual)		3	6.00
Ince and Çevik (2017) [40] Turkey	Music	Exp.	n = 73	Blood draw skills	•	4	6.33
Kahriman et al. (2016) [108] Turkey	Drama	Exp.	n = 48	Empathy	•	6	7.33
Kirklin et al. (2007) [109] UK	Drama	Quasi-exp.	n = 67	Observational skills		4	5.83
Klugman and Beckmann-Mendez (2015) [110] USA	Visual art	Non-exp.	n = 19	Tolerance of ambiguity Attitude toward communication Observational skills		2	4.00
Klugman et al. (2011) [111] USA	Visual art	Non-exp.	n = 32	Tolerance for ambiguity Observational skills	•	4	5.67
Kyle et al. (2023) [112] UK	Drama	Non-exp.	n = 175	Attitudes toward interprofessionalism and nursing advocacy	•	5	6.00

Table 2. Cont.

Author	Intervention	Study Design	Sample	Outcome	PE	No. of QIs Met Abs.	Wt.
Lamet et al. (2011) [113] USA	Visual arts	Quasi-exp.	n = 98	Attitudes toward older people Self-transcendence Willingness to serve		5	6.00
Lesińska-Sawicka (2023) [114] Poland	Comics Graphic novels	Exp.	n = 62	Knowledge of cultural issues	●	4	6.17
Lovell et al. (2021) [115] USA	Visual art	Non-exp.	n = 218	Critical thinking (metacognitive awareness)	●	3	5.17
Moore and Miller (2020) [116] USA	Video storytelling	Non-exp.	n = 88	Knowledge, beliefs, and attitudes related to care for seriously ill people	●	3	5.00
Nash et al. (2020) [117] Australia	Drama	Non-exp. (MMD)	n = 65	Confidence and understanding in challenging situations		3	5.00
Nease and Haney (2018) [118] USA	Visual art	Exp.	n = 36	Observational skills Problem description and identification skills	●	3	5.17
Neilson and Reeves (2019) [119] UK	Drama	Non-exp. (MMD)	n = 100	Communication skills		3	3.67
Özcan et al. (2011) [120] Turkey	Misc.	Non-exp.	n = 48	Empathic skills	●	3	4.50
Park and Cho (2021) [121] South Korea	Movies	Exp.	n = 29	Professional nursing identity Professional nursing values	●	7	7.67
Rashidi et al. (2022) [122] Iran	Poetry	Quasi-exp.	n = 108	Moral sensitivity	●	6	6.83
Röhm et al. (2017) [123] Germany	Movies	Quasi-exp.	n = 51	Attitudes and social distancing toward stigmatized groups		3	5.83
Shieh (2005) [124] USA	Story writing Story-telling	Non-exp. (MMD)	n = 16	Nursing knowledge	●	4	5.50
Sinha et al. (2015) [125] USA	Visual art	Non-exp.	n = 36	Attitudes toward interprofessional collaboration Attitudes toward end-of-life care	●	1	1.83
Slota et al. (2018) [38] USA	Visual art	Non-exp.	n = 9	Observational skills Communication skills		4	5.17
Slota et al. (2022) [56] USA	Visual art	Non-exp.	n = 72	Observational skills Communication skills		3	4.67
Stupans et al. (2019) [126] Australia	Photo-essay	Non-exp. (MMD)	n = 77	Reflective thinking		3	4.83
Tastan et al. (2017) [127] Turkey	Music	Exp.	n = 77	Cardiac resuscitation skills	●	7	7.83
Tokur Kesgin and Hançer Tok (2023) [128] Turkey	Drama	Exp.	n = 78	Attitudes toward violence against women		8	8.00

Table 2. *Cont.*

Author	Intervention	Study Design	Sample	Outcome	PE	No. of QIs Met Abs.	Wt.
Uzun and Cerit (2023) [129] Turkey	Drama	Exp.	n = 70	Postmortem care knowledge and skills	•	6	6.50
Wikström (2001) [130] Sweden	Visual art	Exp.	n = 267	Perception of good nursing care	•	4	5.67
Yamauchi et al. (2017) [131] Japan	Visual art	Non-exp.	n = 307	Attitudes toward people with mental health problems		5	6.67
Zelenski et al. (2020) [132] USA	Drama	Quasi-exp. (MMD)	n = 86	Interprofessional empathy	•	5	6.50

Note. Abbreviations: Misc. = miscellaneous; Exp. = experimental; MMD = mixed-methods design; PE = positive effect; Abs. = absolute; Wt. = weighted. Studies with authors highlighted in italics are considered high-quality based on CEC Standards [74].

2.5. Data Synthesis

To determine if arts-based pedagogy qualifies as an evidence-based practice (EBP), studies beyond the threshold of quality assessment are grouped based on comparable interventions in terms of art form, procedure, and outcome. A differentiated approach is required due to the heterogeneity of studies [133]. The study follows the evidence-based classifications established by CEC [74], and the results are presented in Table A5 in Appendix A.

According to CEC Standards, EBPs must demonstrate positive effects supported by a minimum of two robust group comparison studies with random assignment. As non-random assignment of participants to groups raises the risk of selection bias, the CEC Standards mandate that EBPs show positive effects backed by four methodologically sound group comparison studies [82]. A body of work that fails to meet the criteria for evidence-based practice may be categorized as "potentially EBP", "mixed evidence", "insufficient evidence", or "negative effects" [74].

3. Results

After the screening process, 43 studies were included in the review. Out of these, 13 comparative studies met the criteria for a sound study and were evaluated as an EBP.

3.1. Participants and Settings

Most of the reviewed studies are based on data from undergraduate nursing students at universities or colleges. In six cases, participant groups were interdisciplinary, including medical or social work students [97,111,117,125,131,132]. Two studies took place in a professional training context [118,122]. Sample sizes for group comparison studies range from 40 to 267, while for non-experimental studies they range from 9 to 307.

3.2. Independent Variables

The studies reviewed cover a wide range of intervention designs that are based on various art forms.

A total of 15 interventions utilize the visual arts, with art observation being the most common design. Art observation is typically conducted in a museum (e.g., [56,102,115]). Three interventions engaged participants in creative assignments [95,103,113].

With a total of 10 studies, drama is a well-researched form of arts-based pedagogy [104,128,129]. Students typically participate in role-play or improvisation.

The sample includes five studies that used music as a teaching tool (e.g., [40,105]) or incorporated music into practical care [99]. Four studies examine the effects of cinenurducation [53] using movies as instructional material (e.g., [121,123]).

Other learning environments include photography [126], poetry [122], storytelling (e.g., [116]), comics and graphic novels [114], or a combination of different art forms [106,120].

3.3. Dependent Variables

Sensory perception skills are of particular interest for research (e.g., [56,102,106,107]) with a total of 10 studies. Above all, the impact of art observation on observation skills is examined. Five studies examine cognitive skills (e.g., [115,117,129]). Other studies focus on communication skills (e.g., [56,119]), diagnostic skills [102], or clinical skills [40,127].

Pedagogy that is based on the dramatic arts is often the subject of effectiveness research on attitudes. Ten studies examining the impact of arts-based pedagogy on attitudes toward others were analyzed (e.g., [96,104,116,131]), as well as five studies concerning attitudes toward other nursing issues (e.g., [112,128]). The research also covers complex concepts such as empathy, which is discussed in six studies (e.g., [93,122,132]), and professional identity, which is discussed in three (e.g., [103,121]).

Besides competence development, some studies examine personality traits such as self-efficacy [103], tolerance for ambiguity [110,111], and self-transcendence [95,113]. Five studies have explored the impact of arts-based pedagogy on knowledge acquisition, indicating that this is a peripheral research area (e.g., [114,116,129]).

3.4. Research Designs

Out of the 43 studies examined, 21 were group comparison studies, five of which were conducted as quasi-experiments. The remaining 22 studies were non-experimental. In the entire sample, eight studies utilized a mixed-methods design.

3.5. Methodological Quality

The quality appraisal results are presented in Appendix A in Table A1 for experimental and quasi-experimental studies and in Appendix A in Table A2 for non-experimental studies.

Of the reviewed studies, two experimental studies meet the Qis in full [104,128]. Eleven additional comparative studies score 80% or higher on the Qis [93–95,102,105,108, 121,122,127,129,132]. Thirteen out of the twenty-one comparison studies achieved a high level of methodological quality, with a weighted score of 6.4 Qis or higher. The remaining eight comparison studies were of moderate quality, scoring at least 5.2 Qis.

Non-experimental studies did not meet the 90% threshold specified for this review, with six studies receiving a mediocre rating of 5.6 Qis or higher.

Common methodological shortcomings in all types of studies include inadequate definitions of dependent variables, a lack of reliability, and the absence of evidence of validity. Out of 22 comparison studies, nine lack reliability, and 14 lack evidence of validity (e.g., [114]). Out of the 21 non-experimental studies, 16 rely on measurement tools that use self-developed questionnaires, face validity, or scales that were transferred without reflection (e.g., [56,95,111,116–118]). While some measurement tools lack psychometric data, others require considerable effort to verify because they are referenced in articles that are not available in English [93,103,108,120,121,123,131].

Controlling for internal validity is a common issue in non-experimental studies. Twenty non-experimental studies used a pretest–posttest design, while two studies also conducted a follow-up test [98,125]. Several non-experimental studies have inaccuracies in data analysis and reporting (e.g., [100]). Other studies have problems with reporting implementation fidelity or exposure, or do not provide an in-depth description of the intervention (e.g., [119,125]).

3.6. Effects

Out of the 21 group comparison studies, 14 report significant positive effects on skill levels and attitudes. Three studies show mixed results, lacking significant effects on some dependent variables [95,102,103,113]. Four interventions had no impact [109,123,128]. Although arts-based pedagogy may have a positive impact on students' competencies, it is not necessarily superior to conventional teaching. In two cases, researchers note positive effects but do not identify significant differences in competence development between the experimental and control groups [103,128].

Out of the 22 non-experimental studies, nine reported significant positive effects on nursing knowledge, skills, and attitudes. Another nine studies showed mixed results for changes in skill levels and attitudes. Four interventions failed to achieve an effect [96,97,117,119]. The outcomes are not related to art forms. Even comparable interventions may lead to different results [110,111].

4. Discussion

Out of the 43 studies reviewed, 13 are related to potential EBP as they achieve an 80% score for methodological soundness according to CEC Standards (Appendix A, Table A1). Three of these studies apply a quasi-experimental design [95,122,132], while ten meet the gold-standard of evidence by experimental design [69]. Ten studies describe arts-based interventions with positive effects on knowledge, skills, or attitudes (Appendix A, Table A5).

The sample is heterogeneous in terms of the studies included. It covers a range of different art-based interventions that must be assessed individually for each art form and targeted outcome when classifying research as evidence-based. Due to its variety, arts-based pedagogy needs to be evaluated less by "what works" but by "what works, for whom, and in what circumstances" ([133], p. 218).

4.1. Efficacy of Non-Dramatic Arts

A creative bonding intervention that employed students' collages and other objects in practical care yielded mixed results on self-transcendence and attitudes toward elders [105]. A multi-week Visual Arts Training at a museum significantly improved participants' observational skills but not their diagnostic competency [102]. The sample includes two musical interventions that positively impacted competence development. One intervention aimed to improve auditory skills [105], while the other utilized a disco song as an aid in cardiac resuscitation [127]. Two studies successfully introduced movies to the classroom [94,121]. Both studies screened movies without debriefing, but they differed in the number of movies shown and their duration. The experiments aimed to achieve different outcomes, with one focusing on empathy and the other on professional identity. One intervention that yielded positive effects, is based on poetry [122].

Pedagogical approaches to nursing education that are based on visual arts, music, movies, or poetry cannot be classified as evidence-based because an EBP requires at least one methodologically sound study to support it [82].

The use of visual arts training in museum settings to enhance perceptual abilities is a popular practice in nursing education and has garnered significant attention from researchers [31]. However, this approach has yet to yield robust research findings. Similarly, the incorporation of movies in teaching (cinenurducation) has inspired several studies [54], yet tangible research outcomes remain elusive. Arts-based learning offers interesting opportunities, such as exploring underrepresented art forms like comics, and developing interdisciplinary competencies such as intercultural skills [114]. Dance may enhance communication and collaboration skills [134] and other competencies relevant to clinical leadership [135], but it lacks solid quantitative research representation.

4.2. Efficacy of Creative Drama

Six studies aim to investigate the effects of drama-based pedagogy on nursing competencies [93,108,129,132], with two of them receiving the highest possible quality rating [104,128]. The learning experience was organized in a workshop format using creative drama. All workshops, except for one [129], were led by experienced or certified researchers in creative drama. Participants received training in drama techniques (e.g., [108]) or improvisation techniques [132] and actively applied them by reenacting [128] or role-playing typical care situations (e.g., [93]). One study demonstrates positive effects on postmortem care knowledge and skills [129]. Four studies report positive results on attitudes and empathy, while one intervention was found to be ineffective [128].

Three methodologically sound experimental studies on the use of drama in nursing education have reported positive effects on empathy and involved a total of 183 participants across studies [93,108,132]. These findings suggest that drama-based pedagogy qualifies as an evidence-based practice in nursing education according to the CEC classification [74]. However, it is important to note that these results are limited to empathy as a dependent variable, and there is insufficient evidence to support the effectiveness of creative drama in changing attitudes.

Creative drama is highly significant in nursing education and research because it allows students to explore complex nursing scenarios in a safe and supportive environment [47]. Empathy is an essential nursing competence because it fosters patient trust and the development of a successful therapeutic relationship [136,137]. Identifying creative drama as an EBP in terms of empathy adds to less rigorous research on the potential of drama in nursing education. Drama can enhance understanding of situations in clinical practice and the patient experience through fostering empathy and emotional engagement [48].

4.3. Impact on Professional Identity and Skills

Eight high-quality studies address attitudes reflecting the importance of professional values and their transmission in nursing education [138]. The arts-based teaching interventions documented in these eight studies successfully addressed altruism, empathy, and moral sensitivity (e.g., [93,94,121,122]). For healthcare professionals, prosocial behavior is crucial, and interpersonal competencies are essential in forming their professional identity [138]. As a potential trigger of deep reflection [27], arts-based pedagogy is an effective alternative to common approaches to identity formation, which is predominantly linked to traditional classroom learning [139].

Two high-quality studies focus on perceptual skills. They report positive effects of a music-based approach on auditory skills [105] and mixed effects of visual arts training on observational skills [102]. Together with inconclusive results from less rigorous studies (e.g., [56,107,109]), these findings challenge expectations for arts-based perceptual skills training in nursing education [31,46] and limit the meaningful scope of application to reflectivity. Visual arts have also been used in medical education to improve visual literacy and enhance students' observational and diagnostic skills [140,141]. As in nursing education, there is a lack of robust evidence on the development of competencies [142–146].

4.4. Challenges and Implications for Research

The review supports previous findings that suggest a lack of methodological quality and rigor in research on arts-based nursing education [32,43]. Although there is a substantial body of literature, there is a clear lack of evidence to support the effectiveness of arts-based pedagogy in terms of competency development.

The results suggest a requirement for high-quality research on arts-based teaching methods. Nevertheless, there are various obstacles to implementing evidence-based practice in this area that subpar studies are unable to overcome convincingly. Arts-based practices pose a challenge to the standardization of interventions and replication [147]. Comparative studies may face difficulties in drawing generalizable conclusions due to variability in implementation fidelity, instructor expertise, and student engagement, which can introduce heterogeneity. Arts-based pedagogy is highly context-dependent and influenced by factors such as teachers' attitudes and students' experiences and preferences [27,148]. Contextual variables may interact with the intervention, making it challenging to isolate the effects of arts-based practices. Arts-based pedagogy encompasses a wide variety of artistic mediums, teaching approaches, and instructional strategies. Each practice may have unique characteristics, making direct comparisons between interventions difficult.

To assess the impact of arts-based interventions on competence development, reliable observational data and tested scales are necessary. Sound psychometry is needed to establish contemporary measurement tools for outcomes that arts-based methods typically address [149]. The high-quality studies examined in this review predominantly employ established measurement instruments. In medical education, there are a variety of quantitative scales for assessing observation skills, as well as psychometric scales used to assess the impact of arts-based pedagogies on ambiguity tolerance, communication skills, empathy, and mindfulness [150]. It is recommended that nursing education researchers prioritize the development, validation, and application of robust psychometric instruments tailored to arts-based educational interventions. This will ensure that future studies can more accurately measure and demonstrate the true impact of these pedagogies and their unique characteristics on nursing competencies.

4.5. Requirements and Implications for Educational Practice

Professional standards for nurse educator practice emphasize the importance of employing evidence-based approaches to curriculum design, choice of teaching strategies, and assessment methods [151]. The findings presented in this review suggest that educators expand their teaching repertoire, but integrate arts-based teaching methods with caution. While the potential benefits of arts-based pedagogy cannot be dismissed, the lack of robust evidence necessitates a measured approach. It is recommended that educators engage in ongoing professional development to refine their understanding and implementation of arts-based methods [152]. This should include training on how to effectively integrate these approaches into the curriculum and how to critically evaluate their impact on student learning and competence development. Furthermore, it is of paramount importance for nursing educators to advocate for and adhere to evidence-based practice [151]. This encompasses not only the application of research findings to practice but also the contribution to research itself [153].

4.6. Limitations

The quality appraisal is based on the CEC Standards and categorization scheme for EBP [74,82], with a less rigorous threshold applied [81]. The scope of the review and validity check is limited to English language publications. This approach to quality appraisal is not conclusive. Notably, the selection of quality evaluation tools impacts evaluation findings. Utilizing a different assessment tool and altering the weighting scheme will alter results [154]. Tools for assessing evidence specific to the social sciences are still deficient [75]. The field of education is currently engaged in intense debate about the definition of evidence and the standards that should be applied [91,147,155,156]. The concept of evidence in education extends beyond (quasi-)experimental findings. Unlike in medical science, which provides a variety of assessment tools, comparative studies are rare in educational research. Education is a social system with comparatively weaker validity [156]. As it falls into the category of the "harder-to-do sciences" ([147], p. 424), research on arts-based pedagogy requires specific standards for quality appraisal that do not yet exist.

This review examines the extent to which arts-based pedagogy improves the competencies of nursing students. It does not address the impact of arts-based pedagogy on the learning environment or other factors that contribute to learning success, such as learner engagement [157]. Successful arts-based pedagogy is largely based on disrupting behavior patterns and beliefs that facilitate the learning process [158–160]. Arts-based approaches are believed to benefit from experiential learning, multisensory learning, and emotional engagement [26,161,162]. However, their impact on learners and their influence on competence development require refined quantitative assessment methods and a wider range of methodologically sound comparative studies to build a more definitive evidence base for arts-based pedagogy.

5. Conclusions

Given the increasing recognition of non-traditional teaching methods in nursing education and the necessity to prepare students for the complexities of modern healthcare settings, research on arts-based pedagogy in nursing education is a growing area of interest. This research area is significant because it explores innovative teaching methods that can enhance nursing education and improve patient outcomes. However, there is a lack of evidence regarding the development of competence related to interventions and outcomes relevant to nursing practice, despite the variety of approaches stemming from different art forms.

This review aimed to evaluate whether arts-based approaches to nursing education improve nursing competence and meet the criteria for EBP. The review identified 43 quantitative studies that explored the impact of arts-based pedagogy on the knowledge, skills, and attitudes of nursing students. Thirteen comparative studies met the CEC Standards for high-quality research. Based on the CEC classification scheme, creative drama is considered an EBP, while other forms of arts-based pedagogy do not have enough sound studies to qualify as an EBP.

The findings suggest that the high expectations toward arts-based pedagogy in nursing education should be reconsidered in light of the evidence base. It is important to conduct high-quality research in this field to gain a better understanding of its effectiveness. This effort is critical to advancing arts-based pedagogy from an innovative educational experiment to a foundational, evidence-based practice in nursing education.

Supplementary Materials: The following supporting information can be downloaded at https://www.mdpi.com/article/10.3390/nursrep14020083/s1, Table S1: Database search.

Funding: This research was supported by the University of Applied Sciences Berlin.

Public Involvement Statement: No public involvement in any aspect of this research.

Guidelines and Standards Statement: Reporting follows the Preferred Reporting Items for Systematic reviews and Meta-Analyses (PRISMA) statement [71].

Acknowledgments: The author would like to extend her sincere appreciation to Lilith Merle Meyer, research assistant at the University of Applied Sciences Berlin, for her invaluable assistance in screening, quality assessment, and data extraction throughout the course of this review.

Conflicts of Interest: The author declares no conflicts of interest.

Appendix A

Table A1. Quality assessment results for comparative studies.

Author	1.0	1.1	2.0	2.1	2.2	3.0	3.1	3.2	4.0	4.1	4.2	5.0	5.1	5.2	5.3	6.0	6.1	6.2	6.3	6.4	6.5	6.6	6.7	6.8	6.9	7.0	7.1	7.2	7.3	7.4	7.5	7.6	8.0	8.1	8.2	8.3	No. of QIs Met Absolute	Weighted 80%	Effects Positive	Mixed	Neutral	Negative
Basit et al. (2023) [93]		•		NA	•		•	•		•	•		NA	NA	•		NA	NA	NA	NA	NA	NA	NA	NA	NA		•	•	•	•	•	•		NA	NA	•	6	7.67	•			
Briggs and Abell (2012) [94]		•		NA	•		•	•		•	•		NA	NA	•		NA	NA	NA	NA	NA	NA	NA	NA	NA		•	•	•	•	•	•		NA	NA	•	6	7.33	•			
Chen and Walsh (2009) [95]		•		NA	•		•	•		•	•		NA	•	•		NA	NA	NA	NA	NA	NA	NA	NA	NA		•	•	•		•	•		NA	NA	•	5	7.00		•		
Guo et al. (2021) [102]		•		NA	•		•	•		•	•		NA	•	•		NA	NA	NA	NA	NA	NA	NA	NA	NA		•	•	•	•	•	•		NA	NA	•	7	7.50		•		
HadaviBavili and İlçioğlu (2024) [103]		•		NA	•		•	•		•	•		NA	NA	NA		•	•	•	•	•	•	•	•	•		•		•	•	•			NA	NA	•	4	5.50	•			
Hançer Tok and Cerit (2021) [104]		•		NA	•		•	•		•	•		NA	NA	•		NA	NA	NA	NA	NA	NA	NA	NA	NA		•	•	•	•	•	•		NA	NA	•	8	8.00	•			
Honan Pellico et al. (2012) [105]		•		NA	•		•	•		•	•		NA	NA	•		NA	NA	NA	NA	NA	NA	NA	NA	NA		•	•	•	•	•	•		NA	NA	•	6	7.33	•			
Ince and Çevik (2017) [40]		•		NA	•		•	•		•	•		NA	NA	•		NA	NA	NA	NA	NA	NA	NA	NA	NA		•	•	•	•	•	•		NA	NA	•	4	6.33	•			
Kahrıman et al. (2016) [108]		•		NA	•		•	•		•	•		•	•	•		NA	NA	NA	NA	NA	NA	NA	NA	NA		•	•	•	•	•	•		NA	NA	•	6	7.33	•			
Kirklin et al. (2007) [109]		•		NA	•		•	•		•	•		NA	•	•		NA	NA	NA	NA	NA	NA	NA	NA	NA		•	•	•					NA	NA	•	4	5.83	•			
Lamet et al. (2011) [113]		•		NA	•		•	•		•	•		NA	•	•		NA	NA	NA	NA	NA	NA	NA	NA	NA		•	•	•			•		NA	NA	•	5	6.00		•		
Lesińska-Sawicka (2023) [114]		•		NA	•		•	•		•	•		NA	NA	•		NA	NA	NA	NA	NA	NA	NA	NA	NA		•			•	•			NA	NA	•	4	6.17	•			
Nease and Haney (2018) [118]		•		NA	•		•	•		•	•		NA	NA	•		NA	NA	NA	NA	NA	NA	NA	NA	NA		•	•	•					NA	NA	•	3	5.17	•			
Park and Cho (2021) [121]		•		NA	•		•	•		•	•		NA	NA	•		NA	NA	NA	NA	NA	NA	NA	NA	NA		•	•	•	•	•	•		NA	NA	•	7	7.67	•			
Rashidi et al. (2022) [122]		•		NA	•		•	•		•	•		NA	NA	•		NA	NA	NA	NA	NA	NA	NA	NA	NA		•	•	•	•	•	•		NA	NA	•	6	6.83	•			
Röhm et al. (2017) [123]		•		NA	•		•	•		•	•		NA	NA	•		NA	NA	NA	NA	NA	NA	NA	NA	NA		•	•	•			•		NA	NA	•	3	5.83			•	
Tastan et al. (2017) [127]		•		NA	•		•	•		•	•		NA	NA	•		NA	NA	NA	NA	NA	NA	NA	NA	NA		•	•	•	•	•	•		NA	NA	•	7	7.83	•			
Tokur Kesgin and Hançer Tok (2023) [128]		•		NA	•		•	•		•	•		NA	NA	•		NA	NA	NA	NA	NA	NA	NA	NA	NA		•	•	•	•	•	•		NA	NA	•	8	8.00			•	
Uzun and Cerit (2023) [129]		•		NA	•		•	•		•	•		NA	•	•		NA	NA	NA	NA	NA	NA	NA	NA	NA		•	•	•	•	•			NA	NA	•	6	6.50	•			
Wikström (2001) [130]		•		NA	•		•	•		NA	•		NA	•	•		NA	NA	NA	NA	NA	NA	NA	NA	NA		•	•	•	•				NA	NA	•	4	5.67			•	
Zelenski et al. (2020) [132]		•		NA	•		•	•		•	•		NA	•	•		NA	NA	NA	NA	NA	NA	NA	NA	NA		•	•	•		•			NA	NA	•	5	6.50	•			
Total	21/21	18/21	NA	16/21	20/21	18/21	13/21	10/21	14/21	17/21	21/21	18/21	16/21	NA	NA	NA	14/21	18/21	20/21	16/21	20/21	12/21	8/21	21/21	NA	17/21																

Note. NA = not applicable.

Table A2. Quality assessment results for non-experimental studies.

Author	1.0 1.1	2.0 2.1	2.2	3.0 3.1	3.2	4.0 4.1	4.2	5.0 5.1	5.2	5.3	6.1	6.0 6.2	6.3	6.4	6.5	6.6	6.7	6.8	6.9	7.1	7.0 7.2	7.3	7.4	7.5	7.6	8.1	8.0 8.2	8.3	No. of QIs Met Absolute	Weighted 90%	Effects Positive	Mixed	Neutral	Negative
Dickens et al. (2018) [96]	•	NA	•	•	•			•	NA	NA	•	NA		NA		NA	NA	NA	NA	•	•	•	•			•	•		4	6.33			•	
Dingwall et al. (2017) [97]	•	NA	•	•	•	•	NA	NA	NA	NA	•	NA		NA		NA	NA	NA	NA	•	•	•							2	4.17			•	
Eaton and Donaldson (2016) [98]	•	NA	•	•	•	NA	NA	•	NA	NA	•	NA		NA	•	NA	NA	NA	NA	•	•					•			5	7.00				
Emory et al. (2021) [99]	•	NA	•	•	•	•	NA	•	NA	NA	•	NA		NA		NA	NA	NA	NA	•	•	•							3	5.83	•			
Gazarian et al. (2014) [100]	•	NA	•	•	•	•	NA	•	NA	NA	•	NA		NA		NA	NA	NA	NA	•	•								3	5.00		•		
Grossman et al. (2014) [101]	•	NA	•	•	•			•	NA	NA	•	NA		NA		NA	NA	NA	NA	•	•	•							3	5.33	•			
Honan Pellico et al. (2014) [106]	•	NA	•	•	•			•	NA	NA	•	NA		NA		NA	NA	NA	NA	•	•		•						3	5.67		•		
Honan et al. (2016) [107]	•	NA	•	•	•			•	NA	NA	•	NA		NA		NA	NA	NA	NA	•	•		•						3	6.00	•			
Klugman and Beckmann-Mendez (2015) [110]	•	NA	•	•	•				NA	NA		NA		NA		NA	NA	NA	NA	•	•								2	4.00				
Klugman et al. (2011) [111]	•	NA	•	•	•			•	NA	NA	•	NA		NA		NA	NA	NA	NA	•	•	•							4	5.67	•			
Kyle et al. (2023) [112]	•	NA	•	•	•			•	NA	NA	•	NA		NA		NA	NA	NA	NA	•	•	•							5	6.00	•			
Lovell et al. (2021) [115]	•	NA	•	•	•			•	NA	NA	•	NA		NA		NA	NA	NA	NA	•	•			•					3	5.17	•			
Moore and Miller (2020) [116]	•	NA	•	•	•			•	NA	NA	•	NA		NA		NA	NA	NA	NA	•	•								3	5.00	•			
Nash et al. (2020) [117]	•	NA	•	•	•			•	NA	NA	•	NA		NA		NA	NA	NA	NA	•	•								3	5.00	•			
Neilson and Reeves (2019) [119]	•	NA	•	•	•		NA		NA	NA		NA		NA		NA	NA	NA	NA	•	•								3	3.67			•	
Özcan et al. (2011) [120]	•	NA	•	•	•		NA	•	NA	NA	•	NA		NA		NA	NA	NA	NA	•	•				•				3	4.50	•			
Shieh (2005) [124]	•	NA	•	•	•			•	NA	NA	•	NA		NA		NA	NA	NA	NA	•	•					•	•		4	5.50	•			
Sinha et al. (2015) [125]	•	NA	•	•	•				NA	NA		NA		NA	•	NA	NA	NA	NA	•									1	1.83		•		
Slota et al. (2018) [38]	•	NA	•	•	•		NA	•	NA	NA	•	NA		NA		NA	NA	NA	NA	•	•	•							4	5.17		•		
Slota et al. (2022) [56]	•	NA	•	•	•		NA	•	NA	NA	•	NA		NA		NA	NA	NA	NA	•	•								3	4.67		•		
Stupans et al. (2019) [126]	•	NA	•	•	•			•	NA	NA	•	NA		NA		NA	NA	NA	NA	•	•		•						3	4.83		•		
Yamauchi et al. (2017) [131]	•	NA	•	•	•			•	NA	NA	•	NA		NA		NA	NA	NA	NA	•	•	•		•				•	5	6.67		•		
Total	22/22	12/22	NA	16/22	20/22	18/22	8/22	8/22	12/22	22/22	14/22	22/22	NA	2/22	1/22	0/22	NA	NA	NA	22/22	22/22	10/22	19/22	21/22	6/22	5/22	16/22	1/22	15/22					

Note. NA = not applicable.

Table A3. Summary of comparative studies.

Author	Intervention	Study Design	Participants	Data Collection	Outcome	Measurements	Key Findings	Positive	Mixed	Neutral	Negative	Absolute No. of QIs Met	80% Weighted
Basit et al. (2023) [93] Turkey	Drama Roleplay	Exp.	Nursing students n = 49	Q	Altruism Empathy	Altruism Scale Jefferson Scale of Empathy for Nursing Students (JSENS)	Significant increase in altruism and empathy No enduring effect	•				6	7.67
Briggs and Abell (2012) [94] USA	Movie	Exp.	Junior nursing students n = 49	Q	Empathy	Jefferson Scale of Physician Empathy (JSE)	Significant increase in empathy	•				6	7.33
Chen and Walsh (2009) [95] Taiwan	Visual art	Quasi-exp	Fourth-year nursing students n = 194	Q	Self-transcendence Attitudes toward elders	Self-transcendence scale (STS) Revised Kogan's attitudes toward old people scale (RKAOP)	Significantly more positive attitude toward elders No effect on self-transcendence		•			5	7.00
Guo et al. (2021) [102] China	Visual art	Exp.	First-year nursing students in master program n = 99	Q	Observational skills Diagnostic skills	Clinical image test	Significant increase of observational skills Trend toward improvement of diagnostic skills		•			7	7.50
HadaviBavili and Ilçioğlu (2024) [103] Turkey	Visual art	Exp.	First-year nursing and midwifery students n = 181	Q	Attitudes and self-efficacy toward anatomy courses	Anatomy attitude scale Anatomy self-efficacy scale	No significant effect			•		4	5.50
Hanger Tok and Cerit (2021) [104] Turkey	Drama Roleplay	Exp.	First-year Bachelor of Nursing Science students n = 40	Q	Attitudes toward caring for dying patients	Frommelt Attitude Scale for Caring for Dying (FATCOD)	Significantly more positive attitude toward dying patients	•				8	8.00
Honan Pellico et al. (2012) [105] USA	Music	Exp.	First-year nursing students in master program n = 78	Obs.	Auditory skills	N/A	Significant improvement of organ identification and sound interpretation	•				6	7.33
Ince and Çevik (2017) [40] Turkey	Music	Exp.	First-year nursing students n = 73	Obs.	Blood draw skills	Skill controls list	Significantly decreased anxiety levels Improved blood draw skills	•				4	6.33
Kahriman et al. (2016) [108] Turkey	Drama Roleplay Improvisation	Exp.	Practicing nurses n = 48	Q	Empathy	Empathic Skill Scale (ESS)	Significant increase in empathy	•				6	7.33

Table A3. Cont.

Author	Intervention	Study Design	Participants	Data Collector	Outcome	Measurements	Key Findings	Effects Positive	Effects Mixed	Effects Neutral	Effects Negative	No. of QIs Met Absolute	80% Weighted
Kirklin et al. (2007) [109] UK	Drama	Quasi-exp.	Practicing nurses and doctors n = 68	Obs.	Observational skills	N/A	No significant effect			•		4	5.83
Lamet et al. (2011) [113] USA	Visual arts	Quasi-exp	Junior and senior nursing students n = 98	Q	Attitudes toward older people Self-transcendence Willingness to serve	Self-Transcendence Scale (STS) Attitudes toward Old People Scale	Significant improvement in attitudes toward older people Trend to increased willingness to serve		•			5	6.00
Lesińska-Sawicka (2023) [114] Poland	Comics Graphic novels	Exp.	First-year nursing students n = 62	Q	Knowledge of cultural issues	N/A	Significant increase in knowledge	•				4	6.17
Nease and Haney (2018) [118] USA	Visual art	Exp.	Practicing nurses n = 36	Obs.	Observation skills Problem description and identification skills	N/A	Significant improvement of observation skills Significant improvement of problem description and identification skills	•				3	5.17
Park and Cho (2021) [121] South Korea	Movies	Exp.	Second year undergraduate nursing students n = 29	Q	Professional nursing identity Professional nursing values	Perception of nursing checklist Professional nursing values scale	Significant improvement in perception of nursing and professional nursing values	•				7	7.67
Rashidi et al. (2022) [122] Iran	Poetry	Quasi-exp.	Practicing nurses n = 108	Q	Moral sensitivity	Nursing Moral Sensitivity Questionnaire (MSQ)	Significantly enhanced sensitivity	•				6	6.83
Röhm et al. (2017) [123] Germany	Movies	Quasi-exp.	Bachelor and master students in Rehabilitation Sciences n = 51	Q	Attitudes and social distancing toward stigmatized groups	Social Distance Scale Community Attitudes toward the Mentally Ill (CAMI)	No significant effect			•		3	5.83
Tastan et al. (2017) [127] Turkey	Music	Exp.	Second-year nursing school students n = 77	Obs.	Cardiac resuscitation skills	N/A	Significantly improved performance of cardiac resuscitation	•				7	7.83
Tokur Kesgin and Hançer Tok (2023) [128] Turkey	Drama Roleplay	Exp.	Fourth-year undergraduate nursing science students n = 78	Q	Attitudes toward violence against women	Violence Against Women Attitude Scale (İSKEBE)	No significant effect			•		8	8.00

Table A3. Cont.

Author	Intervention	Study Design	Participants	Data Collection	Outcome	Measurements	Key Findings	Effects: Positive	Effects: Mixed	Effects: Neutral	Effects: Negative	Absolute	80% Weighted	No. of QIs Met
Uzun and Cerit (2023) [129] Turkey	Drama Improvisation Roleplay	Exp.	Third-year undergraduate nursing science students n = 70	Q Obs.	Postmortem care knowledge and skills	Postmortem care knowledge test (PCKT) Postmortem care skills checklist (PCSCL)	Significantly improved postmortem knowledge and skill levels Enduring effect	•				6	6.50	
Wikström (2001) [130] Sweden	Visual art	Exp.	First year nursing students n = 267	Q	Perception of good nursing care	Wheel Questionnaire	Significantly improved understanding of good nursing care	•				4	5.67	
Zelenski et al. (2020) [132] USA	Drama	Quasi-exp. (MMD)	Students in health professions training programs (mainly nursing, pharmacy, medical) n = 86	Q	Interprofessional empathy	Interpersonal Reactivity Index (IRI) Consultative and Relational Empathy (CARE) Ekman Facial Action Coding System	Significant enhancement of interprofessional empathy	•				5	6.50	

Note. Exp. = experimental; MMD = mixed-methods design; N/A = not applicable; Obs. = observation; Q = questionnaire.

Table A4. Summary of non-experimental studies.

Author	Intervention	Study Design	Participants	Data Collection	Outcome	Measurements	Key Findings	Effects Positive	Effects Mixed	Effects Neutral	Effects Negative	No. of QIs Met Absolute	90% Weighted
Dickens et al. (2018) [96] UK	Movies	Non-exp. (MMD)	Undergraduate and postgraduate mental health nursing and counselling students n = 66	Q	Attitudes toward people with PBD Knowledge about people with PBD	Borderline Personality Disorder Questionnaire	Minor changes in knowledge and attitudes			•		4	6.33
Dingwall et al. (2017) [97] UK	Drama	Non-exp. (MMD)	Third-year nursing and social work students n = 63	Q	Attitudes toward older people	Self-developed questionnaire	Significant attitudinal changes among social work students only			•		2	4.17
Eaton and Donaldson (2016) [98] USA	Drama	Non-exp.	Second- and third-semester nursing students n = 12	Q	Attitudes toward older adults	Attitudes Toward Old People Scale (KOP) Refined Version of the Aging Semantic Differential (rASD)	Significant improvement in attitudes	•				5	7.00
Emory et al. (2021) [99] USA	Music	Non-exp. (MMD)	First-year bachelor nursing students n = 18	Q	Attitudes toward older adults	Perspectives on Caring for Older Patients (PCOP) Modified Kogan's Attitudes toward Old People Scale (MKOP)	No significant effect for aggregate variables relating to attitudes toward older adults			•		3	5.83
Gazarian et al. (2014) [100] USA	Digital storytelling	Non-exp.	Senior-level nursing students n = 36	Q	Patient advocacy	Protective Nursing Advocacy Scale (PNAS)	Increase in perceptions of patient advocacy		•			3	5.00
Grossman et al. (2014) [101] USA	Visual art	Non-exp.	Nursing students n = 19	Q	Mindfulness Observational skills	Mindfulness Attention Awareness Scale (MAAS) Clinical Picture Assessment (CPA)	Significant improvement of mindfulness Significant improvement of observational skills		•			3	5.33
Honan Pellico et al. (2014) [106] USA	Visual art Music	Non-exp.	Fourth-year bachelor nursing students n = 23	Obs.	Perceptual aptitude skill (auditory and visual)	N/A	Improved observational skills Significant increase in auscultative interpretive skills		•			3	5.67
Honan et al. (2016) [107] USA	Visual art Music	Non-exp.	Students in an accelerated nursing master's program for non-nursing college graduates n = 39	Obs.	Perceptual aptitude skill (auditory and visual)	N/A	Significantly improvement in most observational skills Significant increase in some auscultative interpretive skills No enduring effects		•			3	6.00

Table A4. Cont.

Author	Intervention	Study Design	Participants	Data Collection	Outcome	Measurements	Key Findings	Effects Positive	Effects Mixed	Effects Neutral	Effects Negative	No. of QIs Met Absolute	90% Weighted
Klugman and Beckmann-Mendez (2015) [110] USA	Visual art	Non-exp.	Undergraduate and graduate nursing students, medical students n = 19	Q Obs.	Tolerance of ambiguity Attitude toward communication Observation skills	Variation of Budner's Tolerance of Ambiguity Scale Communication Skills Attitude Scale (CSAS)	No significant effect on tolerance of ambiguity No significant effect on interest in communication Significant improvement of observational skills		•			2	4.00
Klugman et al. (2011) [111] USA	Visual art	Non-exp.	Undergraduate and graduate nursing students, different level medical students n = 32	Q Obs.	Observational skills Tolerance for ambiguity	Variation of Budner's Tolerance of Ambiguity Scale Communication Skills Attitude Scale (CSAS)	Significant improvement in observational skills Significant increase in tolerance for ambiguity	•				4	5.67
Kyle et al. (2023) [112] UK	Drama	Non-exp.	Undergraduate nursing students n = 175	Q	Attitudes toward interprofessionalism and nursing advocacy	Attitudes toward Healthcare Teams Scale (ATHCTS) Protective Nursing Advocacy Scale (PNAS)	Significant improvement in attitudes toward interprofessionalism and nursing advocacy	•				5	6.00
Lovell et al. (2021) [115] USA	Visual art	Non-exp.	Traditional and accelerated first-year nursing students n = 218	Q	Critical thinking (metacognitive awareness)	Metacognitive Awareness Inventory (MAI)	Significant increase in metacognitive awareness	•				3	5.17
Moore and Miller (2020) [116] USA	Video storytelling	Non-exp.	Second-degree nursing students n = 88	Q	Knowledge, beliefs, and attitudes related to care for seriously ill people	Adapted Story Experience Questionnaire	Significant increase in knowledge, beliefs, and attitudes related to care for seriously ill people	•				3	5.00
Nash et al. (2020) [117] Australia	Drama Roleplay	Non-exp. (MMD)	Students from multiple health professions n = 65	Q	Confidence and understanding in challenging situations	Self-developed questionnaire	Increased confidence and understanding in challenging situations			•		3	5.00
Neilson and Reeves (2019) [119] UK	Drama	Non-exp. (MMD)	First-year nursing students n = 100	Q	Communication skills	Self-developed questionnaire	Improved communication skills			•		3	3.67
Özcan et al. (2011) [120] Turkey	Miscellaneous	Non-exp.	Third class and senior nursing students n = 48	Q	Empathic skills	Empathic Skill Scale	Significant increase in empathic skills	•				3	4.50
Shieh (2005) [124] USA	Story writing Storytelling	Non-exp. (MMD)	Associate Degree in Nursing students n = 16	Q	Nursing knowledge	Self-developed questionnaire	Significant improvement in five areas of nursing knowledge	•				4	5.50

Table A4. Cont.

Author	Intervention	Study Design	Participants	Data Collection	Outcome	Measurements	Key Findings	Effects (Positive/Mixed/Neutral/Negative)	No. of QIs Met (Absolute / 90% Weighted)
Sinha et al. (2015) [125] USA	Visual art	Non-exp.	Mainly third-year nursing and medical students n = 36	Q	Attitudes toward interprofessional collaboration Attitudes toward end-of-life care	Self-developed questionnaire	Significantly improved attitude toward interprofessional collaboration Significantly improved attitude toward end-of-life care	Positive	1 / 1.83
Slota et al. (2018) [38] USA	Visual art	Non-exp.	Post-Master Doctor of Nursing Practice students n = 9	Q	Observation skills Communication skills	Self-developed Visual Intelligence Assessment Tool (VIA)	Significantly improved attitude toward the relevance of observational skills Improved observational skills Deteriorated communication skills	Mixed	4 / 5.17
Slota et al. (2022) [56] USA	Visual art	Non-exp.	Post-Master Doctor of Nursing Practice and Clinical Nurse Leader graduate students n = 72	Q Obs.	Observational skills Communication skills	Self-developed Visual Intelligence Assessment Tool (VIA) Image Assessment	No change in overall visual intelligence scores Significant improvement of observational skills	Mixed	3 / 4.67
Stupans et al. (2019) [126] Australia	Photo-essay	Non-exp. (MMD)	First year Bachelor of Nursing students n = 77	Q	Reflective thinking	Reflective Thinking Questionnaire	Significant increase in understanding and critical reflection Increase in reflection	Mixed	3 / 4.83
Yamauchi et al. (2017) [131] Japan	Visual art	Non-exp.	Nursing students, social work students n = 307	Q	Attitudes toward people with mental health problems	Semantic Differential Attitude Scale regarding people with mental health problems	Significantly improved attitudes toward people with mental health problems	Mixed	5 / 6.67

Note. Exp. = experimental; MMD = mixed-methods design; N/A = not applicable; Obs. = observation; Q = questionnaire.

Table A5. Summary of high-quality studies.

Author	Intervention	Study Design	Participants	Data Collection	Outcome	Measurements	Key Findings	Positive	Mixed	Neutral	Negative	No. of QIs Met Absolute	80% Weighted
Chen and Walsh (2009) [95] Taiwan	Visual art	Quasi-exp.	Fourth-year nursing students n = 194	Q	Self-transcendence Attitudes toward elders	Self-transcendence scale (STS) Revised Kogan's attitudes toward old people scale (RKAOP)	Significantly more positive attitude toward elders No effect on self-transcendence		•			5	7.00
Guo et al. (2021) [102] China	Visual art	Exp.	First-year nursing students in master program n = 99	Q	Observational skills Diagnostic skills	Clinical image test	Significant increase of observational skills Trend toward improvement of diagnostic skills		•			7	7.50
Briggs and Abell (2012) [94] USA	Movies	Exp.	Junior nursing students n = 49	Q	Empathy	Jefferson Scale of Physician Empathy (JSE)	Significant increase in empathy	•				6	7.33
Park and Cho (2021) [121] South Korea	Movies	Exp.	Second year undergraduate nursing students n = 29	Q	Professional nursing identity Professional nursing values	Perception of nursing checklist Professional nursing values scale	Significant improvement in perception of nursing and professional nursing values	•				7	7.67
Honan Pellico et al. (2012) [105] USA	Music	Exp.	First-year nursing students in master program n = 78	Obs.	Auditory skills	N/A	Significant improvement of organ identification and sound interpretation	•				6	7.33
Tastan et al. (2017) [127] Turkey	Music	Exp.	Second-year nursing school students n = 77	Obs.	Cardiac resuscitation skills	N/A	Significantly improved performance of cardiac resuscitation	•				7	7.83
Rashidi et al. (2022) [122] Iran	Poetry	Quasi-exp.	Practicing nurses n = 108	Q	Moral sensitivity	Nursing Moral Sensitivity Questionnaire (MSQ)	Significantly enhanced sensitivity	•				6	6.83

Table A5. Cont.

Author	Intervention	Study Design	Participants	Data Collection	Outcome	Measurements	Key Findings	Effects Positive	Effects Mixed	Effects Neutral	Effects Negative	No. of QIs Met Absolute	80% Weighted
Basit et al. (2023) [93] Turkey	Drama Roleplay	Exp.	Nursing students n = 49	Q	Altruism Empathy	Altruism Scale Jefferson Scale of Empathy for Nursing Students (JSENS)	Significant increase in altruism and empathy No enduring effect	●				6	7.67
Hançer Tok and Cerit (2021) [104] Turkey	Drama Roleplay	Exp.	First-year Bachelor of Nursing Science students n = 40	Q	Attitudes toward caring for dying patients	Frommelt Attitude Scale for Caring for Dying (FATCOD)	Significantly more positive attitude toward dying patients	●				8	8.00
Kahriman et al. (2016) [108] Turkey	Drama Roleplay Improvisation	Exp.	Practicing nurses n = 48	Q	Empathy	Empathic Skill Scale (ESS)	Significant increase in empathy	●				6	7.33
Tokur Kesgin and Hançer Tok (2023) [128] Turkey	Drama Roleplay	Exp.	Fourth-year undergraduate nursing science students n = 78	Q	Attitudes toward violence against women	Violence Against Women Attitude Scale (ISKEBE)	No significant effect			●		8	8.00
Uzun and Cerit (2023) [129] Turkey	Drama Improvisation Roleplay	Exp.	Third-year undergraduate nursing science students n = 70	Q Obs.	Postmortem care knowledge and skills	Postmortem care knowledge test (PCKT) Postmortem care skills checklist (PCSCL)	Significantly improved postmortem knowledge and skill levels Enduring effect	●				6	6.50
Zelenski et al. (2020) [132] USA	Drama	Quasi-exp. (MMD)	Students in health professions training programs (mainly nursing, pharmacy, medical) n = 86	Q	Interprofessional empathy	Interpersonal Reactivity Index (IRI) Consultative and Relational Empathy (CARE) Ekman Facial Action Coding System	Significant enhancement of interprofessional empathy	●				5	6.50

Note. Exp. = experimental; MMD = mixed-methods design; N/A = not applicable; Obs. = observation; Q = questionnaire.

References

Note: References marked with an asterisk (*) indicate studies included in the review.

1. Hirao, M. "The Art of Nursing" by Florence Nightingale, published by Claud Morris Books Limited and printed in 1946, which is considered a draft of "Notes on Nursing". *Nihon Ishigaku Zasshi [J. Jpn. Hist. Med.]* **2000**, *46*, 246–255.
2. Dade, L.; Wolf, L.K. A new approach to the teaching of nursing arts. *AJN Am. J. Nurs.* **1946**, *46*, 404. [CrossRef]
3. Carper, B.A. Fundamental patterns of knowing in nursing. *Adv. Nurs. Sci.* **1978**, *1*, 13–24. [CrossRef] [PubMed]
4. Chan, Z.C. Exploration of artistry in nursing teaching activities. *Nurse Educ. Today* **2014**, *34*, 924–928. [CrossRef] [PubMed]
5. Amendolair, D. Art and science of caring of nursing: Art-based learning. *Int. J. Hum. Caring* **2021**, *25*, 249–255.
6. Badowski, D. Trends in the art and science of nursing education: Responding to the life-changing events of 2020. *Nurs. Educ. Perspect.* **2021**, *42*, 204. [CrossRef] [PubMed]
7. Moseley, S.; Belcher, H.C. Art in the nursing curriculum. *Nurs. Outlook* **1955**, *3*, 86–89. [PubMed]
8. Reed, P.G. Liberal arts and professional nursing education: Integrating knowledge and wisdom. *Nurse Educ.* **1987**, *12*, 37–40. [CrossRef] [PubMed]
9. Darbyshire, P. Understanding caring through arts and humanities: A medical/nursing humanities approach to promoting alternative experiences of thinking and learning. *J. Adv. Nurs.* **1994**, *19*, 856–863. [CrossRef]
10. Vande Zande, G.A. The liberal arts and professional nursing. *J. Nurs. Educ.* **1995**, *34*, 93–94. [CrossRef]
11. Howley, L.; Gaufberg, E.; King, B. *The Fundamental Role of the Arts and Humanities in Medical Education*; Association of American Medical Colleges: Washington, DC, USA, 2020. Available online: https://store.aamc.org/the-fundamental-role-of-the-arts-and-humanities-in-medical-education.html (accessed on 10 January 2024).
12. (WHO) World Health Organization. *Global Competency and Outcomes Framework for Universal Health Coverage*; World Health Organization: Geneva, Switzerland, 2022. Available online: https://www.who.int/publications/i/item/9789240034662 (accessed on 6 January 2024).
13. Staricoff, R.L. Arts in health: The value of evaluation. *J. R. Soc. Promot. Health* **2006**, *126*, 116–120. [CrossRef] [PubMed]
14. McKie, A. Using the arts and humanities to promote a liberal nursing education: Strengths and weaknesses. *Nurse Educ. Today* **2012**, *32*, 803–810. [CrossRef] [PubMed]
15. Archibald, M.M.; Caine, V.; Scott, S.D. Intersections of the arts and nursing knowledge. *Nurs. Inq.* **2017**, *24*, e12153. [CrossRef] [PubMed]
16. Damsgaard, J.B. Integrating the arts and humanities into nursing. *Nurs. Philos.* **2020**, *22*, e12345. [CrossRef]
17. Watson, M.J. *Nursing: The Philosophy and Science of Caring*; Little, Brown and Company: Boston, MA, USA, 1979.
18. McEvoy, L.; Duffy, A. Holistic practice: A concept analysis. *Nurse Educ. Pract.* **2008**, *8*, 412–419. [CrossRef] [PubMed]
19. Frenk, J.; Chen, L.; Bhutta, Z.A.; Cohen, J.; Crisp, N.; Evans, T.; Fineberg, H.; Garcia, P.; Ke, Y.; Kelley, P.; et al. Health professionals for a new century: Transforming education to strengthen health systems in an interdependent world. *Lancet* **2010**, *376*, 1923–1958. [CrossRef] [PubMed]
20. Jones-Schenk, J. Designing education for learning activation. *J. Contin. Educ. Nurs.* **2017**, *48*, 539–540. [CrossRef]
21. Lindström, L. Aesthetic learning about, in, with and through the arts: A curriculum study. *Int. J. Art Des. Educ.* **2012**, *31*, 166–179. [CrossRef]
22. Sotiropoulou-Zormpala, M. Aesthetic teaching: Seeking a balance between teaching arts and teaching through the arts. *Arts Educ. Policy Rev.* **2012**, *113*, 123–128. [CrossRef]
23. Rieger, K.L.; Chernomas, W.M. Arts-based learning: Analysis of the concept for nursing education. *Int. J. Nurs. Educ. Sch.* **2013**, *10*, 53–62. [CrossRef]
24. Møller-Skau, M.; Lindstøl, F. Arts-based teaching and learning in teacher education: "Crystallising" student teachers' learning outcomes through a systematic literature review. *Teach. Teach. Educ.* **2022**, *109*, 103545. [CrossRef]
25. Chisolm, M.S.; Kelly-Hedrick, M.M.; Wright, S.M. How visual arts-based education can promote clinical excellence. *Acad. Med.* **2021**, *96*, 1100–1104. [CrossRef] [PubMed]
26. Rieger, K.L.; Chernomas, W.M.; McMillan, D.E.; Morin, F.L. The arts as a catalyst for learning with undergraduate nursing students: Findings from a constructivist grounded theory study. *Arts Health* **2020**, *12*, 250–269. [CrossRef] [PubMed]
27. Obara, S.; Perry, B.; Janzen, K.J.; Edwards, M. Using arts-based pedagogy to enrich nursing education. *Teach. Learn. Nurs.* **2021**, *17*, 113–120. [CrossRef]
28. Seiler, B. *Wirkfaktoren menschlicher Veränderungsprozesse: Das ModiV in allgemeiner und kunstbezogener Beratung, Psychotherapie und Pädagogik [Effective Factors of Human Change Processes: The ModiV in General and Art-Related Counseling, Psychotherapy and Education]*; Springer: Wiesbaden, Germany, 2018.
29. Evangelista, K.; Macabasag, R.L.A.; Capili, B.; Castro, T.; Danque, M.; Evangelista, H.; Rivero, J.A.; Gonong, M.K.; Diño, M.J.; Cajayon, S. Effects of classical background music on stress, anxiety, and knowledge of Filipino baccalaureate nursing students. *Int. J. Nurs. Educ. Sch.* **2017**, *14*, 20160076. [CrossRef] [PubMed]
30. Jensen, A.; Curtis, M. A descriptive qualitative study of student learning in a psychosocial nursing class infused with art, literature, music, and film. *Int. J. Nurs. Educ. Sch.* **2008**, *5*, 4. [CrossRef] [PubMed]
31. Elhammoumi, C.V.; Kellam, B. Art images in holistic nursing education. *Religions* **2017**, *8*, 103. [CrossRef]

32. Rieger, K.L.; Chernomas, W.M.; McMillan, D.E.; Morin, F.L.; Demczuk, L. Effectiveness and experience of arts-based pedagogy among undergraduate nursing students: A mixed methods systematic review. *JBI Database Syst. Rev. Implement. Rep.* **2016**, *14*, 139–239. [CrossRef]
33. Wit, R.F.; de Veer, A.J.; Batenburg, R.S.; Francke, A.L. International comparison of professional competency frameworks for nurses: A document analysis. *BMC Nurs.* **2023**, *22*, 343. [CrossRef]
34. Hydo, S.K.; Marcyjanik, D.L.; Zorn, C.R.; Hooper, N.M. Art as a scaffolding teaching strategy in baccalaureate nursing education. *Int. J. Nurs. Educ. Sch.* **2007**, *4*, 20. [CrossRef]
35. Frei, J.; Alvarez, S.E.; Alexander, M.B. Ways of seeing: Using the visual arts in nursing education. *J. Nurs. Educ.* **2010**, *49*, 672–676. [CrossRef] [PubMed]
36. Acai, A.; McQueen, S.A.; McKinnon, V.; Sonnadara, R.R. Using art for the development of teamwork and communication skills among health professionals: A literature review. *Arts Health* **2017**, *9*, 60–72. [CrossRef]
37. Lutter, S.L.; Pucino, C.L.; Jarecke, J.L. Arts-based learning strategies in clinical postconference: A qualitative study. *J. Nurs. Educ.* **2018**, *57*, 549–553. [CrossRef] [PubMed]
38. * Slota, M.; McLaughlin, M.; Bradford, L.; Langley, J.F.; Vittone, S. Visual intelligence education as an innovative interdisciplinary approach for advancing communication and collaboration skills in nursing practice. *J. Prof. Nurs.* **2018**, *34*, 357–363. [CrossRef] [PubMed]
39. Suh, E.E.; Ahn, J.; Kang, J.; Seok, Y. The development and application of drama-combined nursing educational content for cancer care. *Int. J. Environ. Res. Public Health* **2021**, *18*, 9891. [CrossRef] [PubMed]
40. * Ince, S.; Çevik, K. The effect of music listening on the anxiety of nursing students during their first blood draw experience. *Nurse Educ. Today* **2017**, *52*, 10–14. [CrossRef] [PubMed]
41. Kinsella Frost, C. Art in debrief: A small-scale three-step narrative inquiry into the use of art to facilitate emotional debriefing for undergraduate nurses. *J. Res. Nurs.* **2019**, *24*, 197–209. [CrossRef] [PubMed]
42. Lake, J.; Jackson, L.; Hardman, C. A fresh perspective on medical education: The lens of the arts. *Med. Educ.* **2015**, *49*, 759–772. [CrossRef] [PubMed]
43. Osman, M.; Eacott, B.; Willson, S. Arts-based interventions in healthcare education. *Med. Humanit.* **2017**, *44*, 28–33. [CrossRef]
44. Byma, E.A.; Lycette, L. An integrative review of humanities-based activities in baccalaureate nursing education. *Nurse Educ. Pract.* **2023**, *70*, 103677. [CrossRef]
45. Moorman, M. The meaning of Visual Thinking Strategies for nursing students. *Humanities* **2015**, *4*, 748–759. [CrossRef]
46. Wikström, B.-M. Works of art as a pedagogical tool: An alternative approach to education. *Creative Nurs.* **2011**, *17*, 187–194. [CrossRef] [PubMed]
47. Arveklev, S.H.; Wigert, H.; Berg, L.; Burton, B.; Lepp, M. The use and application of drama in nursing education: An integrative review of the literature. *Nurse Educ. Today* **2015**, *35*, e12–e17. [CrossRef] [PubMed]
48. Jefferies, D.; Glew, P.; Karhani, Z.; McNally, S.; Ramjan, L.M. The educational benefits of drama in nursing education: A critical literature review. *Nurse Educ. Today* **2020**, *98*, 104669. [CrossRef]
49. Hunter, L.P. Poetry as an aesthetic expression for nursing: A review. *J. Adv. Nurs.* **2002**, *40*, 141–148. [CrossRef] [PubMed]
50. Raingruber, B. Assigning poetry reading as a way of introducing students to qualitative data analysis. *J. Adv. Nurs.* **2009**, *65*, 1753–1761. [CrossRef] [PubMed]
51. Uligraff, D.K. Utilizing poetry to enhance student nurses' reflective skills: A literature review. *Belitung Nurs. J.* **2019**, *5*, 3–8. [CrossRef]
52. Timpani, S.; Sweet, L.; Sivertsen, N. Storytelling: One arts-based learning strategy to reflect on clinical placement: An integrative review. *Nurse Educ. Pract.* **2021**, *52*, 103005. [CrossRef] [PubMed]
53. Oh, J.; Kang, J.; De Gagne, J.C. Learning concepts of cinenurducation: An integrative review. *Nurse Educ. Today* **2012**, *32*, 914–919. [CrossRef]
54. Oh, J.; De Gagné, J.C.; Kang, J. A review of teaching-learning strategies to be used with film for prelicensure students. *J. Nurs. Educ.* **2013**, *52*, 150–156. [CrossRef]
55. Sandberg, B.; Stasewitsch, E.; Prümper, J. Mind the gap: Workshop satisfaction and skills development in art-based learning. *Eur. J. Teach. Educ.* **2022**, *4*, 1–14. [CrossRef]
56. * Slota, M.; McLaughlin, M.; Vittone, S.; Crowell, N. Visual intelligence education using an art-based intervention: Outcomes evaluation with nursing graduate students. *J. Prof. Nurs.* **2022**, *41*, 1–7. [CrossRef] [PubMed]
57. Turton, B.M.; Williams, S.; Burton, C.R.; Williams, L. Arts-based palliative care training, education and staff development: A scoping review. *Palliat. Med.* **2018**, *32*, 559–570. [CrossRef]
58. Höfler, M.; Vasylyeva, T. Studienbewertung in systematischen Reviews der Bildungsforschung: Planungsschritte und Kriterien zur Prüfung der internen Validität von Interventionsstudien [Study evaluation in systematic reviews of educational research: Planning steps and criteria for testing the internal validity of intervention studies]. *Z. Erzieh.* **2023**, *26*, 1029–1051. [CrossRef]
59. Cook, B.G.; Smith, G.J.; Tankersley, M. Evidence-based practices in education. In *APA Educational Psychology Handbook*; Harris, K.R., Graham, S., Urdan, T., McCormick, C.B., Sinatra, G.M., Sweller, J., Eds.; American Psychological Association: Washington, DC, USA, 2012; Volume 1, pp. 495–527.
60. Shavelson, R.; Towne, L. *Scientific Research in Education*; The National Academies Press: Washington, DC, USA, 2002. [CrossRef]

61. Jordan, Z.; Lockwood, C.; Munn, Z.; Aromataris, E. The updated Joanna Briggs Institute Model of Evidence-Based Healthcare. *Int. J. Evid.-Based Health* **2019**, *17*, 58–71. [CrossRef]
62. Gough, D. Appraising evidence claims. *Rev. Res. Educ.* **2021**, *45*, 1–26. [CrossRef]
63. Kirkevold, M. Integrative nursing research: An important strategy to further the development of nursing science and nursing practice. *J. Adv. Nurs.* **1997**, *25*, 977–984. [CrossRef] [PubMed]
64. Paré, G.; Trudel, M.-C.; Jaana, M.; Kitsiou, S. Synthesizing information systems knowledge: A typology of literature reviews. *Inf. Manag.* **2015**, *52*, 183–199. [CrossRef]
65. Ferguson, L.; Day, R.A. Evidence-based nursing education: Myth or reality? *J. Nurs. Educ.* **2005**, *44*, 107–115. [CrossRef]
66. Kitchenham, B.; Charters, S. *Guidelines for Performing Systematic Literature Reviews in Software Engineering*; EBSE Technical Report Version 2.3; Keele University: Keele, UK; University of Durham: Durham, UK, 2007.
67. Nissley, N. Arts-based learning in management education. In *Rethinking Management for the 21st Century*; Wankel, C., DeFillippi, R., Eds.; Information Age Publishing: Greenwich, UK, 2002; pp. 27–61.
68. Parry, S.B. Just what is a competency? (And why should you care?). *Training* **1996**, *35*, 58–64.
69. Kviz, F.J. *Conducting Health Research: Principles, Process, and Methods*; Sage Publications: Thousand Oaks, CA, USA, 2019.
70. Xiao, Y.; Watson, M. Guidance on conducting a systematic literature review. *J. Plan. Educ. Res.* **2019**, *39*, 93–112. [CrossRef]
71. Page, M.J.; McKenzie, J.E.; Bossuyt, P.M.; Boutron, I.; Hoffmann, T.C.; Mulrow, C.D.; Shamseer, L.; Tetzlaff, J.M.; Akl, E.A.; Brennan, S.E.; et al. The PRISMA 2020 statement: An updated guideline for reporting systematic reviews. *Syst. Rev.* **2021**, *10*, 89. [CrossRef]
72. Munn, Z.; Aromataris, E.; Tufanaru, C.; Stern, C.; Porritt, K.; Farrow, J.; Lockwood, C.; Stephenson, M.; Moola, S.; Lizarondo, L.; et al. The development of software to support multiple systematic review types: The Joanna Briggs Institute System for the Unified Management, Assessment and Review of Information (JBI SUMARI). *Int. J. Evid.-Based Health* **2019**, *17*, 36–43. [CrossRef]
73. Belur, J.; Tompson, L.; Thornton, A.; Simon, M. Interrater reliability in systematic review methodology: Exploring variation in coder decision-making. *Sociol. Methods Res.* **2021**, *50*, 837–865. [CrossRef]
74. (CEC) Council for Exceptional Children. Standards for Evidence-Based Practices in Special Education. *Teach. Except. Child.* **2014**, *46*, 206–212. [CrossRef]
75. Lan, H.; Yu, X.; Wang, Z.; Wang, P.; Sun, Y.; Wang, Z.; Su, R.; Wang, L.; Zhao, J.; Hu, Y.; et al. How about the evidence assessment tools used in education and management systematic reviews? *Front. Med.* **2023**, *10*, 1160289. [CrossRef]
76. Moore, T.C.; Maggin, D.M.; Thompson, K.M.; Gordon, J.R.; Daniels, S.; Lang, L.E. Evidence review for teacher praise to improve students' classroom behavior. *J. Posit. Behav. Interv.* **2018**, *21*, 3–18. [CrossRef]
77. Charlton, C.T.; Moulton, S.; Sabey, C.V.; West, R. A systematic review of the effects of schoolwide intervention programs on student and teacher perceptions of school climate. *J. Posit. Behav. Interv.* **2021**, *23*, 185–200. [CrossRef]
78. Fuentealba-Torres, M.; Sánchez, Z.L.; Püschel, V.A.d.A.; Cartagena, D. Systematic reviews to strengthen evidence-based nursing practice. *Aquichan* **2021**, *21*, e2145. [CrossRef]
79. Gersten, R.; Fuchs, L.S.; Compton, D.; Coyne, M.; Greenwood, C.; Innocenti, M.S. Quality indicators for group experimental and quasi-experimental research in special education. *Except. Child.* **2005**, *71*, 149–164. [CrossRef]
80. Horner, R.H.; Carr, E.G.; Halle, J.; McGee, G.; Odom, S.; Wolery, M. The use of single-subject research to identify evidence-based practice in special education. *Except. Child.* **2005**, *71*, 165–179. [CrossRef]
81. Lane, K.L.; Kalberg, J.R.; Shepcaro, J.C. An examination of the evidence base for function-based interventions for students with emotional and/or behavioral disorders attending middle and high schools. *Except. Child.* **2009**, *75*, 321–340. [CrossRef]
82. Cook, B.G.; Buysse, V.; Klingner, J.; Landrum, T.J.; McWilliam, R.A.; Tankersley, M.; Test, D.W. CEC's standards for classifying the evidence base of practices in special education. *Remedial Spec. Educ.* **2015**, *36*, 220–234. [CrossRef]
83. Hirsch, S.E.; Randall, K.; Bradshaw, C.; Lloyd, J.W. Professional learning and development in classroom management for novice teachers: A systematic review. *Educ. Treat. Child.* **2021**, *44*, 291–307. [CrossRef]
84. Criss, C.J.; Konrad, M.; Alber-Morgan, S.R.; Brock, M.E. A systematic review of goal setting and performance feedback to improve teacher practice. *J. Behav. Educ.* **2022**, *31*, 1–22. [CrossRef]
85. Naveenkumar, N.; Georgiou, G.K.; Vieira, A.P.A.; Romero, S.; Parrila, R. A systematic review on quality indicators of randomized control trial reading fluency intervention studies. *Read. Writ. Q.* **2021**, *38*, 359–378. [CrossRef]
86. Wooderson, J.R.; Bizo, L.A.; Young, K. A systematic review of emergent learning outcomes produced by foreign language tact training. *Anal. Verbal Behav.* **2022**, *38*, 157–178. [CrossRef] [PubMed]
87. Park, J.; Gremp, M.; Ok, M.W. Effects of assistive technology instruction on pre-service teachers: A systematic review. *J. Spec. Educ. Technol.* **2023**. Advance online publication. [CrossRef]
88. Döring, N. *Forschungsmethoden und Evaluation in den Sozial- und Humanwissenschaften [Research Methods and Evaluation in the Social and Human Sciences]*, 6th ed.; Springer: Berlin/Heidelberg, Germany, 2023.
89. Lane, K.L.; Common, E.A.; Royer, D.J.; Muller, K. Group Comparison and Single-Case Research Design Quality Indicator Matrix Using Council for Exceptional Children 2014 Standards. March 2021 Version. Available online: http://www.ci3t.org/practice (accessed on 11 February 2024).
90. Carnett, A.; Devine, B.; Ingvarsson, E.; Esch, B. A systematic and quality review of augmentative and alternative communication interventions that use core vocabulary. *Rev. J. Autism Dev. Disord.* **2023**, *10*, 1–17. [CrossRef]

91. Wilkes, T.; Stark, R. Probleme evidenzorientierter Unterrichtspraxis [Problems of an evidence-oriented educational practice]. *Unterrichtswissenschaft* **2023**, *51*, 289–313. [CrossRef]
92. Polit, D.F.; Beck, C.T. *Nursing Research: Generating and Assessing Evidence for Nursing Practice*, 11th ed.; Wolters Kluwer: Philadelphia, MA, USA, 2021.
93. * Basit, G.; Su, S.; Geçkil, E.; Basit, O.; Alabay, K.N.K. The effect of drama-supported, patient role-play experience on empathy and altruism levels in nursing students: A randomized controlled study. *Nurse Educ. Pract.* **2023**, *69*, 103634. [CrossRef] [PubMed]
94. * Briggs, C.L.; Abell, C.H. The influence of film on the empathy ratings of nursing students. *Int. J. Hum. Caring* **2012**, *16*, 59–63. [CrossRef]
95. * Chen, S.; Walsh, S.M. Effect of a creative-bonding intervention on Taiwanese nursing students' self-transcendence and attitudes toward elders. *Res. Nurs. Health* **2009**, *32*, 204–216. [CrossRef] [PubMed]
96. * Dickens, G.L.; Lamont, E.; Stirling, F.J. Student health professionals' attitudes and experience after watching "Ida's Diary", a first-person account of living with borderline personality disorder: Mixed methods study. *Nurse Educ. Today* **2018**, *65*, 128–135. [CrossRef] [PubMed]
97. * Dingwall, L.; Fenton, J.; Kelly, T.B.; Lee, J. Sliding doors: Did drama-based inter-professional education improve the tensions round person-centred nursing and social care delivery for people with dementia: A mixed method exploratory study. *Nurse Educ. Today* **2017**, *51*, 1–7. [CrossRef] [PubMed]
98. * Eaton, J.; Donaldson, G. Altering nursing student and older adult attitudes through a possible selves ethnodrama. *J. Prof. Nurs.* **2016**, *32*, 141–151. [CrossRef] [PubMed]
99. * Emory, J.; Bowling, H.; Lueders, C. Student perceptions of older adults after a music intervention: A mixed approach. *Nurse Educ. Pract.* **2021**, *53*, 103094. [CrossRef]
100. * Gazarian, P.K.; Fernberg, L.M.; Sheehan, K.D. Effectiveness of narrative pedagogy in developing student nurses' advocacy role. *Nurs. Ethics* **2014**, *23*, 132–141. [CrossRef] [PubMed]
101. * Grossman, S.; Deupi, J.; Leitao, K. Seeing the forest and the trees: Increasing nurse practitioner students' observational and mindfulness skills. *Creat. Nurs.* **2014**, *20*, 72. [CrossRef]
102. * Guo, J.; Zhong, Q.; Tang, Y.; Luo, J.; Wang, H.; Qin, X.; Wang, X.; Wiley, J.A. Cultural adaptation, the 3-month efficacy of visual art training on observational and diagnostic skills among nursing students, and satisfaction among students and staff: A mixed method study. *BMC Nurs.* **2021**, *20*, 122. [CrossRef]
103. * HadaviBavili, P.; İlçioğlu, K. Artwork in anatomy education: A way to improve undergraduate students' self-efficacy and attitude. *Anat. Sci. Educ.* **2024**, *17*, 66–76. [CrossRef] [PubMed]
104. * Hançer Tok, H.; Cerit, B. The effect of creative drama education on first-year undergraduate nursing student attitudes toward caring for dying patients. *Nurse Educ. Today* **2021**, *97*, 104696. [CrossRef] [PubMed]
105. * Honan Pellico, L.; Duffy, T.C.; Fennie, K.P.; Swan, K.A. Looking is not seeing and listening is not hearing: Effect of an intervention to enhance auditory skills of graduate-entry nursing students. *Nurs. Educ. Perspect.* **2012**, *33*, 234–239. [CrossRef] [PubMed]
106. * Honan Pellico, H.; Fennie, K.; Tillman, S.; Duffy, T.C.; Friedlaender, L.; Graham, G. Artwork and music: Innovative approaches to physical assessment. *Arts Health* **2014**, *6*, 162–175. [CrossRef]
107. * Honan, L.; Shealy, S.; Fennie, K.; Duffy, T.C.; Friedlaender, L.; Del Vecchio, M. Looking is not seeing and listening is not hearing: A replication study with accelerated BSN Students. *J. Prof. Nurs.* **2016**, *32*, S30–S36. [CrossRef] [PubMed]
108. * Kahriman, I.; Nural, N.; Arslan, U.; Topbas, M.; Can, G.; Kasim, S. The effect of empathy training on the empathic skills of nurses. *Iran. Red Crescent Med. J.* **2016**, *18*, e24847. [CrossRef]
109. * Kirklin, D.; Duncan, J.; McBride, S.; Hunt, S.; Griffin, M. A cluster design controlled trial of arts-based observational skills training in primary care. *Med. Educ.* **2007**, *41*, 395–401. [CrossRef]
110. * Klugman, C.M.; Beckmann-Mendez, D. One thousand words: Evaluating an interdisciplinary art education program. *J. Nurs. Educ.* **2015**, *54*, 220–223. [CrossRef]
111. * Klugman, C.M.; Peel, J.; Beckmann-Mendez, D. Art Rounds: Teaching interprofessional students visual thinking strategies at one school. *Acad. Med.* **2011**, *86*, 1266–1271. [CrossRef]
112. * Kyle, R.G.; Bastow, F.; Harper-McDonald, B.; Jeram, T.; Zahid, Z.; Nizamuddin, M.; Mahoney, C. Effects of student-led drama on nursing students' attitudes to interprofessional working and nursing advocacy: A pre-test post-test educational intervention study. *Nurse Educ. Today* **2023**, *123*, 105743. [CrossRef]
113. * Lamet, A.R.; Sonshine, R.; Walsh, S.M.; Molnar, D.; Rafalko, S. A pilot study of a creative bonding intervention to promote nursing students' attitudes towards taking care of older people. *Nurs. Res. Pract.* **2011**, *2011*, 537634. [CrossRef]
114. * Lesińska-Sawicka, M. Using graphic medicine in teaching multicultural nursing: A quasi-experimental study. *BMC Med. Educ.* **2023**, *23*, 255. [CrossRef] [PubMed]
115. * Lovell, C.; Elswick, R.K.; McKay, S.W.; Robins, J.; Salyer, J. Visual arts in nursing education: An inventive interprofessional initiative to cultivate metacognitive awareness in beginning nursing students. *J. Holist. Nurs.* **2021**, *39*, 135–143. [CrossRef] [PubMed]
116. * Moore, A.K.; Miller, R.J. Video storytelling in the classroom: The role of narrative transportation. *J. Nurs. Educ.* **2020**, *59*, 470–474. [CrossRef] [PubMed]
117. * Nash, L.; Scott, K.; Pit, S.; Barnes, E.; Ivory, K.; Hooker, C. Evaluation of a workshop using verbatim theatre stimuli to address challenging workplace situations: A pilot study. *Clin. Teach.* **2020**, *18*, 43–50. [CrossRef] [PubMed]

118. * Nease, B.M.; Haney, T.S. Evaluating an art-based intervention to improve practicing nurses' observation, description, and problem identification skills. *J. Nurses Prof. Dev.* **2018**, *34*, 2–7. [CrossRef] [PubMed]
119. * Neilson, S.J.; Reeves, A. The use of a theatre workshop in developing effective communication in paediatric end of life care. *Nurse Educ. Pract.* **2019**, *36*, 7–12. [CrossRef]
120. * Özcan, N.K.; Bilgin, H.; Eracar, N. The use of expressive methods for developing empathic skills. *Issues Ment. Health Nurs.* **2011**, *32*, 131–136. [CrossRef]
121. * Park, H.; Cho, H. Effects of nursing education using films on perception of nursing, satisfaction with major, and professional nursing values. *J. Nurs. Res.* **2021**, *29*, e150. [CrossRef]
122. * Rashidi, K.; Ashktorab, T.; Birjandi, M. Impact of poetry-based ethics education on the moral sensitivity of nurses: A semi-experimental study. *Nurs. Ethics* **2021**, *29*, 448–461. [CrossRef]
123. * Röhm, A.; Hastall, M.R.; Ritterfeld, U. How movies shape students' attitudes toward individuals with schizophrenia: An exploration of the relationships between entertainment experience and stigmatization. *Issues Ment. Health Nurs.* **2017**, *38*, 1257672. [CrossRef] [PubMed]
124. * Shieh, C. Evaluation of a clinical teaching method involving stories. *Int. J. Nurs. Educ. Sch.* **2005**, *2*, 30. [CrossRef] [PubMed]
125. * Sinha, P.; Murphy, S.P.; Becker, C.M.; Poarch, H.J.; Gade, K.E.; Wolf, A.T.; Martindale, J.R.; Owen, J.A.; Brashers, V. A novel interprofessional approach to end-of-life care education: A pilot study. *J. Interprofessional Care* **2015**, *29*, 643–645. [CrossRef] [PubMed]
126. * Stupans, I.; Baverstock, K.; Jackson, M. Photo-essay as an assessment strategy for learning about the determinants of health: Students' experiences. *Collegian* **2019**, *26*, 146–150. [CrossRef]
127. * Tastan, S.; Ayhan, H.; Unver, V.; Cinar, F.I.; Kose, G.; Basak, T.; Cinar, O.; Iyigun, E. The effects of music on the cardiac resuscitation education of nursing students. *Int. Emerg. Nurs.* **2017**, *31*, 30–35. [CrossRef] [PubMed]
128. * Tokur Kesgin, M.; Hançer Tok, H. The impact of drama education and in-class education on nursing students' attitudes toward violence against women: A randomized controlled study. *Nurse Educ. Today* **2023**, *125*, 105779. [CrossRef] [PubMed]
129. * Uzun, L.N.; Cerit, B. Effect of postmortem care education using a creative drama method on nursing students' knowledge, skills, and satisfaction: A randomized controlled trial. *Nurse Educ. Today* **2023**, *133*, 106066. [CrossRef] [PubMed]
130. * Wikström, B. Works of art: A complement to theoretical knowledge when teaching nursing care. *J. Clin. Nurs.* **2001**, *10*, 25–32. [CrossRef]
131. * Yamauchi, T.; Takeshima, T.; Hirokawa, S.; Oba, Y.; Koh, E. An educational program for nursing and social work students using artwork created by people with mental health problems. *Int. J. Ment. Health Addict.* **2016**, *15*, 503–513. [CrossRef]
132. * Zelenski, A.B.; Saldivar, N.M.; Park, L.S.; Schoenleber, V.; Osman, F.; Kraemer, S. Interprofessional improv: Using theater techniques to teach health professions students empathy in teams. *Acad. Med.* **2020**, *95*, 1210–1214. [CrossRef]
133. Petticrew, M.; Roberts, H. *Systematic Reviews in the Social Sciences: A Practical Guide*; Blackwell Publishing: Oxford, UK, 2006. [CrossRef]
134. Winther, H.; Grøntved, S.N.; Gravesen, E.K.; Ilkjær, I. The dancing nurses and the language of the body: Training somatic awareness, bodily communication, and embodied professional competence in nurse education. *J. Holist. Nurs.* **2015**, *33*, 182–192. [CrossRef] [PubMed]
135. Mannix, J.; Wilkes, L.; Daly, J. 'Watching an artist at work': Aesthetic leadership in clinical nursing workplaces. *J. Clin. Nurs.* **2015**, *24*, 3511–3518. [CrossRef] [PubMed]
136. Roberts, M. Emotional intelligence, empathy and the educative power of poetry: A Deleuzo-Guattarian perspective. *J. Psychiatr. Ment. Health Nurs.* **2010**, *17*, 236–241. [CrossRef] [PubMed]
137. Moudatsou, M.; Stavropoulou, A.; Philalithis, A.; Koukouli, S. The role of empathy in health and social care professionals. *Healthcare* **2020**, *8*, 26. [CrossRef] [PubMed]
138. Fitzgerald, A. Professional identity: A concept analysis. *Nurs. Forum* **2020**, *55*, 447–472. [CrossRef]
139. Simmonds, A.; Nunn, A.; Gray, M.; Hardie, C.; Mayo, S.; Peter, E.; Richards, J. Pedagogical practices that influence professional identity formation in baccalaureate nursing education: A scoping review. *Nurse Educ. Today* **2020**, *93*, 104516. [CrossRef]
140. Mukunda, N.; Moghbeli, N.; Rizzo, A.; Niepold, S.; Bassett, B.; DeLisser, H.M. Visual art instruction in medical education: A narrative review. *Med. Educ. Online* **2019**, *24*, 1558657. [CrossRef] [PubMed]
141. Dalia, Y.; Milam, E.C.; Rieder, E.A. Art in medical education: A review. *J. Grad. Med. Educ.* **2020**, *12*, 686–695. [CrossRef]
142. Ousager, J.; Johannessen, H. Humanities in undergraduate medical education: A literature review. *Acad. Med.* **2010**, *85*, 988–998. [CrossRef]
143. Perry, M.; Maffulli, N.; Willson, S.; Morrissey, D. The effectiveness of arts-based interventions in medical education: A literature review. *Med. Educ.* **2011**, *45*, 141–148. [CrossRef]
144. Alkhaifi, M.; Clayton, A.; Kangasjarvi, E.; Kishibe, T.; Simpson, J.S. Visual art-based training in undergraduate medical education: A systematic review. *Med. Teach.* **2021**, *44*, 500–509. [CrossRef]
145. Cerqueira, A.R.; Alves, A.S.; Monteiro-Soares, M.; Hailey, D.; Loureiro, D.; Baptista, S. Visual Thinking Strategies in medical education: A systematic review. *BMC Med. Educ.* **2023**, *23*, 536. [CrossRef]
146. Mehta, A.; Agius, S. The use of art observation interventions to improve medical students' diagnostic skills: A scoping review. *Perspect. Med. Educ.* **2023**, *12*, 169–178. [CrossRef]
147. Paul, P.V. Perspectives on Evidence-Based. *Am. Ann. Deaf.* **2019**, *164*, 423–428. [CrossRef] [PubMed]

148. Chemi, T.; Jensen, J.B. Emotions and learning in arts-based practices of educational innovation. In *Dealing with Emotions*; Lund, B., Chemi, T., Eds.; Brill: Leiden, The Netherlands, 2015; pp. 21–36.
149. Katz-Buonincontro, J.; Hass, R.; Perignat, E. Triangulating creativity: Examining discrepancies across self-rated, quasi-expert-rated and verbalized creativity in arts-based learning. *J. Creative Behav.* **2020**, *54*, 948–963. [CrossRef]
150. Ike, J.D.; Howell, J. Quantitative metrics and psychometric scales in the visual art and medical education literature: A narrative review. *Med. Educ. Online* **2021**, *27*, 2010299. [CrossRef] [PubMed]
151. Kalb, K.A.; O'Conner-Von, S.K.; Brockway, C.; Rierson, C.L.; Sendelbach, S. Evidence-based teaching practice in nursing education: Faculty perspectives and practices. *Nurs. Educ. Perspect.* **2015**, *36*, 212–219. [CrossRef]
152. Oreck, B. The artistic and professional development of teachers: A study of teachers' attitudes toward and use of the arts in teaching. *J. Teach. Educ.* **2004**, *55*, 55–69. [CrossRef]
153. Lay, R.P.M.H. Building research capacity: Scaffolding the process through arts-based pedagogy. In *Social Work Research Using Arts-Based Methods*; Huss, E., Bos, E., Eds.; Bristol University Press: Bristol, UK, 2022; pp. 170–180.
154. Zimmerman, K.N.; Ledford, J.R.; Severini, K.E.; Pustejovsky, J.E.; Barton, E.E.; Lloyd, B.P. Single-case synthesis tools I: Comparing tools to evaluate SCD quality and rigor. *Res. Dev. Disabil.* **2018**, *79*, 19–32. [CrossRef]
155. Stark, R. Probleme evidenzbasierter bzw. -orientierter pädagogischer Praxis [Problems of evidence-based or evidence-oriented pedagogical practice]. *Z. Pädagogische Psychol.* **2017**, *31*, 99–110. [CrossRef]
156. Rochnia, M.; Schellenbach-Zell, J.; Steckel, J.; Radisch, F. Eine Taxonomie der Evidenzorientierung im Bildungsbereich: Was, wozu, wo und wie? [A taxonomy of evidence orientation in education: What, why, where and how?]. *PraxisForschungLehrer*InnenBildung* **2022**, *4*, 190–201. [CrossRef]
157. Rieger, K.; Schultz, A.S. Exploring arts-based knowledge translation: Sharing research findings through performing the patterns, rehearsing the results, staging the synthesis. *Worldviews Evid.-Based Nurs.* **2014**, *11*, 133–139. [CrossRef] [PubMed]
158. Barry, D.; Meisiek, S. Seeing more and seeing differently: Sensemaking, mindfulness, and the workarts. *Organ. Stud.* **2010**, *31*, 1505–1530. [CrossRef]
159. Darsø, L. Arts-in-business from 2004 to 2014: From experiments in practice to research and leadership development. In *Artistic Interventions in Organizations: Research, Theory and Practice*; Sköldberg, U.J., Woodilla, J., Antal, A.B., Eds.; Routledge: London, UK, 2016; pp. 18–34.
160. Blackburn Miller, J. Transformative learning and the arts: A literature review. *J. Transform. Educ.* **2020**, *18*, 338–355. [CrossRef]
161. Taylor, S.S.; Ladkin, D.; Martin, L.A.; Edwards, M.; Sayers, J.G.; Hibbert, P.; Beech, N.; Siedlok, F.; Michaelson, C.; Härtel, C.E.J.; et al. Understanding arts-based methods in managerial development. *Acad. Manag. Learn. Educ.* **2009**, *8*, 55–69. [CrossRef]
162. Silverstein, L.B.; Layne, S. *Defining Arts Integration*; The John F. Kennedy Center for the Performing Arts: Washington, DC, USA, 2010.

Disclaimer/Publisher's Note: The statements, opinions and data contained in all publications are solely those of the individual author(s) and contributor(s) and not of MDPI and/or the editor(s). MDPI and/or the editor(s) disclaim responsibility for any injury to people or property resulting from any ideas, methods, instructions or products referred to in the content.

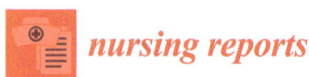

Article

An Exploration of Resilience and Positive Affect among Undergraduate Nursing Students: A Longitudinal Observational Study

L. Iván Mayor-Silva [1], Alfonso Meneses-Monroy [1], Leyre Rodriguez-Leal [2,*] and Guillermo Moreno [1,3,*]

[1] Departamento de Enfermería, Facultad de Enfermería, Fisioterapia y Podología, Universidad Complutense de Madrid, 28040 Madrid, Spain; limayors@ucm.es (L.I.M.-S.); ameneses@ucm.es (A.M.-M.)
[2] Red Cross Nursing University College, Autonomous University of Madrid, 28003 Madrid, Spain
[3] Grupo de Investigación Cardiovascular Multidisciplinar Traslacional (GICMT), Área de Investigación Cardiovascular, Instituto de Investigación Hospital 12 de Octubre (imas12), 28041 Madrid, Spain
* Correspondence: leyre.rodriguez@cruzroja.es (L.R.-L.); guimoren@ucm.es (G.M.)

Abstract: Background: The purpose of this study is to analyze the variation in resilience and emotional state scores in nursing students throughout the four years of training for the nursing degree. Methods: This is a longitudinal observational study of a paired and prospective cohort of 176 nursing students who enrolled in the first year of a bachelor's degree in 2019. The study followed up with the students in 2022 and examined several sociodemographic factors, including sex, marital status, date of birth, living arrangements and occupation. Additionally, the study investigated changes in negative affect, positive affect, and resilience. Results: A total of 176 students participated in the study. The study found that resilience increased from 68.24 ± 10.59 to 70.87 ± 9.06 ($p < 0.001$), positive affect increased from 28.16 ± 4.59 to 33.08 ± 8.00 ($p < 0.001$), and the negative affect score decreased from 25.27 ± 5.12 to 21.81 ± 7.85 ($p < 0.001$). The study also found that married individuals experienced an increase in negative affect ($p = 0.03$) compared to singles or those in open relationships. Furthermore, the change in resilience was greater in men than in women ($p = 0.01$). Conclusions: Throughout their four-year training, nursing students experience an increase in resilience and positive affect, as well as a decrease in negative affect.

Keywords: resilience; positive affect; negative affect; nursing students

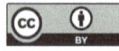

1. Introduction

Resilience and affectivity are two psychological constructs that are highly relevant in the educational field of nursing students, playing a crucial role in their well-being and academic performance [1,2]. Resilience is defined as the ability to cope with adverse situations and is a dynamic process that involves the interaction of individual, social, and environmental factors [3]. Foundational skills for maintaining a healthy state of mind are crucial for meeting the challenges inherent in the nursing profession [4].

Resilience is considered a crucial competency in nursing, as it is related to three diagnoses in the NANDA taxonomy [5]. Furthermore, research suggests that resilience is a necessary characteristic for nurses due to their continuous exposure to human suffering and stressful working conditions [6,7]. Nurses can use resilience to support and motivate patients in coping with the challenges of illness while enhancing their own skills and resources to remain resilient. In addition, higher levels of resilience help them maintain their own health and well-being, ensuring that the physical, emotional, and mental demands of caregiving do not overwhelm them or exhaust their ability to provide care [8]. Resilience can also reduce the symptoms of burnout and its consequences in the nursing profession [9]. Resilience plays a key role in strengthening nursing students by allowing them to bounce back from challenging situations. The range of experiences, whether encouraging or discouraging, profoundly influences their outlook and confidence throughout their clinical education [10].

Affectivity pertains to an individual's subjective emotional state at a particular moment. It is worth noting that affectivity has a significant correlation with an individual's perceived well-being and discomfort [11]. Affective states can range from positive moods, such as happiness and contentment, which increase motivation, satisfaction, and interest in activities, to negative states, such as sadness and anxiety, which generate disinterest, lack of energy, and lack of pleasure in life. The affectivity of nursing students can be influenced by various factors, including academic workload, clinical demands, and emotional experiences associated with patient care [12].

Various studies have explored the relationship between resilience and affectivity. Specifically, in nursing students, resilience can influence how they cope with the academic and emotional challenges associated with their professional training. Several studies have shown a positive correlation between resilience scores and positive affect scores [13–15]. This indicates that nursing students with higher levels of resilience tend to experience more positive emotions. Previous research has explored the correlation between resilience, mood, and stress. The findings suggest that nursing students with higher levels of resilience experience fewer negative emotions, indicating a greater ability to cope with stress and adversity. These results support the notion that resilience is linked to higher positive affect and lower negative impact, which could have significant implications for the well-being and performance of nursing students. For this reason, some authors recommend resilience training starting at the undergraduate level due to its importance for future professionals [16–18].

In the past five years, Spanish universities have implemented various activities to enhance student resilience. These include telephone psychological support programs, clinical simulations, peer mentoring programs, student advocacy, clinical practices with tutors, and participatory conferences on the profession to improve communication among classmates. These strategies have also been incorporated into the formal curriculum at our local university over the past 10 years through participation in clinical programs, simulations, and peer mentoring. The aim of this study is to analyze the variation in resilience and emotional state scores in nursing students throughout the 4 years of training within the nursing degree.

2. Material and Methods

2.1. Design

From September 2019 to October 2022, we conducted a single-center, longitudinal observational study of paired and prospective cohorts using the STROBE statement as a framework [19].

2.2. Participants

The study population comprised 224 nursing students enrolled in the first year of the bachelor's degree in 2019. The researchers used convenience sampling to recruit students through online messages in the academic electronic platform used by professors to communicate with students (virtual campus) in September 2019 and followed up with them in October 2022. None of the students' professors were involved in this study. The data analysis included all students who had completed both assessments.

2.3. Study Variables

Study variables included sociodemographic factors such as sex (male/female), marital status (married/single/open relationship), age, living arrangement (with friends or fellow students/with parents or relatives/as a couple/alone/none of the above), and occupation (sporadic professional activities/continuous and remunerated work/volunteering/none of the above), as well as negative affect, positive affect, and resilience, which were assessed through self-administered online questionnaires sent through the virtual campus:

- The Positive and Negative Affect Schedule (PANAS) [20] questionnaire is a self-report instrument used to evaluate an individual's affective state [11]. It consists of two subscales, each comprising 10 items that are rated on a Likert-type scale with five response options ranging from 1 (little or almost nothing) to 5 (extremely). One scale measures recent positive experiences, which act as a protective element, while the other measures negative experiences, which act as a risk factor for diseases [21]. The scales have demonstrated consistency and stability in the Spanish university population, with good construct validity and a reliability index of Cronbach's alpha >0.87 [22].
- The study collected the Connor–Davidson Resilience Scale (CD-RISC) [23] in the Spanish version [24], which measures resilience using 25 items in a Likert-type response format with five response options (0 = 'not at all', 1 = 'rarely', 2 = 'sometimes', 3 = 'often', and 4 = 'almost always'). The scale ranges from 0 to 100, with higher scores indicating greater resilience. The items are grouped into five dimensions: Persistence, Tenacity, and Self-Efficacy; Control under Pressure; Adaptability and Networking; Control and Purpose; and Spirituality. The thresholds are less than 70 (low), 70 to 87 (intermediate), and greater than 88 (high). The Spanish version has optimal internal consistency, with a Cronbach's alpha of 0.86 [24].

2.4. Data Analysis

Numerical codes were used to match and anonymize participants' personal information to ensure confidentiality. Relative and absolute frequencies were calculated for qualitative variables, while measures of central tendency and dispersion were calculated for continuous variables, with 95% confidence intervals. The normality of the variables was assessed using the Kolmogorov–Smirnov test. Bivariate relationships between sociodemographic variables and the main variables were analyzed using ANOVA and Student t tests, both paired and for independent samples. A statistically significant relationship was recognized when the p-value was less than 0.05. Finally, a correlation analysis was conducted between the main variables of the study. Data analysis was performed using SPSS version 26®.

2.5. Ethical Considerations

This study adhered to the ethical principles for medical research and maintained the confidentiality of data in accordance with Regulation (EU) 2016/679 of the European Parliament and of the Council of 27 April 2016 on Data Protection (GDPR). The Declaration of Helsinki on Biomedical Research Involving Human Subjects was also followed throughout the study. The research team obtained written consent from each student outside of class time, clearly explaining the voluntary and anonymous nature of the study. The project was approved by the Research Committee of the center (approval number: FEFP 20/21).

3. Results

A total of 176 first-year nursing students participated in the study, resulting in a response rate of 78.5%. After four years, 97.15% of the students (n = 171) returned to participate, resulting in a loss of follow-up of only 2.85%. Table 1 displays the sociodemographic characteristics of the sample at the beginning of the study, with 30 (17.5%) male and 145 (82.5%) female participants. The age range was between 21 and 57 years, with a mean age of 23.14 years (SD: 3.97). Out of the participants, 147 (84.8%) were single, 134 (78.4%) did not engage in any work or extracurricular activities outside of the university, and 147 (86.0%) lived with their parents or relatives.

Table 1. Sociodemographic characteristics of the sample at the beginning of the study (2019–2020 academic year, n = 176).

		n	%	Mean	SD
Sex	Male	30	17.5		
	Female	141	82.5		
Age				23.14	3.98
Marital status	Married	5	2.9		
	Single	145	84.8		
	Open relationship	21	12.3		
Living arrangements	With friends or fellow students	13	7.6		
	With parents or relatives	147	86.0		
	As a couple	6	3.5		
	Alone	4	2.3		
	None of the above	1	0.6		
Occupation	Sporadic professional activities	35	20.5		
	Volunteering	15	8.8		
	Continuous and remunerated work	33	19.3		
	None of the above	88	51.54		

3.1. Variation in Resilience

The CD-RISC questionnaire produced an average score of 68.24 (SD: 10.59) points in the first year, which increased to an average of 70.87 (SD: 9.06) points in the fourth year ($p < 0.001$). In the first year, only 0.6% ($n = 1$) of the students exhibited high resilience, while 44.4% ($n = 76$) exhibited intermediate resilience, and 55% ($n = 94$) exhibited low resilience. In the fourth year, 2.9% ($n = 5$) of the students demonstrated a high level of resilience, while 48.5% ($n = 83$) and 48.5% ($n = 83$) demonstrated intermediate and low levels of resilience, respectively. Of the students, 20.5% ($n = 35$) showed an increase in resilience level (from low to intermediate or high resilience and from intermediate to high resilience), 66.7% ($n = 114$) maintained their resilience level, and 12.9% ($n = 22$) showed a decrease in resilience level (from high or intermediate to intermediate or low). This change was statistically significant ($p < 0.001$).

The average score for personal competence increased significantly from 16.44 (SD: 3.77) points in the first year to 17.48 (SD: 2.95) points in the fourth year ($p < 0.001$). Similarly, the average score for tolerance of negative affect and the strengthening effects of stress increased from 16.60 (SD: 3.88) points in the first year to 17.75 (SD: 3.38) points in the fourth year ($p < 0.001$). Positive acceptance of change and secure relationships obtained an average score of 15. The study found that in the first year, the score was 15.70 (SD: 2.78) points, which decreased to 15.66 (SD: 2.27) points in the fourth year ($p = 0.87$). The average score for a sense of control was 8.63 (SD: 2.16) points in the first year, which increased to 9.16 (SD: 1.58) points in the fourth year ($p < 0.001$). Spiritual influence had an average score of 4.30 (SD: 2.20) points in the first year, which decreased to 4.22 (SD: 2.06) points in the fourth year ($p < 0.001$). Table 2 displays the change in specific items.

Table 2. Results of the CD-RISC questionnaire by items and dimensions in the first and fourth year.

	1st Year		4th Year		Change			
	Mean	SD	Mean	SD	Mean	SD	t *	p **
CD-RISC items								
1. I'm able to adapt when changes occur	3.00	0.89	2.94	0.70	−0.06	1.01	0.84	0.40
2. I have one close and secure relationship	3.39	0.81	3.39	0.64	−0.01	0.86	0.09	0.93
3. Sometimes fate or God helps me	1.43	1.35	1.57	1.23	0.15	1.16	−1.65	0.10
4. I can deal with whatever comes my way	2.86	0.81	2.84	0.68	−0.02	0.85	0.36	0.72
5. Past successes give me confidence	3.34	0.87	3.36	0.80	0.02	1.01	−0.30	0.76
6. I try to see the humorous side of things	2.68	1.00	3.00	0.80	**0.32**	1.01	−4.17	**<0.001**
7. Having to cope with stress makes me stronger	2.71	1.05	2.74	0.88	0.03	1.22	−0.31	0.75
8. I tend to bounce back after illness, injury or other hardships	3.11	0.87	3.14	0.73	0.04	1.01	−0.45	0.65
9. I believe most things happen for a reason	2.88	1.32	2.64	1.21	**−0.23**	1.22	2.50	**0.01**
10. I make my best effort, no matter what	3.25	0.80	3.18	0.69	−0.08	0.88	1.13	0.26
11. I believe I can achieve my goals, even if there are obstacles	3.08	0.79	3.11	0.59	0.02	0.88	−0.35	0.73
12. Even when hopeless, I do not give up	2.89	0.90	2.95	0.73	0.06	1.05	−0.80	0.43
13. In times of stress, I know where to find help	2.97	1.09	3.19	0.81	**0.22**	1.16	−2.51	**0.01**
14. Under pressure, I stay focused and think clearly	2.26	1.19	2.63	0.94	**0.36**	1.24	−3.82	**<0.001**
15. I prefer to take the lead in problem-solving	2.71	1.12	2.91	0.81	**0.20**	1.06	−2.52	**0.01**
16. I am not easily discouraged by failure	1.74	1.17	2.24	0.90	**0.50**	1.31	−5.03	**<0.001**
17. I think of myself as a strong person when dealing with life's changes and difficulties	2.40	1.17	2.83	0.89	**0.43**	1.10	−5.14	**<0.001**
18. I make unpopular or difficult decisions	2.19	0.91	2.18	0.86	−0.01	0.98	0.16	0.88
19. I am able to handle unpleasant or painful feelings like sadness, fear and anger	2.49	1.01	2.65	0.79	**0.16**	1.02	−2.10	**0.04**
20 I have to act on a hunch	1.57	1.01	1.65	0.88	0.09	1.13	−1.01	0.31
21. I have a strong sense of purpose in life	2.88	0.85	3.09	0.62	**0.20**	1.00	−2.68	**0.01**
22. I feel like I am in control	2.78	0.99	2.88	0.75	0.10	1.09	−1.19	0.23
23. I like challenges	2.73	1.01	2.78	0.86	0.05	0.93	−0.74	0.46
24. I work to attain goals	3.54	0.67	3.49	0.57	−0.05	0.78	0.89	0.38
25. I take pride in my achievements.	3.44	0.85	3.50	0.68	0.06	0.80	−0.95	0.34
CD-RISC dimensions								
Personal competence	16.44	3.77	17.48	2.95	**2.61**	3.23	−4.03	**<0.001**
Tolerance of negative affect and the strengthening effects of stress	16.60	3.88	17.75	3.38	**3.00**	3.73	−4.23	**<0.001**
Positive acceptance of change and secure relationships	15.70	2.78	15.66	2.27	2.05	2.47	0.16	0.87
Sense of control	8.63	2.16	9.16	1.58	**1.40**	1.78	−2.87	**<0.001**
Spiritual influence	4.30	2.20	4.22	2.06	1.87	2.23	0.68	0.50

* Note: Student t test for paired samples. ** Note: Significant results ($p < 0.05$).

3.2. Variation of Affective State at the Beginning and End of the Degree

The PANAS questionnaire revealed a statistically significant increase in positive affect score from a mean of 28.16 (SD: 4.59) points in year one to a mean of 33.08 (SD: 8.00) points in year four ($p < 0.001$). Additionally, the negative affect score decreased from a mean of 25.27 (SD: 5.12) in the first year to 21.81 (SD: 7.85) in the fourth year ($p < 0.001$). Table 3 presents a comparison of specific items from the PANAS questionnaire in the first and fourth years. The data indicates a statistically significant increase in interest, distress, excitement, upset, strength, pride, alertness, and attention and a decrease in guiltiness, hostility, nervousness, and jitteriness.

Table 3. Results of the PANAS questionnaire in first and fourth years and their change.

	1st Year		4th Year		Change			
	Mean	SD	Mean	SD	Mean	SD	t *	p **
Interested	3.27	0.92	3.69	0.97	**0.41**	1.24	−4.42	<0.001
Distressed	2.49	1.2	2.9	1.21	**0.86**	1.514	7.51	<0.001
Excited	2.93	1.07	3.45	0.99	**0.44**	1.28	4.49	<0.001
Upset	2.23	1.06	2.47	1.21	**0.24**	1.53	2.08	0.04
Strong	3.16	0.97	3.44	1.06	**0.26**	1.23	1.96	0.01
Guilty	1.88	1.17	1.65	0.98	−0.23	1.55	6.30	0.05
Scared	1.95	1.03	2.03	1.11	0.10	1.41	0.97	0.33
Hostile	1.97	0.99	1.65	0.97	**−0.32**	1.42	−2.94	<0.001
Enthusiastic	3.44	0.93	3.36	1.09	−0.09	1.29	−0.88	0.38
Proud	3.37	0.94	3.78	1.11	**0.41**	1.37	3.92	<0.001
Irritable	2.39	1.07	2.51	1.15	0.12	1.36	1.17	0.24
Alert	3.02	1.01	3.29	0.97	**0.28**	1.27	2.86	0.01
Ashamed	1.78	1.02	1.62	0.92	0.17	1.21	−1.82	0.07
Inspired	2.74	0.98	2.9	1.03	0.15	1.33	1.48	0.14
Nervous	3.25	1.11	2.94	1.22	**−0.30**	1.53	−2.58	0.01
Determined	3.21	0.97	3.3	0.93	0.08	1.10	0.96	0.34
Attentive	3.01	0.94	3.18	0.92	**−0.20**	1.21	−2.12	0.04
Jittery	1.92	1.07	2.28	1.1	**−0.20**	1.52	0.09	<0.001
Active	3.39	0.93	3.52	0.96	0.13	1.25	1.40	0.16
Afraid	2.03	1.08	2.02	1.12	0.06	1.28	0.65	0.52

* Note: Student t test for paired samples. ** Note: Significant results ($p < 0.05$).

3.3. Changes According to Sociodemographic Characteristics

Table 4 shows statistically significant differences in the change of negative affect. It is observed that married individuals experience an increase in negative affect ($p = 0.03$). Furthermore, the change in resilience is greater in men than in women ($p = 0.01$). No statistically significant differences were observed in the remaining sociodemographic variables.

Table 4. Change in resilience and positive and negative affect according to sociodemographic variables.

		Change Positive Affect			Change Negative Affect			Change CD-RISC		
		Mean	SD	p *	Mean	SD	p *	Mean	SD	p *
Sex	Man	6.83	8.90	0.15	−4.00	8.63	0.85	6.57	11.12	0.01 **
	Woman	4.36	8.42		−3.68	8.27		1.72	9.37	
Marital status	Married	3.40	13.16	0.91	3.80	8.41	0.03 **	−4.20	11.45	0.26
	Single	4.78	8.57		−4.36	8.17		2.92	9.63	
	Open relationship	5.24	7.42		−1.24	8.28		1.76	10.79	
Living arrangements	With friends or fellow students	5.69	9.93	0.53	−3.15	8.37	0.71	6.92	7.29	0.17
	With parents or relatives	4.80	8.44		−3.80	8.09		2.52	9.60	
	As a couple	0.50	10.03		−1.67	15.11		1.50	17.03	
	Alone	9.50	4.80		−8.00	4.55		−6.50	10.08	
	None of the above	0.00	0.00		3.00	0.00		−4.00	0.00	
Occupation	Sporadic professional activities	4.00	7.84	0.89	−2.66	8.16	0.66	3.63	11.32	0.71
	Continuous and remunerated work	4.76	10.87		−5.18	9.48		2.21	9.29	
	Volunteering	4.13	6.40		−3.67	6.69		0.13	9.95	
	None of the above	5.24	8.23		−3.64	8.21		2.69	9.48	

* Note: One-factor ANOVA. ** Note: Significant results ($p < 0.05$)

4. Discussion

The aim of this study was to investigate changes in resilience and affect during the four-year bachelor's degree in nursing program to determine if the students improved in these areas for their future clinical practice. It is important to note that this study focused solely on resilience and affect and did not investigate other factors that may impact student success. Our findings indicate that 55% of students begin the program with low resilience, which is consistent with the findings of other authors [2]. Over the course of the four-year program, just over 20% of students demonstrated an increase in their resilience score. The data generally indicate that students exhibit greater resilience, although the most significant variations were observed between low and intermediate resilience levels without reaching high scores. Therefore, there is still room for improvement. In addition, compared to their resilience levels in the first year, some students showed a decrease in resilience. This fact is significant because various studies have demonstrated that the university population generally exhibits medium to high levels of resilience [16,25].

In terms of resilience, personal competence, tolerance of negative affect, and the strengthening effects of stress and sense of control, there is an increase during the four-year period. This may be a normal aspect of academic development, given the complexity of the degree, the difficulty of the subjects, the practical clinical training, and the need to balance work and personal life. The results indicate that the academic and clinical training process provided during the bachelor's degree in nursing can contribute to the development of resilience in students, similar to other professions [26].

However, this decrease in positive acceptance of change and secure relationships, as well as spiritual influence, is negative since these factors are the ones that most protect nursing professionals against burnout syndrome and other difficult situations typical of the nursing role [27,28], such as post-traumatic stress [29]. Several studies have associated spiritual influence with resilient behaviors, which can improve quality of life and act as a protective factor against suicidal ideation [30,31]. Spiritual influence also appears to be a good modulator of the effects of burnout on mental health [32]. Additionally, extroversion and secure relationships have been found to be associated with greater satisfaction with nursing work [33].

Although hospital practice can contribute to the development of nursing students' resilience, studies have shown that their resilience scores are moderate overall [34]. This work is consistent with those findings. This shows that these difficult situations posed by clinical practice will strengthen the student as long as there is support from the tutor, support from peers, and better management of these experiences by the student [15,35–37].

It is important to consider that the students may have been impacted by the COVID-19 pandemic in both positive and negative ways, affecting their resilience. Additionally, the social environment before the pandemic may differ greatly from the post-pandemic world, particularly in areas such as technology, social relationships, and personal fulfillment [38,39]. Therefore, the variations observed in the scores may be attributed to this event and the resulting social change. In the post-pandemic era, it is important to implement pedagogical interventions that have been proven effective in developing resilience in nursing students [40,41] to prevent future risks to the mental health of future professionals.

In terms of affect, positive affect increased while negative affect decreased over the four-year period. The observed changes included an increase in distress, excitement, upset, strength, pride, alertness, and attention, as well as a decrease in guiltiness, hostility, nervousness, and jitteriness. These changes may act as protective or risk factors in the development of diseases among new professionals. These findings may reflect the fact that, overall, nursing students are generally satisfied with their clinical learning experiences [42] and demonstrate that students are positively influenced by professors and their clinical practices, as other studies have suggested [43]. Despite evidence suggesting that confinement during COVID-19 had a negative impact on mood [39], our students were able to increase positive affect and decrease negative affect by the end of their training period, indicating that the influence of confinement was mitigated in the following years.

The study has shown that sex and marital status are factors that affect the development of these variables. Single individuals experience a greater increase in negative affect compared to married individuals or those in an open relationship. Some studies suggest that marriage may have a positive impact on well-being by reducing negative effects in the short term. However, this beneficial effect may diminish in the long term, particularly for women [44]. This could explain why negative affect changes more in married couples compared to single or open relationships. Our findings indicate that men experience a greater increase in resilience levels than women. Other studies on students have found results similar to ours, where men exhibit significantly higher levels of resilience than women. In contrast, women score higher in their perception of stress and social support [45]. Male adolescents scored significantly higher in resilience than females, which may be related to the brain maturing as adolescents grow [46]. Men and women cope differently with adversity. This may be because certain resilience factors are more effective for one gender than the other [47]. Exposure to stress during puberty tends to have more immediate and significant consequences for girls, heightening the likelihood of mood and stress disorders like depression, anxiety, and PTSD. The hormonal shifts that occur with menopause influence emotional regulation in women. Moreover, early life hardships can also modify the influence of estradiol on brain functions [48].

Although no other sociodemographic variable has been found to contribute to influence resilience and affect, other studies have reported that self-esteem, family support, subjective well-being, psychological well-being [49], regular sleep, perceived stress, well-being [50], empathy, responsibility, optimism, hope and interpersonal skills (communication, self-efficacy, self-control, autonomy, problem-solving) [51] may influence resilience levels. On the other hand, perceived teaching quality and professors' communication technology competence [52], self-regulatory capacity (boredom, awareness, goal, and emotion control) [53], self-efficacy [54], bedtime procrastination, and mobile phone addiction [55] may influence positive and negative emotions in students. Future studies should include these and new factors to control for changes in resilience and positive/negative effects over time.

4.1. Practical Implications

Based on our main findings, it is important to note that the demands of nursing education, such as schedules, classes, and clinical practice, may not be adequate for developing the required level of resilience for future professional practice. In fact, this approach may even diminish resilience factors. Our findings suggest that promoting support from colleagues and tutors, teaching coping skills, and emphasizing the significance of spirituality could lead to more resilient professionals. This is important to attain the required levels for professional practice and compensate for current deficits in educational plans.

According to the recommendations elaborated by Margaret Mcallister and Jessica McKinnon [56], enhancing resilience in health professional education settings can be achieved through immersive learning experiences that focus on building work endurance, coping mechanisms, and developing strengths and leadership skills to navigate increased work demands. In addition, the learning and practice context should provide opportunities for reflection and assimilation of practice and peer knowledge. Increasing exposure to role models who teach adaptive strategies for success in healthcare settings is invaluable. Nurses who demonstrate resilience and post-traumatic growth can have a profound influence on aspiring students. It is important to engage in dialogue, critical analysis, and practical application of the valuable lessons learned from challenging situations. This approach should include collaborative decision-making training, reflective practice through clinical supervision, mentoring, or group support. Resilient nurses can motivate students by sharing their experiences through interactive methods such as seminars, conferences, or publications. Additional tools may include the establishment of cross-year forums for senior students to encourage critical thinking and constructive dialogue.

4.2. Limitations

One of the main strengths of this study is its longitudinal design over four years, which evaluates changes in resilience and affect during the bachelor's degree in nursing. The study had high participation and minimal loss of follow-up among subjects. However, we identified some limitations that should be considered. For instance, the sociodemographic information collected was limited to prevent the identification of students. Additionally, the sample selection was based on convenience, which may hinder the generalizability of the results. Finally, the categorization of sociodemographic variables, such as the over-representation of females in the sample, may lead to an underestimation or overestimation of the results. It is important to note that these limitations are inherent to our profession and the time of the study. In addition, this study was conducted in a single center, which may limit the generalizability of the main findings of this study. Future studies could replicate the design of this study on an international level to account for differences between different university programs and cultural influences. Also, adding a qualitative component to the design would enhance and extend the quantitative findings.

5. Conclusions

Nursing students experience an increase in resilience and positive affect, as well as a decrease in negative affect, throughout their 4-year training, despite events such as the COVID-19 pandemic in 2020. However, there is still room for improvement, particularly in the resilience levels of nursing students. These results must be considered as they would enable students to enter the job market with all the necessary adaptations, reducing the dropout rate and discomfort of nurses during their initial years of professional practice. Therefore, it is crucial to cultivate resilience during university studies. In addition, promoting peer and tutor support, teaching coping skills, and emphasizing the importance of spirituality could lead to more resilient professionals. This would compensate for current deficits in education plans.

Author Contributions: L.I.M.-S., conceptualization, methodology, writing—original draft preparation; A.M.-M., conceptualization, methodology, writing—original and editing; L.R.-L., data curation, visualization, software, validation; G.M., translation, validation, writing—reviewing and editing. All authors have made substantial contributions to all of the following: (1) the conception and design of the study, or acquisition of data, or analysis and interpretation of data, (2) drafting the article or revising it critically for important intellectual content, (3) final approval of the version to be submitted. All authors have read and agreed to the published version of the manuscript.

Funding: This research did not receive any specific grant from funding agencies in the public, commercial, or not-for-profit sectors.

Institutional Review Board Statement: The authors assert that all procedures contributing to this work comply with the ethical standards of the relevant national and institutional committees on human experimentation and with the Helsinki Declaration of 1975, as revised in 2008. The Ethics and Research Committee of the Faculty of Nursing, Physiotherapy and Podiatry approved all procedures involving human subjects/patients (approval number: FEFP 20/21, on 4 November 2020). All participants included in the study were informed, verbally and in writing, of the study objectives and conditions. Written informed consent was obtained from all participants.

Informed Consent Statement: Informed consent was obtained from all subjects involved in the study.

Data Availability Statement: The datasets generated and/or analyzed during the current study are not publicly available due to data protection policy but are available from the corresponding author upon reasonable request.

Public Involvement Statement: No public involvement in any aspect of this research.

Guidelines and Standards Statement: This manuscript was drafted against the STROBE for observational research.

Acknowledgments: We would like to thank the students for their generosity.

Conflicts of Interest: The authors declare that they have no competing interests.

References

1. Amzil, A. Academic Resilience and its Relation to Academic Achievement for Moroccan University Students During the Covid19 Pandemic. *Int. Educ. Stud.* **2022**, *16*, 1. [CrossRef]
2. Sood, S.; Sharma, A. Resilience and Psychological Well-Being of Higher Education Students During COVID-19: The Mediating Role of Perceived Distress. *J. Health Manag.* **2020**, *22*, 606–617. [CrossRef]
3. Cabanyes Truffino, J. Resilience: An approach to the concept. *Rev. Psiquiatr. Salud. Ment.* **2010**, *3*, 145–151. [CrossRef] [PubMed]
4. Tusaie, K.; Dyer, J. Resilience: A historical review of the construct. *Holist. Nurs. Pract.* **2004**, *18*, 3–10. [CrossRef] [PubMed]
5. NANDA. *Nursing Diagnoses: Definitions and Classifications*; Elsevier: Amsterdam, The Netherlands, 2018.
6. Arrogante, O.; Aparicio-Zaldívar, E. Tools to Face Burnout in Nursing: Social Support, Resilience and Coping Strategies. *Rev. Enferm.* **2017**, *40*, 10–17.
7. McCann, C.M.; Beddoe, E.; McCormick, K.; Huggard, P.; Kedge, S.; Adamson, C.; Huggard, J. Resilience in the health professions: A review of recent literature. *Int. J. Wellbeing* **2013**, *3*, 60–81. [CrossRef]
8. McAllister, M.; Brien, D.L. Resilience in Nursing. In *Empowerment Strategies for Nurses*; Springer: Berlin/Heidelberg, Germany, 2019; pp. 1–28.
9. Guo, Y.-F.; Luo, Y.-H.; Lam, L.; Cross, W.; Plummer, V.; Zhang, J.-P. Burnout and its association with resilience in nurses: A cross-sectional study. *J. Clin. Nurs.* **2018**, *27*, 441–449. [CrossRef] [PubMed]
10. Huang, H.-M.; Fang, Y.-W.; Liao, S.-J. The process and indicators of resilience among nursing students in clinical practicum in Taiwan: A qualitative study. *Heliyon* **2023**, *9*, e225242023. [CrossRef] [PubMed]
11. Lopez-Gomez, I.; Hervas, G.; Vazquez, C. Adaptación de las "Escalas de afecto positivo y negativo" (PANAS) en una muestra general española. *Behav. Psychol. Conduct.* **2015**, *23*, 529–548.
12. Alves Apóstolo, J.L.; Alves Rodrigues, M.; Pineda Olvera, J. Evaluación de los estados emocionales de estudiantes de enfermería. *Index de Enfermería* **2007**, *16*, 26–29. [CrossRef]
13. Cleary, M.; Visentin, D.; West, S.; Lopez, V.; Kornhaber, R. Promoting emotional intelligence and resilience in undergraduate nursing students: An integrative review. *Nurse Educ. Today* **2018**, *68*, 112–120. [CrossRef] [PubMed]
14. Tugade, M.M.; Fredrickson, B.L. Resilient individuals use positive emotions to bounce back from negative emotional experiences. *J. Pers. Soc. Psychol.* **2004**, *86*, 320–333. [CrossRef] [PubMed]
15. Smith, G.D.; Yang, F. Stress, resilience and psychological well-being in Chinese undergraduate nursing students. *Nurse Educ. Today* **2017**, *49*, 90–95. [CrossRef] [PubMed]
16. Caldera Montes, J.F.; Aceves Lupercio, B.I.; Reynoso González, Ó.U. Resilience in university students. A comparative study among different careers. *Psicogente* **2016**, *19*, 229–241. [CrossRef]
17. Li, Z.-S.; Hasson, F. Resilience, stress, and psychological well-being in nursing students: A systematic review. *Nurse Educ. Today* **2020**, *90*, 104440. [CrossRef] [PubMed]
18. Rísquez, M.; Garcia, C.; Tebar, E. Resilience and burnout syndrome in nursing students and its relationship with sociodemographic variables and interpersonal relationship. *Int. J. Psychol. Res.* **2012**, *5*, 88–95. [CrossRef]
19. von Elm, E.; Altman, D.G.; Egger, M.; Pocock, S.J.; Gøtzsche, P.C.; Vandenbroucke, J.P. The Strengthening the Reporting of Observational Studies in Epidemiology (STROBE) statement: Guidelines for reporting observational studies. *Lancet* **2007**, *370*, 1453–1457. [CrossRef] [PubMed]
20. Watson, D.; Clark, L.A.; Tellegen, A. Development and validation of brief measures of positive and negative affect: The PANAS scales. *J. Pers. Soc. Psychol.* **1988**, *54*, 1063–1070. [CrossRef] [PubMed]
21. Krijthe, B.P.; Walter, S.; Newson, R.S.; Hofman, A.; Hunink, M.G.; Tiemeier, H. Is positive affect associated with survival? A population-based study of elderly persons. *Am. J. Epidemiol.* **2011**, *173*, 1298–1307. [CrossRef]
22. Sandín, B. Escalas Panas de afecto positivo y negativo para niños y adolescentes (PANAS). *Rev. Psicopatol. Psicol. Clin.* **2003**, *8*, 173–182. [CrossRef]
23. Connor, K.M.; Davidson, J.R.T. Development of a new resilience scale: The Connor-Davidson Resilience Scale (CD-RISC). *Depress. Anxiety* **2003**, *18*, 76–82. [CrossRef]
24. García-León, M.Á.; González-Gómez, A.; Robles-Ortega, H.; Padilla, J.L.; Peralta-Ramírez, M.I. Psychometric properties of the connor-davidson resilience scale (CD-RISC) in the Spanish population. *An. Psicol.* **2019**, *35*, 33–40. [CrossRef]
25. Ríos-risquez, M.I.; Carrillo-garcía, C.; Ángeles, E.D.L. Resilencia, Síndrome de estar quemado en el trabajo y malestar psicológico en estudiantes de enfermería. *Ansiedad Estrés* **2014**, *20*, 115–126.
26. Aryuwat, P.; Asp, M.; Lövenmark, A.; Radabutr, M.; Holmgren, J. An integrative review of resilience among nursing students in the context of nursing education. *Nurs. Open* **2023**, *10*, 2793–2818. [CrossRef] [PubMed]
27. Liao, T.; Liu, Y.; Luo, W.; Duan, Z.; Zhan, K.; Lu, H.; Chen, X. Non-linear association of years of experience and burnout among nursing staff: A restricted cubic spline analysis. *Front. Public Health* **2024**, *12*, 1343293. [CrossRef] [PubMed]
28. Jackson, D.; Firtko, A.; Edenborough, M. Personal resilience as a strategy for surviving and thriving in the face of workplace adversity: A literature review. *J. Adv. Nurs.* **2007**, *60*, 1–9. [CrossRef]

29. Zhang, D.; Qin, L.; Huang, A.; Wang, C.; Yuan, T.; Li, X.; Yang, L.; Li, J.; Lei, Y.; Sun, L.; et al. Mediating effect of resilience and fear of COVID-19 on the relationship between social support and post-traumatic stress disorder among campus-quarantined nursing students: A cross-sectional study. *BMC Nurs.* **2023**, *22*, 164. [CrossRef] [PubMed]
30. Wahl, R.A.; Cotton, S.; Harrison-Monroe, P. Spirituality, adolescent suicide, and the juvenile justice system. *South Med. J.* **2008**, *101*, 711–715. [CrossRef]
31. Walker, B.H.; Abel, N.; Anderies, J.M.; Ryan, P. Resilience, Adaptability, and Transformability in the Goulburn-Broken Catchment, Australia. *Ecol. Soc.* **2009**, *14*, 12. [CrossRef]
32. Arrogante, Ó. Mediator effect of resilience between burnout and health in nursing staff. *Enferm. Clin.* **2014**, *24*, 283–289. [CrossRef]
33. Arrogante, O.; Pérez-García, A.M. Is subjective well-being perceived by non-health care workers different from that perceived by nurses? Relation with personality and resilience. *Enferm. Intensiv.* **2013**, *24*, 145–154. [CrossRef]
34. Suliman, M.; Warshawski, S. Nursing students' satisfaction with clinical placements: The contribution of role modeling, epistemic authority, and resilience-a cross- sectional study. *Nurse Educ. Today* **2022**, *115*, 105404. [CrossRef]
35. Flott, E.A.; Linden, L. The clinical learning environment in nursing education: A concept analysis. *J. Adv. Nurs.* **2016**, *72*, 501–513. [CrossRef]
36. Chan, M.-K.; Snell, L.; Philibert, I. The education avenue of the clinical learning environment: A pragmatic approach. *Med. Teach.* **2019**, *41*, 391–397. [CrossRef] [PubMed]
37. Nordquist, J.; Hall, J.; Caverzagie, K.; Snell, L.; Chan, M.-K.; Thoma, B.; Razack, S.; Philibert, I. The clinical learning environment. *Med. Teach.* **2019**, *41*, 366–372. [CrossRef]
38. Zager Kocjan, G.; Kavčič, T.; Avsec, A. Resilience matters: Explaining the association between personality and psychological functioning during the COVID-19 pandemic. *Int. J. Clin. Health Psychol.* **2021**, *21*, 100198. [CrossRef]
39. Mayor-Silva, L.I.; Romero-Saldaña, M.; Moreno-Pimentel, A.G.; Álvarez-Melcón, Á.C.; Molina-Luque, R.; Meneses-Monroy, A. Psychological Impact during Confinement by COVID-19 on Health Sciences University Students-A Prospective, Longitudinal, and Comparative Study. *Int. J. Environ. Res. Public Health* **2022**, *19*, 9925. [CrossRef] [PubMed]
40. Jiménez-Rodríguez, D.; Molero Jurado, M.D.M.; Pérez-Fuentes, M.D.C.; Arrogante, O.; Oropesa-Ruiz, N.F.; Gázquez-Linares, J.J. The Effects of a Non-Technical Skills Training Program on Emotional Intelligence and Resilience in Undergraduate Nursing Students. *Healthcare* **2022**, *10*, 866. [CrossRef] [PubMed]
41. Mayor-Silva, L.I.; Romero-Saldaña, M.; Moreno-Pimentel, A.G.; Álvarez-Melcón, Á.; Molina-Luque, R.; Meneses-Monroy, A. The role of psychological variables in improving resilience: Comparison of an online intervention with a face-to-face intervention. A randomised controlled clinical trial in students of health sciences. *Nurse Educ. Today* **2021**, *99*, 104778. [CrossRef]
42. Al-Daken, L.; Lazarus, E.R.; Al Sabei, S.D.; Alharrasi, M.; Al Qadire, M. Perception of Nursing Students About Effective Clinical Teaching Environments: A Multi-Country Study. *SAGE Open Nurs.* **2024**, *10*, 23779608241233144. [CrossRef]
43. Longo, D.; Gili, A.; Ramacciati, N.; Morcellini, R.; Ramacciati, N. How Teaching and Internship Influence the Evidence-Based Practice Approach of Nursing Students: A Longitudinal Study. *Florence Nightingale J. Nurs.* **2023**, *31*, 194–202. [PubMed]
44. Huntington, C.; Stanley, S.M.; Doss, B.D.; Rhoades, G.K. Happy, healthy, and wedded? How the transition to marriage affects mental and physical health. *J. Fam. Psychol. JFP J. Div. Fam. Psychol. Am. Psychol. Assoc.* **2022**, *36*, 608–617. [CrossRef] [PubMed]
45. Yalcin-Siedentopf, N.; Pichler, T.; Welte, A.-S.; Hoertnagl, C.M.; Klasen, C.C.; Kemmler, G.; Siedentopf, C.M.; Hofer, A. Sex matters: Stress perception and the relevance of resilience and perceived social support in emerging adults. *Arch. Womens Ment. Health* **2021**, *24*, 403–411. [CrossRef]
46. Pan, N.; Yang, C.; Suo, X.; Shekara, A.; Hu, S.; Gong, Q.; Wang, S. Sex differences in the relationship between brain gray matter volume and psychological resilience in late adolescence. *Eur. Child Adolesc. Psychiatry*, **2023**; *Epub ahead of print*.
47. Fallon, I.P.; Tanner, M.K.; Greenwood, B.N.; Baratta, M.V. Sex differences in resilience: Experiential factors and their mechanisms. *Eur. J. Neurosci.* **2020**, *52*, 2530–2547. [CrossRef] [PubMed]
48. Hodes, G.E.; Epperson, C.N. Sex Differences in Vulnerability and Resilience to Stress Across the Life Span. *Biol. Psychiatry* **2019**, *86*, 421–432. [CrossRef]
49. Martín, M.H.; Moriña, A. Resilience Factors in Students with Disabilities at a Portuguese State University. *Pedagogika* **2022**, *146*, 110–128. [CrossRef]
50. Al Omari, O.; Al Yahyaei, A.; Wynaden, D.; Damra, J.; Aljezawi, M.; Al Qaderi, M.; Al Ruqaishi, H.; Shahrour, L.A.; ALBashtawy, M. Correlates of resilience among university students in Oman: A cross-sectional study. *BMC Psychol.* **2023**, *11*, 2. [CrossRef] [PubMed]
51. Elena, B. Protective Factors for Student Resilience. *Rev. Românească Pentru Educ. Multidimens.* **2023**, *15*, 185–197.
52. Shao, K.; Kutuk, G.; Fryer, L.K.; Nicholson, L.J.; Guo, J. Factors influencing Chinese undergraduate students' emotions in an online EFL learning context during the COVID pandemic. *J. Comput. Assist. Learn.* **2023**, *39*, 1465–1478. [CrossRef]
53. Li, S.; Wu, H.; Wang, Y. Positive emotions, self-regulatory capacity, and EFL performance in the Chinese senior high school context. *Acta Psychol.* **2024**, *243*, 104143. [CrossRef]
54. Wang, Z.; Zheng, B. Achievement Emotions of Medical Students: Do They Predict Self-regulated Learning and Burnout in an Online Learning Environment? *Med. Educ. Online* **2023**, *28*, 2226888. [CrossRef] [PubMed]

55. Zhu, Y.; Liu, J.; Wang, Q.; Huang, J.; Li, X.; Liu, J. Examining the Association between Boredom Proneness and Bedtime Procrastination among Chinese College Students: A Sequential Mediation Model with Mobile Phone Addiction and Negative Emotions. *Psychol. Res. Behav. Manag.* **2023**, *16*, 4329–4340. [CrossRef] [PubMed]
56. McAllister, M.; McKinnon, J. The importance of teaching and learning resilience in the health disciplines: A critical review of the literature. *Nurse Educ. Today* **2009**, *29*, 371–379. [CrossRef] [PubMed]

Disclaimer/Publisher's Note: The statements, opinions and data contained in all publications are solely those of the individual author(s) and contributor(s) and not of MDPI and/or the editor(s). MDPI and/or the editor(s) disclaim responsibility for any injury to people or property resulting from any ideas, methods, instructions or products referred to in the content.

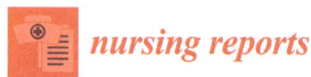 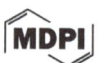

Article

Addressing a Critical Voice in Clinical Practice: Experiences of Nursing Students, Teachers, and Supervisors—A Qualitative Study

Ingrid Rachel Strand *, Unni Knutstad, Anton Havnes and Mette Sagbakken

Faculty of Health, OsloMet—Oslo Metropolitan University, 0130 Oslo, Norway; unnikn@oslomet.no (U.K.); anton@oslomet.no (A.H.); metsa@oslomet.no (M.S.)
* Correspondence: ingfi@oslomet.no

Abstract: Aim: Our goal was to explore how power asymmetry manifests within the relationships between students, teachers, and supervisors, and how it influences students' ability for critical reflection. Design: This study has an explorative qualitative design. Methods: Thirty in-depth interviews with nursing students (15), teachers (9), and supervisors (6) were conducted in addition to 16 observations of mid-term assessments during clinical practice. The analysis was conducted using Braun and Clarke's thematic analysis. Results: The students described being a student as a balancing act between humility, conforming to the supervisor's expectations, and speaking their minds. The view expressed by the teachers and supervisors is that training for the nursing profession is closely linked to the students' ability to act independently. Due to the supervisors' hierarchical position, however, students are hesitant to voice any criticism regarding insufficient supervision or unsatisfactory performance of clinical tasks while at the same time being evaluated on their ability to critically reflect on their own and others' clinical performance. This study was prospectively registered with the Norwegian Centre for Research Data on the 15th of August 2017 with the registration number 54821.

Keywords: clinical practice; student–supervisor relationship; asymmetry in power; critical reflection

Citation: Strand, I.R.; Knutstad, U.; Havnes, A.; Sagbakken, M. Addressing a Critical Voice in Clinical Practice: Experiences of Nursing Students, Teachers, and Supervisors—A Qualitative Study. *Nurs. Rep.* **2024**, *14*, 788–800. https://doi.org/10.3390/nursrep14020061

Academic Editors: Antonio Martínez-Sabater, Elena Chover-Sierra and Carles Saus-Ortega

Received: 23 January 2024
Revised: 20 March 2024
Accepted: 25 March 2024
Published: 29 March 2024

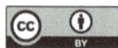

Copyright: © 2024 by the authors. Licensee MDPI, Basel, Switzerland. This article is an open access article distributed under the terms and conditions of the Creative Commons Attribution (CC BY) license (https://creativecommons.org/licenses/by/4.0/).

1. Introduction

Nursing students in Norway undergo a period of supervised clinical practice in their bachelor programme. They are supervised by a Registered Nurse (RN) in clinical practice and a faculty member from the university (teachers). The teachers are either assistant professors or associate professors in the bachelor program in nursing at the university. The supervisors are RNs; employees either in clinical wards, hospitals, nursing homes, home-based care, or psychiatric units; and not employees at the university. The supervisors play a crucial role in evaluating the students' clinical competence and readiness for independent practice. Approval from a supervisor or teacher (or both) is usually necessary for students to progress in their clinical training or to pass their clinical rotations. This evaluation process is important to ensure that the students have the knowledge, skills, and critical thinking abilities required to provide safe and high-quality patient care. Clinical competence is defined by Liou et al. [1] as "The ability to apply critical thinking, problem solving and clinical decision-making skills in patient care" [1] p. 2654). We lean on the definition of Griffiths and Tann on critical reflection, where they argue that critical reflection can be both spontaneous and a more systematic reflection [2]. The significance of being able to assess and reflect on one's clinical competencies, as well as those of others, is well documented in research as a critical factor in enhancing patient safety [3–5]. Thus, critical thinking is seen as a crucial part of clinical competence in nursing. However, a challenge highlighted in prior research is that the capacity for self-reflection and assessment typically grows with experiences, a quality that nursing students pursuing a bachelor's programme may possess to varying degrees [6]. Previous studies focusing on students' learning experiences in clinical practice have identified several factors that influence their learning process. These include the necessity of a close and trustful relationship with their supervisors [7–14]. A safe relationship supports students' professional development, protects, and assists them in times of difficulty, and guides their learning throughout clinical practice [8]. Honkavuo's qualitative study of the perspective of Finnish nursing students regarding a caring relationship with their supervisor revealed that a relationship built on mutual respect and having supervisors well versed in research-based pedagogical techniques was of utmost significance. This implied that supervisors possessed insight into optimizing students' learning experiences [8].

In the evaluating process, there are three defined roles: the student, the Registered Nurse in clinical practice, and the teacher. Both Rees et al. and Johnson [5,15] underline the importance of power asymmetry as manifested by defined roles.

Power imbalances may emerge in both the student–supervisor and student–teacher relationship. In their role, both supervisors and teachers will be wielding greater authority compared to the students [5,15]. Besides defined roles, several influencing factors, including age, knowledge, experience, language proficiency, and hierarchical position, can create or increase this discrepancy in power [15]. Thus, the discrepancy can be understood as an imbalance within the relationship, often referred to as power asymmetry.

In *Discipline and Punish: The birth of the prison*, Foucault examines the development of disciplinary mechanisms and the exercise of power within various institutions, including schools and hospitals. Foucault argues that these institutions are not merely places of education and healing, but also sites where power is exercised and normalized. He suggests that disciplinary power operates through a variety of techniques, such as surveillance, normalization, and examination, to regulate individual behaviour and enforce conformity to social norms. In the context of educational institutions, Foucault explores how disciplinary practices, including hierarchical structures, strict schedules, and surveillance mechanisms, are employed to mould students into obedient subjects [16].

In our point of view, understanding power asymmetry in this context of education and supervision is essential for ensuring fairness, accountability, and effective mentorship. This asymmetry can also influence students and supervisors' communications and collaboration. Haugan highlights the need to address power dynamics for creating a supportive and productive learning environment, which can help the students to express their critical perspectives in various educational settings [13].

A study conducted in Norway concerning the student–supervisor relationship in clinical practice found that a lack of continuity and inadequate supervision led to students feeling uncertain about their own capabilities [13]. One of the primary objectives in examining the student–supervisor relationship within the context of power asymmetry is to heighten awareness of potential power-related challenges that might hinder students' learning, such as instances where supervisors fail to provide constructive feedback. Rees emphasizes the critical need for a balanced relationship to facilitate student development and learning, while recognizing that a power imbalance could potentially obstruct effective communication and feedback [5], p. 1150. At its essence, Philling and Roth claim that supervision aims to support learners in their professional development, and supervisors can achieve this by adopting a relationship-based approach to education and training [17]. Conversely, power imbalances can lead to abuse, as seen in a study on undergraduate nursing students' clinical experiences conducted in South Africa [10]. Examples included supervisors making disparaging comments on students' assessment, stifling, or suppressing students' expression and opinions, and subjecting them to verbal mistreatment in front of peers. While cultural norms may vary, promoting belongingness is crucial across contexts, empowering students to advocate for themselves, engage in self-assessment, and enhance their learning experiences.

However, both students and supervisors can wield power, and students may respond to and utilize this power in various ways. Rees et al. revealed that students might exercise their own power by, for instance, actively seeking feedback from supervisors and engaging in discussions about such feedback with both the supervisor and fellow students, particularly when they are dissatisfied with the supervisor's communication style [5].

Perry et al. conducted a comprehensive review aimed at identifying factors that enhance student accountability for learning in clinical practice, including countries such as Sweden, Canada, the UK, and the USA. In their review, they established that a crucial aspect contributing to this accountability is the sense of belongingness. Belongingness, as defined by Perry et al., refers to the presence of a nurturing relationship with a supportive supervisor who fosters an environment with support throughout the learning process. Importantly, if the relationship is defined by belonging, it is also a relationship experienced as a partnership, emphasized by both Perry et al. and Dysthe as implying an exchange of reflections and ideas [18–20].

Several studies have explored the dynamics of student–supervisor interactions within clinical practice, spanning various countries such as Norway [7,12,13], Finland [8], Denmark [9], Australia [5], South Africa [10], England [11], and Sweden [14]. However, few studies have delved into the student–supervisor relationship's power asymmetry and its repercussions for their interactions, including its impact on students' ability to reflect on both their own and others' clinical performances.

As stated above, while there is a wealth of research on the experiences of students and supervisors in clinical practice, only a limited number of studies have explored how power imbalances among students, supervisors, and teachers affect interaction patterns. This study aims to explore how power asymmetry may manifest within the relationships between students, teachers, and supervisors (RNs), and how it may influence students' ability for critical reflection, with data from actual assessment situations and mid-term assessment.

Research Questions

1. What are the experiences and perceptions of students, teachers, and supervisors regarding their relationships and the dynamics of power asymmetry?
2. How may potential power asymmetry influence students' ability to critically reflect?

2. Method

2.1. Study Design

This study adopts a qualitative, exploratory design with the primary goal of enhancing our comprehension of power imbalances between students and supervisors and how it influences students' ability to critically reflect. This research incorporates 30 in-depth interviews conducted with students, teachers, and supervisors within a bachelor's degree program at a Norwegian university. Additionally, 16 mid-term assessment observations were included as a method to gain deeper understanding of the contextual dynamics and interactions among the involved parties [21,22].

To ensure maximum variation, inspired by Patton, this study encompassed all three academic years of the program, spanning placements in diverse healthcare settings such as homecare, nursing homes, surgery wards, medical wards, and psychiatric units. Variation was also secured by encompassing individuals of different genders and ages, as well as students, teachers, and supervisors (see Table 1) [23].

2.2. Setting

This study, comprising both interviews and observations, was carried out in various clinical settings where students underwent their clinical placements. The mid-term assessment (MTA) of the students served as a pivotal context for observing the interactions between the students, their program teacher, and the clinical supervisor. The MTA typically occurs approximately four to five weeks into the clinical placement and involves the student, a teacher from the bachelor programme, and the supervisor representing the clinical setting.

Table 1. Participant sample (F—female, M—male).

Sample	Observed	Participated in Interview	Year of Program 1st/2nd/3rd yr.	Age Range
Teachers	9 (7F/2M)	9 (7F/2M)	3/3/3	57–70
Students	16 13F/3M	15 (11F/4M)	4/3/8	20–58
Supervisors	13 13F	6 6F	1/2/3	25–59
Total	38	30	30	20–70

To ensure an uninterrupted environment, a separate room within the ward is utilized for the MTA, which typically lasts between 45 and 60 min. During the MTA, an assessment form is utilized, encompassing a list of predefined learning outcomes, with the performance being scored as "as expected" or "below expected". This MTA can be viewed as a tripartite discussion involving the student, the teacher, and the clinical supervisor, with the student receiving both formal and summative feedback on their performance and clinical competencies related to the specified learning outcomes.

2.3. Recruitment

The participants for this study were recruited with the assistance of teachers from the bachelor program in nursing who served as gatekeepers. A total of 44 teachers were approached for participation in this study, either via email or during a teacher's meeting. Thirteen teachers agreed and consented to participate. During a pre-clinical practice meeting, this study was presented to students (totalling 161) of these 13 teachers, resulting in 74 students signing consent forms. To accommodate the timing and the mid-term assessments (MTAs) and to encompass various clinical placements for data collection, 16 students were selected to participate in the observations. Subsequently, the supervisors of these 16 students were approached and invited to join this study, and they all agreed and signed consent forms. The teachers participating in this study were either assistant professors or associate professors in the bachelor program in nursing at the current university. The supervisors participating in this study were RNs; employees in either clinical wards, hospitals, nursing homes, home-based care, or psychiatric units; and not employees at the current university. We did not address whether the supervisors and/or teachers had participated in any formal education in student clinical assessment beyond their bachelor's degree in nursing.

All the observed participants were also invited to take part in interviews, and fifteen students, nine teachers, and six supervisors agreed to do so. Teachers and supervisors who declined to participate in the interviews cited time constraints as their reason for non-participation. One student who did not participate in the interview declined due to personal challenges encountered during clinical practice.

2.4. Participants

To ensure maximum variation [23], we included different genders and ages, as well as a sample comprising students, teachers, and supervisors (see Table 1). The number of potential participants that received information about this study and signed the consent form totalled 100, including teachers, students, and supervisors (Table 1). However, due to organizational limits and the timing of the mid-term assessment, a strategic sample was made to include participants in all types of clinical placements. The sample included 9 teachers, 16 students, and 13 supervisors.

2.5. Data Collection

To gain a more comprehensive understanding of the interactions between students, teachers, and supervisors during the assessment process, observations and interviews were chosen as methods. The MTA was selected for observation due to an assumption that this setting might reveal situations where potential power imbalances in the interactions among the participants become evident. A total of 16 MTA observations were conducted, with a specific focus on the verbal and nonverbal interaction patterns among the participants. The notes and reflections from the observations were typed on a computer by the first author during the observation process.

Approximately two to three weeks after the MTA, 30 in-depth interviews were conducted in private settings, either at the university or within clinical settings. These interviews followed a semi-structured interview guide. Students were questioned about their experiences of assessment (including MTA), their relationship with their supervisor, how they perceived their role as students in clinical practice, and their overall clinical experiences. Similarly, teachers and supervisors were asked questions about their experiences in supervising and assessing students in clinical practice, including the MTA.

2.6. Analysis

This study is part of a larger research project that centres on the assessment of nursing students in clinical practice, exploring the experiences of students, teachers, and supervisors. For the analysis of the data, Braun and Clarke's six-step thematic analysis framework [24] was employed.

The initial data analysis began during the transcription of the interviews, with comments and codes being recorded as interviews were transcribed and observational notes were revised. To structure and organize the text systematically, all data pages were imported into the qualitative analysis tool NVIVO, version 12 PRO. A second comprehensive reading was conducted manually, where each line of the text was carefully reviewed. Key text passages pertaining to different facts of interaction patterns during supervision and assessment in clinical practice, including potential power imbalances among students, teachers, and supervisors, and their impact on students' ability to engage in critical reflection, were analysed using NVIVO. An inductive approach to the data characterized the initial part of the analysis.

During the coding process, the recognition of power asymmetry in the relationship among the three parties involved prompted the formulation of a more refined research question: "How may potential power asymmetry influence students' ability to critically reflect?". This research question guided the subsequent abductive phase of the analysis. Excerpts providing insights into the relationship, interaction, and consequences of supervisors and teachers' methods of supervision; power asymmetry; reactions to power asymmetry; the exercise of power asymmetry; and how power asymmetry manifested in the relationship, and students' ability to critically reflect, were assigned new codes.

The following phase involved successive rounds of condensing codes that were relevant to the research question, resulting in the emergence of patterns related to power asymmetry and its diverse impacts on the students' ability to critical reflect. Throughout this process, themes were progressively abstracted into overarching themes. These overarching themes served as a guide to ensure consistency in all phases of the analysis and theme abstraction, aligning with the research question. Ultimately, the data were condensed into three overarching themes: (i) different expectations, (ii) socialized into servility, (iii) daring to critically reflect. The analytical process was characterized by a dynamic interplay between meaningful entities, condensed meaning units, abstraction, code development, and theme generation. During the process of analysis, codes and themes were discussed with the researchers of this study and members within the research group as a validation of findings. As this study progressed, all four authors collectively agreed upon these three final themes.

2.7. Ethical Considerations

This study received approval from the Norwegian Centre for Research Data in August 2017, case number 54821. This study also gained approval from the university's department head and the program coordinators for the first, second, and third years of the bachelor program in nursing. The directors and department managers of various healthcare institutions and departments also provided their approval for this study.

All participants, including students, teachers, and supervisors, were provided with both verbal and written information about this study's objectives and purpose. They were informed of their right to withdraw from this study at any time without facing any adverse consequences. All participants signed a consent form.

To ensure data security and privacy, a risk and vulnerability analysis was conducted. Subsequently, data were stored on an encrypted memory stick, which was placed in a locked drawer, and access was restricted to the researcher alone.

3. Findings

3.1. Different Expectations

The results reveal that the assessment process was influenced by the individual expectations of teachers and supervisors regarding what they anticipated from the students. This encompassed their expectations of student behaviour and performance in interactions with colleagues and patients across different departments. The findings suggest that when supervisors and teachers assert influence over student conduct, these personal expectations may be perceived as a form of control or even disciplinary measures. An illustrative incident during a mid-term assessment further exemplifies this phenomenon. This pertains to an adult nursing student with relevant knowledge, who answered a professional question posed by a co-worker, a nurse. This was interpreted as arrogant behaviour and inappropriate coming from a student. The issue was brought up during the mid-term evaluation, on observation, and the following was expressed by the teacher:

"You should be yourself, but don't demand too much attention" (at the ward).

Different expectations from the educational institution and from the clinical placement were illustrated by a second-year teacher during an interview:

"In this regard, I wish that we were much more ideologically visionary and ideologically based in our education, in facing a field of practice that would be willing to play along. However, how do you get thousands of practical contacts and fields of practice to engage with us on matters they have no interest in?"

The teacher seemed to have a specific view on the supervisors as not visionary. The supervisors, however, had some views on limits in the nursing education, as stated by a supervisor in clinical practice:

"Perhaps the university should swallow that bitter pill and simply write it out plainly on paper, thus sparing the students from trembling like leaves and feeling as though they are about to discuss matters they do not comprehend in the slightest".

Although the supervisor and teacher may not intentionally communicate their expectations to express their authority, students often interpreted the communication of expectations as asymmetrical. Even though the expectations outlined by teachers and supervisors were deemed to be pertinent, the way they were conveyed was crucial. This was exemplified when a teacher, during an interview, contemplated the anticipated skills for the nursing profession while also considering the hierarchical position of the student within the ward:

"My impression is that students, well, they may feel like they're a nuisance, and they may feel that they cannot ask, but at the same time, I feel that it is a skill in a busy working day to be able to know when I can ask questions and when I have to wait, because not all questions require immediate answers".

This contemplation positions the student within a hierarchical framework, whether consciously or subconsciously, possibly serving as a means of their initiation into the profession or establishing expectations regarding student conduct. Data based on the interviews with students indicated that students often passively accepted their position as a student and their role within the ward hierarchy, conforming to supervisors' expectations when observed. Students also expressed a sort of acceptance of the ongoing adaptation of expectations and set of standards they experienced from different supervisors in different clinical placements during their bachelor program. New clinical placements required new insights into the new supervisors' expectations. One student commented on different expectations during their interview, and said:

"What do you expect today? I need to know what is expected of me. Everybody has different expectations".

This quote reflects the frustration expressed by multiple students during clinical practice, feeling the need to conform to their supervisors' varying expectations.

3.2. Socialised into Servility

Several students articulated their experience as a delicate balance between demonstrating humility, conforming to their supervisors' expectations, and having the courage to voice their opinions. A first-year student reflected during their interview on how they were met the first day in clinical practice, and how that first meeting made them feel unimportant and inferior:

"They were unaware that we were coming... it was a case of "oh, are you coming today... and why were we not informed?", which resulted in an unpleasant atmosphere."

Furthermore, the same student described a lack of training in nursing skills during clinical practice in nursing homes, and that it was difficult to question the task and activities they were left in charge of:

"I had expected to be given more responsibility than we were. . .that we would be tested more in relation to typical nursing tasks. However, we were more or less assigned a role of activity coordinators, with a great deal of focus being placed on that."

Similar reflections were communicated by several other students regarding their first day in clinical practice. As a result, students often found themselves feeling relegated to the bottom of the hierarchy, with their expectations and desires regarding their role often going unfulfilled. This perceived asymmetry appeared to hinder their acquisition of clinical skills, leading to a diminished sense of autonomy. In an interview, a third-year student shared the sentiment of feeling burdensome in relation to their supervisor and colleagues:

"You often feel you are a burden [. . .], and then there may be some people who show that it's exhausting having students (laughs) [. . .] I've just accepted that this is a part of the student's role".

Most students stated that they were "aware" of their position or status in the clinical ward hierarchy, and, consequently, in their learning environment, and that this position required some degree of subservience. On the other hand, students emphasized factors such as trust and consistent feedback from their supervisor as essential elements in their relation and the development of the necessary clinical competencies. Additionally, teachers discussed the process of students assimilating into the nursing profession and how both they and their supervisors passed on knowledge and clinical skills to the students through imitation. A second-year teacher expressed this during an interview:

"I experience way too much imitation of what's going on at the ward [. . .] learning is about much more than just imitation, so I would prefer to see a more active way of acquiring clinical competencies."

A second-year teacher connected the act of imitation to a lack of confidence in students and their approach to acquiring competencies during an interview:

"I think it's about a lack of trust in the student, in them being capable of finding their own way. That we sort of do a quality assurance, almost like a meat inspection, instead of thinking the opposite, giving them (the students) optimal opportunities."

Moreover, the data indicated that supervisors' expectations regarding students' adaptation to the nursing profession were linked to their capacity for independence within the clinical setting, as elucidated by a third-year supervisor during an interview:

> "What we are working towards is that they should be as independent as possible [...] if they take responsibility for the patient, and several patients, and use their supervisors as a consultant, that's great."

Findings derived from both observations and interviews show that both teachers and supervisors stressed the importance of students demonstrating independence in their execution of clinical tasks and activities. Nevertheless, the data also suggest that supervisors and teachers resorted to disciplinary measures to maintain control over students, while students emulated their supervisors to achieve what was perceived as vital clinical competence by the supervisor. This disparity, along with the resulting imbalance in the student–supervisor, student–teacher dynamic, appeared to be linked to supervisory and teaching roles rather than actual knowledge.

Data from the student interviews indicated that students often passively accepted their position as a student and their role within the ward hierarchy, conforming to supervisors' expectations when observed.

During an interview, a second-year teacher conveyed this sentiment while responding to inquiries about how students were adopted into the nursing profession, supporting the perceptions of many students:

> "They (the students) are in a way socialized into a form of servility."

When asked about students' integration into the nursing profession, this teacher's response aligns with the perceptions of numerous students. The implication is that, instead of openly engaging in critical reflection, students tend to unquestioningly embrace the views and practices of their supervisors.

3.3. Daring to Critically Reflect

Based on both observational and interview data, it became evident that some students hesitated to openly discuss negative perceptions or experiences related to the competence of their clinical colleagues and supervisors. They feared that expressing such viewpoints might result in not passing clinical practice. Similarly, the students were cautious about sharing critical feedback regarding the adequacy of the supervision. In an interview, a third-year student expressed fear, during an interview, of not being taken seriously if they complained about the supervision:

> "It's one person's words against the other—who are they going to listen to?".

Consequently, students refrained from expressing critiques of the leadership, supervisors' performance in clinical tasks, and inadequate supervision due to being apprehensive about potential consequences. As articulated by a third-year student in an interview, this fear of repercussions was a significant factor in their reluctance to voice such concerns:

> "You're afraid of speaking out as a student. I just grit my teeth and get through it" (clinical practice).

Students described how such interactions consumed valuable time that could otherwise be dedicated to learning activities during clinical practice. They expressed concerns about not being heard or taken seriously by their teachers, supervisors, or the head of the department. Although supervisors encouraged students to improve their clinical and professional skills through self-reflection and constructive feedback, students perceived the use of such feedback as "risky".

4. Discussion

In this study, we examined the experiences and perceptions of students, teachers, and supervisors regarding their relationships and the dynamics of power asymmetry in an assessment and evaluation setting. Additionally, we explored how such asymmetry might influence students' ability to engage in critical reflection. Students frequently described challenges in expressing critical perspectives within clinical practice due to hierarchical structures, fearing potential negative reactions from supervisors. Teachers experienced that students often imitate their supervisors excessively. They attributed this behaviour to the imbalance in power dynamics in the relationship, resulting in students behaving in accordance with what they perceived as supervisors' expectations and demands. Supervisors observed a deficiency in students' independence in pursuing their learning outcomes.

However, they did not express specific concerns about potential consequences stemming from an imbalanced power dynamic in the student–supervisor relationship, such as students seldom critically reflecting and openly assessing and discussing performances and practices at the clinical ward.

Previous research has shown that essential nursing skills include the capacity to engage in reflective practices, the ability to critically analyse, and the evaluation of various aspects of nursing [10,25]. Other studies have identified challenges in sharing reflections, often attributed to power imbalances between teachers and students [26], or students being inhibited from expressing their opinions due to an abuse of authority [10]. Due to the hierarchical position of the supervisor, students hesitated to offer constructive feedback regarding inadequate supervision or a substandard execution of clinical duties. This discovery presents a paradox, as the desired learning outcomes emphasize the importance of students' ability to critically reflect on their clinical experiences. According to our findings, it was the personal expectations of the individual supervisors rather than the typical ward-level expectations that primarily influenced the comments and expectations regarding students' clinical performance. This subjective approach by supervisors regarding key clinical competencies and their emphasis on student evaluation based on these abilities makes it challenging to convey clear expectations to students before their clinical placements.

In our study, teachers noted how supervisors tended to pass on their own methods for performing clinical tasks, which was interpreted as a lack of trust in the students' ability to develop their own learning paths. This lack of student independence aligns with Foucault's argument that disciplinary measures often result from a lack of trust in students' capacity to acquire new skills independently [16].

The role of a supervisor or teacher as a guide for students entering the nursing profession can also be viewed as an embodiment of tradition. In this context, traditions encompass the preservation and transmission of assessment knowledge, clinical competencies, and institutional understanding [27], p. 70. However, as our findings indicate, students' imitation and adjustment to the established norms and practices in institutional settings could be seen as a socialization into the profession, following a traditional form of learning of the nursing profession. This again could limit their learning process rather than facilitate it, restraining the students from critical thinking and independence. When knowledge is merely handed down or passively transmitted to students, they might be prevented from actively and critically acquiring the knowledge necessary to become professional nurses. This process of imitation can inadvertently perpetuate outdated practices or even lead to malpractice. To aid students in cultivating a critical perspective on their own and their colleagues' clinical task performance, process evaluation becomes essential, enabling students to assess their current standing and map out their course for further learning [28–32].

Adopting an assessment framework for the clinical learning environment, as suggested by Ozga et al., as a routine procedure for evaluating students' experiences during clinical practice could offer valuable insights. This approach allows supervisors and educators to scrutinize and contemplate the dynamics of their supervisory relationships and the role of the nursing teacher and direct attention towards the pedagogical environment [33].

As illustrated in our findings, asymmetric relations and hierarchical systems tended to prevent students to voice concerns about what they perceived as irregularities in supervision. Consequently, our results suggest that students' hesitancy regarding offering critical feedback on the clinical performance of supervisors or colleagues, including their supervisory abilities, may be related to teachers and supervisors' disciplinary inclinations. These findings align with those of a Norwegian study by Christiansen et al., which revealed that supervisors' anticipations of student conduct influenced the assessment process, including the anticipation of independence in the learning process. Additionally, it was observed that supervisors predominantly based their assessments on their personal judgments of what comprised critical nursing skills [7].

According to our study, students appear to conform and adapt to their supervisors' current expectations, despite having encountered different standards from previous supervisors or educators. This adaptability may be attributed to students quickly adapting to their position or role within the existing hierarchy, or, as Foucault (p. 123) emphasizes, to the status or role of being a student. In institutional settings, such as hospitals or universities, shared norms and hierarchies, like the ward hierarchy, exemplify the power structures that students must acclimatize to [16]. These power dynamics can vary across different institutions [34]. In general, a doctor holds the highest status within a hospital due to superior expertise and skills [16,35]. Similarly, a nurse holds a higher rank than an auxiliary nurse, and depending on their progress in training, nursing students fall somewhere between the status of a nurse and an auxiliary nurse.

Students embark on a transformative journey to become nurses and enter the field of nursing. In this process, teachers and supervisors play a pivotal role in guiding students and providing feedback on various aspects such as their conduct, interactions with colleagues and patients in the ward, and their overall professional engagement. When supervisors, whether consciously or unconsciously, instil obedience in students, it may result in future nurses conforming to the system rather than critically evaluating and reflecting on professional standards.

Drawing on Foucault's insight [16], the exertion of power by teachers and supervisors can subjectify students, forming them to behave in accordance with the supervisors' expectations, essentially leading to socialization into subservience. A recognized Danish researcher who focuses on the student–supervisor relationship and feedback argues that students should rely on themselves and their own learning process to acquire the essential competencies, but self-reliance is contingent on the presence of a trusting relationship between the student and the supervisor [9]. In a parallel manner, data based on the student interviews emphasize the importance of fostering a relationship founded on mutual trust and providing trustworthy, consistent feedback. This aligns with findings from prior research, e.g., Ref. [18], highlighting the importance of providing students with opportunities for autonomy and accountability in clinical practice. It also emphasizes the necessity for supervisors to utilize pedagogical approaches that foster the cultivation of independent learning. Dysthe's partnership model [19] offers a valuable perspective on the supervisor–student relationship. According to this model, feedback is conveyed through dialogue, allowing for an open discussion and negotiation of the feedback. Dysthe emphasizes that the relationship does not assume symmetry in terms of students and supervisors possessing identical knowledge or insight. Instead, the supervision process fosters a dialogic space where both parties can initiate and advocate for their perspectives. A partnership-oriented connection, as outlined by this model, has the potential to facilitate the development of students' critical thinking and independence, rather than attempting to assimilate the students into a traditional mould or encouraging them to imitate the supervisor. This approach can be effectively employed to rectify or balance existing asymmetry and improve the overall learning environment, as highlighted by previous research [5,9,15].

From our perspective, the use of disciplinary measures by supervisors or teachers as a form of authority may exacerbate the existing asymmetry, potentially hindering students from freely expressing themselves. However, a supervisor or teacher may find it necessary to exercise a degree of restraint and discipline to guide a nursing student's journey into the profession, somewhat akin to providing institutional "parenting" to the student. Thus, a complete lack of disciplinary measures, without any form of quality assurance for students transitioning into the nursing profession, may pose a risk to the integrity of both the profession and the institutions where they practice. Nevertheless, it is crucial for supervisors and educators to be mindful of the potential drawbacks of asymmetry in the student–supervisor relationship, ensuring that students can fully harness their learning potential and openly articulate their critical reflections on supervision and other clinical matters.

5. Conclusions

In conclusion, the insight shared by teachers and supervisors underlines the close connection between training for the nursing profession, students' critical thinking skills, and their ability to function independently. Nevertheless, the hierarchical position of supervisors appeared to inhibit students from voicing critiques concerning inadequate supervision or subpar clinical task performances, even though they were simultaneously being assessed on their capacity to critically evaluate both their own and their colleagues' clinical performance. This apparent contradiction arises from the evaluation criteria, which entail an expectation that students actively engage in critical reflection and assessment of their co-workers and peers. Despite the potential power imbalances that could suppress or disempower students, our findings revealed that students frequently accepted their hierarchical position and adapted to their role as a student.

To gain a more comprehensive understanding of the power asymmetry in student–supervisor relationships, we recommend that future research should concentrate on institutional dynamics and involve leaders in clinical practice. Additionally, we propose conducting student and supervisor observations in diverse clinical settings, followed by in-depth interviews focusing on their perceptions of their own authority and its potential impact on others. Such investigations can provide valuable insights into the complexities of the power dynamics within the student–supervisor and student–teacher relationship.

6. Limitations

The data for this study were collected from one university and one bachelor program in nursing in Norway. However, due to the similarity of findings from previous studies, we believe the findings have transfer value to other nursing and health education programs in similar contexts. We acknowledge that the data utilized in this study are from 2017 and 2018. However, it is important to note that the regulation of clinical placements and associated assessment procedures has remained unchanged since 2016. There is still a need for the further exploration of assessment in clinical practice, particularly focusing on the asymmetry in the relationship between supervisors and students. This aspect remains relevant and warrants further exploration.

Author Contributions: Conceptualization: I.R.S., U.K., A.H. and M.S.; Methodology: I.R.S., U.K., A.H. and M.S.; Validation: I.R.S., U.K., A.H. and M.S.; Formal Analysis: I.R.S., U.K., A.H. and M.S.; Writing—Original Draft Preparation: I.R.S., U.K., A.H. and M.S.; Writing—Review and Editing: I.R.S., U.K., A.H. and M.S.; Supervision: M.S., U.K. and A.H.; Project Administration: I.R.S., U.K., A.H. and M.S. All authors have read and agreed to the published version of the manuscript.

Funding: This research received no external funding.

Institutional Review Board Statement: The study was conducted according to the guidelines of the Declaration of Helsinki and approved by the Norwegian Centre for Research Data; Approval Code: 54821, Approval Date: 17 August 2017.

Informed Consent Statement: Informed consent was obtained from all subjects involved in the study.

Data Availability Statement: Dataset available on request from the authors. The raw data supporting the conclusions of this article will be made available by the authors on request.

Public Involvement Statement: No public involvement in any aspect of this research.

Guidelines and Standards Statement: This manuscript was drafted against the consolidated criteria for reporting qualitative research (COREQ) for qualitative research.

Acknowledgments: The authors thank all students, teachers, and supervisors that participated in the study.

Conflicts of Interest: The authors declare no conflicts of interest.

References

1. Liou, S.-R.; Liu, H.-C.; Tsai, S.-L.; Chu, T.-P.; Cheng, C.-Y. Performance competence of pregraduate nursing students and hospital nurses: A comparison study. *J. Clin. Nurs.* **2020**, *29*, 2652–2662. [CrossRef] [PubMed]
2. Griffiths, M.; Tann, S. Using reflective practice to link personal and public theories. *J. Educ. Teach.* **1992**, *18*, 69–85. [CrossRef]
3. Coster, S.; Watkins, M.; Norman, I.J. What is the impact of professional nursing on patients' outcomes globally? An overview of research evidence. *Int. J. Nurs. Stud.* **2018**, *78*, 76–83. [CrossRef] [PubMed]
4. Laurant, M.; van der Biezen, M.; Wijers, N.; Watananirun, K.; Kontopantelis, E.; van Vught, A. Nurses as substitutes for doctors in primary care. *Cochrane Database Syst. Rev.* **2018**, *7*, CD001271. [CrossRef] [PubMed]
5. Rees, C.E.; Davis, C.; King, O.A.; Clemans, A.; Crampton, N.J.; McKeown, T.; Morphet, J.; Seear, K. Power and resistance in feedback during work-integrated learning: Contesting traditional student supervisor asymmetries. *Assess. Eval. High. Educ.* **2019**, *45*, 1136–1154. [CrossRef]
6. Taylor, I.; Bing-Jonsson, P.; Wangensteen, S.; Finnbakk, E.; Sandvik, L.; McCormack, B.; Fagerström, L. The self-assessment of clinical competence and the need for further training: A crosssectional survey of advanced practice nursing students. *J. Clin. Nurs.* **2020**, *29*, 545–555. [CrossRef]
7. Christiansen, B.; Averlid, G.; Baluyot, C.; Blomberg, K.; Eikeland, A.; Finstad IR, S.; Larsen, M.; Lindeflaten, K. Challenges in the assessment of nursing students in clinical placements: Exploring perceptions among nurse mentors. *Nurs. Open* **2021**, *8*, 1069–1076. [CrossRef] [PubMed]
8. Honkavuo, L. Nursing students' perspective on a caring relationship in clinical supervision. *Nurs. Ethics* **2020**, *27*, 1225–1237. [CrossRef] [PubMed]
9. Jorgensen, B.M. Investigating Non-Engagement with Feedback in Higher Education as a Social Practice. *Assess. Eval. High. Educ.* **2019**, *44*, 623–635. [CrossRef]
10. Donough, G.; Van der Heever, M. Undergraduate nursing students' experience of clinical supervision. *Curationis* **2018**, *41*, e1–e8. [CrossRef]
11. Bifarin, O.; Stonehouse, D. Clinical supervision: An important part of every nurse's practice. *Br. J. Nurs.* **2017**, *26*, 331–335. [CrossRef] [PubMed]
12. Amsrud, K.E.; Lyberg, A.; Severinsson, E. The influence of clinical supervision and its potential for enhancing patient safety—Undergraduate nursing students views. *J. Nurs. Educ. Pract.* **2015**, *5*, 87–96. [CrossRef]
13. Haugan, G. Relasjonen til veilederen betyr mye for sykepleierstudenter i sykehuspraksis. *Sykepl. Forsk.* **2012**, *7*, 152–158. [CrossRef]
14. Severinsson, E.; Sand, Å. Evaluation of the clinical supervision and professional development of student nurses. *J. Nurs. Manag.* **2010**, *18*, 669–677. [CrossRef] [PubMed]
15. Johnson, M. Feedback Effectiveness in Professional Learning Contexts. *Rev. Educ.* **2016**, *4*, 195–229. [CrossRef]
16. Foucault, M. *Discipline and Punish: The Birth of the Prison*; Vintage Books: New York, NY, USA, 1979.
17. Philling, S.; Roth, A.D. The competent clinical supervisor. In *The Wiley International Handbook of Clinical Supervision*; Watkins, C.E., Jr., Milne, D.L., Eds.; John Wiley and Sons Ltd.: London, UK, 2014; Chapter 2, pp. 20–37.
18. Perry, C.; Henderson, A.; Grealish, L. The behaviours of nurses that increase student accountability for learning in clinical practice: An integrative review. *Nurse Educ. Pract.* **2018**, *65*, 177–186. [CrossRef]
19. Dysthe, O. Professors as Mediators of Academic Text Cultures. An Interview Study with Advisors and Master's Degree Students in Three Disciplines in a Norwegian University. *Writ. Commun.* **2002**, *19*, 493–544. [CrossRef]
20. Liljedahl, M.; Bjorck, E.; Kalen, S.; Ponzer, S.; Bolander Laksov, K. To belong or not to belong: Nursing students' interactions with clinical learning environments–an observational study. *BMC Medic. Educ.* **2016**, *16*, 197. [CrossRef] [PubMed]
21. Kvale, S. *Det Kvalitative Forskningsintervju (Qualitative Research Interview)*; Gyldendal Norsk Forlag: Oslo, Norway, 2015.
22. Fangen, K. *Deltagende Observasjon (Participant Observation–in Norwegian)*, 2nd ed.; Fagbokforlaget: Bergen, Norway, 2017.
23. Patton, M.Q. *Qualitative Research and Evaluation Methods. Integrating Theory and Practice*, 4th ed.; The SAGE Dictionary: Thousand Oaks, CA, USA, 2002.
24. Braun, V.; Clarke, V. Using thematic analysis in psychology. *Qual. Res. Psychol.* **2006**, *3*, 77–101. [CrossRef]
25. Rega, M.L.; Telaretti, F.; Alvaro, R.; Kangasniemi, M. Philosophical and theoretical content of the nursing discipline in academic education: A critical interpretive synthesis. *Nurse Educ. Today* **2017**, *57*, 74–81. [CrossRef]
26. Zhan, Y. Conventional or Sustainable? Chinese University Students' Thinking about Feedback. *Assess. Eval. High. Educ.* **2019**, *44*, 973–986. [CrossRef]
27. Cavalcante Schuback, M.S. Being without Heidegger. *Gather. Heidegger Circ. Annu.* **2017**, *7*, 70–83. [CrossRef]
28. Boud, D. Sustainable assessment: Rethinking assessment for the learning society. *Stud. Contin. Educ.* **2000**, *22*, 151–167. [CrossRef]
29. Nicol, D.J.; Macfarlane-Dick, D. Formative assessment and self-regulated learning: A model and seven principles of good feedback practice. *Stud. High. Educ.* **2006**, *31*, 199–218. [CrossRef]

30. Boud, D.; Molly, E. Rethinking models of feedback for learning: The challenge of design. *Assess. Eval. High. Educ.* **2013**, *38*, 698–712. [CrossRef]
31. Nicol, D.; Thomson, A.; Breslin, C. Rethinking feedback practices in higher education: A peer review perspective. *Assess. Eval. High. Educ.* **2014**, *39*, 102–122. [CrossRef]
32. Carless, D. *Excellence in University Assessment: Learning from Award-Winning Practice*; Routledge: London, UK, 2015.
33. Ozga, D.; Gutysz-Wojnicka, A.; Lewandowski, B.; Dobrowolska, B. The clinical learning environment, supervision and nurse teacher scale (CLES+T): Psychometric properties measured in the context of postgraduate nursing education. *BMC Nurs.* **2020**, *19*, 61. [CrossRef] [PubMed]
34. Emerson, R.M. Power-dependence relations. *Am. Sociol. Rev.* **1962**, *27*, 31–41. [CrossRef]
35. O'shea, A.; Boaz, A.L.; Chambers, M. A hierarchy of power: The place of patients and public involvement in health care service development. *Med. Sociol.* **2019**, *4*, 38. [CrossRef]

Disclaimer/Publisher's Note: The statements, opinions and data contained in all publications are solely those of the individual author(s) and contributor(s) and not of MDPI and/or the editor(s). MDPI and/or the editor(s) disclaim responsibility for any injury to people or property resulting from any ideas, methods, instructions or products referred to in the content.

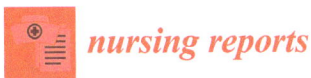

Communication

Positive Aspects and Potential Drawbacks of Implementing Digital Teaching/Learning Scenarios in Health Professions Using Nursing Education as an Example: A Research Report from Germany

Lydia Pfeifer [1,*], Sophia Fries [1], Alexander Stirner [1], Lisa Nagel [1], Christian Cohnen [2], Leona Aschentrup [1,3,4], Marleen Schönbeck [1], Annette Nauerth [1], Patrizia Raschper [1], Tim Herzig [1,3] and Kamil J. Wrona [1,3,*]

[1] Faculty of Health, Hochschule Bielefeld University of Applied Sciences and Arts, 33619 Bielefeld, Germany; lisa.nagel@hsbi.de (L.N.); leona.aschentrup@hsbi.de (L.A.); marleen@schoenbeck.de (M.S.); annette.nauerth@hsbi.de (A.N.); patrizia.raschper@hsbi.de (P.R.); tim_christian.herzig1@hsbi.de (T.H.)

[2] Faculty of Educational Science, Bielefeld University, 33615 Bielefeld, Germany; christian.cohnen@uni-bielefeld.de

[3] Faculty of Engineering and Mathematics, Hochschule Bielefeld University of Applied Sciences and Arts, 33619 Bielefeld, Germany

[4] School of Public Health, Bielefeld University, 33615 Bielefeld, Germany

* Correspondence: lydia.pfeifer@hsbi.de (L.P.); kamil.wrona@hsbi.de (K.J.W.); Tel.: +49-52110670907 (L.P.); +49-52110670087 (K.J.W.)

Abstract: Background: Learning arrangements in health care profession education are increasingly taking place in digital environments. Virtual reality (VR) in nursing education, as a digital element, is the subject of controversial debate. On one hand, it supports the authenticity of case studies by adding realistic perspectives and information. On the other hand, the costs of developing and maintaining software and hardware hinder its long-term implementation. Based in the German context, our aim is to promote the adoption of innovative digital methods in nursing education and to offer invaluable experiences from the field. Methods: In this paper, we describe our findings and insights from two different research projects focused on the incorporation of digital tools, particularly VR, into nursing education. Results: Starting with a brief recapitulation of the projects, we elucidate pedagogical strategies for embedding VR-driven scenarios in nursing education. Based on our experiences during the projects, we identify various positive aspects, such as changing perspective and simulating acute situations. Key findings: Although potential drawbacks remain, we advocate the long-term implementation and specific use of VR at the interface between theory and practice. Nevertheless, it is crucial to establish regular evaluation, observing the value of digitalisation, especially VR, for nursing education.

Keywords: virtual reality; 360-degree video; digital tools; nursing education; VR-driven scenarios; pedagogical strategies; digital methodologies; immersion; collaboration

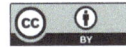

1. Introduction

In addition to a shortage of qualified professionals and regional supply shortfalls, current challenges in healthcare professions also include demographic change, which is accompanied by an increasing proportion of chronically ill people and people in need of nursing care [1]. Digital transformation has the potential to address these challenges [2]. It should enable faster and more comprehensive access to high-quality healthcare, uncomplicated communication between service providers and relief for employees in the health sector through the optimisation of processes, such as simple and secure access to health data or digital support for routine activities. In particular, effective relief for employees contributes to raising the attractiveness of the professional field and might counteract the shortage of qualified staff [3]. The changes brought about by digitalisation in the occupational field also have an impact on professional education in healthcare professions, thus demanding curricular integration combined with the educational objective of competent handling of digital media and technologies by health professionals. Additionally, 19 current developments at universities show that, encouraged by online teaching during the pandemic, face-to-face teaching is increasingly complemented by blended learning formats and the use of digital media and technologies [4]. This changing teaching/learning culture is also prominent in education for health professions. Here, too, the use of digital media is increasing. However, their use often does not follow a systematic structure or evaluated pedagogical (subject-related) didactical concepts (ibid). Although digitalisation is integrated into the curricula of health professions in Germany, there is a lack of understanding of digital competence as cross-cutting competence. Against this backdrop, healthcare professionals struggle to actively shape the potential of digitalisation in their work processes [5,6]. To achieve this, educational staff in schools and companies must also be appropriately qualified [7]. Virtual reality (VR) technology can support the aforementioned competence development in the education of health professionals at various points [8]. Due to their design principles, VR glasses offer the phenomenon of immersion and, depending on the design of the experienced scenario, the experience of presence as well [8]. This can reduce visual and acoustic distractions to allow for focused learning in a safe space. Furthermore, a strong experience of presence can evoke emotions in learners that need to be processed and reflected upon in an evaluation discussion or during debriefing in practice or in class. As a result, VR scenarios offer a complement to traditional learning in all learning venues, including the seminar room, simulation environment and practical field [9,10].

Based on the results and experiences of two research and development projects on the topic of the digitalisation of nursing education, this article examines how different forms of VR can be justified in the context of teaching/learning theory and which challenges and possibilities arise with the use of digital teaching/learning scenarios in health professions, using nursing education as an example. This paper is intended to serve both researchers and educational staff in the health sector in the conception of further digitalisation approaches as well as in the design of digital teaching/learning situations in the education of health professionals.

2. Theoretical Background

This chapter addresses the current state of research on the topic. This includes both theoretical and empirical findings. However, we do not claim to provide a comprehensive review of the literature on the topic. This chapter, therefore, serves as a brief overview and transition towards our findings. In general, working with problem-oriented case studies is recommended for education in all health professions [11]. Case work and case-based learning are associated with strong practice orientation, increased motivation to learn and the development of analytical, problem-solving and reflective skills [12,13]. Digitally supported case work can enable location-independent, self-directed learning in clinical practice and education. This can also promote interprofessional collaboration between medicine and nursing. If cases are embedded in a learning management system (LMS), further case-relevant, interactively prepared information can be made available in addition to video and audio files. The large amount of additional information is accompanied by greater authenticity of the cases [13]. As a result, in addition to a differentiated view of the case, the computer-supported learning environment promotes in particular the adoption of perspectives and linking with theoretical knowledge [13]. At the same time, the learning medium can bring advantages for both teachers and learners. In addition to increased levels of motivation and engagement [14], learning in the virtual world can help facilitate practical exercises by conserving resources (e.g., material consumption) or repeatedly testing situations that would be costly to recreate in the real world. To achieve this, it is important that what is learned in the virtual exercise is transferred to a practical exercise and thus to a real situation. This is supported on one hand by the realistic interaction with the learning material in VR [15] and on the other hand by the associated addressing of several sensory channels during learning [16]. Additionally, VR can be linked to simulation-based learning, which is often associated with the learning environment skills lab, which is recommended in healthcare profession education and specifically in nursing education [17]. In addition to case-based learning, one aim of simulation-based learning, among others, is the transfer from theoretical knowledge to practical skill during nursing education. VR is often portrayed as an alternative means of simulation which enables more flexibility for the learning process [18].

Against this background, learning arrangements in virtual learning environments are increasingly finding their way into medical, nursing and therapeutic education (or health professions), but at the same time, their development and dissemination is only just beginning [7]. Estimates of the degree of future establishment in nursing education range from short-term hype to a fundamental transformation of nursing education [19,20]. According to the current literature, the following benefits are attributed to the use of VR technology in nursing education [21–26]:

- Realistic discussions of rare or dangerous nursing situations;
- Safe training in a virtual learning environment;
- Authentic learning experience with reduced pressure to act;
- Immediate feedback on actions in virtual reality;
- Resource-saving practice with action sequences;
- Learning that is independent of time and place;
- Personalised learning;
- Increased motivation and enjoyment;
- Improved integration of theory and practice;
- The ability to plan the learning experience;
- An improved ability to analyse the learning experience.

Despite these advantages, the nursing and media didactic as well as the learning theory underpinning of the use of VR technology are regarded as controversial [7]. The costs associated with the use of VR technology for the development, acquisition and maintenance of hardware and software, as well as the "not inconsiderable psychophysiological requirements" [23] for learning in virtual learning environments, mean that VR technology currently leads a "shadowy existence" [27]. Additionally, VR is negatively associated with technical problems, cumbersome interfaces and entertainment-driven development [23,27].

In order to minimise the aforementioned costs and development efforts, and to enable educators to create content, an alternative technique can be used instead of the usual creation of digital objects or characters based on geometric modelling: 360° video technology [28]. Such videos are recorded with a 360° camera. These cameras continuously record their entire environment and allow users to view the recording while actively changing their perspective. If several such recordings are available, they can be enriched with interaction icons and linked to a 360° VR scenario. This allows users to interact with people or objects in the scenario and actively change the scenario. It should be noted that here, the range of action is limited. There is no free movement in virtual space, and the options for interaction are more limited than in reality [7]. However, transfer from theory to practice is not yet supported in connection with other learning formats, such as simulation-based learning in the skills lab, for example. This is crucial as the transfer of the VR simulation to reality is of great importance for learning success [13].

3. Materials and Methods

Based on the guiding principle that learning with media cannot be ascribed an added value per se compared to conventional learning arrangements but that the media unfold their potential in a coherent didactical design [29], it is important to identify the educational purpose that is being pursued with the use of VR technology. Such an educational purpose may be to promote self-directed and/or cooperative learning, as well as social exchange, or the temporal and spatial flexibility of learning and thus the consideration of heterogeneous learning prerequisites through the use of the digital medium [29,30]. Against this background, the projects "Digital and Virtually Supported Casework in the Health Professions" (DiViFaG) and "Virtual Reality-based Digital Reusable Learning Objects in Nursing Education" (ViRDiPA) tested didactical designs that combine established teaching/learning arrangements with the possibilities of digital and virtual elements.

3.1. DiViFaG

The DiViFaG project, funded by the German Federal Ministry of Education and Research (BMBF) in the funding line "Digital Higher Education" (01/2020-12/2022), is an interdisciplinary joint project under the consortium leadership of the Bielefeld University of Applied Sciences and Arts (HSBI) with the participation of the Emden/Leer University of Applied Sciences, Osnabrück University of Applied Sciences and Bielefeld University with its Educational Science and Medicine faculties. The aim of the DiViFaG project is to develop and implement a didactical concept for university education for health professions that combines problem-oriented case studies [31] with innovative human–technology interactions, including virtual reality [32]. For this purpose, the originally text-based case work was enriched with the concepts of cognitive apprenticeship [33] and the learning of social–communicative action competences [32,34].

The project developed, tested and evaluated in total ten case-based, digitally supported teaching/learning scenarios for university education for health professions, in particular medicine and nursing. The case scenarios focus on different practical, communicative and interactive skills. Thus, they strongly address the interface between theoretical learning and practical skills. The digital teaching/learning scenarios were developed as a blended learning concept in which both digital and established teaching/learning methods were linked in classroom and online phases [35]. Due to its immersive character, VR technology was conceptually implemented between the cognitive acquisition of the action steps and the first practical exercise in the skills lab during the presence phase. Through the realistic representation of the action situation (Figure 1), the use of VR has a preparatory effect on learning in the skills lab. The combination of didactical approaches and concepts with digital media and simulative teaching/learning environments facilitates the comprehensive development of students' competences [32]. All teaching/learning scenarios, including the VR tasks, were evaluated using qualitative and quantitative methods. Approximately 170 students participated in the implementation: 86 of them completed the quantitative online questionnaire, and 31 students participated in qualitative group interviews.

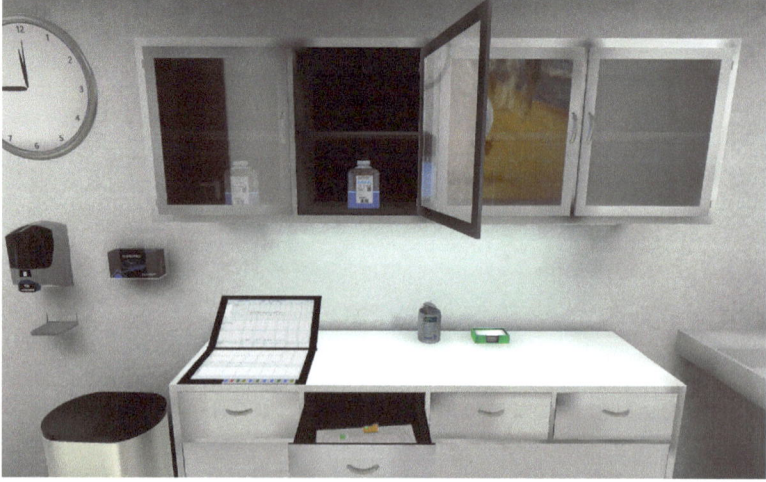

Figure 1. Fully animated ward room from a first-person perspective (DiViFaG).

3.2. ViRDiPA

Within the framework of the research project ViRDiPA, which was also funded by the BMBF, the University of Bielefeld, the University of Applied Sciences Emden/Leer and an organization with a focus on digital teaching and learning participated in the project period (March 2020–August 2023) under the consortium leadership of the Bielefeld University of Applied Sciences and Arts. An interdisciplinary consortium consisting of actors from nursing didactics, media pedagogy and computer science connected, for the first time, the learning task framework, a proven pedagogical approach in nursing [36], with VR scenarios. Previously analogue learning tasks were digitally prepared and enriched with various media such as images, audio files, videos and tasks. The resulting novel didactical tools enable deep learning by integrating multimodal elements and, in particular, VR applications to promote engagement with the content, thus increasing vividness, situatedness and application orientation. The use of problem-oriented methods such as concrete case studies promotes the cognitive and emotional activation of the learner. In addition, the digital provision of digitally supported learning tasks allows for a flexible organisation of learning in terms of time, space and social interaction. For example, teaching/learning content can be viewed and worked on at home or in the practice facility. In addition, it is possible to work at one's own pace, which allows for the different needs of learning groups [29].

In order to integrate VR technology into education, a training concept was developed, tested and evaluated in order to promote the media-pedagogical competence of educational staff in schools and workplaces with regard to teaching and learning in an immersive learning environment. This educational course enhanced the media and technology skills of 14 teachers and practical instructors. Simultaneously, the participant's existing subject and nursing pedagogical expertise was combined. In order to transfer learning outcomes (what has been learnt) into everyday working life, the educators developed digitally supported learning tasks with 360° VR scenarios. This particular type of VR scenario is particularly suitable for development by educational staff themselves as no specific programming skills are required. Instead, the authors use the paneoVR authoring kit developed in the project to link 360° videos and enrich them with interaction symbols. See Figure 2 for an example of a 360° VR scenario. The learning tasks and 360° VR scenarios developed in the project were piloted with 114 student nurses. The trials were accompanied by a quantitative and qualitative evaluation, the results of which have been submitted for publication [10]. The development of digitally supported learning tasks with VR scenarios was based on the expectation that they would be highly reusable so that they could be used beyond the context of the project in the cooperating institutions and also be made available to the general public as an open educational resource. Against the background of both projects presented, the didactical designs developed and tested are presented below and analysed with regard to their positive aspects and thus possibilities.

Both projects developed, implemented and evaluated different kinds of VR scenarios and their use in blended learning scenarios in context of linking theory with practice. Both projects published the scenarios and their data as open access material. In addition, the responsible researchers generated various forms of experiences and insights which are delineated in the following chapters. As an example of the use of our VR scenarios in nursing education, specifically in both research projects, a learning unit on dehydration is briefly summarized here. After familiarising themselves with the basics of the subject, learners are presented with a case study relating to dehydration. The learners then reflect on their previous experience of the topic and discuss the options for action in the event of dehydration. As one possible course of action, they practise preparing an infusion in the VR scenario. Then, using a simulated patient, they practise formulating nursing diagnoses, plans and goals. This example shows that VR can only be one building block in a complex learning unit.

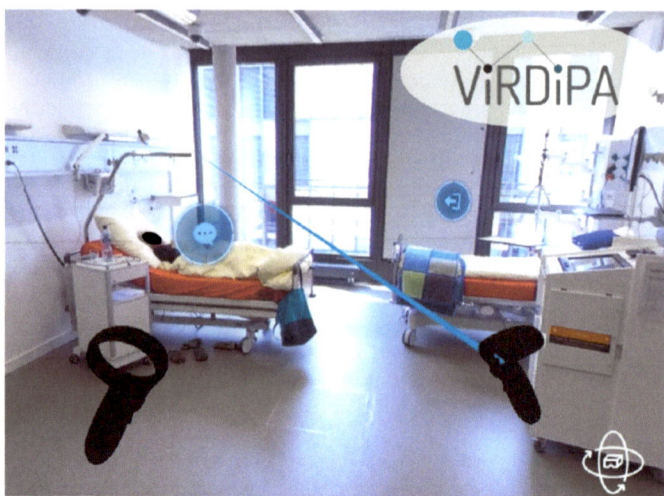

Figure 2. Perceived environment from a first-person perspective with interaction elements (ViRDiPA).

4. Results: Description of the Major Positive Aspects of Using VR for Education

VR currently presents a special form of learning and teaching. Learning takes place through interaction in recorded nursing situations and creates a feeling of immersion in the care situation. A learning unit in virtual space, therefore, has many potential qualities that can be used in the context of nursing education and can prepare an individual for nursing practice. In both projects, the VR scenarios were treated as additional components to the usual tools in the teaching and learning process. VR was most often used between theoretical and practical learning processes in both methods (case-based scenarios and learning tasks). In general, the students first acquired the theoretical content and discussed possible courses of action in relation to the case example. They then trained the actions in VR in different ways (360° or fully immersive). After that, it was very important to enhance the VR training by practising the actions with a simulated patient in the skills lab or in professional practice. In the following subsections, positive aspects and therefore possibilities are identified as the two projects, ViRDiPA and DiViFaG, are presented. A detailed and broad presentation of the collected data can be found, e.g., in Strecker et al. [37].

4.1. Increasing Immersion

VR simulations with a high degree of immersion enable the experience of so-called presence in VR, i.e., the subjective feeling of actually being in the virtual space [8]. Thus, experiencing situations from the perspectives of other actors can feel very real and evoke emotions that are also evoked when actually experiencing the real situation. Thus, by appropriately supplementing subject–didactical methods with animated and 360° VR scenarios, the possibilities for teaching, activating and supporting learners are expanded. According to [29], learning takes place in a situational context, meaning it is linked to social situations. Hence, knowledge acquired in the theoretical setting of an educational institution cannot always be ideally applied in practical situations [29]. However, immersive learning scenarios allow for the provision of targeted learning opportunities in a simulated practice environment in different locations. In addition, immersive scenarios have a high degree of impact due to the potentialities of visual illustration. Constant interaction with the learning content, subjects such as avatars and filmed people and contexts enhance the immersive experience. Application relevance is immediately apparent in immersive learning environments as practice can be carried out in a simulated practical situation. Case descriptions can also help familiarise oneself with patients in advance. To illustrate this, an example of a 360° VR scenario is given below.

In the VR scenario "I didn't know what to do", Mrs. Müller's patient file can be viewed at the nurses' station. After a little while, Mrs. Müller calls for assistance using the bell system. Upon entering the room, the learner finds Mrs. Müller lying on the floor in front of the bed, moaning and calling for help to get up so she can go to the toilet. The learner now has to decide whether to accompany Mrs. Müller to the toilet or to ask a colleague for help. They are faced with an unexpected situation that requires careful consideration and quick decision making. The confrontation with a helpless person lying on the floor causes consternation, shame and the impulse to help immediately in many learners, but due to the design principles in this scenario, one's own inability to act in a challenging situation must be endured. The experiences in the 360° VR scenario are prepared and followed up with by reflection questions and discussions within the framework of a learning task. In addition to the VR scenario, the skills lab can be used to practise appropriate actions to take after a fall. For example, an assessment for fractures and serious internal injuries and a transfer from the floor back to the bed can be practised. The vivid and application-oriented representation of learning content makes complex or abstract topics accessible to learners. Direct experience and self-direction contribute to the communication of learning content [38,39]. On one hand, there is a "spatialisation" in which learners have the impression of being in a virtual world. On the other hand, haptic and auditive sensory perceptions are addressed in addition to the visual channels [39]. Learning environments designed according to these principles are actively explored in a self-directed manner whereby new ways of imparting knowledge are created through interaction [40].

4.2. Extending Professional Nursing Action through a Change of Perspective

Changing perspectives with other people can be ideally implemented in a 360° VR scenario. A scene can be filmed from the perspective of a fictional person wherein the 360° camera acts as a placeholder for that person. Later, the person's own perspective can be captured in a 360° VR scenario. This change of perspective, combined with a high degree of immersion, allows important nursing components such as empathy to be trained in interpersonal scenarios. Empathy is an important component of effective communication in the nursing profession and the basis for high-quality, person-centred nursing care. Empathic nursing care has a positive impact not only on the health outcomes of the person being cared for but also on the professional satisfaction of the nurse. One way to promote empathy in learners can be through simulations in which learners take on the role of the person being cared for [41]. Furthermore, changing perspective is not only possible in terms of the client or their relatives but also in terms other professions and actors in the healthcare system. In a multi-player scenario, location-independent collaborative learning is possible in the didactical context of roleplay. For example, an interprofessional ward round or case discussion can be implemented, or interprofessional topics (e.g., hygiene in care) can be integrated into teaching. Communication between learners works directly through the hardware's voice input and output and can be implemented without additional equipment. The degree of learner self-direction is variable through external teacher intervention or teacher participation in the role play (e.g., as a patient). The high degree of immersion in VR makes both the immersion in the new role and the experience of the situation seem more present and real [37]. On one hand, interprofessionality is a frequently requested building block in the care context to reduce current problems and the duplication of structures; on the other hand, the implementation and permanent integration of interprofessional cooperation in the care context prove to be difficult and challenging. By renewing communication skills and developing interprofessional competences through VR, a further contribution to professional nursing care is made.

4.3. Intra- and Interprofessional Collaboration in VR Scenarios

In addition to the initiation of interprofessional competences by adopting the perspectives of other professions in the simulation, collaborative working and learning is possible in VR. Joint learning can initiate shared awareness, mutual trust and respect between health professions and counteract ignorance, prejudice and rivalry [42]. Consequently, interprofessional collaboration and communication, as demanded by experts, is already integrated into education continuously and in addition to existing learning content [43,44]. Interprofessional learning is a prerequisite for later interprofessional work [45]. The central intention of interprofessional learning is to develop the competences required for interprofessional action as part of professional socialisation during education [46]. Interprofessional learning is not about blurring the boundaries between individual professions but rather about working through a common problem by sharing expectations, experiences and perspectives from different roles as part of a collaborative and interactive process [42]. Using roleplay, a treatment plan was developed collaboratively, creating a shared understanding of treatment approaches and perspectives on the same health problem. In principle, collaborative learning in VR can also take place in an intraprofessional context, depending on the objectives of the teaching/learning situation. Here, the focus can be on social–communicative and teamwork skills.

4.4. Preparation for Acute Situations

According to Kirkevold (2002) [47], acute situations are characterised by the fact that they occur suddenly, that the situation can take a dramatic course and that quick and correct action is necessary to prevent damage to people's health. This involves a rapid and appropriate assessment of the situation and a quick decision regarding the immediate action to be taken. In addition, the professional nurse's own composure and ability to act should be maintained. In addition to working calmly and safely, professional nurses also need to be able to offer their clients an interpretation of their condition and explain interventions and measures [47].

VR scenarios are ideally suited for experiencing acute situations due to several favourable characteristics of the medium. Acute situations are usually difficult to practise in clinical settings because they occur unexpectedly. In a VR scenario, however, all learners can be exposed to a specific simulated acute situation at the push of a button. Experiencing an acute situation in a VR scenario provides a simulated first confrontation with the situation and can allow feelings and emotions to be brought forward into the action-relieved framework of the VR experience. Time for briefing and debriefing can be planned in advance. Although the acute situation is only simulated, VR goggles provide a strong immersion experience [8] so that the learner's focus is entirely on the simulated acute situation and stimuli from the environment are largely blocked out. Three-hundred-sixty-degree VR scenarios achieve the immersion effect through a filmed environment, while animated VR scenarios use a computer-generated environment. This results in different options for visualisation and interaction. For example, the facial expressions and gestures of filmed persons in 360° VR scenarios can be intuitively recognised, which increases the feeling of authenticity of the situation and thus the affective involvement [10]. With computer-generated avatars, facial expressions and gestures cannot be displayed in the same differentiated way. Animated VR scenarios create additional scope for action or interaction and thus allow necessary steps to be practised in emergency situations in the VR environment.

4.5. Observation and Action without Decision-Making Pressure

In VR scenarios, scenes of professional nursing practice can be observed without the pressure of time and action. Due to the realistic depiction of the filmed environment, 360° VR scenarios are ideal for learning by observing. Three-hundred-sixty-degree video recordings can be filmed in an individual practice setting for the familiarisation or recognition of spatial and organisational circumstances. This can increase identification with the content being viewed. Unlike watching videos on a screen, viewing a 360° VR scenario through VR goggles fully immerses the learner in the scenario. The visual and acoustic barrier to the real environment helps avoid distractions. High levels of immersion can be achieved. In the action-free VR environment, the focus can be on observation without the pressure of time and action. Original observation tasks, such as observing an epileptic seizure, are suitable for this, as is the observation of nursing situations, e.g., to reflect the communication of nursing staff. Methodologically, observation-oriented VR scenarios can be prepared for comparison. In this way, learners can watch several similar versions of a scene one after the other and compare them. This also provides the opportunity to observe processes in acute situations (e.g., with experienced nursing staff) without any pressure to act. Animated VR scenarios, on the other hand, are suitable for the repeated practice of concrete, predefined procedures. While in the skills lab, a high level of material consumption is necessary for repetitive exercises, e.g., the preparation of an infusion, learning these action steps in VR has only a low level of resource consumption and is also independent of time and space.

A particular pressure situation arises with action sequences that must be recalled in acute situations. Therefore, for nursing students, this is particularly useful in direct connection with the acquisition of psychomotor skills in the skills lab [40]. With the help of VR scenarios, not only can action situations be practised without time pressure but the learners' fear of contact can also be reduced through first practical tasks. In the interest of theory–practice transfer, learners are thus prepared for various placements in the healthcare context or are introduced to new areas of application. Typical sounds and minor procedures can be experienced or tried out. Basic nursing measures can be observed, and decisions can be made about the process.

5. Discussion: A Critical Reflection on the Use of Digital VR Learning Scenarios in Nursing Education

This section reflects the critical aspects of using VR learning scenarios in nursing education based on the results above by exploring the resource requirements for developing and implementing VR learning scenarios, including costs, hardware and software needs. This document emphasizes the future relevance and reusability of VR scenarios as digital reusable learning objects (DRLOs), accessible as open educational resources (OERs). This section also touches on the challenges of using VR, such as a high initial investment, data protection and the need for continuous updates and adaptations. The suitability of 360° VR scenarios for achieving cognitive and affective learning outcomes is highlighted. In addition, limitations for psychomotor learning are noted. Moreover, the potential for cognitive overload when using VR technology in education is discussed, suggesting the need for structured preparation and follow-up processes.

5.1. Resource Requirements for Development, Implementation and Application

In addition to the description of positive aspects of using VR learning scenarios, they must also be critically reflected upon. Regarding the planning and development effort, as well as costs for the procurement of hardware and software, important design principles should be observed when developing a VR scenario. Monetary and personnel costs are considered to be in a reasonable proportion if "future relevance" and "exemplarity" are the guiding didactical design principles in the development of VR scenarios. This means that VR scenarios are developed to address topics which will likely be relevant in the coming years. In addition, the VR scenarios should be suitable for delivering basic learning content in nursing education so that they can be used in different contexts with regard to educational level and teaching topic. Designing such elaborate learning objects should also follow the aim of a "high degree of reusability" [48]. The construction of such reusable digital learning modules with VR technology was the central aim of the projects described here. The VR scenarios developed in the projects were designed as digital reusable learning objects (DRLOs) so that they should be reusable across institutions. They are published as open educational resources (OERs) in an openly accessible form and can thus be used by educational staff at other institutions [7].

As a special form of VR technology, 360° VR scenarios can be produced with less time and money. Even inexperienced teachers can develop these scenarios on their own after a training period, which reduces the resource burden of development. However, when an educational institution decides to use VR technology, the initial investment is high because of the hardware and software that need to be purchased. During the acquisition process, the existing Internet infrastructure must be assessed. A stable and powerful Internet connection is an important prerequisite for the use of VR technology. In addition, especially when learning with VR in health professions, strict data protection regulations must be observed by health institutions when using their internet Infrastructure. Last but not least, the use of VR requires a high level of individual support.

When using VR technology for educational purposes, it is important to remember that it is an innovative technology that is subject to rapid change. Updates from the manufacturers the head-mounted displays require the adaptation of self-developed applications or scenarios to new circumstances. Teaching/learning materials that have already been developed may also lose their relevance and thus their usability.

5.2. Three-Hundred-Sixty-Degree VR Scenarios Are Not Suitable for Psychomotor Learning Outcomes

It should be emphasised that 360° VR scenarios can primarily be used to target affective and cognitive learning outcomes. By appealing to the visual and auditory senses, it is possible to evoke emotions which then can be reflected upon during briefing and debriefing. In this way, values and attitudes can be brought to mind and, if the individual so wishes, changed. Cognitive learning outcomes can also justify the use of 360° VR scenarios. For example, knowledge of action sequences or understanding of contexts can be communicated. The key is to combine this with a suitable subject–didactical method that is also geared towards achieving the relevant learning outcomes and allows for comprehensive briefing and debriefing. Due to design principles, a 360° VR scenario can only be viewed from one point of view. There is no freedom of movement in space. Interaction is also limited to the activation of specific interaction icons. Therefore, no motor sequences can be practised. 360° VR scenarios are therefore not suitable for achieving psychomotor learning outcomes. However, it has been shown that the design principles of 360° VR scenarios offer promising possibilities for achieving affective and cognitive learning objectives. Other forms of VR, such as fully immersive scenarios, can be used for psychomotor learning outcomes. It is necessary to include direct perceptible feedback in the VR, e.g., motion tracking, to improve the outcomes of the students.

5.3. Cognitive Overload

Students and teachers perceive VR technology as innovative and associate it with entertainment media. This contributes to a high level of attention and motivation when learning with VR. However, enthusiasm for the technology can distract from the subject matter, especially if there is no previous experience with VR technology. Only after a few VR learning sessions and the onset of a habituation effect is it possible to concentrate fully on the learning object. The coordination of the elements used for the scenario is also important. However, a mismatch between the learning and gaming elements is referred to as chocolate-covered broccoli [49].

Although the advantages of VR technology should be used specifically for nursing education, and the attractiveness of VR technology can certainly be used for motivation, it is only by embedding it in subject–didactically designed situations that it is possible to map the nursing process.

In addition, the VR experience should be accompanied by structured, guided preparation and follow-up processes which should also be reflected in the didactically chosen method, such as working with learning tasks. Furthermore, a frustration effect or a certain negative attitude can quickly arise if flawlessness and intuitiveness are not guaranteed. As a result, VR will not promote the desired learning outcomes.

6. Conclusions

The didactical use of virtual reality is particularly suitable at the interface between theory and practice. Due to the high degree of immersion, the situation experienced by the learner is close to reality and serves as good preparation for clinical periods in the course of professional education. However, such an application is also conceivable in the context of further education since new fields of action are usually opened up by students in further education. Our report highlights the importance of balancing the innovative potential of VR in nursing education, with its positive aspects and potential drawbacks as listed below (Table 1).

Table 1. Overview of the positive aspects and potential drawbacks of using VR-based scenarios in nursing education.

Positive Aspects	Potential Drawbacks
Resource Efficiency: Less resource-intensive 360° VR scenarios can be developed even by inexperienced teachers. Reusability and Accessibility: VR scenarios are designed as digital reusable learning objects (DRLOs) available as open educational resources (OERs) for widespread use. Educational Impact: Suitable for cognitive and affective learning, VR can enhance knowledge and understanding, evoke emotions and influence attitudes and values.	High Initial Investment: Significant upfront costs for hardware and software. Infrastructure Needs: Requires a stable and powerful internet connection, and compliance with strict data protection regulations. Rapid Technological Changes: Frequent updates and adaptations are necessary due to the evolving nature of VR technology. Limited Psychomotor Learning: 360° VR scenarios are not suitable for psychomotor learning outcomes due to limited interaction and movement capabilities.

In both projects, the embedding of VR in simulation-based procedures (skills lab) and/or action-oriented teaching procedures (learning tasks and case work) has proved successful. Nevertheless, it is of fundamental importance that the use of VR in the teaching/learning context is accompanied and justified by didactic methods. VR should basically be seen as a digital medium and therefore has an impact on the outcomes, content and methods of a teaching/learning situation. These interdependencies need to be analysed and taken into account. Due to the novelty of VR, a long-term and continuous embedding of this medium in terms of curriculum design seems to be sensible, as it has been shown that learners get used to the degree of immersion and thus the intended learning successes only occur after repeated use. Therefore, it is vital to use VR as well as other digital tools beyond themes and contents of various learning processes to minimize the barriers of VR. In addition, the initiation of digital literacy should be considered, and systematically prepared teachers should be responsible for this. The challenges for appropriate didactics in higher education lie, among other factors, in making digitality the subject of learning processes in studies and education and, in addition, in using digital media—as described here using the example of VR—to design learning situations. It is recognised that digital media serve to support learning and that the actual learning topics will continue to be at the forefront of educational processes. Nonetheless, VR has to be adapted to the intended learning outcomes, the didactical methods, themes and topics as well as the group of learners to integrate it successfully into the curriculum of nursing education. It is crucial to enhance the understanding of digital competence as cross-cutting competence among educational staff and health professionals.

As already stated at the beginning, the current challenges in the health sector, such as a shortage of skilled workers, regional supply bottlenecks and demographic change, underline the urgency for change and adaptation in the health professions. Digitalisation, especially in the context of nursing education, can be perceived as a promising tool for meeting these challenges. As described, the introduction of VR in nursing education offers an innovative learning tool. However, the following points need to be considered for its successful integration.

There should be greater curricular integration of digitalisation and digital literacy into the education of health professionals. This should go beyond the mere use of digital media, and digital competence should be seen as cross-cutting competence.

Regular evaluation and feedback loops should be established to ensure the effectiveness and added value of digitalisation and the use of VR in education.

To optimise the use of VR and other digital teaching/learning scenarios, universities and other educational institutions should work closely with research institutions.

In the long term, the findings obtained from these projects should be transferred to and implemented in professional practice with a particular focus on the stated positive aspects, as well as potential drawbacks, followed by a scientific evaluation. Altogether, digitalisation and the use of VR in nursing education offer significant opportunities to improve education and address current challenges in the health sector. It is crucial to take advantage of these opportunities and to continuously evaluate and optimise the process.

Author Contributions: L.P., S.F., A.S., L.N. and C.C. drafted the manuscript; K.J.W., T.H., L.A. and M.S. contributed to the drafting process; A.N. and P.R. were in charge of the research project; T.H. and K.J.W. supervised the project's publication as senior authors. All authors discussed and revised the manuscript critically for important intellectual content and approved the final version. All authors have read and agreed to the published version of the manuscript.

Funding: This publication is funded by the German Federal Ministry of Education and Research (BMBF). The sole responsibility for the content of this publication lies with the authors.

Institutional Review Board Statement: The Ethics Committee of Bielefeld University reviewed both research projects in accordance with the ethical guidelines of the German Psychological Society and the Professional Association of German Psychologists and found them to be ethically unobjectionable. The application for ViRDiPA was filed under the number EUB 2020-050. The application for DiViFaG was filed under the number EUB 2021-170.

Informed Consent Statement: Not applicable.

Data Availability Statement: Research data is not yet publically available.

Public Involvement Statement: The public was involved in the study solely for testing the virtual scenarios. No research was conducted on humans.

Guidelines and Standards Statement: Not applicable.

Conflicts of Interest: The authors declare no conflict of interest.

References

1. Weyland, U.; Reiber, K. Entwicklungen und Perspektiven in den Gesundheitsberufen—Aktuelle Handlungs- und Forschungsfelder. 2017 by Bundesinstitut für Berufsbildung, Bonn. Available online: https://www.bibb.de/dienst/publikationen/en/download/8474 (accessed on 21 August 2023).
2. Fischer, U.H.P.; Müller, M.; Neumüller, M. Digitalisierung in der Pflegebranche fördern. *Pflegezeitschrift* **2021**, *74*, 57–61. [CrossRef]
3. Boll-Westermann, S.; Hein, A.; Heuten, W.; Krahn, T. Pflege 2050—Wie die technologische Zukunft der Pflege aussehen könnte. In *Pflege und Digitale Technik*; Zentrum für Qualität in der Pflege (ZQP): Berlin, Germany, 2021; pp. 10–15.
4. Darmann-Finck, I.; Wolf, K.D.; Schepers, C.; Küster, J. Digital unterstütztes Lernen in der Pflegeausbildung. MedienPädagogik: Zeitschrift für Theorie und Praxis der Medienbildung. *Jahrb. Medien.* **2016**, *16*, 317–345. [CrossRef]
5. Walkenhorst, U.; Herzig, T. Relevanz der Medienkompetenz in der Lehrer*innenbildung für die Digitalisierung in den Humandienstleistungsberufen. In *Care Work 4.0. Digitalisierung in Personenbezogenen Dienstleistungsberufen*; Friese, M., Ed.; wbv: Bielefeld, Germany, 2021; pp. 32–44.
6. Mohr, J.; Riedlinger, I.; Reiber, K. Die Bedeutung der Digitalisierung in der Neuausrichtung der pflegerischen Ausbildung—Herausforderungen für die berufliche Pflege im Kontext der Fachkräftesicherung. In *Jahrbuch der Berufs- und Wirtschaftspädagogischen Forschung*; Wittmann, E., Frommberger, D., Weyland, U., Eds.; Verlag Barbara Budrich: Leverkusen, Germany, 2020.
7. Bartolles, M.; Kamin, A.M.; Meyer, L.; Pfeiffer, T. VR-basierte Digital Reusable Learning Objects. *Medien. Z. Theor. Prax. Medien.* **2022**, *47*, 138–156. [CrossRef]
8. Dörner, R.; Broll, W.; Grimm, P.; Jung, B. *Virtual und Augmented Reality (VR/AR)*; Springer: Berlin/Heidelberg, Germany, 2019.
9. Freina, L.; Ott, M. A Literature Review on Immersive Virtual Reality in Education: State of the Art and Perspectives. In Proceedings of the International Scientific Conference eLearning and Software for Education (eLSE), Bucharest, Romania, 23–24 April 2015. [CrossRef]

10. Pfeifer, L.; Fries, S.; Freese, C.; Nauerth, A.; Raschper, P. Virtual Reality didaktisch fundiert in der Pflegeausbildung einsetzen—Erfahrungen aus dem Projekt ViRDiPA. In *Berufsbildung im Zeichen von Fachkräftesicherung und Versorgungsqualität*; Reiber, K., Evans, M., Mohr, J., Eds.; Wbv Reihe Berufsbildung, Arbeit und Innovation; wbv: Bielefeld, Germany, 2023.
11. Frenk, J.; Chen, L.; Bhutta, Z.A.; Cohen, J.; Crisp, N.; Evans, T.; Fineberg, H.; Garcia, P.; Ke, Y.; Kelley, P.; et al. Health professionals for a new century: Transforming education to strengthen health systems in an interdependent world. *Lancet* 2010, 376, 1923–1958. [CrossRef] [PubMed]
12. Bergjan, M. Mediengestütztes, Problemorientiertes Lernen in der Ausbildung von Pflegeberufen. Entwicklung und Lernforschung zum Blended Learning. Ph.D. Thesis, Universität Osnabrück, Osnabrück, Germany, 2007.
13. Olleck, R. *Mediengestützte Fallarbeit in Computerunterstützten Lernumgebungen: Technische Anforderungen und Funktionalitäten für Einzelarbeit, Gruppenarbeit und Blended Learning-Szenarien, Mediengestützte Fallarbeit. Konzepte, Erfahrungen und Befunde zur Kompetenzentwicklung von Erwachsenenbildnern*; Schrader, J., Hohmann, R., Hartz, S., Eds.; EB Buch; W. Bertelsmann Verlag: Bielefeld, Germany, 2010; Volume 31, pp. 191–209.
14. Concannon, B.J.; Esmail, S.; Roberts, M.R. Head-Mounted Display Virtual Reality in Post-secondary Education and Skill Training. *Front. Educ.* 2019, 4, 80. [CrossRef]
15. Lindwedel-Reime, U.; Plotzky, C.; Scheurer, A.; Kunze, C.; König, P. *SituCare—Situative Unterstützung und Krisenintervention in der Pflege: Abschlussbericht zum Verbundvorhaben*; Hochschule Furtwangen: Furtwangen, Germany, 2019. [CrossRef]
16. Schwan, S.; Buder, J. Virtuelle Realität und E-Learning. 2006. Available online: https://www.e-teaching.org/materialien/literatur/schwan-buder-2005 (accessed on 23th March 2023).
17. Waxmann, K.T. The development of evidence-based clinical simulation scenarios: Guidelines for nurse educators. *J. Nurs. Educ.* 2010, 49, 29–35. [CrossRef] [PubMed]
18. Plotzky, C.; Lindwedel, U.; Sorber, M.; Loessl, B.; König, P.; Kunze, C.; Kugler, C.; Meng, M. Virtual reality simulations in nurse education: A systematic mapping review. *Nurse Educ. Today* 2021, 101, 104868. [CrossRef] [PubMed]
19. Schlegel, C.; Weber, U. Lernen mit Virtual Reality: Ein Hype in der Pflegeausbildung. *Pädagogik Gesundheitsberufe* 2019, 3, 182–186.
20. Pottle, J. Virtual reality and the transformation of medical education. *Future Healthc. J.* 2019, 6, 181–185. [CrossRef] [PubMed]
21. Bartolles, M.; Kamin, A.-M. Virtual Reality basierte Digital Reusable Learning Objects in der Pflegeausbildung—Rahmenbedingungen, Anforderungen und Bedarfe aus medienpädagogischer Perspektive. In *Innovative Lehr-/Lernszenarien in den Pflege- und Gesundheitsberufen*; Working Paper-Reihe der Projekte DiViFaG und ViRDiPA 1; Universität Bielefeld: Bielefeld, Germany, 2021. [CrossRef]
22. Kavanagh, S.; Luxton-Reilly, A.; Wuensche, B.; Plimmer, B. A systematic review of Virtual Reality in Education. *Themes Sci. Technol. Educ.* 2017, 10, 85–119.
23. Dyrna, J.; Liebscher, M.; Fischer, H.; Brade, M. Implementierung von VR-basierten Lernumgebungen. Theoretischer Bezugsrahmen und praktische Anwendung. In *Seamless Learning. Lebenslanges, Durchgängiges Lernen Ermöglichen*; Müller Werder, C., Erlemann, J., Eds.; Waxmann Verlag GmbH: Münster, Germany, 2020; pp. 59–68.
24. Hebbel-Seeger, A.; Kopischke, A.; Riehm, P.; Baranovskaa, M. LectureCast als 360°-Video. Welchen Einfluss haben Immersion und Präsenzerleben auf die Lernleistung? In *Teilhabe in der Digitalen Bildungswelt*; Hafer, J., Mauch, M., Schumann, M., Eds.; Waxmann: Münster, Germany; New York, NY, USA, 2019; pp. 110–127.
25. Wu, S.-H.; Huang, C.-C.; Huang, S.-S.; Yang, Y.-Y.; Liu, C.-W.; Shulruf, B.; Chen, C.-H. Effect of virtual reality training to decreases rates of needle stick/sharp injuries in new-coming medical and nursing interns in Taiwan. *J. Educ. Eval. Health Prof.* 2020, 17, 1149154. [CrossRef] [PubMed]
26. Foronda, C.L.; Fernandez-Burgos, M.; Nadeau, C.; Kelley, C.N.; Henry, M.N. Virtual Simulation in Nursing Education: A Systematic Review Spanning 1996 to 2018. *Simul. Healthc. J. Soc. Simul. Healthc.* 2020, 15, 46–54. [CrossRef] [PubMed]
27. Hellriegel, J.; Čubela, D. Das Potenzial von Virtual Reality für den schulischen Unterricht Eine konstruktivistische Sicht. *Medien. Z. Theor. Prax. Medien.* 2018, 58–80. [CrossRef]
28. Eiris, R.; Gheisari, M.; Esmaeili, B. PARS: Using Augmented 360-Degree Panoramas of Reality for Construction Safety Training. *Int. J. Environ. Res. Public Health* 2018, 15, 2452. [CrossRef] [PubMed]
29. Kerres, M. *Mediendidaktik*; De Gruyter: Berlin, Germany, 2018. [CrossRef]
30. Bundesministerium für Gesundheit, Digitalisierungsstrategie. 2022. Available online: https://www.bundesgesundheitsministerium.de/themen/digitalisierung/digitalisierungsstrategie.html (accessed on 15 March 2023).
31. Kaiser, F.-J. *Die Fallstudie. Theorie und Praxis der Fallstudiendidaktik, Forschen und Lernen*; Klinkhardt: Bad Heilbrunn, Germany, 1983; Volume 6.
32. Freese, C.; Nagel, L.; Makowsky, K.; Nauerth, A. *Digitale und Virtuell Unterstützte Fallarbeit in den Gesundheitsberufen—Digitale Fallarbeit in der Hochschulischen Pflegebildung*; Universität Bielefeld: Bielefeld, Germany, 2023. [CrossRef]
33. Collins, A.; Brown, J.S.; Newman, S.E. Cognitive Apprenticeship: Teaching the Crafts of Reading, Writing, and Mathematics. In *Knowing, Learning, and Instruction. Essays in Honor of Robert Glaser*; Resnick, L.B., Ed.; Lawrence Erlbaum Associates: Hillsdale, MI, USA, 1989.
34. Euler, D. Manche lernen es aber warum? Lerntheoretische Fundierung zur Entwicklung von sozial-kommunikativen Handlungskompetenzen. *Z. Berufs Wirtsch.* 2001, 97, 346–374.
35. Erpenbeck, J.; Sauter, S.; Sauter, W. *E-Learning und Blended Learning*; Springer Fachmedien: Wiesbaden, Germany, 2015. [CrossRef]
36. Müller, K. Lernaufgaben. Pflegepädagogik. In *Pflegedidaktische Handlungsfelder*; Ertl-Schmuck, R., Greb, U., Eds.; Beltz Juventa: Weinheim, Germany, 2023; pp. 278–287.

37. Strecker, M.; Oldak, A.; Lätzsch, R.; Falk-Dulisch, M.; Eickelmann, A.K.; Liebau, L.; Nagel, L.; Hejna, U.; Pieper, M.; Stirner, A.; et al. Digitale und virtuell unterstützte fallbasierte Lehr-/Lernszenarien in den Gesundheitsberufen—Implementierung, Evaluation, Reflexion. In *Innovative Lehr-/Lernszenarien in den Pflege- und Gesundheitsberufen*; Working Paper-Reihe der Projekte DiViFaG und ViRDiPA 5; Universität Bielefeld: Bielefeld, Germany, 2023. [CrossRef]
38. Engel, B. Immersion oder Versinken in der Virtuellen Realität—Auch ein Thema für die Arbeitsmedizin? *ASU Arbeitsmedizin Sozialmedizin Umweltmedizin Z. Med. Prävention* **2019**, *54*, 600–603. Available online: https://www.researchgate.net/publication/338557874_ZUR_DISKUSSION_GESTELLT_Immersion_oder_Versinken_in_der_virtuellen_Realitat_-auch_ein_Thema_fur_die_Arbeitsmedizin_Immersion_or_falling_into_virtual_reality_-another_issue_for_occupational_medicine_Im (accessed on 7 June 2023).
39. Aichinger, S. Ausgewählte digitalisierte Elemente in der Hochschullehre. *Weiterentwicklung Unterrichtspraxis* **2018**, *7*, 33–43. [CrossRef]
40. Schöllan, L. Chancen und Herausforderungen von Virtual Reality in ausgewählten Bildungskontexten. *Online Mag. Ludwigsburger Beiträge Medien.* **2019**, *20*, 1–25. [CrossRef] [PubMed]
41. Holland, T. Educational Strategies to Foster Empathy Utilizing Simulation Pedagogy. *Int. J. Caring Sci.* **2020**, *3*, 1589–1595.
42. Barr, H.; Gray, R.; Helme, M.; Low, H.; Reeves, S.; CAIPE. Interprofessional Education Guidelines. 2016. Available online: https://www.caipe.org/resources/publications/caipe-publications/barr-h-gray-r-helme-m-low-h-reeves-s-2016-interprofessional-education-guidelines# (accessed on 7 November 2023).
43. Kälble, K. Interprofessionalität in der gesundheitsberuflichen Bildung im Spannungsfeld von beruflicher Identitätsentwicklung und Professionalisierung. In *Interprofessionelles Lernen, Lehren und Arbeiten. Gesundheits- und Sozialprofessionen auf dem Weg zu kooperativer Praxis*; Ewers, M., Paradis, E., Herinek, D., Eds.; Beltz Verlag: Weinheim, Germany, 2019; pp. 70–84.
44. Canadian Interprofessional Health Collaborative. *A National Interprofessional Competency Framework*; Canadian Interprofessional Health Collaborative: Vancouver, BC, Canada, 2010. Available online: http://www.cihc-cpis.com/publications1.html (accessed on 3 May 2022).
45. Räbiger, J.; Beck, E.-M. *Interprofessionelles Lernen als Voraussetzung für Interprofessionelle Zusammenarbeit, Professionsbezogene Qualitätsentwicklung im Interdisziplinären Gesundheitswesen. Gestaltungsansätze, Handlungsfelder und Querschnittbereiche*; Hensen, P., Stamer, M., Eds.; Springer VS: Wiesbaden, Germany, 2018; pp. 157–170.
46. Fleischmann, N.; Eichner, I.; Simmenroth, A.; Zarnack, F.; Müller, C. Interprofessionelle Ausbildung in den Gesundheitsberufen: Auszubildende der Gesundheits- und Krankenpflege leiten Medizinstudierende in der Curricularen Lehreinheit „Diabetes Mellitus" an. 2017. Available online: https://www.researchgate.net/publication/321651517_Interprofessionelle_Ausbildung_in_den_Gesundheitsberufen_Auszubildende_der_Gesundheits-_und_Krankenpflege_leiten_Medizinstudierende_in_der_curricularen_Lehreinheit_Diabetes_mellitus_an (accessed on 9 September 2022).
47. Kirkevold, M. *Pflegewissenschaft als Praxisdisziplin (Pflegewissenschaft, 1. Aufl.)*; Huber: Bern, Switzerland; Göttingen, Germany; Toronto, ON, Canada; Seattle, WA, USA, 2022.
48. Baumgartner, P.; Kalz, M. Wiederverwendung von Lernobjekten aus didaktischer Sicht, Medien in der Wissenschaft. In *Auf zu neuen Ufern! E-Learning Heute und Morgen*; Tavangarian, D., Ed.; Waxmann: München, Germany, 2005; Volume 34, pp. 97–106.
49. Hopkins, I.; Roberts, D. Chocolate-covered Broccoli? Games and the Teaching of Literature. *Chang. Engl.* **2015**, *22*, 222–236. [CrossRef]

Disclaimer/Publisher's Note: The statements, opinions and data contained in all publications are solely those of the individual author(s) and contributor(s) and not of MDPI and/or the editor(s). MDPI and/or the editor(s) disclaim responsibility for any injury to people or property resulting from any ideas, methods, instructions or products referred to in the content.

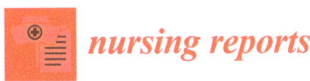

Systematic Review

Umbrella Review: Stress Levels, Sources of Stress, and Coping Mechanisms among Student Nurses

Leodoro J. Labrague

Marcella Neihoff School of Nursing, Loyola University Chicago, Chicago, IL 60611, USA; leo7_ci@yahoo.com

Abstract: Prelicensure nursing students face significant stress from their education and clinical placements, highlighting the crucial need for the development of effective coping mechanisms with which to manage both academic and clinical responsibilities, ultimately enhancing the wellbeing and academic performance of these students. This umbrella review aims to evaluate and synthesize existing review articles that examine stress levels and coping mechanisms among student nurses during their education and training. Five databases (PsycINFO, PubMed, CINAHL, Scopus and Web of Science) were searched for review articles published from 2010 onwards. This review includes twelve articles, encompassing 189 studies. The review findings demonstrate that student nurses experience moderate-to-high levels of stress during their nurse education. Major sources of stress include academic demands, patient care responsibilities, and interactions with nursing staff and faculty. Commonly utilized coping skills involve problem-solving behaviors, transference, and maintaining an optimistic outlook. Given the adverse consequences of stress, nurse educators play a critical role in the development of strategies with which to reduce stress and enhance coping skills among student nurses. This study was not registered.

Keywords: stress; coping; nursing; education; students; integrative review; systematic review

Citation: Labrague, L.J. Umbrella Review: Stress Levels, Sources of Stress, and Coping Mechanisms among Student Nurses. *Nurs. Rep.* **2024**, *14*, 362–375. https://doi.org/10.3390/nursrep14010028

Academic Editors: Antonio Martínez-Sabater, Elena Chover-Sierra and Carles Saus-Ortega

Received: 18 November 2023
Revised: 3 February 2024
Accepted: 4 February 2024
Published: 5 February 2024

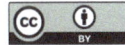

Copyright: © 2024 by the author. Licensee MDPI, Basel, Switzerland. This article is an open access article distributed under the terms and conditions of the Creative Commons Attribution (CC BY) license (https://creativecommons.org/licenses/by/4.0/).

1. Introduction

Stress and coping during nurse education and training are widely recognized as important areas of research, as nursing students often experience high levels of stress due to academic demands, clinical placements, and personal life stressors [1,2]. Stress, universally defined, is a physiological and psychological response to a perceived threat or challenge. It involves the body's adaptive reactions aimed at mobilizing resources to cope with the demands of a situation. Stress can manifest as a complex interplay of physical, emotional, and behavioral changes, and its intensity varies based on individual perceptions and coping mechanisms [3,4]. Although stress in general is often considered harmful, when maintained at manageable levels, it can potentially offer benefits by serving as a motivational force for students, fostering resilience, and encouraging the development of effective coping strategies [5].

Numerous studies have identified common stressors in nursing students, including heavy academic workloads, time pressures, clinical placements, and personal life challenges such as financial problems and family issues [4,6]. Prolonged exposure to excessively high stress levels can have detrimental effects on the psychological health, academic performance, and overall wellbeing of student nurses [5,6]. Therefore, effective coping strategies are essential for reducing stress, promoting wellbeing, and fostering academic success among nursing students.

When faced with stress, nursing students commonly employ a combination of problem-centered coping strategies and emotion-centered coping mechanisms [7,8]. Problem-centered coping mechanisms involve seeking social support, managing time effectively, and engaging in active problem-solving. These strategies target the root causes of stress and provide long-term stress relief [8,9]. On the other hand, emotion-focused coping strategies encompass positive reinterpretation, acceptance, and mindfulness. While these strategies may help mitigate and manage the behavioral responses to stress, they offer only short-term stress reduction as they do not directly address the underlying causes of stress [9,10].

This umbrella review is guided by Lazarus and Folkman's transactional model of stress and coping [9]. This influential framework emphasizes that individuals engage in coping strategies based on their appraisal of stressors, employing both problem-centered and emotion-centered mechanisms [9]. In the context of nursing students, the model provides a comprehensive lens through which to understand how they navigate stress, addressing not only the identification of stress levels and sources but also shedding light on the effectiveness of the coping mechanisms employed. By utilizing this theoretical foundation, the research aims to explore the dynamic interplay between stressors and coping strategies, offering insights applicable to the development of targeted interventions in nursing education and practice.

Over the past three decades, stress and coping in student nurses have been extensively researched, resulting in a substantial volume of individual studies and literature reviews [11,12]. Guided by the Joanna Briggs Institute (JBI) methodology, this umbrella review aims to examine the current state of knowledge on stress and coping in student nurses during their prelicensure programs [13,14].

In the context of nurse education and training, the results of this umbrella review are crucial for several reasons in the context of nursing practice for students. Firstly, understanding the specific stressors encountered by student nurses and the sources of their stress is essential for the development of targeted interventions by which to promote mental wellbeing during their education. By comprehensively synthesizing existing literature, this review aims to identify common stressors, such as academic pressures, clinical demands, and interpersonal challenges, and thus provide valuable insights for educators and institutions to tailor support mechanisms. Moreover, a detailed examination of coping mechanisms utilized by student nurses is vital for informing evidence-based strategies that can be incorporated into nursing education programs. Identifying effective coping strategies is not only beneficial for students' mental health but also crucial for enhancing their resilience and their ability to manage stressors in their future nursing careers. This review aims to contribute to the ongoing efforts in nursing education to create environments that foster student wellbeing, reduce burnout, and ultimately cultivate a workforce that is better equipped to provide high-quality and compassionate patient care. The findings from this umbrella review have the potential to guide policy decisions, curriculum development, and support services, ultimately shaping the landscape of nursing education and practice. Despite the abundance of literature reviews examining stress and coping in students, no umbrella review synthesizing findings from previous reviews has been found to date.

The aim of this research was to conduct an umbrella review to systematically synthesize and analyze existing literature on stress levels, sources of stress, and coping mechanisms among student nurses. This overarching review seeks to provide a comprehensive understanding of the multifaceted aspects of stress experienced by student nurses during their education. Specifically, the research aimed to identify common stressors, explore variations in stress levels across different educational settings, and critically evaluate the effectiveness of coping mechanisms employed by students.

2. Materials and Methods

2.1. Design

An umbrella review is a systematic review that summarizes and evaluates the findings of multiple systematic reviews and research syntheses on a specific topic [15]. An umbrella review synthesizes and evaluates the quality, quantity, and consistency of evidence from multiple reviews, providing a broader and more reliable understanding of a specific research question or topic [13]. By integrating and summarizing the findings from various reviews, an umbrella review offers a more comprehensive and nuanced perspective on a particular field of study [16]. This type of review can be particularly valuable when guiding clinical practice and decision-making, informing clinical guidelines, public health policies, and future research directions [15,17].

Belbasis et al. [15] have provided a guideline for conducting an umbrella review. Their guideline includes steps such as clearly defining the research question, establishing inclusion and exclusion criteria, conducting a literature search, extracting, and analyzing data, evaluating the strength of evidence, and summarizing and presenting the data. Their result was presented using the Preferred Reporting Items for Systematic Reviews and Meta-Analyses (PRISMA).

2.2. Sources of Data and Search Strategy

To locate relevant literature reviews, five databases (SCOPUS, Web of Science, PubMed, CINAHL and PsychINFO) were searched using the following search terms: "student nurses" OR "prelicensure student nurses" AND "stress" OR "psychological distress" AND "coping mechanisms" OR "coping skills" AND "nurse education" OR "clinical practice" AND "integrative review" OR "systematic review" OR "scoping review" OR "literature review". The inclusion criteria for articles were as follows: (a) peer-reviewed quantitative reviews of original studies assessing stress and coping among prelicensure nursing students, (b) published in the English language and (c) published from 2010 onwards. For the purpose of homogeneity, this review was limited to quantitative reviews. Focusing exclusively on quantitative studies in this umbrella review ensures a rigorous and systematic analysis of objective, numerical data related to stress levels, sources of stress, and coping mechanisms among student nurses. This approach allows for a standardized synthesis of evidence, enabling the identification of patterns, trends, and statistically significant associations that contribute to a more robust and generalizable understanding of the topic.

2.3. Search Outcomes

The initial search identified a total of 189 articles examining stress and coping in student nurses. These studies were then screened and filtered for duplicates, resulting in the removal of 91 reviews. The remaining 98 articles were further evaluated based on the inclusion criteria, leading to the exclusion of an additional 71 articles. The full texts of the remaining 27 articles were read, and 12 articles were found to be relevant for the review (Figure 1).

2.4. Quality Appraisal

The JBI Critical Appraisal Checklist for Systematic Review and Research Syntheses was used to assess the quality of the gathered evidence. This checklist consists of 11 items that can be answered with yes (1), no (0) or unclear (0), with a maximum score of 11. The quality of each review was categorized as low (<5.5), moderate (5.5–8), or high (9–11).

2.5. Data Extraction and Synthesis

Data extraction and synthesis were conducted by two researchers. The primary researcher, who was also the author of the study, worked alongside a second independent researcher not affiliated with the study to enhance objectivity and reliability in the process. This dual-researcher approach aimed to enhance the robustness and validity of the data extraction and synthesis process, contributing to the comprehensive analysis of stress levels, sources, and coping mechanisms among student nurses. To facilitate result comparison, a matrix table was created, and the following information was extracted: author, country, review type, databases used, number of studies included, key findings, and the quality appraisal checklist employed. The results of each review were synthesized based on the formulated research questions.

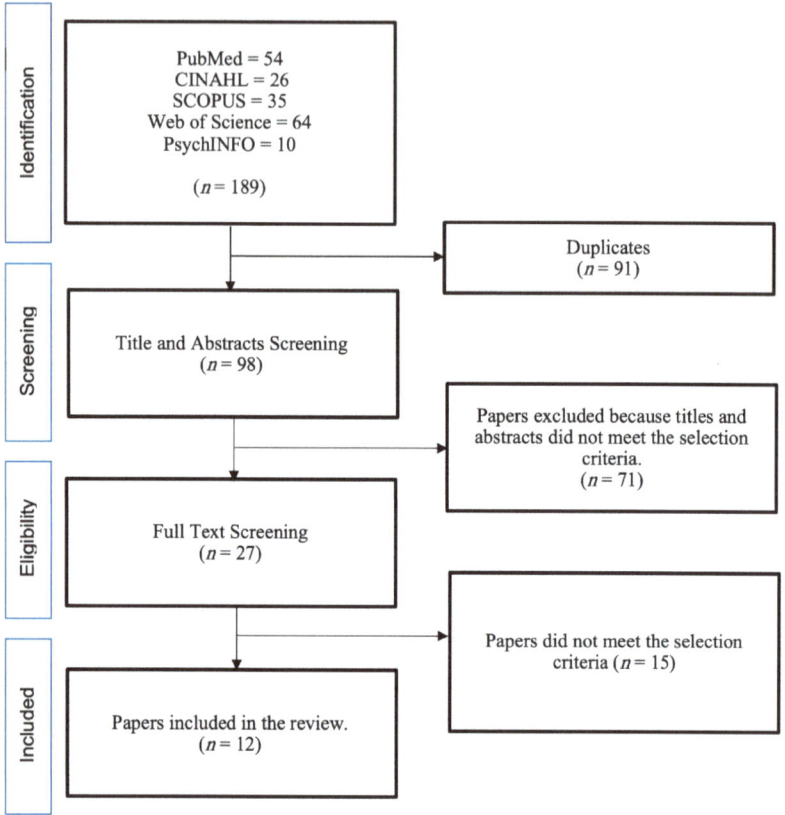

Figure 1. Diagram of the process used to identify references for the review.

3. Results

3.1. Characteristics of the Included Review Articles

Twelve reviews were included in this umbrella review. Among these, six utilized an integrative review design [3,8,18–21], three employed a systematic review design [5,22,23], two used a scoping review design [24,25], and one conducted a systematic review with a meta-analysis [11]. The number of studies included in each review ranged from 8 to 27, resulting in a total of 189 studies (Table 1). The most commonly used databases for retrieving relevant articles were CINAHL, MEDLINE, Scopus and PubMed. Seven studies reported the quality appraisal checklist used to assess the methodological rigor of the reviews, with the Critical Appraisal Skills Programme (CASP) being employed in three of them. Among the 12 reviews, 2 were deemed to have moderate quality, while the remaining 10 were rated as high quality (Table 2).

Table 1. Summary of studies included.

Author	Country	Review Type	Databases Used	Number of Studies	Key Findings	Quality Appraisal Checklist
Alatawi et al. [24]	Saudi Arabia	Scoping review	PubMed, CINAHL, EBSCO, ProQuest and Medline	22	• Stress level: moderate to high. • Sources of stress: academic stressors (academic loads, time management, fear of examination), clinical stressors (nursing staff expectations, caring for patients), and personal stressors (financial distress, death of family).	NR
Alzayyat et al. [18]	Jordan	Integrative review	MEDLINE, CINAHL, PsycINFO and PubMed	13	• Sources of stress: academic demands, relations in the clinical environment and caring for patients and families. • Academic year level was not associated with stress levels.	NR
Bhurtun et al. [21]	Finland	Integrative review	MEDLINE, CINAHL, PsycINFO and PubMed	13	• Stress level: moderate to high levels of stress during their clinical training. • Sources of stress: teachers and nursing staff were a strong stressor. • Top coping skills: problem solving and transference the most common coping techniques.	NR
Labrague et al. [3]	Oman	Integrative review	PsycINFO, PubMed, CINAHL, MEDLINE and Scopus	27	• Top coping skills: problem focuses coping strategies—problem solving behaviors, self-confident behaviors. • Least frequently used coping skills: avoidance.	QualSysts
Labrague et al. [8]	Oman	Integrative review	CINAHL, MEDLINE, PsycINFO and PubMed	13	• Stress level: moderate levels of stress. • Sources of stress: caring for patients, assignments and workloads, and negative interactions with staff and faculty. • Top coping skills: problem-solving strategies such as developing objectives to resolve problems, adopting various strategies to solve problems, and finding the meaning of stressful events.	Critical Appraisal Checklist

Table 1. Cont.

Author	Country	Review Type	Databases Used	Number of Studies	Key Findings	Quality Appraisal Checklist
Labrague et al. [22]	Oman	Systematic review	SCOPUS, CINAHL, PubMed and Ovid	11	• Stress level: moderate-to-high stress levels. • Sources of stress: heavy workloads, taking care of patients. • Top coping skills: problem solving behaviors. • Least frequently used coping skills: avoidance. • Higher level students experiencing higher stress levels.	Critical Appraisal Checklist
Majrashi et al. [25]	Saudi Arabia	Scoping review	CINAHL, MEDLINE and PubMed,	13	• Sources of stress: stress from distance learning, stress from assignment and workloads, clinical training, stress from COVID-19 infection. • Top coping skills: seeking information, staying optimistic, transference.	Hawker's Quality Assessment Tool
McCarthy et al. [19]	Ireland	Integrative review	CINAHL, PubMed and PsycINFO	25	• Sources of stress: caring for patients, relationship with clinical colleagues and faculty, academic environment, examinations, and assignments. • Top coping skills: problem solving, staying optimistic, transference, and social support.	Critical Appraisal Tool
Pulido-Martos et al. [23]	Spain	Systematic review	MEDLINE and PsycInfo	23	• Sources of stress: academics (reviews, workload and problems associated with studying, among others). • Other sources of stress include clinical sources (such as fear of unknown situations, mistakes with patients or handling of technical equipment). • No changes occur at the different years of the student's education.	NR
Younas [20]	Canada	Integrative review	PubMed, EMBASE, Cochrane, CINHAL, ASSIA, PsycInfo, Science Direct and Google Scholar	9	• Stress level: moderate stress levels. • Sources of stress: assignment workloads, lack of clinical knowledge, inadequate training, long clinical hours. • Top coping skills: problem solving behaviors, transference, optimism, seeking family, and professional support.	NR

Table 1. Cont.

Author	Country	Review Type	Databases Used	Number of Studies	Key Findings	Quality Appraisal Checklist
Zheng et al. [11]	China	Systematic Review with meta-analysis	PubMed, Cochrane, Web of Science, CNKI and China Biomedical Literature Service System	8	• The prevalence of stress among practicing nursing students was estimated to be 61.97%, suggesting a high prevalence of psychological stress among practicing nursing students.	Agency for Healthcare Quality and Research (AHRQ)
Li & Hasson [5]	Ireland	Systematic Review	CINAHL, Web of Science, Medline (OVID), PsycInfo, CNKI, WanFang Data, VIP and CMB	12	• Stress level: moderate-to-high stress levels. • Interaction between resilience and stress and wellbeing was high. • Resilience and low stress were found to better predict wellbeing.	Critical Appraisal Skills Programme (CASP)

NR = not reported.

Table 2. JBI Critical Appraisal Checklist Criteria for Systematic Review and Research Syntheses.

Reference	1	2	3	4	5	6	7	8	9	10	11	Total
Alatawi et al. [24]	1	1	1	1	1	0	1	1	0	1	1	9
Alzayyat et al. [18]	1	1	1	1	1	0	1	1	0	1	1	9
Bhurtun et al. [21]	1	1	1	1	1	1	1	1	0	1	1	10
Labrague et al. [3]	1	1	1	1	1	1	0	1	0	1	1	9
Labrague et al. [8]	1	1	1	1	1	1	1	1	0	1	1	10
Labrague et al. [22]	1	1	1	1	1	1	1	1	0	1	1	10
Majrashi et al. [25]	1	1	1	0	1	1	1	1	0	1	1	9
McCarthy et al. [19]	1	1	1	0	1	1	1	1	0	1	1	9
Pulido-Martos et al. [23]	1	1	1	0	1	0	1	1	0	1	1	8
Younas [20]	1	1	1	1	1	0	0	1	0	1	1	8
Zheng et al. [11]	1	1	1	1	1	1	1	1	1	1	1	11
Li & Hasson [5]	1	1	1	1	1	1	1	1	0	1	1	10

Note: yes = 1; no/unclear = 0; 1 = is the review question clearly and explicitly stated?; 2 = were the inclusion criteria appropriate for the review question?; 3 = was the search strategy appropriate?; 4 = were the sources and resources used to search for studies adequate?; 5 = were the criteria for appraising studies appropriate?; 6 = was critical appraisal conducted by two or more reviewers independently?; 7 = were there methods to minimize errors in data extraction?; 8 = were the methods used to combine studies appropriate?; 9 = was the likelihood of publication bias assessed?; 10 = were recommendations for policy and/or practice supported by the reported data?; 11 = were the specific directives for new research appropriate?

3.2. Major Findings

The results of the data synthesis were categorized into four themes: (a) moderate-to-severe stress levels, (b) sources of stress, (c) frequently used coping skills, and (d) stress in relation to academic levels.

3.2.1. Moderate-to-Severe Stress Levels

Seven reviews reported stress levels in student nurses ranging from moderate [3,20] to severe [5,11,21,22,24]. Three of these reviews utilized an integrative design, two employed a systematic design, one used a scoping review, and one conducted a systematic review with a meta-analysis. All reviews analyzed articles on stress among students from various countries, except for the work of Labrague et al. [22], which focused specifically on Saudi Arabian student nurses, and the work of Younas [20], which included studies conducted only in Asia. Qualitative synthesis of the review results was conducted in all reviews except for that of Zheng et al. [11], who performed a meta-analysis to estimate the prevalence of psychological stress in practicing student nurses. The meta-analysis revealed a prevalence rate of 61.97%, indicating a higher prevalence of psychological stress among pre-licensure nursing students.

3.2.2. Sources of Stress

Under this theme, stress in the context of nursing education is defined as the psychological and emotional strain [9] experienced by students due to the demanding nature of academic coursework, clinical training, and interpersonal dynamics within educational settings, potentially impacting their overall wellbeing and academic performance. The top sources of stress identified in student nurses during nurse education and training were 'academic demands', 'caring for patients' and 'interaction with nursing staff and faculty'.

Academic Stress

This subtheme pertains to the psychological strain experienced by nursing students in response to the demanding nature of their coursework, examinations, and high academic expectations, collectively referred to as academic stress [9]. Seven reviews identified 'academic demands' as the primary source of stress for student nurses during their education and training. Three integrative reviews identified heavy academic workloads [3,18,19] as the main stressor, while two systematic reviews [23,24] reported unreasonable assignments, tests, and examinations as major stressors for students. Similar findings were observed in reviews assessing stress and coping among Saudi Arabian student nurses [22] and in select Asian countries [20]. A scoping review examining stress and coping during the height of the pandemic identified academic demands and virtual learning as major stressors [25].

Stress from Caring for Patient

This subtheme encompasses the emotional and psychological strain experienced by nursing students, due to the challenges and responsibilities associated with providing care to individuals who are ill or in need of medical attention—referred to as stress from caring for patients [10]. Six reviews identified 'caring for patients' as the second most common source of stress for student nurses. Three integrative reviews identified caring for ill patients and dealing with families as the main sources of stress [8,18,19]. This finding was supported by a systematic review by Labrague et al. [22], in which Saudi Arabian students reported heightened psychological stress levels when caring for patients. Two scoping reviews, one conducted before the pandemic [24] and one during the pandemic crisis [25], examined clinical sources of stress among pre-licensure students. Both reviews identified stress associated with patient care as a common challenge during their clinical placements.

Stress from Interaction with Staff and Faculty

Under this subtheme, stress from interactions with staff and faculty in the context of nursing education is characterized by the emotional and psychological strain experienced by students due to challenging or negative encounters, expectations, or dynamics with nursing faculty and staff members during their academic and clinical training [9]. 'Interaction with nursing staff and faculty' was reported as the third most common source of stress for students during their nursing program. This stressor was identified in three integrative reviews and one scoping review. In a scoping review of 13 studies, in addition to unreasonable academic workloads, many pre-licensure students reported elevated levels of stress when interacting with nursing staff and clinical instructors [24]. This finding was supported by three integrative reviews, where interaction with nursing staff and faculty was regarded as one of the top stressors for students [8,19,21].

3.2.3. Frequently Used Coping Skills

Coping skills in the context of nursing education refer to the adaptive strategies and mechanisms employed by students to effectively manage and navigate the various stressors, challenges, and demands inherent in their academic coursework, clinical training, and interactions with faculty and staff [10]. Three distinct coping strategies were identified: problem-solving behaviors, transference, and staying optimistic.

Problem Solving Behaviors

Under this subtheme, problem-solving behaviors, as a coping strategy in nursing education, refer to the deliberate and systematic approach employed by nursing students to identify, analyze, and resolve challenges or stressors encountered during their academic and clinical training [9]. Seven review articles reported 'problem-solving behaviors' as the top coping strategy employed by student nurses to deal with and manage their stressors. Three of these were integrative reviews, one was a systematic review, and the remaining three were scoping reviews. These reviews, which analyzed global studies, consistently identified problem-solving behaviors as the most frequently used coping skill among nursing students [3,8,21]. A systematic review focusing on stress and coping among nursing and midwifery students found that both groups were more inclined to use desirable coping skills, including problem-solving [19]. Another systematic review conducted during the pandemic also identified seeking information, a problem-solving skill, as the most frequently used coping mechanism [25]. Two of these reviews had a narrower scope, one specific to Saudi students [22], and the work of Younas [20] focusing on Asian nursing students. In the systematic review of 13 studies conducted in Saudi Arabia, problem-solving behaviors were identified as the most frequently used coping skills, while avoidance was the least frequently used [22]. Younas [20] also found problem-solving behaviors to be the top-rated coping skills among Asian nursing students based on the analysis and appraisal of nine studies.

Transference

Transference as a coping strategy in nursing education involves the unconscious redirection of feelings, attitudes, and expectations from past experiences or relationships onto current interactions with faculty, staff, or peers [10]. Four review articles identified 'transference' as the second most frequently used coping strategy among student nurses. Bhurtun et al. [21] appraised and synthesized 13 studies, identifying transference as the second most frequently used coping strategy after problem-solving behaviors. Younas [20], in a study analyzing stress and coping studies in an Asian context, found that student nurses used problem-solving behaviors and transference as coping skills. McCarthy et al. [19], analyzing 25 studies, found that both midwifery and nursing students utilized transference as a way of managing academic and clinical stress. A scoping review of 13 studies conducted during the pandemic [25] also identified transference as frequently used coping during the height of the pandemic crisis.

Staying Optimistic

Staying optimistic as a coping skill involves maintaining a positive and hopeful outlook, even in the face of challenges or stressful situations [9]. This includes adopting a mindset that focuses on positive possibilities, finding silver linings, and cultivating resilience to navigate difficulties with a hopeful attitude. Three review articles reported 'being optimistic' as the third most frequently used coping skill when confronted with stressors during clinical placements. Staying optimistic was identified as one of the main coping skills utilized by Asian students in an integrative review by Younas [20]. Similar results were obtained in a literature review of 25 studies that measured stress and coping in nursing and midwifery students [19]. In a study examining stress and coping among student nurses during the height of the COVID-19 crisis, Majrashi et al. [25] identified staying optimistic as one of the most frequently used coping skills, alongside seeking information.

3.2.4. Stress in Relation to Academic Year Level

Three review articles assessed how stress levels change according to academic year levels. Two reviews found no apparent changes in stress levels across academic year levels [18,23], while one review [22] found that academic year levels were associated with heightened stress levels in students. A systematic review of 23 studies found no apparent changes in stress levels as student nurses progressed to higher academic year levels [23]. Similarly, an integrative review by Alzayyat et al. [18] found no statistical difference in stress levels among student nurses across different year levels. In contrast, a systematic review of stress and coping studies in Saudi Arabia showed higher stress levels in student nurses in higher academic year levels compared with those in lower year levels [22].

4. Discussion
4.1. Key Findings

The literature has consistently identified stress as a common experience among health-related professions, with studies indicating a high prevalence of stress among this population. Earlier studies have reported that up to 80% of health profession students experience a high amount of stress during their academic years, which is supported by the findings of Liu et al. [1] and Ayaz-Alkaya and Simones [2]. Nursing students, in particular, face personal life challenges during their adolescent stage, and the nursing program itself exposes them to various stressors throughout their pre-licensure program [4,6]. Balancing academic studies with clinical rotations, which often involve long hours and unpredictable schedules, further contributes to the higher stress experience in student nurses. Across countries, the umbrella review reveals a relatively uniform intensity of stress, consistent sources of stress, and common coping mechanisms among student nurses. These findings underscore the global nature of challenges faced by nursing students during education and clinical training. In light of this, the implications for nursing education globally are significant, necessitating collaborative efforts to establish standardized support measures, culturally sensitive interventions, and the integration of flexible learning technologies with which to address the shared stressors experienced by nursing students worldwide.

This review identified the top stressors in student nurses, including academic demands, caring for patients, and interactions with nursing staff and faculty. Academic demands are expected to be the top stressor in nursing students due to the heavy workload of lectures, labs, clinical rotations, and assignments [5]. Clinical experiences, including caring for patients, can be emotionally and physically demanding, especially for students and new nurses. The responsibility of caring for sick and dying patients and the emotional toll of witnessing patients' suffering can overwhelm nursing students [26]. Interactions with nursing staff and faculty can also be a potential source of stress if students feel unsupported and lack guidance in their clinical training [5,21]. Nursing students may feel intimidated, particularly when faced with experienced staff nurses [27]. Student nurses may perceive interactions with faculty and nursing staff as stressful due to a variety of reasons. Firstly, a lack of clear communication and expectations can create uncertainty, leading to heightened anxiety among students [7]. Additionally, disparities in power dynamics, with students often perceiving faculty and staff as authority figures, may contribute to feelings of intimidation and hinder open communication [8,9]. Moreover, inadequate feedback and support in clinical settings can exacerbate stress, as students may struggle to navigate challenges without sufficient guidance [10]. Addressing these issues through clear communication, supportive mentorship, and constructive feedback can help alleviate stress and enhance the overall learning experience for student nurses. This result provides support to earlier research that has identified academic demands, caring for patients, and interactions with nursing staff and faculty as top sources of stress [9,18,20].

To effectively manage and deal with these stressors, individuals should utilize coping skills that provide long-term resolutions to stress, such as problem-solving behaviors rather than emotion-focused strategies [28]. This review identified three coping strategies frequently used by student nurses: problem-solving behaviors, staying optimistic, and transference. Problem-solving behaviors and staying optimistic have been shown to be effective coping mechanisms in managing stress and challenging circumstances [9,10]. Optimism, which involves maintaining a positive outlook on life, helps student nurses remain motivated and resilient in difficult circumstances [10,28]. Problem-solving involves identifying issues, developing action plans, and implementing them, in turn enabling individuals to reduce stress and regain control [9]. These findings support prior reports that have identified problem-solving behaviors and optimism as important coping strategies for nursing and non-nursing students [4,6]. These findings coincide with earlier research, wherein student nurses identified these coping mechanisms as useful for dealing with and managing their stressors during nursing education and training [18,21,24]

In addition to problem-focused coping strategies, an emotion-focused strategy, including transference, was also identified as a coping mechanism used by students to deal with stressors. Transference is a psychological phenomenon that occurs when individuals unconsciously transfer feelings, attitudes, and expectations from one person or situation to another. Transference, however, is considered an undesirable coping mechanism as it can prevent individuals from developing healthy coping skills and addressing the root causes of stress [9,10]. Overreliance on transference can be counterproductive [25]. In nursing education, students often face demanding academic and clinical challenges that may be beyond their immediate control. Emotion-focused coping strategies become crucial as they navigate stressors like heavy workloads and high-pressure situations in healthcare settings. By teaching nursing students techniques such as mindfulness, self-care, and seeking peer support, educators can help them effectively manage their emotional responses, promoting resilience and wellbeing in the demanding context of nursing education.

Nurse faculty can promote problem-solving behaviors in nursing students by providing constructive feedback, encouragement, and modeling the use of problem-solving skills. By assisting students in identifying the root causes of their stress and brainstorming potential solutions, nurse faculty can help them effectively handle their stressors instead of projecting their emotions onto others or situations.

4.2. Limitations of the Study

A limitation of this study is that it exclusively focused on quantitative studies, thereby excluding valuable qualitative insights that could provide a deeper understanding of the subjective experiences related to stress, sources of stress, and coping mechanisms among nursing students. Additionally, the decision to restrict the review to studies published in the English language may introduce language bias, potentially omitting relevant findings from non-English literature that could offer diverse perspectives on the topic. Another limitation lies in the exclusion of articles published before 2010, which may overlook earlier research that could contribute historical context and highlight potential changes or trends in stress among nursing students over time. These limitations collectively underscore the need for future research to adopt a more inclusive approach, considering both qualitative and non-English literature, and exploring a broader timeframe to ensure a comprehensive understanding of stress in nursing education.

4.3. Future Research Directions

This umbrella review identified several critical points that can guide future literature reviews. Firstly, of the 12 reviews analyzed, 5 did not evaluate the methodological rigor of the included studies. Assessing the quality of evidence is crucial for determining the reliability and validity of research findings [29]. Without analyzing the quality of the studies, it becomes challenging to make informed decisions based on the review findings.

Meta-analysis is a powerful tool that can improve the reliability and quality of research findings, informing evidence-based practice and policy decisions [30]. In this umbrella review, only one review utilized meta-analysis to analyze the data, partly due to the heterogeneity of the included studies, such as variations in scales used. Future research synthesis should consider statistical pooling or meta-analysis for a comprehensive evaluation of the evidence.

Although this umbrella review provides evidence regarding the prevalence of stress among nursing students across countries, the studies included often lack in-depth discussions considering specific contextual nuances related to each country. Consequently, due to this limited contextual analysis, comparing differences across countries that might affect stress and coping in students becomes challenging. Recognizing the influence of varying cultural, educational, and healthcare system factors on student experiences is crucial for a comprehensive understanding of stress in nursing education, emphasizing the need for future studies to adopt a more nuanced approach in exploring and reporting results within diverse international contexts. Therefore, to advance our understanding of the nuanced factors contributing to stress among nursing students, future studies should delve into the specific contextual nuances, considering the diverse educational, cultural, and healthcare landscapes across countries, to facilitate more meaningful cross-cultural comparisons and inform tailored interventions.

Furthermore, there is a need for reviews examining the interaction between stress and coping, specifically identifying which coping skills are most effective for nursing students in dealing with their stressors. Different coping strategies may be effective depending on the situation and individual characteristics and resources [9,10,28]. This knowledge is essential to assist nurse educators in identifying potential coping strategies that could effectively reduce stress in students. Overall, enhancing the methodological rigor of reviews, conducting meta-analyses when appropriate, and exploring the specific coping skills that best assist nursing students in managing their stressors will contribute to a deeper understanding of stress and coping in this population and inform evidence-based interventions and support strategies.

5. Relevance to Nurse Education

Stress during nurse education and clinical training can potentially exacerbate the current shortage experienced by healthcare institutions worldwide. Consequently, nurse educators play a crucial role in the development of stress reduction measures and enhancing coping skills in nursing students. Given that academic demands have been identified as the primary stressor among student nurses, it is vital for nurse educators to implement measures that assist students in effectively managing their workloads and reducing stress [31]. This may involve prioritizing essential coursework and assignments, increasing flexibility, and providing academic support [31]. By strengthening coping and social support, engaging in stress-reducing activities, and seeking professional help when needed, student nurses can effectively deal with stress related to patient care and improve their overall health and wellbeing [18,23]. The literature has identified several theoretically based interventions that are equally effective in reducing stress among students, including mindfulness-based interventions [32], behavioral-based stress management programs [33], and evidence-based resilience interventions [34].

To strengthen positive coping skills, nurse educators should focus on building and fostering problem-focused coping strategies in students to help them effectively deal with their stressors. Evidence has shown the importance of structured orientation programs for new students and structured faculty–student mentoring programs to assist students in developing active coping skills [35,36]. Social support, derived from family, relatives, and friends, should be strengthened as it has been found to be helpful in protecting students from the long-term effects of stress [36]. Additionally, nurse educators can model positive coping behaviors and share their own experiences of managing stress in a healthy way, leading to improved wellbeing and increased retention [37]. Collectively, these strategies can assist student nurses in bolstering their coping abilities and effectively managing the numerous stressors encountered during nurse education and training.

6. Conclusions

This umbrella review provides a new understanding of stress in nurse education by synthesizing evidence from multiple reviews and research syntheses. Globally, the intensity of stress and coping mechanisms among student nurses exhibits variation, yet the identified sources of stress remain remarkably consistent. While stress levels range from moderate to severe across different regions, the overarching themes of academic demands, patient care responsibilities, and interactions with nursing staff and faculty persist as primary stressors for students worldwide. Commonly used coping strategies included problem-solving behaviors, transference, and maintaining optimism. This review did not establish a relationship between academic levels and stress experience among pre-licensure nursing students. This suggests a universal need for targeted interventions and support strategies to address common stressors and enhance coping mechanisms among student nurses on a global scale.

Funding: This research received no external funding.

Institutional Review Board Statement: Not applicable.

Informed Consent Statement: Not applicable.

Public Involvement Statement: No public involvement in any aspect of this research.

Guidelines and Standards Statement: This manuscript was drafted against the Preferred Reporting Items for Systematic Reviews and Meta-Analyses.

Conflicts of Interest: The author declare no conflict of interest.

References

1. Liu, J.; Yang, Y.; Chen, J.; Zhang, Y.; Zeng, Y.; Li, J. Stress and coping styles among nursing students during the initial period of the clinical practicum: A cross-section study. *Int. J. Nurs. Sci.* **2022**, *9*, 222–229. [CrossRef] [PubMed]
2. Ayaz-Alkaya, S.; Simones, J. Nursing education stress and coping behaviors in Turkish and the United States nursing students: A descriptive study. *Nurse Educ. Pract.* **2022**, *59*, 103292. [CrossRef] [PubMed]
3. Thomas, L.M.B. Stress and depression in undergraduate students during the COVID-19 pandemic: Nursing students compared to undergraduate students in non-nursing majors. *J. Prof. Nurs.* **2022**, *38*, 89–96. [CrossRef] [PubMed]
4. Lavoie-Tremblay, M.; Sanzone, L.; Aubé, T.; Paquet, M. Sources of stress and coping strategies among undergraduate nursing students across all years. *Can. J. Nurs. Res.* **2022**, *54*, 261–271. [CrossRef] [PubMed]
5. Li, Z.S.; Hasson, F. Resilience, stress, and psychological well-being in nursing students: A systematic review. *Nurse Educ. Today* **2020**, *90*, 104440. [CrossRef] [PubMed]
6. Labrague, L.J.; McEnroe-Petitte, D.M.; Gloe, D.; Thomas, L.; Papathanasiou, I.V.; Tsaras, K. A literature review on stress and coping strategies in nursing students. *J. Ment. Health* **2017**, *26*, 471–480. [CrossRef] [PubMed]
7. Chaabane, S.; Chaabna, K.; Bhagat, S.; Abraham, A.; Doraiswamy, S.; Mamtani, R.; Cheema, S. Perceived stress, stressors, and coping strategies among nursing students in the Middle East and North Africa: An overview of systematic reviews. *Syst. Rev.* **2021**, *10*, 136. [CrossRef]
8. Lazarus, R.S.; Folkman, S. Transactional theory and research on emotions and coping. *Eur. J. Pers.* **1987**, *1*, 141–169. [CrossRef]
9. Labrague, L.J.; McEnroe-Petitte, D.M.; Al Amri, M.; Fronda, D.C.; Obeidat, A.A. An integrative review on coping skills in nursing students: Implications for policymaking. *Int. Nurs. Rev.* **2018**, *65*, 279–291. [CrossRef]
10. Biggs, A.; Brough, P.; Drummond, S. Lazarus and Folkman's psychological stress and coping theory. In *The Handbook of Stress and Health: A Guide to Research and Practice*; John Wiley & Sons: Hoboken, NJ, USA, 2017; pp. 349–364.
11. Zheng, Y.X.; Jiao, J.R.; Hao, W.N. Stress levels of nursing students: A systematic review and meta-analysis. *Medicine* **2022**, *101*, e30547. [CrossRef]
12. Fitzgibbon, K.; Murphy, K.D. Coping strategies of healthcare professional students for stress incurred during their studies: A literature review. *J. Ment. Health* **2023**, *32*, 492–503. [CrossRef]
13. Aromataris, E.; Fernandez, R.S.; Godfrey, C.; Holly, C.; Khalil, H.; Tungpunkom, P. *Methodology for JBI Umbrella Reviews*; The Joanna Briggs Institute: Adelaide, Australia, 2014.
14. Munn, Z.; Barker, T.H.; Moola, S.; Tufanaru, C.; Stern, C.; McArthur, A.; Stephenson, M.; Aromataris, E. Methodological quality of case series studies: An introduction to the JBI critical appraisal tool. *JBI Evid. Synth.* **2020**, *18*, 2127–2133. [CrossRef] [PubMed]
15. Gessler, M.; Siemer, C. Umbrella review: Methodological review of reviews published in peer-reviewed journals with a substantial focus on vocational education and training research. *Int. J. Res. Vocat. Educ. Train.* **2020**, *7*, 91–125. [CrossRef]
16. Papatheodorou, S.I.; Evangelou, E. Umbrella reviews: What they are and why we need them. In *Meta-Research: Methods and Protocols*; Humana: New York, NY, USA, 2022; pp. 135–146.

17. Belbasis, L.; Bellou, V.; Ioannidis, J.P. Conducting umbrella reviews. *BMJ Med.* **2022**, *1*, e000071. [CrossRef] [PubMed]
18. Alzayyat, A.; Al-Gamal, E. A review of the literature regarding stress among nursing students during their clinical education. *Int. Nurs. Rev.* **2014**, *61*, 406–415. [CrossRef] [PubMed]
19. McCarthy, B.; Trace, A.; O'Donovan, M.; Brady-Nevin, C.; Murphy, M.; O'Shea, M.; O'Regan, P. Nursing and midwifery students' stress and coping during their undergraduate education programmes: An integrative review. *Nurse Educ. Today* **2018**, *61*, 197–209. [CrossRef]
20. Younas, A. Levels of stress and coping strategies used by nursing students in Asian countries: An integrated literature review. *J. Middle East. N. Afr. Sci.* **2016**, *2*, 50–57. [CrossRef]
21. Bhurtun, H.D.; Azimirad, M.; Saaranen, T.; Turunen, H. Stress and coping among nursing students during clinical training: An integrative review. *J. Nurs. Educ.* **2019**, *58*, 266–272. [CrossRef] [PubMed]
22. Labrague, L.J.; McEnroe–Petitte, D.M.; De Los Santos, J.A.A.; Edet, O.B. Examining stress perceptions and coping strategies among Saudi nursing students: A systematic review. *Nurse Educ. Today* **2018**, *65*, 192–200. [CrossRef]
23. Pulido-Martos, M.; Augusto-Landa, J.M.; Lopez-Zafra, E. Sources of stress in nursing students: A systematic review of quantitative studies. *Int. Nurs. Rev.* **2012**, *59*, 15–25. [CrossRef]
24. Alatawi, A.O.; Morsy, N.M.; Sharif, L.S. Relation between resilience and stress as perceived by nursing students: A scoping review. *Evid.-Based Nurs. Res.* **2022**, *4*, 19-9. [CrossRef]
25. Majrashi, A.; Khalil, A.; Nagshabandi, E.A.; Majrashi, A. Stressors and coping strategies among nursing students during the COVID-19 pandemic: Scoping review. *Nurs. Rep.* **2021**, *11*, 444–459. [CrossRef] [PubMed]
26. Onieva-Zafra, M.D.; Fernández-Muñoz, J.J.; Fernández-Martínez, E.; García-Sánchez, F.J.; Abreu-Sánchez, A.; Parra-Fernández, M.L. Anxiety, perceived stress and coping strategies in nursing students: A cross-sectional, correlational, descriptive study. *BMC Med. Educ.* **2020**, *20*, 370. [CrossRef] [PubMed]
27. Ahmed, W.A.; Mohammed, B.M. Nursing students' stress and coping strategies during clinical training in KSA. *J. Taibah Univ. Med. Sci.* **2019**, *14*, 116–122. [CrossRef] [PubMed]
28. Kupcewicz, E.; Grochans, E.; Kadučáková, H.; Mikla, M.; Jóźwik, M. Analysis of the relationship between stress intensity and coping strategy and the quality of life of nursing students in Poland, Spain and Slovakia. *Int. J. Environ. Res. Public. Health* **2020**, *17*, 4536. [CrossRef] [PubMed]
29. Remington, R. Quality appraisal. In *A Step-by-Step Guide to Conducting an Integrative Review*; Springer International Publishing: Cham, Switzerland, 2020; pp. 45–55.
30. Borenstein, M.; Hedges, L.V.; Higgins, J.P.; Rothstein, H.R. *Introduction to Meta-Analysis*; John Wiley & Sons: Hoboken, NJ, USA, 2021.
31. Abdullah, N.A.; Shamsi, N.A.; Jenatabadi, H.S.; Ng, B.K.; Mentri, K.A.C. Factors affecting undergraduates' academic performance during COVID-19: Fear, stress and teacher-parents' support. *Sustainability* **2022**, *14*, 7694. [CrossRef]
32. Garmaise-Yee, J.S.; LeBlanc, R.G. Reducing stress and increasing mindfulness in nursing students: An online mindfulness intervention study. *Nurs. Educ. Perspect.* **2022**, *43*, 375–377. [CrossRef] [PubMed]
33. Terp, U.; Hjärthag, F.; Bisholt, B. Effects of a cognitive behavioral-based stress management program on stress management competency, self-efficacy and self-esteem experienced by nursing students. *Nurse Educ.* **2019**, *44*, E1–E5. [CrossRef]
34. Lanz, J.J. Evidence-based resilience intervention for nursing students: A randomized controlled pilot trial. *Int. J. Appl. Posit. Psychol.* **2020**, *5*, 217–230. [CrossRef]
35. Turner, K.; McCarthy, V.L. Stress and anxiety among nursing students: A review of intervention strategies in literature between 2009 and 2015. *Nurse Educ. Pract.* **2017**, *22*, 21–29. [CrossRef]
36. Labrague, L.J. Psychological resilience, coping behaviours and social support among health care workers during the COVID-19 pandemic: A systematic review of quantitative studies. *J. Nurs. Manag.* **2021**, *29*, 1893–1905. [CrossRef] [PubMed]
37. Henderson, D.; Sewell, K.A.; Wei, H. The impacts of faculty caring on nursing students' intent to graduate: A systematic literature review. *Int. J. Nurs. Sci.* **2020**, *7*, 105–111. [CrossRef] [PubMed]

Disclaimer/Publisher's Note: The statements, opinions and data contained in all publications are solely those of the individual author(s) and contributor(s) and not of MDPI and/or the editor(s). MDPI and/or the editor(s) disclaim responsibility for any injury to people or property resulting from any ideas, methods, instructions or products referred to in the content.

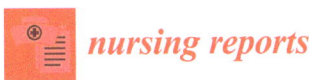

Article

Challenges Faced by University of Limpopo Learner Nurses during Psychiatry Clinical Exposure: A Qualitative Study

L. S. Hlahla *, C. Ngoatle, M. N. Kgatla and E. M. Mathapo-Thobakgale

Department of Nursing Sciences, University of Limpopo, Polokwane 0700, South Africa
* Correspondence: sebolaisi.hlahla@ul.ac.za

Abstract: Clinical exposure of learner nurses to psychiatric hospitals is a requirement by the South African Nursing Council. Clinical experience helps learner nurses build cognitive and affective skills, cultural acculturation, and professional identity. The clinical placement also aids nursing learner nurses in making decisions regarding future career paths. The goal of psychiatric nursing practice is to enhance mental and physical health and improve the patient's quality of life and rehabilitation. A qualitative research approach was followed, and a descriptive, explorative, and contextual design was used in this study to explore the challenges faced by University of Limpopo learner nurses during psychiatry clinical exposure. The population included learner nurses from level two to level four who registered for psychiatric nursing science practice. Convenience sampling was adopted. Semi-structured interviews were used to collect data, and the data were analyzed using the Tesch open coding method. Measures to ensure trustworthiness were adhered to, and ethical considerations were observed. The findings of this study indicated that learner nurses go through challenges and discomfort in the form of mental health care users, clinical environment matters, and the attitude of clinical staff in the hospital. Proper preparation of the learner nurses and clinical areas can assist in reducing the challenges that learner nurses go through.

Keywords: challenges; learner nurses; psychiatry; clinical exposure

1. Introduction

The South African Nursing Council [1] specifies that in order to register as professional nurses, learner nurses must possess the necessary practical and clinical competencies. Therefore, nursing education institutions must provide learner nurses with opportunities for clinical learning through clinical placements before they graduate. The South African Nursing Council [1] further states that if a learner nurse does not receive 80% of clinical exposure hours in psychiatric nursing, that learner nurse will not be permitted to perform the final clinical assessment of a patient.

Clinical placement of learner nurses is an important part of nursing education and training. It gives learner nurses the chance to apply the knowledge and abilities they have learned in the classroom to real patients while under the supervision of professional nurses [2]. The development of their identities as future professional nurses depends on quality clinical exposure [3]. When the learner nurses are placed in the clinical area, they get an opportunity to apply theoretical knowledge learned in the classroom to practice [4]. Additionally, it helps them build their cognitive and affective skills, cultural acculturation, and professional identity. The clinical placement also aids learner nurses in making decisions regarding future career paths [5].

Nursing clinical training takes place in a complicated clinical learning environment that is influenced by a variety of factors, unlike education in a classroom. This setting offers learner nurses the chance to learn through experimentation and apply theoretical information to a range of required nursing skills that are important for psychiatric patient care. One of the key elements influencing the quality of clinical education is how learner

Citation: Hlahla, L.S.; Ngoatle, C.; Kgatla, M.N.; Mathapo-Thobakgale, E.M. Challenges Faced by University of Limpopo Learner Nurses during Psychiatry Clinical Exposure: A Qualitative Study. *Nurs. Rep.* **2024**, *14*, 164–173. https://doi.org/10.3390/nursrep14010014

Academic Editors: Antonio Martínez-Sabater, Elena Chover-Sierra and Carles Saus-Ortega

Received: 26 October 2023
Revised: 4 January 2024
Accepted: 5 January 2024
Published: 9 January 2024

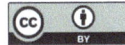

Copyright: © 2024 by the authors. Licensee MDPI, Basel, Switzerland. This article is an open access article distributed under the terms and conditions of the Creative Commons Attribution (CC BY) license (https://creativecommons.org/licenses/by/4.0/).

nurses are exposed to, and prepared for, the clinical environment [6]. Because an optimal clinical learning environment promotes the professional development of the learner nurses, a poor learning environment can be detrimental to their professional development. The unpredictability of the clinical training environment might cause challenges for learner nurses [6].

Psychiatric nursing is an area in nursing education and practice that brings specialized knowledge from nursing. Psychiatric nursing focuses on the mental health and wellbeing of individuals [7]. The goal of psychiatric nursing practice is to enhance mental and physical health and improve the patient's quality of life and rehabilitation. The main aim of psychiatric nursing is to assist patients to realize their problems and needs. Psychiatric and mental health nursing, in particular, is based on a trusted nurse–patient relationship [2].

While clinical placement gives the learner nurses a chance to build themselves professionally, it does, however, go without saying that learner nurses in clinical areas have challenges meeting their learning objectives during psychiatric clinical placements [8]. Learner nurses cannot naturally transfer knowledge from the classroom to a clinical setting; rather, their growth is influenced by their encounters and relationships with nurses and other professionals when they interact with actual patients [3].

Most learner nurses have their first encounter with psychiatric patients during their clinical placement in the hospital. Regardless of what they are taught in class, they have a tendency to maintain a belief that psychiatric patients are violent, dangerous, and hostile. These beliefs contribute to stress and anxiety in learner nurses regarding psychiatry clinical exposure. The stress and anxiety cause them to limit their interaction with the psychiatric patients [9].

A study conducted in Turkey indicated that students experience emotional challenges, such as fear, concern, anxiety, alienation, and loneliness, during mental health clinical education [10]. In South Arabia, it was discovered that poor preclinical exposure preparation makes students frustrated when they go for psychiatry clinical exposure [7]. A study conducted in Malawi showed that students have no confidence when they have to nurse psychiatric patients because of the stigma attached to mental illness [11]. Another study conducted in Gauteng Province, South Africa, reported that students do not receive the needed support from nurses in the hospital when they go for clinical exposure [12].

This study aimed to explore the challenges that learner nurses encounter when they are allocated for clinical exposure in psychiatric nursing institutions. This study is the first study at the University of Limpopo to explore the challenges facing learner nurses when they are placed in a psychiatric hospital for clinical exposure. The findings of this study will aid lecturers and nurses in hospital to assist students to adjust and perform their psychiatric clinical duties competently with minimal or no challenges.

2. Methods

A qualitative research approach was used in this study to help explain the challenges faced by University of Limpopo learner nurses during psychiatry clinical exposure. A descriptive, explorative, and contextual design was followed in this study. An explorative design was used to gather views from learner nurses regarding the challenges they face during psychiatry clinical exposure. The descriptive design was used by creating a diagram that showed the themes and the sub-themes, and the study was conducted in the context of the University of Limpopo.

2.1. Study Site

This study was conducted at the University of Limpopo, Mankweng, Limpopo Province. The University is approximately 36 km away from Polokwane city. Nursing programme is offered for four years at the University of Limpopo. When this study was conducted, the students were allocated for psychiatry clinical exposure from level 2 to level 4 of study. The students are taken through theoretical teaching and simulation before they can be taken to the hospital for psychiatric clinical exposure.

2.2. Population and Sampling

2.2.1. Population

The population for this study was University of Limpopo learner nurses enrolled for the psychiatric nursing science practice module. The total number of learner nurses who were eligible to be part of the study was 228 in 2022. That is 67 learner nurses at the 2nd level, 85 at the 3rd level, and 76 at the 4th level of study. All these learner nurses from the University of Limpopo were once allocated for psychiatric clinical exposure in mental health institutions so the researchers hoped they would provide the needed relevant information.

2.2.2. Sampling

The researchers used a non-probability sampling method to select participants for this study from the study population. The researchers chose readily available participants [13], and convenience sampling technique was used in this study.

Inclusion Criteria and Exclusion Criteria

Inclusion: All the learner nurses at the 2nd, 3rd, and 4th levels who were registered for psychiatric nursing science practice were included in the study. These learner nurses were included because they had been exposed to mental health/psychiatric institutions.

Exclusion: This study excluded all the learner nurses at the 2nd, 3rd, and 4th levels who registered for the psychiatric nursing science practice but were not available during data collection.

2.3. Data Collection

The primary author collected data at University of Limpopo. Private offices were used for data collection to ensure privacy. The interviews lasted from 45 min to 1 h. Data in this study were collected using semi-interviews, whereby a voice recorder was utilized to record the interviews, and the field notes were written down during the interview process. A consent form was signed during the briefing session before the interview, and the participants were informed that a tape recorder would be used in the interview process. An interview guide was used to direct the interviews, with the central question being, "What are the challenges you face as a learner nurse during psychiatry clinical exposure". Follow-up questions were then asked based on the participants' response. Data saturation was reached at participant number 22 where no further new information arose.

2.4. Data Analysis

Data were analysed using Tesch's eight-step open coding method as follows [14]: 1. The researchers read through the transcriptions and then continued to write ideas to obtain a sense of the whole picture. 2. Then, they started with the most exciting shortest interviews, considering the underlying meaning of information while writing views in the margins. 3. They further made a list of all topics coming from the transcript. 4. Then, they listed back to abbreviate the topics as codes and wrote the codes next to the relevant segment of the text. 5. They then identified descriptive phrasing for the topics and turned them into categories. 6. Abbreviations for each category were made, and researchers arranged the codes in alphabetical order. 7. Introductory analysis was made by collecting the data material belonging to each category in one place. 8. The researchers lastly summarized the themes and sub-themes developed, and then the raw data were sent to an independent coder who assisted with coding.

2.5. Measures to Ensure Trustworthiness

The following measures of trustworthiness were adhered to: credibility, dependability, transferability, confirmability, authenticity, and reliability. Credibility was ensured by the researchers spending more time in the field. Dependability was achieved by the researchers through the use of an independent coder. Transferability was adhered to by explaining the methodology in depth. Confirmability was achieved through an audit trail. Authenticity was achieved through a deep, vivid description of the methodology used [14].

2.6. Ethical Considerations

Ethical clearance to conduct research was requested and received from the University of Limpopo Turfloop Research Ethics Committee (TREC/318/2022:UG-26 June 2022). Permission to conduct the study using University of Limpopo learner nurses was obtained from the Director of the School of Health Care Sciences and the Head of the Department of Nursing Science department. After receiving information about the study, the learner nurses voluntarily consented to participate in the study. A consent form was provided to learner nurses to sign before interviews. The researchers assured the learner nurses of confidentiality, privacy, and anonymity, and the principle of justice was also adhered to.

3. Results

3.1. Demographic Data

The number of learner nurses who participated in this study was twenty-two. There were seventeen female learner nurses who participated in this study, and there were five male learner nurses. The gender discrepancy is mainly because most learners who enroll for the profession at the University of Limpopo are females. The participants were from level two of study to level four. Data were collected until saturation was reached at participant 22. Table 1 below indicates the demographics of the learner nurses who participated in the study.

Table 1. Demographics.

	Characteristics	Number
Gender	Female	17
	Male	5
Level of study	Level 2	5
	Level 3	8
	Level 4	9

3.2. Themes and Sub-Themes

The responses provided by the learner nurses during the process of collecting data led to the formation of themes and sub-themes, as tabulated below. Table 2 provides a presentation of themes and sub-themes that came out of the study.

Table 2. Themes and sub-themes.

Theme	Subtheme
1. Discomfort towards the mental health care users	1.1. Fear of mental health care users
	1.2. Uncertainty about learned psychiatry skills
2. Clinical environment matters	2.1. Different clinical environment
	2.2. The limited time of exposure
3. The attitude of clinical staff at the psychiatric hospital	3.1. Failure to supervise learner nurses
	3.2. Non-engagement of learner nurses in psychiatric procedures

Theme 1: Discomfort towards mental healthcare users

This theme yielded two sub-themes, which were fear of mental healthcare users and uncertainty about their learned psychiatry skills.

Sub-Theme 1.1. Fear of mental healthcare users

The learner nurses reported that when they allocated to a psychiatric institution, they find themselves afraid of the mental healthcare users. The responses below are evidence:

Participant 3 mentioned the following:

"When interacting with patients we get scared that the patients may hit us or something like that..."

Participant 5 added, by saying the following:

"Um, I had fear, to be honest. I already had stories about nurses being killed by healthcare users or being sexually assaulted. So I had that fear that what if I don't come back that day? What if I go to the wrong corner? And then a mental healthcare user comes after me? That was my greatest".

Participant 8 said that because of the stories they heard about mental healthcare users, they felt unsafe.

"Okay, when we are at Thabamoopo, we are having an emotional problem because we are not safe. After all, there are people who kill other people, and then meaning that we are not safe because we feel like those people will also kill us or rape other people. So that's why we are saying it affects me emotionally. Because sometimes I feel like I don't want to be close with them due to their threat to us that I have that a challenge....then the police or security must be available anytime or four to five police. Not only one".

Sub-Theme 1.2: Uncertainty about learned psychiatry skills

The learner nurses reported that they were not comfortable being around mental healthcare users because even if they had learned about them in the classroom, they were not sure how to handle them. They voiced their opinions, as stated below, to confirm that they were not sure of the learned skills in the classroom.

Participant 18 reported that, at times, what they are taught in class does not correspond with what they find in the hospital.

"...what we are taught in class and what we see at the psychiatric institution do not always correlate, for example in class, we are taught that each ward must have a therapeutic ward program; then when we get there some wards do not have those programs".

Participant 20 gave a report that what they learn in the classroom does not seem through enough.

"I refrain from interacting with mental health care users. I am not able to apply theory into practice, hence am saying we do not learn enough....We tend not to know how to interact with mental health care users. What we learn is not enough".

Participant 11 added the following:

"We do not have all the skills we will need to can use in the future to see if we can get this done so we are limited in the way we must learn".

Theme 2: Clinical environment matters

The theme addressing clinical environment matters yielded two sub-themes, which were different clinical environment and limited time of exposure.

Sub-Theme 2.2. Different clinical environment

The learner nurses reported that they found the psychiatric nursing clinical environment to be rather different from the general nursing environment they were used to. They gave the accounts below to describe the psychiatric clinical environment.

Participant 11 found out that the way patient care is rendered in a psychiatric hospital is different to the patient care in a general hospital.

"The challenge that I could say we encountered during psychiatric clinical allocation is that we don't get to do much patient care like the way we do in the general hospital. All we do is just to interact with the patients the whole day, and give them medications".

Participant 3 added the following:

"okay, I feel like it affects us when it comes to learning. Because, like I said that we don't get to do too much. And most of the time, we are just sitting outside and interacting with the patients. So, we are not exposed as to what is done during psych, and that it's a public or a government facility for treating people with mental illness".

Participant 20 further said the following:

"I expected to meet severely ill mental health care users. To be able to implement a lot of theory into practice but I found the patients mostly stable and communicating well".

Participant 11 added the following:

"Honestly, I didn't know what to expect. But I could say I did not expect the environment to be the way I saw it. So, I just thought maybe it was supposed to be like a normal hospital or it was going to be something else that of which is not what I saw in terms of arrangements, the way they sleep, how they eat and dress".

Sub-Theme 2.2: The limited time of exposure

The learner nurses reported that they were only allocated to the psychiatric hospitals for a limited time and that this came as a challenge to their learning. They gave information through the quotes below.

Participant 6 reported that time they were given at the psychiatric hospital was limited.

"uh, the challenges, one of the challenges is that we have uh one uh closer hospital of psychiatry around which limits the number of learner nurses to go there for clinical exposure whereby you find that you go there once or twice in the whole of the allocation so the exposure is very much limited".

Participant 08 confirmed this, saying the following:

"Oh, the time of exposure to the psychiatric hospital is limited and we are not exposed to all the wards. With the limited time of exposure, we end-up not having more knowledge about psychiatry".

Participant 19 relayed

"I was exposed to one unit, and therefore could not learn more about another user in different units....I could not learn how to manage patients in other units because of limited time allocation. I was not able to learn enough without the assistance of the nurses".

Theme 3: The attitude of clinical staff

This theme yielded two sub-themes regarding the attitude of the clinical staff in psychiatric institutions. The sub-themes were failure to supervise learner nurses and non-engagement of learner nurses in psychiatric procedures.

Sub-Theme 3.1: Failure to supervise learner nurses

The learner nurses reported that nurses in the psychiatric hospital did not supervise them. They spent most of their time alone without the supervision of professional nurses. They gave the below responses in talking about the lack of supervision from nurses:

Participant 16 said that they are not supervised in their nursing activities.

"The first challenge is that the nurses at the psychiatric institution are rude to us. Another challenge is that we are not learning anything there; we just sit with patients the whole day until it is time to knock off...I expected that the nurses would involve us in the nursing care of the patients, to learn more about the psychiatric patients and their conditions".

Participant 19 also added that

"I was exposed to one unit and could not learn more about other users in different units. The staff does not give attention to the learner nurses...I could not learn how to manage patients in the other units, I was not able to learn enough without the assistance of the nurses".

Participant 5 reported that the nurses did not look after them:

"I wouldn't say so as much were normally. . .In my case, I feel like we don't get enough monitoring, or even really been getting monitored, to be honest. And the reality because most of the time you find that they're the staff nurses are in there where they normally sit, and we're outside with the patients like literally were the ones will you get to explain the patient alone without them explaining to us, like I said, before my challenges, we don't know this patient and their conditions. We just have to learn it by ourselves. Sometimes. Yes, we do check the files, of course. But if you're there with us, I feel like it'll be easier for us because why people write and really what they see or interact with, is much more different. So, we don't really get monitoring from the nurses who are in charge of us".

Sub-Theme 3.2: Non-engagement of learner nurses in psychiatric procedures

The learner nurses reported that the nurses in the hospital were not engaging with them when they were performing psychiatric nursing procedures, and this led to the learner nurses feeling left out. The learner nurses gave the accounts below:

Participant 06 reported that

"When we go to the hospital uhm, those Nurses, most of the time when we are there, they do not even give us the attention. . .".

Participant 06 further added

"We don't do anything, we do not even give medication, we don't even fill form or something, so they only call us maybe when they want us to take vital signs only when the doctors came there to check the patients".

Participant 04 mentioned that

"I also think of this one of the nurses not being able to, like, you know, they just do not teach us what we are supposed to do, like they do not".

Participant 16 said this regarding non-engagement:

"I expected that the nurses would involve us in the nursing care of the patients, to learn more about the psychiatric patients and their conditions".

4. Discussion

This research aimed to explore the challenges that learner nurses faced during psychiatric clinical exposure. This study discovered that the challenges that the learner nurses go through include their discomfort towards mental healthcare users: the clinical environment they find themselves in and the attitude of clinical staff working in the psychiatric hospital. A study conducted in Iran confirmed that learner nurses face challenges in clinical areas when dealing with patients during clinical placement and when they have to interact with staff in the clinical environment [6].

The learner nurses reported that they were afraid of psychiatric patients. This could be because there are common mental illness stereotypes, including psychiatric patients being dangerous and aggressive [9]. There is a tendency of exaggerated crime rates and aggression of psychiatric patients, which makes learner nurses avoid them; this public discrimination against psychiatric patients may also be seen in the news and movies [15]. The learning objectives of learner nurses must focus on building the confidence of learner nurses and reducing their anxiety towards psychiatric patients [16].

The results of this study show that learner nurses have uncertainties about their learned psychiatric skills. This was supported by a study conducted in China by [15], who reported that it is common for learner nurses to feel nervous and afraid about taking care of psychiatric patients because some think they lack the necessary knowledge and abilities. The study further stated that the main reason for the learner nurses' worry and anxiety was their concern over how to handle patients with mental health problems. Due to fear, the learner nurses find themselves not knowing what to do when they are faced with psychiatric patients; they do not know how to act or interact with the individual [16].

The findings of the study indicated that learner nurses had issues with the psychiatric clinical environment. They found the psychiatric nursing environment to be different from the general nursing environment that they were used to. Psychiatric hospitals are specialized hospitals that are unique in that they are mostly in an isolated environment, with complicated patient conditions, heavy workloads, and high risks, necessitating higher professional skills and physical demands for nurses [17]. Proper orientation of the learner nurses to the setting can be useful in helping the learner nurses adapt to the environment [9].

The learner nurses reported that they are given a limited time in the psychiatric hospital; as such, they are unable to master the clinical skills related to psychiatric nursing. This was supported by [10], who said training and the type of clinical environment are significant factors influencing learner nurse competence in mental health clinical practice. The findings of their study reported that learner nurses failed to complete the practice and assessment phases of the nursing process and were unable to provide clients with holistic care because of the limited time exposure in the clinical area. The emphasis of the findings is that learner nurses need to be allocated a longer time in certain clinical areas for the learner nurses to be able to deliver competent nursing care.

The study findings show that the learner nurses met with the negative attitude of the staff at the psychiatric hospital. They were in the hospital without supervision, and they were not engaged in the procedures related to psychiatric nursing. When the learner nurses try to adjust to the psychiatric clinical setting smoothly, they face challenges. The adjustment of learner nurses is seriously hampered by feelings of abandonment and helplessness from the nursing staff. This is because the learner nurses felt like they were a burden on the nursing staff since they were rarely listened to and were neglected [18].

The learner nurses reported that they were not engaged in the psychiatric procedures by the nurses. The neglect of the learner nurses by the nursing staff in the clinical area is a constant struggle for learner nurses. This is observable when the nurses in the ward do not show interest in the learner nurses and choose not to supervise them. It is also observable when learner nurses are never given feedback to foster their learning in wards [17]. The learner nurses face challenges in the clinical areas where there are no preceptors when the learner nurses need them to assist them with practical nursing skills and the care of psychiatric patients. At times when the learner nurses go to clinical areas, nurses are not aware of their presence in the clinical setting, which leads to tensions in clinical settings. The majority of learner nurses thought the clinical environments were unwelcoming and they rarely felt welcomed [17,18].

5. Recommendations

Based on the findings of this study, it is evident that the learner nurses go through various challenges when they are allocated to a psychiatric hospital. Proper orientation of the learners, when they go to the psychiatric hospital, can be helpful to assist them to get used and adapt to the psychiatric hospital environment. The learning objectives of the learner nurses should be such that the fear of learner nurses is reduced, even before they go to the psychiatric hospital. Regular meetings between the university and psychiatric hospitals about the learning objectives of the learner nurses can be helpful in helping the nurses to understand why the learner nurses are in the hospital and what can be done to enhance their learning while they are in the hospital. The learner nurses need to be given enough time in the psychiatric nursing institution so that they learn and get used to the environment.

A study [16] recommended that nurse educators assist learner nurses in recognizing themselves, building awareness of the patient–nurse relationship, and good communication skills before their initial exposure to a psychiatric environment. The use of standardized patients can also be adopted during simulation to improve the learner nurses' relationship with patients. This means that the learner nurses will learn how to approach patients suffering from mental illness, and they will also learn how to communicate with them in preparation for the clinical environment [19]. Thus, the simulation of psychiatric skills for learner nurses before clinical exposure should be comprehensive so that the learner nurses are ready emotionally and physically to work in a psychiatric hospital.

6. Limitations of the Study

The study was conducted on learner nurses at the University of Limpopo. Therefore, the results cannot be generalized to other learner nurses at other universities.

7. Conclusions

The findings of this study show that the learner nurses go through various challenges during psychiatric clinical exposure. The challenges they face range from discomfort towards mental healthcare users, which include fear of mental healthcare users to uncertainty about the learned psychiatric skills. Clinical environment matters were also raised as a challenge. Learner nurses found the psychiatric institution to be a different clinical environment from what they had been exposed to, and they were only exposed for a limited time. The other challenge was the attitude of clinical staff towards the learner nurses where the professional nurses failed to supervise the learner nurses and were not involving the learner nurses in psychiatric activities. The said challenges can be addressed through proper preparations before the learner nurses can be taken to the clinical institutions. Learner nurses need to be thoroughly prepared before they are exposed to the clinical areas. The hospitals where the learners are allocated must also be prepared to receive learner nurses so that learning continues in the institutions without fail.

Author Contributions: Conceptualization, L.S.H. and C.N.; methodology, M.N.K.; validation, C.N.; formal analysis E.M.M.-T.; investigation, L.S.H. and E.M.M.-T.; resources, C.N. and M.N.K.; data curation, L.S.H.; writing—original draft preparation, L.S.H.; writing—review and editing, L.S.H., C.N., M.N.K. and E.M.M.-T.; visualization, M.N.K.; supervision, E.M.M.-T. and L.S.H. All authors have read and agreed to the published version of the manuscript.

Funding: This research received no external funding.

Institutional Review Board Statement: The study was conducted by the Declaration of Helsinki and approved by the Institutional Review Board (or Ethics Committee) of the Turfloop Research Ethics Committee (TREC/305/2018:PG, University of Limpopo).

Informed Consent Statement: Informed consent was obtained from all learner nurses involved in the study.

Data Availability Statement: The data used backing the findings of this study are available from the corresponding author upon request.

Public Involvement Statement: Participants in the study were the learner nurses from the University of Limpopo. Consent was obtained from all participants to use their personal stories as data.

Guidelines and Standards Statement: This manuscript was drafted against the Consolidated criteria for reporting qualitative research (COREQ) for Qualitative research.

Acknowledgments: The authors acknowledge all the students who took part in this study.

Conflicts of Interest: The authors declare no conflicts of interest.

References

1. Republic of South Africa. *Nursing Act, 2005 (Act No. 33 of 2005; Notice No. 492 of 2006)*; Government Gazette 491(28883); Government Printers: Cape Town, South Africa, 2006.
2. Sunnqvist, C.; Karlsson, K.; Lindell, L.; Fors, U. Virtual patient simulation in psychiatric care—A pilot study of digital support for collaborate learning. *Nurse Educ. Pract.* **2016**, *17*, 30–35. [CrossRef] [PubMed]
3. Ewertsson, M.; Bagga-Gupta, S.; Allvin, R.; Blomberg, K. Tensions in learning professional identities-nursing students' narratives and participation in practical skills during their clinical practice: An ethnographic study. *BMC Nurs.* **2017**, *16*, 48. [CrossRef]
4. Al-Ghareeb, A.; McKenna, L.; Cooper, S. The influence of anxiety on student nurse performance in a simulated clinical setting: A mixed methods design. *Int. J. Nurs. Stud.* **2019**, *98*, 57–66. [CrossRef] [PubMed]
5. Tuvesson, H.; Andersson, E.K. Registered nurse preceptors' perceptions of changes in the organisation of clinical placements in psychiatric care for undergraduate nursing students: A mixed-methods study. *Nurse Educ. Pract.* **2021**, *57*, 103295. [CrossRef] [PubMed]
6. Jamshidi, N.; Molazem, Z.; Sharif, F.; Torabizadeh, C.; Kalyani, M.N. The Challenges of Nursing Students in the Clinical Learning Environment: A Qualitative Study. *Sci. World J.* **2016**, *2016*, 1846178. [CrossRef] [PubMed]

7. Kamel, N.F.; Alshowkan, A.A.; Mohamed, N.; Kamel, F. Nursing Student Experiences of Psychiatric Clinical Practice: A Qualitative Study Emotional intellegence View project comparative of Osce and clinical practical exam View project Nursing Student Experiences of Psychiatric Clinical Practice: A Qualitative. *IOSR J. Nurs. Health Sci.* **2016**, *5*, 60–67. [CrossRef]
8. Lee, C.T.; Padilla-Walker, L.M.; Memmott-Elison, M.K. The role of parents and peers on adolescents' prosocial behavior and substance use. *J. Soc. Pers. Relat.* **2017**, *34*, 1053–1069. [CrossRef]
9. Demir, S.; Ercan, F. The first clinical practice experiences of psychiatric nursing students: A phenomenological study. *Nurse Educ. Today* **2018**, *61*, 146–152. [CrossRef] [PubMed]
10. Günaydin, N.; Arguvanli Çoban, S. Experiences of nursing students during clinical education in mental health clinics: A phenomenological qualitative study. *Nurse Educ. Pract.* **2021**, *54*, 103113. [CrossRef] [PubMed]
11. Bvumbwe, T. Student nurses' preparation for psychiatric nursing practice: Malawian experiences. *J. Ment. Health Train. Educ. Pract.* **2016**, *11*, 294–304. [CrossRef]
12. Motsaanaka, M.N.; Makhene, A.; Ally, H. Student nurses' experiences regarding their clinical learning opportunities in a public academic hospital in Gauteng province, South Africa. *Health SA Gesondheid* **2020**, *25*, 1217. [CrossRef] [PubMed]
13. Gray, J.R.; Grove, S.K. *Burns and Grove's the Practice of Nursing Research-E-Book: Appraisal, Synthesis, and Generation of Evidence*; Elsevier Health Sciences: Amsterdam, The Netherlands, 2020; ISBN 9780323779258.
14. Creswell, J. *Research Design: Qualitative, Quantitative, and Mixed Methods Approaches-John W. Creswell-Google Books*, 4th ed.; Markanich, M., Ed.; SAGE Publications, Inc: Los Angeles, CA, USA, 2014; ISBN 978-1-4522-2609-5.
15. Zhang, X.; Wu, Y.; Sheng, Q.; Shen, Q.; Sun, D.; Wang, X.; Shi, Y.; Cai, C. The clinical practice experience in psychiatric clinic of nursing students and career intention in China: A qualitative study. *J. Prof. Nurs.* **2021**, *37*, 916–922. [CrossRef] [PubMed]
16. Sarikoc, G.; Ozcan, C.T.; Elcin, M. The impact of using standardized patients in psychiatric cases on the levels of motivation and perceived learning of the nursing students. *Nurse Educ. Today* **2017**, *51*, 15–22. [CrossRef] [PubMed]
17. Younas, A.; Essa, C.D.; Batool, S.I.; Ali, N.; Albert, J.S. Struggles and adaptive strategies of prelicensure nursing students during first clinical experience: A metasynthesis. *J. Prof. Nurs.* **2022**, *42*, 89–105. [CrossRef] [PubMed]
18. Laugaland, K.; Kaldestad, K.; Espeland, E.; McCormack, B.; Akerjordet, K.; Aase, I. Nursing students' experience with clinical placement in nursing homes: A focus group study. *BMC Nurs.* **2021**, *20*, 159. [CrossRef] [PubMed]
19. Doolen, J.; Giddings, M.; Johnson, M.; de Nathan, G.G.; Badia, L.O. An Evaluation of Mental Health Simulation with Standardized Patients. *Int. J. Nurs. Educ. Scholarsh.* **2014**, *11*, 55–62. [CrossRef] [PubMed]

Disclaimer/Publisher's Note: The statements, opinions and data contained in all publications are solely those of the individual author(s) and contributor(s) and not of MDPI and/or the editor(s). MDPI and/or the editor(s) disclaim responsibility for any injury to people or property resulting from any ideas, methods, instructions or products referred to in the content.

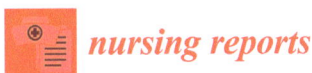

Article

Virtual Active Learning to Maximize Knowledge Acquisition in Nursing Students: A Comparative Study

Guillermo Moreno [1,2], Alfonso Meneses-Monroy [1,*], Samir Mohamedi-Abdelkader [1], Felice Curcio [3], Raquel Domínguez-Capilla [4], Carmen Martínez-Rincón [1], Enrique Pacheco Del Cerro [1,5] and L. Iván Mayor-Silva [1]

[1] Department of Nursing, Faculty of Nursing, Physiotherapy and Podiatry, Universidad Complutense de Madrid, 28040 Madrid, Spain; guimoren@ucm.es (G.M.); samirmoh@ucm.es (S.M.-A.); nutrias@ucm.es (C.M.-R.); quique@ucm.es (E.P.D.C.); limayors@ucm.es (L.I.M.-S.)
[2] Translational Multidisciplinary Cardiovascular Research Group (ICMT), Cardiovascular Research Area, Hospital 12 de Octubre Research Institute (imas12), 28041 Madrid, Spain
[3] Department of Nursing, Faculty of Medicine and Nursing, University of Córdoba, 14004 Córdoba, Spain; felicecrc@gmail.com
[4] La Fe University and Polytechnic Hospital, 46026 Valencia, Spain; raqueldominguezcapilla94@gmail.com
[5] Processes Research Innovation and Information Systems Unit, Directorate of Nursing, Instituto de Investigación Sanitaria San Carlos (San Carlos Health Research Institute-IDISSC), Hospital Clínico San Carlos (San Carlos Clinical Hospital), 28040 Madrid, Spain
* Correspondence: ameneses@ucm.es

Abstract: Background: Nursing students need to acquire knowledge through active methods that promote critical thinking and decision making. The purpose of this study is to analyze whether there are differences in the acquisition of knowledge by nursing students between active face-to-face or virtual teaching methods. Methods: In this comparative study, nursing students enrolled in the psychology course were divided into two groups: a face-to-face group that received active teaching methods and a virtual group. The virtual group was exposed to the Effective Learning Strategy (ELS), which included seminars based on video content through the Virtual Campus and answering questions using the H5P tool. In addition, participants engaged in reflection tasks on the content. Covariate data were collected, and knowledge tests were administered to both groups before and after the course. After three months, subjects were re-evaluated with a final exam to assess content retention. Results: A total of 280 students were randomized. No differences were found in students' scores at the end of the knowledge test or in their final grades in the subject. Having study habits (b = 0.12, $p = 0.03$) and social support from relevant people (b = 0.09; $p = 0.03$) were associated with better post-intervention scores, and inversely with social support from friends (b = −0.12, $p < 0.01$). Final grades were inversely associated with digital safety literacy (b = −0.101, $p = 0.01$). No factors were associated with the scores of each group separately. Conclusions: The ELS virtual active learning model is as effective as face-to-face active learning methods for teaching psychology to first-year nursing students. This study was not registered.

Keywords: competencies; nursing; education; seminars; virtual campus; H5P

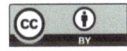

1. Introduction

Nursing education requires the development of critical thinking, initiative in decision making, and analytical skills [1]. Active learning methods have been shown to promote the development of critical thinking [1]. This encourages students to reflect on the content they are learning and to develop decision-making skills. Active learning generally refers to "Any instructional method that engages students in the learning process beyond listening and passive note taking. Active learning approaches focus on developing students' skills and higher-order thinking through activities such as reading, writing, and/or discussion" [2]. The learning process requires the active participation of the student as the main actor in one's own learning [3], allowing the student to learn how to learn, which favors the development of the individual's autonomy [1,4]. In the case of nursing, active learning helps to integrate theory and practice, promotes students' self-confidence, and makes them better prepared for the job market, more empathetic, confident, and creative [1]. Active group learning develops communication skills, evaluation of individual and group learning, and awareness of individual and collective limitations and needs [5]. In addition, the use of artificial intelligence (AI) in facilitating learning outcomes has been shown to improve students' efficiency in active learning and help them solve difficult questions in test scores in combination with flipped classroom [6]. Alternative active learning methodologies, such as hands-on art and 3D atlas-based educational methods employed in anatomy education, have demonstrated notable enhancements in self-efficacy. These approaches foster creative abilities, rendering complex concepts more accessible and comprehensible [7]. Certain active learning methods have been shown to increase students' reported confidence, particularly in the acquisition of specific skills, such as bedside cardiac assessment for medical students [8]. Buzz sessions, an active learning method, make class more interesting, interactive, and help students to enhance their communication and reasoning skills and promote collaborative learning among students [9]. Clinical simulation, an active learning method commonly used in contemporary nursing education, enhances the acquisition of communication skills. Using this technique to train students in palliative care is proving effective in helping them develop meaningful relationships with end-of-life patients and their families [10]. The online problem-based active learning course, utilizing Norton's five-step process for nursing students, resulted in notable changes in educational practices. This not only contributed to enriching the academic experience but also provided opportunities for enhancing the curriculum development process, fostering collaborative learning in a community setting [11]. Recent systematic reviews indicate that active learning increases satisfaction and knowledge acquisition and generally outperforms traditional lecture-based approaches when assessed by both direct and indirect outcome measures [12]. In teaching psychology to undergraduate students using active learning methods, it has been observed that active learning is an effective tool for improving higher-level thinking and knowledge [13]. Students in perceived psychology courses responded favorably to active learning, indicating its effectiveness in achieving its intended goals. Specifically, students expressed positive views of it as an innovative approach to assessing their understanding of course content. They appreciated its role in promoting classroom interactivity, maintaining interest, engagement, and concentration, ultimately contributing to a more enjoyable learning experience [14].

The change in the COVID-19 pandemic has made it possible to implement active educational strategies based on the use of virtual platforms and the development of digital skills [15]. These platforms have been shown to encourage communication between students and teachers, and to promote self-discipline by requiring students to manage and distribute their time in order to carry out the various virtual activities proposed [16]. Despite some inconveniences associated with virtual learning, studies show that students can adapt by using protective coping strategies. This adaptation has led them to appreciate the positive elements of virtual learning, such as flexibility [17]. In a national survey of plastic surgery residents and fellows, the virtual learning format for training was found to be more time-efficient and conducive to expression of opinions compared to an in-person format [18]. Besides, some studies have shown positive effects of virtual learning on nursing knowledge, skills, and attitudes [19]. And it extends to other health care disciplines such as oral and maxillofacial surgery [20], occupational therapy, physiotherapy [21], or medicine [22]. Studies have shown that student satisfaction, performance, and evaluations are similar to those of face-to-face students when teaching psychology [23]. Moreover, online learning in teaching psychology meet the personalized requirements of the students and encourage their learning potential if it is suitable for the students' abilities [24].

The active learning methods used during the COVID-19 pandemic (H5P, infographics, videos, and scape rooms) proved to be effective in engaging nursing students in their learning process [25,26]. However, there is a lack of studies comparing the effectiveness of a face-to-face active learning methodology versus virtual active learning methodologies.

Therefore, the objectives of this study are to analyze whether there are differences in the acquisition of knowledge by nursing students between the two teaching methods.

2. Materials and Methods

2.1. Design

Comparative study of two randomized parallel groups (1:1 ratio) with students of the Bachelor of Nursing program belonging to a University in Madrid (Spain) during the academic year 2022–2023.

2.2. Population

All first-year undergraduate nursing students (N = 280) were included in the study. All students were enrolled in the psychology subject in which this study was conducted. Students were assigned to both groups by simple randomization in a 1:1 ratio. One group (Face-to-face Active Learning Group) received the content (which can be seen in Supplementary Table S1) under the active teaching methodology in the format of case resolution, discussion in small groups (6 participants), presentation of conclusions, explanation, and direct feedback from the teacher. The other group (Virtual Active Learning Group) received the same content virtually under a methodology that we designed and called Effective Learning Strategy (ELS). Inclusion criteria included obtaining written informed consent, while exclusion criteria included not completing all course baseline questionnaires and examinations. A total of 280 first-year nursing students were recruited. After randomization, 38 participants in the virtual group and 14 in the face-to-face group were excluded from the analysis due to noncompliance with baseline questionnaires and examinations (Figure 1).

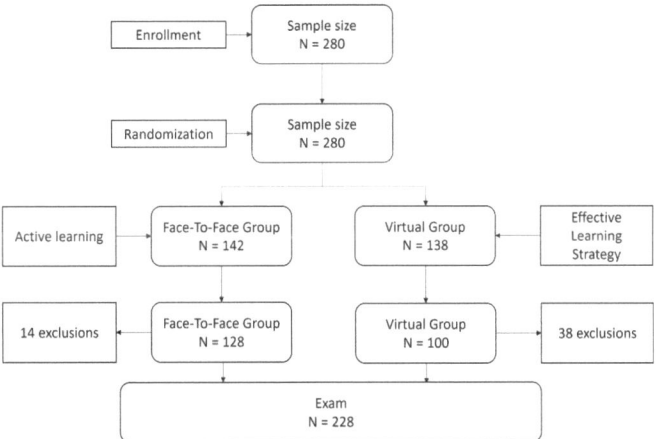

Figure 1. Flowchart.

2.3. Protocol

For the virtual group, five videos were recorded with the content of the subject and edited with the H5P tool, adding multiple choice questions (with three answer choices) related to the content in the same video. The videos were 45 min long and the questions were distributed throughout the videos every 10 min. Students were required to watch the videos and answer questions related to the content. Until the student answered the question correctly, they could not continue watching the video. At the end of watching each video, the student had to complete three tasks: summarize the main idea, justify the usefulness, and argue the application of the content to their future professional role. The aim of these tasks was to improve the student's autonomous thinking and reflection.

Both groups received the content simultaneously in different classrooms at the center. To ensure participation and viewing of the videos, the virtual active learning group was supervised by one of the researchers. The face-to-face group was also supervised, and the students' attendance was closely monitored.

The duration of the study was five sessions of 1 h per day. A prior knowledge test was administered at the beginning of the first session, and knowledge was reassessed with the same test at the end of the last session, in each group. The test consisted of ten multiple-choice questions with three possible answers. The questions were identical for both groups (Table 1). After 3 months, the participants of both groups were evaluated on the content of the interventions in the final examination of the subject.

Table 1. Ten questions of the pre-post knowledge test.

(1) The stimulus that signals to a subject that his behavior will be reinforced is called:
   (a) Excitatory conditioned stimulus.
   (b) Discriminative stimulus (correct).
   (c) Excitatory unconditioned stimulus.

(2) A learning process by classical conditioning in children would be... (points to True option):
   (a) Acquire dislikes, attitudes, phobias, and fears (correct).
   (b) Acquire study habits.
   (c) Eliminate bad habits.

(3) Which of these varieties of learning is known as negative reinforcement?
   (a) Escape or avoidance (correct).
   (b) Positive punishment.
   (c) Extinction.

(4) When the mother picks up the crying child, eliminating what for her is an annoying and unpleasant sound, this is a type of reinforcement:
   (a) Positive reinforcement for the mother.
   (b) Negative reinforcement for the mother (correct).
   (c) A negative punishment for the child.

(5) Maria is a 10-year-old girl who is afraid of dogs, so she avoids going to parks where she can find them. The operant response is:
   (a) Maria's fear when she sees a dog.
   (b) Maria's fear of parks.
   (c) Park avoidance behavior (correct).

(6) A learning process by classical conditioning in children would be... (points to True option):
   (a) Acquire dislikes, attitudes, phobias, and fears (correct).
   (b) Acquire study habits.
   (c) Eliminate bad habits.

(7) The token economy technique is based on a program of:
   (a) Interval.
   (b) Reason (correct).
   (c) Vicarious reinforcement.

(8) The subject who has a hobby of fishing (points to the True option):
   (a) It is being reinforced by a fixed-interval program.
   (b) It is being reinforced by a variable interval program (correct).
   (c) It is being reinforced by a fixed-rate program.

(9) The Time-Out Technique:
   (a) It is based on a negative reinforcement programme.
   (b) It is based on a positive punishment programme.
   (c) It is based on an extinction program (correct).

(10) Positive punishment consists of:
   (a) Tell the subject about their accomplishments and positives before giving them the punishment.
   (b) In applying a very negative stimulus when a behavior that we want to correct is emitted (correct).
   (c) To say that punishment will have a positive purpose for the subject.

2.4. Variables

The independent variable was the type of active learning method (face-to-face vs. virtual). The dependent variables were the final answers to the knowledge test (Table 1) and the grades obtained in the final subject exam (we extract the qualifications from the questions of the exam related to the topics addressed in the interventions). As covariates, before the first session, sociodemographic data and psychosocial aspects were collected through different self-administered questionnaires in order to analyse their possible influence on the outcome of the intervention and on the acquisition of knowledge:

- Sociodemographic data: age, sex, and employment status.
- Learning strategies: measured by the ACRA scale. This is a self-administered instrument designed to assess learning strategies (Román and Gallego, 1994). It consists of forty-four items based on the cognitive theory and made up of three dimensions (cognitive and face-to-face learning strategies, learning support strategies and study habits). It has adequate reliability indices, $\alpha = 0.88$. It is scored on a 4-point Likert scale (1 = never, 2 = sometimes, 3 = almost always, and 4 = always). This scale has not cut-off points, the higher the student scores on each subscale, the more the student uses the learning strategy [27].
- Perceived Social Support: this variable was measured using The Multidimensional Scale of Perceived Social Support (MPSS) was administered (Zimet, 1988). It is a 12-item self-administered instrument that collects information on the individual's perception of the level of social support received in three domains: family, friends, and significant others. Each item is rated on a Likert scale (from 1—strongly disagree to 7—strongly agree). This scale has adequate psychometric indices, with an overall internal consistency of 0.89 and for each of the subscales: family (0.89), friends (0.92), and significant others (0.89). This scale does not have any cut-off points; the higher the person's score on each of the subscales, the higher the person's perceived social support [28].
- Perceived Academic stress: this variable was measured using the Academic Stressors Scale of the Academic Stress Questionnaire (ECEA) (Canabach, Valle, Rodríguez, & Piñeiro, 2008), in its latest version (Cababach, 2016), was administered. It is a self-administered instrument that assesses perceived academic stress through the degree to which major academic stressors affect college students. The scale is composed of fifty-four items grouped into eight dimensions (methodological deficiencies of the teachers, student academic overload, beliefs about academic performance, public interventions, negative social climate, examinations, content value gap, participation difficulties). Each item is rated on a 5-point Likert scale (1 = never, 2 = sometimes, 3 = quite often, 4 = almost always, and 5 = always). The scale has very good psychometric indices (total alpha of the scale of 0.96, with factors ranging from 0.79 to 0.93). This scale does not have any cut-off points; the higher the student's score on each of the subscales, the higher the student's perceived stress from that academic stressor [29].
- Perceived Digital literacy: this variable was measured using the Digital Literacy Questionnaire—IKANOS (Moscoso et al., 2022): The information collection instrument that includes the descriptors of the digComp framework validated by the European Commission in 2013. This self-administered instrument consists of 30 items related to the five competency areas analyzed by digComp (information, communication, content creation, security, and problem solving). Each item is rated on a 5-point Likert scale (1 = seldom or never, 2 = rarely or almost never, 3 = sometimes, 4 = often or almost always, 5 = very often or always). Cronbach's alpha for each of the dimensions ranged from 0.63 to 0.783. This scale has no cut-off points; the higher the person's score on each of the subscales, the higher the person's perceived digital literacy competence [30].

2.5. Statistical Analysis

Descriptive statistics were used by means with standard deviation or median plus interquartile range for quantitative variables and absolute and relative frequencies for qualitative variables. The Shapiro–Wilks test was used to compare normality of quantitative variables. The Student's *t*-test and the ANOVA test were used for paired and independent samples, respectively, to assess within-group differences and between-group differences in knowledge test scores and final subject exam grades. The Chi-Squared test was used for qualitative variables. Repeated measures tests (general linear model) were used to assess differences in scores obtained at each time point. Finally, the association between the covariates and the scores obtained was analysed using stepwise multiple linear regression models. Significance was defined for a 95% confidence interval and a *p*-value < 0.05. Statistical analyses were performed with the SpSS statistical tool (version 25.0).

2.6. Ethical and Legal Considerations

Participants' personal information was anonymized using numerical codes to ensure confidentiality. Data collection took place in October 2022, and surveys were administered anonymously. None of the researchers who participated in the data collection for the study were directly involved in the psychology course to avoid hierarchical relationships with the students. The resulting data were transcribed into a database using the anonymous identification codes previously used for each participant. The tenets of the Declaration of Helsinki on Biomedical Research Involving Human Subjects were followed at all times. Written consent to participate in the study was obtained from each student by the research team outside of class time. The voluntary and anonymous nature of the study was explained. It was also explained that their refusal to participate in the study would have no effect on the psychology subject or any other subject. This study was approved by the University Ethics Committee (internal code: CE_20220915-12_SAL).

3. Results

3.1. Baseline Differences between Groups

The face-to-face group consisted of a final sample of 128 first-year nursing students (81.2% female, 18.8% male) with a mean age of 21.08 (7.01) years; and the virtual group consisted of a final sample of 100 students (81.0% female, 19.0% male) with a mean age of 20.34 (5.43) years.

There were no differences in age ($p = 0.39$) or sex ($p = 0.55$) between the groups. Sociodemographic data are shown in Table 2.

Table 2. Sociodemographic differences between groups.

		Face-to-Face Group N (%)/M (SD)	Virtual Group N(%)/M (SD)	*p*-Value *
Age		21.08 (7.01)	20.34 (5.4)	$p = 0.39$
Sex	Woman	104 (81.2%)	24 (18.8%)	$p = 0.55$
	Man	24 (18.8%)	19 (19.0%)	
Employment status (working)		33 (25.8%)	19 (19.0%)	$p = 0.15$
Marital status	Married	95 (74.2%)	79 (79.0%)	
	Single	10 (7.8%)	4 (4.0%)	$p = 0.47$
	In a relationship (not married)	23 (18.0%)	17 (17.0%)	

* Note: Chi-Squared test used.

Differences in covariate scores between the two groups were analysed to contrast whether both groups were similar in terms of learning strategies (ACRA), perceived social support (MPSS), perceived academic stress (ECEA), and perceived digital health literacy (IKANOS). No statistically significant differences were found between the groups except for three subscales of ECEA with higher perceived stress in the face-to-face group, meaning that both groups are similar in terms of use of learning strategies, social support, and digital literacy (Table 3).

Table 3. Baseline differences in intergroup covariates.

	Face-to-Face Group M (SD)	Virtual Group M (SD)	p-Value *
Cognitive and Face-to-Face Learning Strategies (ACRA)	78.98 (10.38)	81.02 (11.08)	$p = 0.15$
Learning Support Strategies (ACRA)	44.13 (6.38)	43.79 (6.42)	$p = 0.69$
Study Habits (ACRA)	15.64 (3.16)	15.60 (3.13)	$p = 0.92$
Family Social Support (MPSS)	23.24 (4.59)	23.94 (4.23)	$p = 0.24$
Friends Social Support (MPSS)	24.16 (4.47)	24.31 (4.58)	$p = 0.79$
Other Social Support (MPSS)	24.84 (4.01)	24.40 (4.73)	$p = 0.45$
Methodological Deficiencies of Teachers (ECEA)	44.20 (9.98)	41.40 (11.25)	$p = 0.048$
Student Academic Overload (ECEA)	34.17 (9.91)	32.54 (10.12)	$p = 0.22$
Beliefs About Academic Performance (ECEA)	35.26 (11.55)	32.24 (11.62)	$p = 0.045$
Public Interventions (ECEA)	26.86 (9.99)	25.28 (9.92)	$p = 0.24$
Negative Social Climate (ECEA)	13.39 (6.14)	13.75 (6.29)	$p = 0.67$
Examinations (ECEA)	14.16 (3.97)	13.04 (3.99)	$p = 0.035$
Content Value Gap (ECEA)	10.43 (4.09)	10.99 (4.43)	$p = 0.32$
Participation Difficulties (ECEA)	7.71 (3.21)	7.41 (3.46)	$p = 0.49$
Information (IKANOS)	20.61 (4.77)	20.16 (4.48)	$p = 0.47$
Communication (IKANOS)	20.85 (3.69)	21.07 (3.32)	$p = 0.64$
Content Creation (IKANOS)	11.76 (5.20)	12.04 (4.92)	$p = 0.68$
Security (IKANOS)	18.84 (4.34)	18.35 (4.84)	$p = 0.42$
Problem Solving (IKANOS)	20.95 (4.14)	20.24 (4.10)	$p = 0.20$

Note: ACRA: Learning strategies; MPSS: Multidimensional Scale of Perceived Social Support; ECEA: Academic Stressors Scale of the Academic Stress Questionnaire; IKANOS: Digital Literacy Questionnaire. * Student's t-test for independent samples.

3.2. Differences in Pre-Intervention, Post Intervention, Final Scores, Within-Group, and Between-Group Scores

The differences in the pre-intervention and post-intervention scores on the knowledge tests in both groups and in the final exam scores are shown in Figure 2.

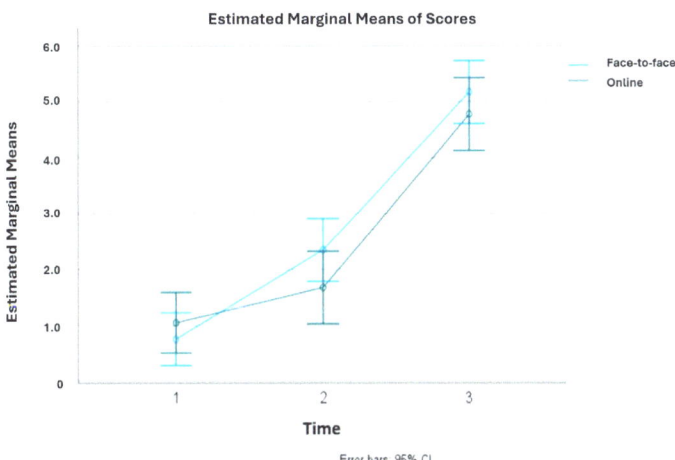

Figure 2. Pre-post knowledge test and final exam grade differences between groups (face-to-face and virtual). Time 1: Pre-intervention; Time 2: Post-intervention; Time 3: Final exam of the subject.

Although the face-to-face group generally showed better results, no statistically significant differences were observed between the groups in pre-intervention test scores (CG: 0.74 ± 2.25 vs. GI: 0.79 ± 2.15, $p = 0.87$), post-intervention scores (CG: 2.20 ± 2.56 vs. GI: 1.55 ± 2.74, $p = 0.10$), or final exam scores (CG: 5.12 ± 2.46 vs. GI: 4.75 ± 2.76, $p = 0.32$). Pre-post improvements were observed in both groups, with a higher mean score improvement in the face-to-face group (mean improvement in CG: 1.72; mean improvement in IG: 0.65, $p = 0.03$).

3.3. Repeated Measures Linear Models

In the general linear model, no statistically significant differences were observed in the interaction time by group, as the lines of both groups crossed from the pre-intervention to the post-intervention period ($p = 0.059$). There were also no significant changes between the groups from the pre-intervention to the final grades of the subject ($p = 0.198$). No overall differences were found between the two groups ($p = 0.35$) (Table 4).

Table 4. Repeated measures linear models.

		Sum of Squares	F	p
Test within-subjects contrasts	Interaction time × group (time pre vs. post)	32.703	3.635	0.059
	Interaction time × group (time post vs. exam)	16.776	1.675	0.198
Test of between-subjects effects	Overall differences between groups	380.871	0.878	0.350

3.4. Predictors of Post-Intervention and Final Grades

To evaluate the influence of the covariates on the post-intervention scores and the subjects' final grades, the variables that predicted the scores in both groups at the post-intervention and final grades were first analysed. According to the multiple linear regression model, in both groups, study habits and social support from relevant people were associated with better post-intervention scores. A non-significant trend was found for employment status (not working). This model explains 11.0% of the variability of the post-test scores (R = 0.33) with the selected variables (Table 5). Regarding the final grades, only the safety variable (IKANOS) was inversely associated with the subject's final exam scores, explaining 2.8% of the variability of the scores (R = 0.181). No associations were found in each group separately for each of the evaluation moments.

Table 5. Multiple linear regression model of post-intervention grades and final subject grades.

		Coefficients B	Std. Error	p
Post-intervention	Does not work	0.734	0.383	0.057
	Study Habits (ACRA)	0.116	0.052	0.026
	Social Support: Friends (MPSS)	−0.123	0.042	0.004
	Social Support: Other Relevant (MPSS)	0.099	0.044	0.026
Exam Notes	Security (IKANOS)	−0.105	0.041	0.012

Note: ACRA: Learning strategies; MPSS: Multidimensional Scale of Perceived Social Support; IKANOS: Digital Literacy Questionnaire.

4. Discussion

Although there is an improvement in knowledge acquisition in the experimental group between the pre-intervention and post-intervention period (mean improvement in IG: 0.65), our results of the linear model of repeated measures comparing knowledge acquisition between groups (F = 0.878; p = 0.350) lead us to conclude that the virtual active learning methodology, based on conducting seminars with audiovisual material created with the H5P tool, does not allow us to obtain better knowledge acquisition. Therefore, it is not more effective as a learning strategy than the face-to-face active learning model. The results of the two methods for teaching psychology in nursing students are similar. Our results do not necessarily mean that H5P and the ELS methodology that we have developed cannot be used to teach psychology to nursing students; in fact, it can be used as it is equally effective in improving learning through knowledge acquisition. Despite the fact that the H5P tool and the virtual active learning methodology it uses have been developed as a methodology to improve active learning [31], not many studies have been conducted with students to evaluate the effectiveness of this tool/methodology. The group of Wehling et al. tested this methodology in the teaching of otolaryngology and concluded that the use of interactive H5P tools through the Moodle LMS provides a great benefit to the teaching process by allowing the easy adaptation of pre-existing video material into appropriate online content [32]. However, these authors do not provide data on the evidence of this tool in improving knowledge acquisition, and therefore our data are not comparable with this study.

According to our findings, students' knowledge would be directly related to students' study habits (β = 0.116; p = 0.026), perceived social support from relevant people (β = 0.099; p = 0.026), and inversely related to friends' support (β = -0.123; p = 0.004) and digital literacy in terms of security (β = -0.105; p = 0.012). There may also be a direct relationship between knowledge acquisition and employment status (β = 0.734; p = 0.057). Although data published in the literature indicate that students who work part-time study fewer hours, this does not affect participation in academic activities or absenteeism [33]. Our findings may differ from those of other recent studies, such as those by Warner et al., who found that employment status was not associated with poorer academic outcomes among nursing students, whereas ethnicity, race, and number of sleep hours were associated with poorer academic outcomes [34]. However, there is controversy on this point, as more classical studies have shown that nursing students who work while studying have worse academic performance, although it has been shown that academic results depend more on the number of hours worked per week than on the actual fact of working, which, as other authors have commented, would not affect part-time workers [35].

We did not find associations with the level of academic stress and the level of knowledge acquired. However, these results should be interpreted with caution, as both groups have baseline differences in perceived academic stress, with higher academic stress in some areas in the face-to-face group, which may have influenced our results.

Our findings regarding social support as a determinant of academic performance (friends' support: β = -0.123; p = 0.004 and relevant people: β = 0.099; p = 0.026) are both consistent and contradictory to other studies, which have found that low social support from friends and family predicts poor academic performance [36], whereas, according to our results, academic performance would only be associated with a lack of support from relevant people and high social support from friends. An alternative explanation for this phenomenon may be related to the use of social applications that students use to connect with their friends. The increase in the number of hours students spend on social media has a negative impact on study habits and academic performance [37,38]. Therefore, social support from friends may interfere with academic performance if students spend too much time on social networks and neglect their academic responsibilities, rather than building social support relationships, which is a predictor of good academic performance [39].

To our knowledge, there are no studies that have examined the role of digital literacy in academic performance (digital literacy in terms of security: β = -0.105; p = 0.012). However, the use of digital learning based on gamification (which is related to high digital literacy) has been associated with better academic performance [40,41]. However, this association does not fully explain the negative association we found between digital literacy in security and academic performance, so these results should be confirmed in future studies.

4.1. Practical Implications

Given that there is evidence that mandatory face-to-face attendance can be counterproductive to academic performance and that student motivation is one of the most important predictors of academic success [42], the results of this study open up the possibility of working with other types of audiovisual learning methods that allow students greater freedom and, as our data show, do not result in a decrease in their academic performance. Conversely, the use of such methods is advisable in specific situations where traditional face-to-face modalities are impractical, such as cases of student overcrowding, insufficient classroom space, or a shortage of teaching staff.

4.2. Limitations

The data in this study came from a single academic centre and a small sample of nursing students. Other studies with more students, including other programs, and with more content should be conducted to contrast and expand our findings regarding the usefulness of using active learning methods to develop educational materials and their impact on students' academic performance. On the other hand, this study did not include student satisfaction with both methodologies, and therefore it was not possible to analyse the influence of motivation.

5. Conclusions

The ELS virtual active learning teaching method through video creation with H5P has shown similar effectiveness to face-to-face active learning methods in knowledge acquisition in psychology among nursing students, so its use in other disciplines could be explored and considered. This opens the possibility of implementing more virtual methods in university environments, allowing students to explore other modalities without compromising their academic performance. Future studies should investigate the influence of student motivation on knowledge acquisition in virtual and face-to-face active methods.

Supplementary Materials: The following supporting information can be downloaded at: https://www.mdpi.com/article/10.3390/nursrep14010011/s1, Table S1: Contents taught in both groups.

Author Contributions: G.M.: Conceptualization, Methodology, Writing—Reviewing and Editing. A.M.-M.: Writing—Reviewing and Editing. C.M.-R.: Data curation, Visualization, Software, Validation. R.D.-C.: Writing—Reviewing and Editing. F.C.: Writing—Reviewing and Editing. S.M.-A.: Writing—Reviewing and Editing. E.P.D.C.: Writing—Reviewing and Editing. L.I.M.-S. All authors have read and agreed to the published version of the manuscript.

Funding: This research received no external funding.

Institutional Review Board Statement: The authors declare that all procedures contributing to this work complied with the ethical standards of the relevant national and institutional committees on human experimentation and with the Helsinki Declaration of 1975 as revised in 2008. All procedures involving human subjects/patients were approved by the Ethics and Research Committee of the Faculty of Nursing, Physiotherapy and Podiatry (approval number: CE_20220915-12_SAL). All participants enrolled in the study were informed verbally and in writing about the objectives and conditions of the study. Written informed consent was obtained from all participants.

Informed Consent Statement: Informed consent was obtained from all subjects involved in the study.

Data Availability Statement: The data presented in this study are available on request from the corresponding author. The data are not publicly available due to data protection policy.

Public Involvement Statement: No public involvement in any aspect of this research.

Guidelines and Standards Statement: This manuscript was drafted against the STROBE for Observational research.

Acknowledgments: We would like to thank the students for their generosity and contribution.

Conflicts of Interest: The authors declare no conflicts of interest.

References

1. Ghezzi, J.F.S.A.; Higa, E.d.F.R.; Lemes, M.A.; Marin, M.J.S. Strategies of active learning methodologies in nursing education: An integrative literature review. *Rev. Bras. Enferm.* **2021**, *74*, e20200130. [CrossRef]
2. Bonwell, C.C.; Eison, J.A. *Active Learning: Creating Excitement in the Classroom*. ASHE-ERIC Higher Education Report No. 1; Washington University, School of Education and Human Development: Washington, DC, USA, 1991.
3. Ledesma, V. El Cambio de Paradigma Educativo y sus Repercusiones en las Instituciones De Educación Superior. *Rev. Electron. Desarro. Competencias* **2011**, *1*, 6–31. Available online: http://redec.utalca.cl/index.php/redec/article/view/56/59 (accessed on 1 October 2023).
4. Escobar-Castellanos, B.; Concha, P.J. Filosofía de Patricia Benner, aplicación en la formación de enfermería: Propuestas de estrategias de aprendizaje. *Educación* **2019**, *28*, 182–202. [CrossRef]
5. Donnelly, P.; Frawley, T. Active learning in Mental Health Nursing—Use of the Greek Chorus, dialogic knowing and dramatic methods in a university setting. *Nurse Educ. Pract.* **2020**, *45*, 102798. [CrossRef]
6. Sanchez-Gonzalez, M.; Terrell, M. Flipped Classroom With Artificial Intelligence: Educational Effectiveness of Combining Voice-Over Presentations and AI. *Cureus* **2023**, *15*, e48354. [CrossRef]
7. HadaviBavili, P.; Ilçioğlu, K. Artwork in anatomy education: A way to improve undergraduate students' self-efficacy and attitude. *Anat. Sci. Educ.* **2023**, *17*, 66–76. [CrossRef]
8. Meisel, J.L.; Chen, D.C.R.; Cohen, G.M.; Bernard, S.A.; Carmona, H.; Petrusa, E.R.; Opole, I.O.; Navedo, D.; Valtchinov, V.I.; Nahas, A.H.; et al. Listen Before You Auscultate: An Active-Learning Approach to Bedside Cardiac Assessment. *Mededportal J. Teach. Learn. Resour.* **2023**, *19*, 11362. [CrossRef]
9. Gilkar, S.A.; Jaan, I.; Arawa, S.; Nyiem, M.P.; Bashir, M. Buzz Session as an Active Learning Method in Medical Undergraduate Physiology Teaching—An Institutional-Based Study. *Med. Sci. Educ.* **2023**, *33*, 1215–1220. [CrossRef]
10. Abad-Corpa, E.; Guillén-Ríos, J.F.; Pastor-Bravo, M.d.M.; Jiménez-Ruiz, I. Assessment of high fidelity simulation with actors in palliative care in nursing students: A mixed methods study. *Enferm. Clin.* **2023**, *33*, 401–411. [CrossRef]
11. Murakami, K.; Ito, M.; Nagata, C.; Tsutsumi, M.; Tanaka, A.; Stone, T.E.; Conway, J. Japanese nurse academics' pedagogical development using collaborative action research. *Nurse Educ. Today* **2023**, *132*, 106001. [CrossRef]
12. Perez, A.; Green, J.; Moharrami, M.; Gianoni-Capenakas, S.; Kebbe, M.; Ganatra, S.; Ball, G.; Sharmin, N. Active learning in undergraduate classroom dental education—A scoping review. *PLoS ONE* **2023**, *18*, e0293206. [CrossRef]
13. Richmond, A.S.; Hagan, L.K. Promoting Higher Level Thinking in Psychology: Is Active Learning the Answer? *Teach. Psychol.* **2011**, *38*, 102–105. [CrossRef]
14. Ioannou, A.; Artino, A.R. Using a classroom response system to support active learning in an educational psychology course: A case study. *Int. J. Instr. Media* **2010**, *37*, 315+. Available online: https://link.gale.com/apps/doc/A273901559/AONE?u=anon~5e1496f4&sid=googleScholar&xid=624b437f (accessed on 1 October 2023).
15. Palomé-Vega, G.; Escudero-Nahón, A.; Lira, A.J. Impacto de una estrategia b-learning en las competencias digitales y estilos de aprendizaje de estudiantes de enfermería. *RIDE Rev. Iberoam. Investig. Y El Desarro. Educ.* **2020**, *11*, e118. [CrossRef]
16. Li, W.; Gillies, R.; He, M.; Wu, C.; Liu, S.; Gong, Z.; Sun, H. Barriers and facilitators to online medical and nursing education during the COVID-19 pandemic: Perspectives from international students from low- and middle-income countries and their teaching staff. *Hum. Resour. Health* **2021**, *19*, 64. [CrossRef]
17. Ollen-Bittle, N.; Sivajohan, A.; Jesin, J.; Gasim, M.; Watling, C. Examining the Effect of Virtual Learning on Canadian Pre-Clerkship Medical Student Well-Being During the COVID-19 Pandemic. *Perspect. Med. Educ.* **2023**, *12*, 488–496. [CrossRef]
18. Arora, J.S.B.; Pham, J.T.B.; Alaniz, L.B.; Khoshab, N.; Tang, C.J. The Implications of Virtual Learning on Plastic Surgery Education: A National Survey of Plastic Surgery Residents and Fellows. *Plast. Reconstr. Surg.-Glob. Open* **2023**, *11*, e5373. [CrossRef]
19. Siah, C.-J.R.; Huang, C.-M.; Poon, Y.S.R.; Koh, S.-L.S. Nursing students' perceptions of online learning and its impact on knowledge level. *Nurse Educ. Today* **2022**, *112*, 105327. [CrossRef]
20. Pandya, R.; AbdelRahman, A.; Fowell, C.; Elledge, R.O. Virtual learning in maxillofacial surgery in the post-COVID world: Where are we now? *Br. J. Oral Maxillofac. Surg.* **2023**, *61*, 623–627. [CrossRef]
21. Smith-Turchyn, J.; Hamilton, J.; Harris, J.E.; Wojkowski, S. Evaluation of virtual problem-based tutorials in healthcare professional education. *Disabil. Rehabil.* **2023**, *14*, 1–8. [CrossRef]
22. Botha, R.; Breedt, D.S.; Barnard, D.; Couper, I. Lessons from innovation in medical education during the COVID-19 pandemic: Student perspectives on distributed training. *Rural Remote Health* **2023**, *23*, 8257. [CrossRef]
23. Waschull, S.B. The Online Delivery of Psychology Courses: Attrition, Performance, and Evaluation. *Teach. Psychol.* **2001**, *28*, 143–147. [CrossRef]
24. Wei, X.; Sun, S.; Wu, D.; Zhou, L. Personalized Online Learning Resource Recommendation Based on Artificial Intelligence and Educational Psychology. *Front. Psychol.* **2021**, *12*, 767837. [CrossRef]

25. Meneses-Monroy, A.; Rivas-Paterna, A.B.; Orgaz-Rivas, E.; García-González, F.J.; González-Sanavia, M.J.; Moreno, G.; Pacheco, E. Use of infographics for facilitating learning of pharmacology in the nursing degree. *Nurs. Open* **2022**, *10*, 1611–1618. [CrossRef]
26. Lackmann, S.; Léger, P.-M.; Charland, P.; Aubé, C.; Talbot, J. The Influence of Video Format on Engagement and Performance in Online Learning. *Brain Sci.* **2021**, *11*, 128. [CrossRef]
27. De la Fuente Arias, J.; Justicia, F.J. Escala de estrategias de aprendizaje ACRA-Abreviada para alumnos universi-tarios. *Rev. Electrónica Investig. Psicoeduc. Y Psicopedag.* **2003**, *1*, 20. Available online: http://www.investigacion-psicopedagogica.org/revista/articulos/2/espannol/Art_2_16.pdf%0Ahttp://www.redalyc.org/pdf/2931/293152877008.pdf (accessed on 10 October 2023).
28. Zimet, G.D.; Dahlem, N.W.; Zimet, S.G.; Farley, G.K. The Multidimensional Scale of Perceived Social Support. *J. Persinal. Assess.* **1988**, *52*, 30–41. [CrossRef]
29. Cabanach, R.G.; Souto-Gestal, A.; Franco, V. Escala de Estresores Académicos para la evaluación de los estresores académicos en estudiantes universitarios. *Rev. Iberoam. Psicol. Y Salud* **2016**, *7*, 41–50. [CrossRef]
30. Paucarchuco, K.M.M.; Espíritu, M.M.B.; Villegas, M.A.N.; Trigos, J.C.S. Competencias digitales y rendimiento académico en estudiantes universitarios: Una mirada desde la educación no presencial: ISBN: 978-0-3110-0019-7, EAN: 9780311000197, UPC: 978031100019, BIC: JNQ. Editor. Tecnocintífica Am. **2023**, 1–135. [CrossRef]
31. Amali, L.N.; Kadir, N.T.; Latief, M. Development of e-learning content with H5P and iSpring features. *J. Phys. Conf. Ser.* **2019**, *1387*, 012019. [CrossRef]
32. Wehling, J.; Volkenstein, S.; Dazert, S.; Wrobel, C.; van Ackeren, K.; Johannsen, K.; Dombrowski, T. Fast-track flipping: Flipped classroom framework development with open-source H5P interactive tools. *BMC Med. Educ.* **2021**, *21*, 135. [CrossRef]
33. Clynes, M.; Sheridan, A.; Frazer, K. Ref: NET_2019_1563: Working while studying: The impact of term-time employment on undergraduate nursing students' engagement in the Republic of Ireland: A cross-sectional study. *Nurse Educ. Today* **2020**, *92*, 104513. [CrossRef]
34. Warner, A.; Barrow, J.; Berken, J.; Williams, A.; Davis, A.; Hurst, H.; Riddle, K. The relationship among BSN students' employment, educational, and health-related characteristics and semester grades: A multi-site study. *J. Prof. Nurs. Off. J. Am. Assoc. Coll. Nurs.* **2020**, *36*, 308–316. [CrossRef]
35. Rochford, C.; Connolly, M.; Drennan, J. Paid part-time employment and academic performance of undergraduate nursing students. *Nurse Educ. Today* **2009**, *29*, 601–606. [CrossRef]
36. Chan, M.-K.; Sharkey, J.D.; Nylund-Gibson, K.; Dowdy, E.; Furlong, M.J. Social support profiles associations with adolescents' psychological and academic functioning. *J. Sch. Psychol.* **2022**, *91*, 160–177. [CrossRef]
37. Shen, J. Social-media use and academic performance among undergraduates in biology. *Biochem. Mol. Biol. Educ.* **2019**, *47*, 615–619. [CrossRef]
38. Sampasa-Kanyinga, H.; Chaput, J.-P.; Hamilton, H.A. Social Media Use, School Connectedness, and Academic Performance Among Adolescents. *J. Prim. Prev.* **2019**, *40*, 189–211. [CrossRef]
39. MacCann, C.; Jiang, Y.; Brown, L.E.R.; Double, K.S.; Bucich, M.; Minbashian, A. Emotional intelligence predicts academic performance: A meta-analysis. *Psychol. Bull.* **2020**, *146*, 150–186. [CrossRef]
40. Tavares, N. The use and impact of game-based learning on the learning experience and knowledge retention of nursing undergraduate students: A systematic literature review. *Nurse Educ. Today* **2022**, *117*, 105484. [CrossRef]
41. Yeh, Y.; Ting, Y. Comparisons of creativity performance and learning effects through digital game-based creativity learning between elementary school children in rural and urban areas. *Br. J. Educ. Psychol.* **2023**, *93*, 790–805. [CrossRef]
42. Mackintosh-Franklin, C. An evaluation into the impact of undergraduate nursing students classroom attendance and engagement with online tasks on overall academic achievement. *Nurse Educ. Today* **2018**, *61*, 89–93. [CrossRef] [PubMed]

Disclaimer/Publisher's Note: The statements, opinions and data contained in all publications are solely those of the individual author(s) and contributor(s) and not of MDPI and/or the editor(s). MDPI and/or the editor(s) disclaim responsibility for any injury to people or property resulting from any ideas, methods, instructions or products referred to in the content.

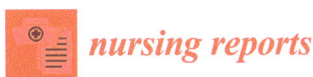

Article

Nomophobia and Its Relationship with Social Anxiety and Procrastination in Nursing Students: An Observational Study

Irene Tárrega-Piquer [1], María Jesús Valero-Chillerón [1,*], Víctor Manuel González-Chordá [1,*], Irene Llagostera-Reverter [1], Águeda Cervera-Gasch [1], Laura Andreu-Pejo [1], Víctor Pérez-Cantó [2], Víctor Ortíz-Mallasén [1], Guillem Blasco-Palau [1] and Desirée Mena-Tudela [1]

[1] Nursing Department, Universitat Jaume I, Avda Sos Baynat s/n, 12071 Castelló de la Plana, Spain; al387383@uji.es (I.T.-P.); llagoste@uji.es (I.L.-R.); cerveraa@uji.es (Á.C.-G.); pejo@uji.es (L.A.-P.); ortizv@uji.es (V.O.-M.); al225789@uji.es (G.B.-P.); dmena@uji.es (D.M.-T.)

[2] Nursing Department, University of Alicante, Carretera San Vicente del Raspeig s/n, 03080 Alicante, Spain; victor.pc@ua.es

* Correspondence: chillero@uji.es (M.J.V.-C.); vchorda@uji.es (V.M.G.-C.)

Abstract: Nomophobia is a phenomenon that describes the fear of not having one's mobile phone accessible. This study aimed to evaluate the presence of nomophobia among nursing students as well as its relationship with procrastination and social anxiety. Methods: An observational, descriptive, cross-sectional study was conducted in a sample of 308 nursing students. Data were collected using the Nomophobia Questionnaire, Academic Procrastination Scale-Short Form, and Social Anxiety Questionnaire for Adults. Additionally, sociodemographic variables related to academic performance and smartphone use were collected. We performed a descriptive, bivariate, and multivariate analysis of the Nomophobia Questionnaire score. Results: 19.5% ($n = 60$) of the students presented with or were at high risk of nomophobic behaviour. Moreover, nomophobic behaviour was positively correlated with high levels of social anxiety ($p < 0.001$), longer daily smartphone usage time ($p < 0.001$), and a high frequency of smartphone checking in class ($p < 0.001$). The predictive variables for nomophobic behaviour included age, variables related to smartphone use, social anxiety levels, work, procrastination tendency, sex, and self-reported average grade. Conclusion: One out of five students in the sample studied presented with or were at high risk of nomophobic behaviour. Additionally, nomophobic behaviour was associated with social anxiety and variables related to smartphone use. This study was not registered.

Keywords: nursing students; Nomophobia; social anxiety; procrastination

1. Introduction

Worldwide, especially in developed countries, there have been recent major digital transformations at the societal level, with the development of Information and Communication Technologies (ICTs) being a major driving factor [1].

Mobile phones and the Internet were introduced at the user level in 1994, followed by a dramatic increase in their use. In 2019, for the first time, the number of mobile phone subscriptions exceeded the number of people. In 2022, there were 8.6 billion mobile subscribers worldwide [2]. Moreover, people aged 15–24 years use the Internet 1.24 times more than the rest of the population [3].

The wide range of possibilities offered by smartphones with Internet access and the worldwide widespread use of these technologies have altered social interactions, work/study environments, and other aspects of daily living, including shopping and banking. However, misuse or abuse of ICTs may have adverse consequences [4], including mobile phone addiction, which is defined as "compulsive mobile phone usage" [5], or nomophobia, which is defined as "the fear of being unable to use or being unreachable via one's smartphone" [6].

Nomophobia, which is derived from "no mobile phone phobia", is a relatively recent concept [7]. Accordingly, it remains in the early research stages [8]. One of the most cited consequences of nomophobia in the literature is anxiety about not having a phone nearby [9,10]. This anxiety can cause continuous distractions [11] and have a negative impact on academic performance [12] due to procrastination derived from inappropriate use of the smartphone, causing dysfunctional behaviours [13,14].

Studies have indicated that nomophobia is more prevalent among women [15] and young people, especially those aged <24 years [7,8,16], which is consistent with the profile of nursing students [17].

Moderate-to-high levels of nomophobia have been reported in nursing students [16,18–20]. Additionally, mobile phone abuse and nomophobia can negatively affect the academic and learning environments of nursing students [21]. The intensive use of smartphones has been related to a decrease in concentration, which leads to an increase in academic procrastination [22], thus increasing distractions [18] and leading to poor academic performance [8,23].

The presence of nomophobia in nursing students acquires special relevance, not only because of the consequences derived from this phenomenon that may have repercussions on the care provided during clinical practice but also because of its proximity to their practice as nursing professionals. Among these consequences, previous studies have observed that the presence of nomophobia leads to poorer communication with patients [24] and with other healthcare professionals [25], an increased risk of dysfunctional attitudes [26], as well as increased distractions [18,27,28], which may compromise patient safety [22]. Accordingly, it is important to address the problem of nomophobia in the academic sphere. Therefore, this study aimed to evaluate the presence of nomophobia in nursing undergraduate students at the Universitat Jaume I, as well as to explore related factors.

2. Materials and Methods

2.1. Design and Sample

This descriptive and cross-sectional observational study was conducted between January and June 2022. We included nursing students at Universitat Jaume I (Castellón de la Plana; Spain).

The study population comprised 480 nursing students (120 students per academic course). The selection criteria were to have an electronic device from which to fill in the data collection booklet and to participate voluntarily and anonymously. Non-probabilistic convenience sampling was conducted by taking advantage of the scheduled classes of the degree program.

2.2. Variables and Instruments

We collected the following variables: sociodemographic variables (age, sex, work activity, and self-reported average grade), variables related to smartphone use (daily smartphone usage time and frequency of smartphone checking in class), and questionnaire-related variables (procrastination tendency, nomophobia, and social anxiety).

Procrastination tendency was measured using the Academic Procrastination Scale-Short Form (APS-SF), which has been adapted for nursing students and validated in Spanish [29]. This instrument comprises five items measured on a 5-point Likert scale (1 = totally agree, 5 = totally disagree). The APS-SF showed internal consistency within the population sample ($\alpha = 0.842$). Given the lack of cut-off values for the questionnaire scores, cluster analysis was performed to determine the number of groups in the sample. A cluster analysis of the APS-SF scores was performed using Ward's method of grouping and using the squared Euclidean distance as a measure. Once the clustering was performed and the resulting categorised variable scores were saved, differences between groups were confirmed by ANOVA test. APS-SF scores of 5–8, 9–16, and 17–25 points correspond to a low, moderate, and high procrastination tendency, respectively.

Nomophobia was assessed using the Nomophobia Questionnaire (NMP-Q). Specifically, we used the Spanish version adapted for nursing students and validated by Gutiérrez-

Puertas et al. [12]. This questionnaire comprises 20 items measured on a 7-point Likert scale (1 = totally agree, 7 = totally disagree). The items were grouped into four dimensions: (1) fear of inability to have immediate access to information; (2) fear of giving up the convenience provided by mobile devices; (3) emotions produced by being unable to remain online; and (4) fear or nervousness for being unable to communicate with other people. The NMP-Q showed global internal consistency in the studied sample (α = 0.945); moreover, the internal consistency of its dimensions was as follows: (1) α = 0.839; (2) α = 0.799; (3) α = 0.937; (4) α = 0.818. This questionnaire has three cut-off points related to the 15th, 80th, and 95th percentiles [30], which yielded four categories (no nomophobia, low risk of nomophobic behaviour, moderate risk of nomophobic behaviour, and nomophobic behaviour).

Finally, social anxiety was measured using the Social Anxiety Questionnaire for Adults (CASO-A30), which has been validated for university students and translated into Spanish [31]. It comprises 30 items measured with a 5-point Likert scale (1 = no discomfort, 5 = a lot of discomfort) and encompasses five dimensions: (1) interaction with the opposite sex; (2) embarrassment or ridicule; (3) interaction with strangers; (4) public speaking/interaction with people in authority; (5) assertive expression of annoyance, displeasure, or anger. The internal consistency for our sample was α = 0.928; additionally, the internal consistency of its dimensions was as follows: (1) α = 0.835; (2) α = 0.680; (3) α = 0.855; (4) α = 0.874; (5) α = 0.774. Given the lack of cut-off values for the questionnaire scores, cluster analysis was performed to determine the number of groups in the sample. The cluster analysis procedure was the same as described for the APS-SF instrument. For the study sample, scores of 44–75, 76–101, and 102–145 points indicate low, moderate, and high anxiety levels, respectively.

2.3. Data Collection

Data were collected through online forms in February 2022, after the first semester exams, which allowed the collection of the average academic grades while the students could still remember them. The study was presented to students in scheduled undergraduate classes, where students were informed of the study's purpose as well as its voluntary and anonymous nature.

2.4. Statical Analysis

Quantitative variables are presented as the mean and standard deviation, while qualitative variables are presented as absolute and relative frequencies. For bivariate analysis, the applicability conditions of the parametric tests were initially checked using the Kolmogorov–Smirnov normality test and the Levene test to study the homoscedasticity. Differences were tested using the Chi-square test for qualitative variables and the Mann–Whitney U test, ANOVA test, or Kruskal–Wallis test, as appropriate, depending on the nature of the variables.

Multivariate ordinal regression analysis was performed to explore the effect of variables on nomophobic behaviour. Due to the absence of previous multivariate regression models in this field of study, this model included variables significantly associated with the outcome variable in bivariate analysis. Next, we performed a bivariate analysis to examine the association between the variables included in the model and the remaining variables. Finally, we designed a location model to study the main effects of all variables and significant bivariate interactions among the included variables in the model. The negative log–log link function was used since the univariate analysis indicated that the lower categories were the most probable. The goodness-of-fit indicators and Nagelkerke's R-squared values were used to determine the quality of the resulting model.

Statistical analyses were performed using the Statistical Package for Social Sciences (SPSS) version 25. Statistical significance was set at $p < 0.05$.

3. Results

3.1. Description of the Sample

The mean age of the overall population was 21.63 ($\pm$5.249) years. Moreover, 88.6% (n = 273) of the students were female, and 15.6% (n = 48) were employed. Notably, 57.5% (n = 177) of the students owned their first smartphone at the age of 12 or 13 years. Additionally, 41.6% (n = 128) of the students reported a daily smartphone usage time of 3–5 h, while 27.9% (n = 86) reported that they checked their smartphones eight or more times during class. Finally, 78.6% (n = 242) of the students reported having notable academic grades (Table 1).

Table 1. Sociodemographic variables and variables related to smartphone use.

Variable/Category	n [1]	% [2]
Sex		
Male	35	11.4
Female	273	88.6
Active in employment		
No	260	84.4
Yes	48	15.6
Self-reported average academic record		
Sufficient	49	15.9
Notable	242	78.6
Excellent	17	5.5
Age at which the first smartphone was owned		
<10	11	3.6
10	12	3.9
11	35	11.4
12	116	37.7
13	61	19.8
14	31	10.1
15	18	5.8
16	12	3.9
17	3	1
$\geq$18	9	2.9
Daily cell phone usage time		
<1	15	4.9
1–3	113	36.7
3–5	128	41.6
>5	52	16.9
Times the smartphone is checked during class		
0–3	107	34.7
4–7	115	37.3
$\geq$8	86	27.9

[1] Absolute frequencies; [2] Relative frequencies.

We found that 22.1% (n = 68) of the students showed a high tendency to procrastinate. Based on the overall NMP-Q score, 4.9% (n = 15) presented nomophobia, and 14.6% (n = 45) were at high risk of nomophobic behaviour, which is consistent with the results obtained in the analysis by dimensions. Regarding social anxiety, 39% (n = 120) and 16.6% (n = 51) of the students presented a high and low risk of developing anxious behaviour, respectively (Table 2).

Table 2. Descriptive analysis of questionnaires.

Questionnaire/Category	n [1]	% [2]
Academic Procrastination Scale-Short Form (APS-SF)		
Low procrastination tendency	70	22.7
Middle procrastination tendency	170	55.2
High procrastination tendency	68	22.1
Nomophobia Questionnaire (NMP-Q)		
No nomophobic behaviour	48	15.6
Low risk of nomophobic behaviour	200	64.9
High risk of nomophobic behaviour	45	14.6
Nomophobic behaviour	15	4.9
Social Anxiety Questionnaire for Adults (CASO-A30)		
Low risk of anxious behaviour	51	16.6
Middle risk of anxious behaviour	137	44.5
High risk of anxious behaviour	120	39

[1] Absolute frequencies; [2] Relative frequencies.

3.2. Bivariate Analysis Results

As shown in Table 3, nomophobic behaviour was positively associated with the daily smartphone usage time and frequency of smartphone checking in class (both $p < 0.001$). In fact, the number of students with nomophobia or at high risk of nomophobic behaviour increases if the number of hours of daily smartphone use increases. Similarly, the number of students with nomophobia or at high risk of nomophobic behaviour also increases if students consult their smartphones more often during lessons. Additionally, the incidence of nomophobic behaviour or high risk of nomophobic behaviour was relatively higher in students aged 21 or 22 years. Nomophobic behaviour showed a significant positive correlation with social anxiety levels (CASO-A30 scores; $p < 0.001$); however, it was not correlated with the tendency to procrastinate ($p = 0.073$).

Table 3. Relationships between nomophobic behaviour and variables under study.

	No Nomophobic Behaviour		Low Risk of Nomophobic Behaviour		High Risk of Nomophobic Behaviour		With Nomophobic Behaviour		p-Value
	n [1]	% [2]	n	%	n	%	n	%	
Daily cell phone usage hours									<0.001 [3]
<1	7	46.7	8	53.3	-	-	-	-	
1–3	24	21.2	75	66.4	11	9.7	3	2.7	
3–5	14	10.9	86	67.2	23	18	5	3.9	
>5	3	5.8	31	59.6	11	21.2	7	13.5	
Times the smartphone is consulted in class									<0.001 [3]
0–3	30	28	69	64.5	5	4.7	3	2.8	
4–6	12	12.4	67	69.1	14	14.4	4	4.1	
7–9	2	5.4	22	59.5	10	27	3	8.1	
≥10	4	6	42	62.7	16	23.9	5	7.5	
Age categorized by percentiles (years old)									0.009 [3]
18–19	8	8.5	68	72.3	16	17	2	2.1	
20	12	17.4	45	65.2	10	14.5	2	2.9	
21–22	13	13.5	59	61.5	14	14.6	10	10.4	
≥23	15	30.6	28	57.1	5	10.2	1	2	
Age at which the first smartphone was owned (years old)									<0.001 [3]
<10	-	-	4	36.4	6	54.5	1	9.1	
10	2	16.7	8	66.7	2	16.7	-	-	
11	3	8.6	19	54.3	12	34.3	1	2.9	
12	22	19	78	67.2	10	8.6	6	5.2	
13	7	11.5	42	68.9	9	14.8	3	4.9	

Table 3. Cont.

	No Nomophobic Behaviour		Low Risk of Nomophobic Behaviour		High Risk of Nomophobic Behaviour		With Nomophobic Behaviour		
	n [1]	% [2]	n	%	n	%	n	%	p-Value
14	4	12.9	24	77.4	3	9.7	-	-	
15	1	5.6	13	72.2	1	5.6	3	16.7	
16	5	41.7	4	33.3	2	16.7	1	8.3	
17	-	-	3	100	-	-	-	-	
≥18	4	44.4	5	55.6	-	-	-	-	
	m [4]	sd [5]	m	sd	m	sd	m	sd	p-Value
Social anxiety	82.5	22.4	96.09	20.42	103.67	17.29	114.07	17.86	<0.001 [6]
Procrastination	11.21	4.83	12.99	4.66	13.20	4.52	12.13	5.01	0.073 [6]

[1] Absolute frequencies; [2] Relative frequencies; [3] Chi-square test; [4] Mean; [5] Standard deviation; [6] Kruskal-Wallis.

Although no differences were observed between the level of procrastination and nomophobic behaviour, it was possible to observe that those students with a higher level of procrastination used their smartphones a greater number of hours daily ($p < 0.001$), as well as a greater number of times during classes ($p = 0.016$). Similarly, social anxiety was associated with the daily smartphone usage time and frequency of smartphone checking in class (both $p < 0.001$) (Table 4).

Table 4. Relationship of smartphone-related variables with procrastination tendency and social anxiety.

	Social Anxiety			Procrastination		
	m [1]	sd [2]	p-Value [3]	m	sd	p-Value [3]
Daily cell phone usage hours			<0.001			<0.001
<1	79.60	25.63		8.93	4.92	
1–3	91.27	21.12		12.15	4.94	
3–5	98.84	21.07		13.35	4.44	
>5	103.77	16.69		13.38	4.21	
Times the smartphone is consulted in class			<0.001			<0.016
0–3	91.63	21.54		11.54	4.78	
4–6	100.95	20.85		12.39	4.50	
7–9	93.19	22.41		14.12	4.37	
≥10	97.16	20.10		14.22	4.56	

[1] Mean; [2] Standard deviation; [3] Kruskal-Wallis.

3.3. Multivariate Analysis Results

Table 5 presents the design of the ordinal logistic regression model and shows the variables included as the main effects and the interactions indicated by the bivariate analysis. The global fit test confirmed improvement of the final model compared with the model in which only the intersection was considered (chi-square test: 271.058; $p < 0.001$). The goodness-of-fit was confirmed using Pearson's test (chi-square:1063.806, $p < 0.001$) and chi-squared test (chi-square: 343.880, $p = 1$). The non-significant deviation indicated no significant difference between the predicted and observed values. Nagelkerke's pseudo-R-square value was 0.677, which indicated that the included variables accounted for 67.7% of the variance.

Despite the good results of the model, only some categories of the "self-reported average academic grade" showed a significant negative correlation with nomophobia severity ($p < 0.001$). Consistent with the bivariate analysis, multivariate analysis indicated no significant relationship between the tendency of procrastination and nomophobia ($p = 0.114$), despite the positive correlation with daily smartphone usage time and frequency of smartphone checking in class (both $p < 0.001$). Additionally, the level of social anxiety was not positively correlated with the number of nomophobic behaviour categories ($p = 0.906$).

Table 5. Ordinal logistic regression model for nomophobic behaviour.

	Location Model	Link Function: Negative Log-Log	
Main Effects			
	Age categorised by percentiles		
	Age at which the first smartphone was owned		
	Times the smartphone is consulted in class		
	Daily cell phone usage hours		
	Social anxiety		
	Active in employment		
	Procrastination		
	Sex		
	Self-reported average academic record		
Interactions included in the model from the bivariate analysis			*p*-Value
	Social anxiety × Active in employment		<0.001 [1]
	Social anxiety × Daily cell phone usage hours		<0.001 [1]
	Times the smartphone is consulted in class × Age categorised by percentiles		<0.001 [2]
	Times the smartphone is consulted in class × Daily cell phone usage hours		<0.001 [2]
	Times the smartphone is consulted in class × Procrastination		<0.001 [1]
	Daily cell phone usage hours × Age categorised by percentiles		<0.001 [2]
	Daily cell phone usage hours × Age with the first smartphone		<0.001 [2]
	Daily cell phone usage hours × Procrastination		0.002 [1]
	Social anxiety × Sex		0.003 [3]
	Daily cell phone usage hours × Self-reported average academic record		0.004 [2]
	Social anxiety × Times the smartphone is consulted in class		0.016 [1]
	Social anxiety × Age categorised by percentiles		0.017 [1]
	Daily cell phone usage hours × Active in employment		0.019 [2]
	Times the smartphone is consulted in class × Age with the first smartphone		0.034 [2]
	Procrastination × Self-reported average academic record		0.044 [4]
Results	Logarithm of the likelihood: 343,880 Chi-square test: 271,058; Pearson Chi: 1063,806 Deviation Chi: 343,880 1 Nagelkerke R-square: 0.677		<0.001

[1] Kruskal–Wallis; [2] Chi-square test; [3] U de Mann–Whitney; [4] ANOVA.

4. Discussion

Nomophobia is a common phenomenon among young people [32] that negatively affects academic performance or social interactions [8,33]. Therefore, it is important to study the prevalence of nomophobia among students to mitigate these negative consequences.

In our study, most students fell within the low-risk percentile for nomophobic behaviour, which is inconsistent with similar reports from previous studies. For example, Gutiérrez-Puertas et al. [12] and Gutiérrez-Puertas et al. [21] reported high nomophobia levels among nursing students, while Çatiker et al. [34] reported moderate levels of nomophobic behaviour. Notably, Gutiérrez-Puertas et al. [12] and Gutiérrez-Puertas et al. [21] did not apply standardised categorisation as proposed by González-Cabrera et al. [30], which was used in the present study. Instead, they simply relied on the mean score being above the median of the possible range of questionnaire scores. Çatiker et al. [34] based their categorisation of the different levels of nomophobia on an ad hoc predetermined classification methodology. In the validation process of an instrument, it is useful to establish cut-off points that facilitate the comparability of the results of different studies, since it is in the lack of use of the cut-off points of the NMP-Q where the potential difference between the results described lies. It would be interesting to advance the validation process of the instrument in future studies, so that cut-off points could be established using consistent methodological tests such as the area under the curve.

Regarding the relationship between anxious behaviour and nomophobia, Mir and Akhtar [11] observed a positive correlation between anxiety levels and nomophobic behaviour, which is consistent with our findings. Additionally, they found that nomophobia in individuals with certain cognitive and sensory distractions worsened their anxiety levels. This could be attributed to a fear of missing out on things (FOMO) resulting from not having a mobile phone, which causes a feeling of nervousness and leads to anxious behaviour [35].

Consistent with the reports by Rengifo-Acho and Arapa-Turpo [36], we observed no relationship between the tendency to procrastinate and levels of nomophobia. This could be attributed to the fact that procrastination is not only related to mobile phone addiction but also may occur for other reasons, including excessive social activities. Consistent with the results by Estremadoiro-Parada and Schulmeyer [37], most students exhibited a low-to-moderate tendency to procrastinate. Additionally, in line with the reports by Gutiérrez-Puertas et al. [21] and Ortega Sanz and Dominguez Lara [38], intensive smartphone use during the day and specifically during classes reduces students' attention and increases procrastination, which negatively affects academic performance [39].

Consistent with the findings by Gutiérrez-Puertas et al. [16] and Çatiker et al. [34], the daily smartphone usage time and frequency of smartphone checking in class were related to nomophobia levels. This is further indicated by the fact that none of the students who used their mobile phones for < 1 h presented nomophobic behaviour.

An integrative literature review conducted by Ramjan et al. [14] showed that one study observed positive correlations between smartphone addiction and anxiety. Nonetheless, there have been inconsistent reports regarding the relationship of smartphone-related variables with anxiety and nomophobia. Future studies are warranted to elucidate the interactions.

Regarding academic performance, the self-reported average academic grade was not related to nomophobia levels. However, Mendoza et al. [39], Rodríguez-García et al. [8], and Gutiérrez-Puertas et al. [21] observed a significant relationship between nomophobia levels and academic performance.

Furthermore, Rodríguez-García et al. [8] suggested that variables such as sex and age are predictors of nomophobia; specifically, they observed high levels of nomophobia among nursing students, which is inconsistent with our findings. This suggests that sex is not correlated with the level of nomophobia.

No previous study on nomophobia levels among nursing studies has performed multivariate analysis, which impedes comparisons of our findings to previous ones. Nonetheless, our findings indicated that the development of nomophobic behaviour is a multifactorial phenomenon. Future well-designed studies are warranted to establish causal relationships. For example, large-scale longitudinal studies are warranted to explore the variables involved and the interactions between them in order to inform interventions for mitigating the development of nomophobic behaviour in nursing students.

It seems interesting to incorporate, from the academic sphere, awareness-raising sessions on the misuse and abuse of technology. Monitoring the use of technology in general and of smartphones, in particular, could be a good starting point from which to become aware of actual individual use. In addition, it would be appropriate to introduce tools that make it easier to manage tasks properly, allowing, for example, temporary distraction blockers to be set up in order to reduce the risk of procrastination through technology. Similarly, in a world that is increasingly connected through technology, appropriate policies on the use of technology in both academic and clinical settings should be established, and access to self-assessments of emotional and mental well-being in relation to technology use should be made available to assess the prevalence of nomophobia.

Limitations

First, this single-centre study was conducted using a non-randomised sample, which limits the generalisability of our findings. Second, we did not perform a longitudinal analysis of the students throughout the program. Therefore, it was not possible to confirm whether the presence of nomophobia negatively affects the learning environment of nursing students, so it would be interesting to explore this hypothesis in future, more methodologically rigorous studies. Similarly, future studies should consider other variables related to nomophobia levels and smartphone use, including sleep quality, self-esteem, loneliness, and communication skills. Despite these limitations, our findings could inform interventions for nomophobic behaviour among young people, which can have negative effects that extend to the professional stage, and thus affect patient care in healthcare practice.

5. Conclusions

Our findings indicated that one in five students nursing undergraduate students in Universitat Jaume I presented with or were at high risk of nomophobic behaviour. Additionally, we identified the following as potential risk factors for nomophobic behaviour: high levels of social anxiety, daily smartphone usage time > 1 h, frequency of smartphone checking in class > 8 times, age of 21 or 22 years, and age at onset of smartphone use of 11–13 years.

Author Contributions: Conceptualization, I.T.-P., M.J.V.-C. and V.P.-C.; methodology, M.J.V.-C., V.M.G.-C. and D.M.-T.; software, I.T.-P., I.L.-R. and V.O.-M.; formal analysis, I.L.-R., V.O.-M. and L.A.-P.; investigation, I.T.-P. and G.B.-P.; data curation, I.T.-P., I.L.-R. and V.O.-M.; writing—original draft preparation, I.T.-P., V.P.-C., G.B.-P. and M.J.V.-C.; writing—review and editing, D.M.-T., V.M.G.-C. and Á.C.-G.; visualization, D.M.-T., V.O.-M. and L.A.-P.; supervision, D.M.-T. and V.M.G.-C. All authors have read and agreed to the published version of the manuscript.

Funding: This work has been funded by the Recognition of Educational Innovation Groups Program of Universitat Jaume I in 2022 (reference 46117).

Institutional Review Board Statement: The study was conducted in accordance with the Declaration of Helsinki and approved by the Deontological Commission of Universitat Jaume I (Spain) with the file number CD/14/2022 on January 2022.

Informed Consent Statement: Informed consent was obtained from all subjects involved in the study.

Data Availability Statement: Data are available upon reasonable request. All necessary data are supplied and available in the manuscript; however, the corresponding author will provide the dataset upon request. All data relevant to the study are included in the article.

Public Involvement Statement: No public involvement in any aspect of this research.

Guidelines and Standards Statement: Not applicable.

Conflicts of Interest: The authors declare no conflict of interest.

References

1. Perron, B.E.; Taylor, H.O.; Glass, J.E.; Margerum-Leys, J. Information and Communication Technologies in Social Work. *Adv. Soc. Work* **2010**, *11*, 67–81. [CrossRef] [PubMed]
2. Taylor, P. Statista Number of Mobile (Cellular) Subscriptions Worldwide from 1993 to 2022. Available online: https://www.statista.com/statistics/262950/global-mobile-subscriptions-since-1993/ (accessed on 1 October 2023).
3. International Telecommunication Union. Measuring Digital Development: Facts and Figures 2021. Available online: https://www.itu.int/en/ITU-D/Statistics/Documents/facts/FactsFigures2021.pdf (accessed on 1 October 2023).
4. Gökçearslan, Ş.; Mumcu, F.K.; Haşlaman, T.; Çevik, Y.D. Modelling Smartphone Addiction: The Role of Smartphone Usage, Self-Regulation, General Self-Efficacy and Cyberloafing in University Students. *Comput. Human Behav.* **2016**, *63*, 639–649. [CrossRef]
5. Kim, S.J.; Byrne, S. Conceptualizing Personal Web Usage in Work Contexts: A Preliminary Framework. *Comput. Human Behav.* **2011**, *27*, 2271–2283. [CrossRef]
6. Notara, V.; Vagka, E.; Gnardellis, C.; Lagiou, A. The Emerging Phenomenon of Nomophobia in Young Adults: A Systematic Review Study. *Addict. Health* **2021**, *13*, 120–136. [CrossRef] [PubMed]
7. Bragazzi, N.L.; Del Puente, G. A Proposal for Including Nomophobia in the New DSM-V. *Psychol. Res. Behav. Manag.* **2014**, *7*, 155–160. [CrossRef] [PubMed]

8. Rodríguez-García, A.-M.; Moreno-Guerrero, A.-J.; López Belmonte, J. Nomophobia: An Individual's Growing Fear of Being without a Smartphone-A Systematic Literature Review. *Int. J. Environ. Res. Public Health* **2020**, *17*, 580. [CrossRef] [PubMed]
9. King, A.L.S.; Valença, A.M.; Silva, A.C.O.; Baczynski, T.; Carvalho, M.R.; Nardi, A.E. Nomophobia: Dependency on Virtual Environments or Social Phobia? *Comput. Human Behav.* **2013**, *29*, 140–144. [CrossRef]
10. Sharma, M.; Mathur, D.M.; Jeenger, J. Nomophobia and Its Relationship with Depression, Anxiety, and Quality of Life in Adolescents. *Ind. Psychiatry J.* **2019**, *28*, 231. [CrossRef]
11. Mir, R.; Akhtar, M. Effect of Nomophobia on the Anxiety Levels of Undergraduate Students. *J. Pak. Med. Assoc.* **2020**, *70*, 1492–1497. [CrossRef]
12. Gutiérrez-Puertas, L.; Márquez-Hernández, V.V.; Aguilera-Manrique, G. Adaptation and Validation of the Spanish Version of the Nomophobia Questionnaire in Nursing Studies. *CIN Comput. Inform. Nurs.* **2016**, *34*, 470–475. [CrossRef]
13. Ge, J.; Liu, Y.; Cao, W.; Zhou, S. The Relationship between Anxiety and Depression with Smartphone Addiction among College Students: The Mediating Effect of Executive Dysfunction. *Front. Psychol.* **2023**, *13*, 103304. [CrossRef] [PubMed]
14. Ramjan, L.M.; Salamonson, Y.; Batt, S.; Kong, A.; McGrath, B.; Richards, G.; Roach, D.; Wall, P.; Crawford, R. The Negative Impact of Smartphone Usage on Nursing Students: An Integrative Literature Review. *Nurse Educ. Today* **2021**, *102*, 104909. [CrossRef] [PubMed]
15. Işcan, G.; Yildirim Baş, F.; Özcan, Y.; Özdoğanci, C. Relationship between "Nomophobia" and Material Addiction "Cigarette" and Factors Affecting Them. *Int. J. Clin. Pract.* **2021**, *75*, e13816. [CrossRef] [PubMed]
16. Gutiérrez-Puertas, L.; Márquez-Hernández, V.V.; São-Romão-Preto, L.; Granados-Gámez, G.; Gutiérrez-Puertas, V.; Aguilera-Manrique, G. Comparative Study of Nomophobia among Spanish and Portuguese Nursing Students. *Nurse Educ. Pract.* **2019**, *34*, 79–84. [CrossRef]
17. Chan, Z.C.; Chan, Y.T.; Lui, C.W.; Yu, H.Z.; Law, Y.F.; Cheung, K.L.; Hung, K.K.; Kei, S.H.; Yu, K.H.; Woo, W.M.; et al. Gender Differences in the Academic and Clinical Performances of Undergraduate Nursing Students: A Systematic Review. *Nurse Educ. Today* **2014**, *34*, 377–388. [CrossRef] [PubMed]
18. Aguilera-Manrique, G.; Márquez-Hernández, V.V.; Alcaraz-Córdoba, T.; Granados-Gámez, G.; Gutiérrez-Puertas, V.; Gutiérrez-Puertas, L. The Relationship between Nomophobia and the Distraction Associated with Smartphone Use among Nursing Students in Their Clinical Practicum. *PLoS ONE* **2018**, *13*, e0202953. [CrossRef]
19. Bartwal, J.; Nath, B. Evaluation of Nomophobia among Medical Students Using Smartphone in North India. *Med. J. Armed Forces India* **2020**, *76*, 451–455. [CrossRef]
20. Farooqui, I.A.; Pore, P.; Gothankar, J. Nomophobia: An Emerging Issue in Medical Institutions? *J. Ment. Health* **2018**, *27*, 438–441. [CrossRef]
21. Gutiérrez-Puertas, L.; Márquez-Hernández, V.V.; Gutiérrez-Puertas, V.; Granados-Gámez, G.; Aguilera-Manrique, G. The Effect of Cell Phones on Attention and Learning in Nursing Students. *CIN Comput. Inform. Nurs.* **2020**, *38*, 408–414. [CrossRef]
22. Eskin Bacaksiz, F.; Tuna, R.; Alan, H. Nomophobia, Netlessphobia, and Fear of Missing out in Nursing Students: A Cross-Sectional Study in Distance Education. *Nurse Educ. Today* **2022**, *118*, 105523. [CrossRef]
23. Dasgupta, P.; Bhattacherjee, S.; Dasgupta, S.; Roy, J.; Mukherjee, A.; Biswas, R. Nomophobic Behaviors among Smartphone Using Medical and Engineering Students in Two Colleges of West Bengal. *Indian J. Public Health* **2017**, *61*, 199. [CrossRef] [PubMed]
24. Cerit, B.; Çıtak Bilgin, N.; Ak, B. Relationship between Smartphone Addiction of Nursing Department Students and Their Communication Skills. *Contemp. Nurse* **2018**, *54*, 532–542. [CrossRef] [PubMed]
25. Katz-Sidlow, R.J.; Ludwig, A.; Miller, S.; Sidlow, R. Smartphone Use during Inpatient Attending Rounds: Prevalence, Patterns and Potential for Distraction. *J. Hosp. Med.* **2012**, *7*, 595–599. [CrossRef] [PubMed]
26. Lee, S.; McDonough, I.M.; Mendoza, J.S.; Brasfield, M.B.; Enam, T.; Reynolds, C.; Pody, B.C. Cellphone Addiction Explains How Cellphones Impair Learning for Lecture Materials. *Appl. Cogn. Psychol.* **2021**, *35*, 123–135. [CrossRef]
27. Cho, S.; Lee, E. Distraction by Smartphone Use during Clinical Practice and Opinions about Smartphone Restriction Policies: A Cross-Sectional Descriptive Study of Nursing Students. *Nurse Educ. Today* **2016**, *40*, 128–133. [CrossRef] [PubMed]
28. Zarandona, J.; Cariñanos-Ayala, S.; Cristóbal-Domínguez, E.; Martín-Bezos, J.; Yoldi-Mitxelena, A.; Hoyos Cillero, I. With a Smartphone in One's Pocket: A Descriptive Cross-Sectional Study on Smartphone Use, Distraction and Restriction Policies in Nursing Students. *Nurse Educ. Today* **2019**, *82*, 67–73. [CrossRef]
29. Brando-Garrido, C.; Montes-Hidalgo, J.; Limonero, J.T.; Gómez-Romero, M.J.; Tomás-Sábado, J. Academic Procrastination in Nursing Students. Spanish Adaptation of the Academic Procrastination Scale-Short Form (APS-SF). *Enfermería Clínica* **2020**, *30*, 371–376. [CrossRef]
30. González-Cabrera, J.; León-Mejía, A.; Pérez-Sancho, C.; Calvete, E. Adaptación Al Español Del Cuestionario Nomophobia Questionnaire (NMP-Q) En Una Muestra de Adolescentes. *Actas Españolas Psiquiatr.* **2017**, *45*, 137–144.
31. Caballo, V.E.; Arias, B.; Irurtia, M.J.; Marta Calderero y Equipo de Investigación CISO-A España. Validación Del "Cuestionario de Ansiedad Social Para Adultos" (CASO-A30) En Universitarios Españoles: Similitudes y Diferencias Entre Carreras Universitarias y Comunidades Autónomas. *Behav. Psychol.* **2010**, *18*, 5–34.
32. Yildirim, C.; Correia, A.P. Exploring the Dimensions of Nomophobia: Development and Validation of a Self-Reported Questionnaire. *Comput. Human Behav.* **2015**, *49*, 130–137. [CrossRef]

33. Moreno-Guerrero, A.J.; Hinojo-Lucena, F.J.; Trujillo-Torres, J.M.; Rodríguez-García, A.M. Nomophobia and the Influence of Time to REST among Nursing Students. A Descriptive, Correlational and Predictive Research. *Nurse Educ. Pract.* **2021**, *52*, 103025. [CrossRef] [PubMed]
34. Çatiker, A.; Bulucu Büyüksoy, G.D.; Özdil, K. Correlation between Nomophobia, Fear of Missing Out and Academic Success. *Bağımlılık Derg.* **2022**, *23*, 283–291. [CrossRef]
35. Farchakh, Y.; Hallit, R.; Akel, M.; Chalhoub, C.; Hachem, M.; Hallit, S.; Obeid, S. Nomophobia in Lebanon: Scale Validation and Association with Psychological Aspects. *PLoS ONE* **2021**, *16*, e0249890. [CrossRef] [PubMed]
36. Rengifo-Acho, D.; Arapa-Turpo, F. *Nomofobia y Procrastinación Académica En Estudiantes Del Cuarto y Quinto Del Nivel Secundario de Una Institución Educativa Pública de La Ciudad de Juliaca*; Universidad Peruana Unión: Juliaca, Peru, 2021.
37. Estremadoiro-Parada, B.; Schulmeyer, M.K. Procrastinación Académica En Estudiantes Universitarios. *Rev. Aportes Comun. Cult.* **2021**, *30*, 51–66. [CrossRef]
38. Ortega Sanz, M.P.; Dominguez Lara, S.A. *Relación Entre El Uso Excesivo de Los Smartphones y La Procrastinación Académica En Estudiantes de Una Universidad Privada*; Universidad San Ignació de Loyola: Lima, Perú, 2020.
39. Mendoza, J.S.; Pody, B.C.; Lee, S.; Kim, M.; McDonough, I.M. The Effect of Cellphones on Attention and Learning: The Influences of Time, Distraction, and Nomophobia. *Comput. Human Behav.* **2018**, *86*, 52–60. [CrossRef]

Disclaimer/Publisher's Note: The statements, opinions and data contained in all publications are solely those of the individual author(s) and contributor(s) and not of MDPI and/or the editor(s). MDPI and/or the editor(s) disclaim responsibility for any injury to people or property resulting from any ideas, methods, instructions or products referred to in the content.

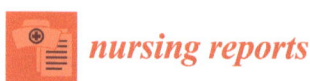

Article

Locus of Control and Self-Directed Learning Readiness of Nursing Students during the COVID-19 Pandemic: A Cross-Sectional Study from Saudi Arabia

Hanan A. Alkorashy [1,2,*] and Hanan A. Alotaibi [3]

[1] Nursing Administration & Education Department, College of Nursing, King Saud University, Riyadh 11362, Saudi Arabia
[2] Nursing Administration Department, Faculty of Nursing, Alexandria University, Alexandria 21526, Egypt
[3] Maternal and Child Health Nursing Department, College of Nursing, King Saud University, Riyadh 11362, Saudi Arabia; halotaibib@ksu.edu.sa
* Correspondence: halkorashy@ksu.edu.sa; Tel.: +96-611-805-0835

Abstract: Background: Coronavirus disease (COVID-19) has caused one of the worst global pandemics in recent decades. It has disrupted education systems worldwide, leading to a forced shift from traditional face-to-face to blended or fully distanced learning, requiring a higher level of student readiness for self-directed learning (SDL) and a more internal locus of control (LOC). Objective: This study explored the relationship between locus of control and level of readiness for SDL among Saudi nursing students and whether the COVID-19 pandemic has impacted this relationship. Methods: A cross-sectional correlational descriptive study was conducted to survey 277 Saudi nursing students enrolled in the bachelor program at one of the reputable universities in Saudi Arabia. An E-questionnaire containing two scales, the Self-Directed Learning Readiness Scale for Nursing Education, and the Locus of Control Scale, was used to collect data in addition to the selected participants' characteristics. Results: Nursing students had a moderate-to-low level of readiness for SDL (mean = 144.0), and the majority had an external LOC. There was a significant association between locus of control and level of readiness for self-directed learning ($r = 0.19 *, p = 0.001$), and the internal locus of control was more significantly associated with self-directed learning ($r = 0.22 *, p = 0.0001$) than with external locus of control. Conclusion: The study findings indicate a propensity of respondents indicating an external locus of control, whereas most of the respondents' reported levels of readiness ranged between low and moderate across all dimensions of self-directed learning. This study was not registered.

Keywords: locus of control; self-directed learning readiness; nursing students; Saudi Arabia; undergraduates; COVID-19 pandemic

Citation: Alkorashy, H.A.; Alotaibi, H.A. Locus of Control and Self-Directed Learning Readiness of Nursing Students during the COVID-19 Pandemic: A Cross-Sectional Study from Saudi Arabia. *Nurs. Rep.* **2023**, *13*, 1658–1670. https://doi.org/10.3390/nursrep13040137

Academic Editors: Antonio Martínez-Sabater, Elena Chover-Sierra, Carles Saus-Ortega and Richard Gray

Received: 14 November 2023
Revised: 22 November 2023
Accepted: 28 November 2023
Published: 30 November 2023

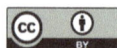

Copyright: © 2023 by the authors. Licensee MDPI, Basel, Switzerland. This article is an open access article distributed under the terms and conditions of the Creative Commons Attribution (CC BY) license (https://creativecommons.org/licenses/by/4.0/).

1. Introduction

As a result of the global Coronavirus disease (COVID-19) pandemic, education has undergone dramatic changes, including in Saudi Arabia. Following COVID-19, academic institutions were forced to shift their efforts to facilitate an abrupt and unexpected transition to online education and assessment [1]. Due to these efforts, e-learning has grown significantly, and nursing education is also now available via digital platforms [2]. The abrupt closure of educational institutions negatively affected students' academic performance and achievement [3,4]. Additionally, it had an adverse effect on university students' lives in all areas [5,6], including nursing students. Students' educational requirements have been affected by heightened stress and anxiety due to COVID-19 [3,7,8]. Saudi Arabian universities had to take immediate action to contain the Coronavirus' spread after unscheduled closures, which began on 9 March 2020.

Similar to other universities around the world, the College of Nursing at the targeted Saudi university was urged to develop online courses with reformatted content and innovative teaching methods within a relatively short timeframe in order to remain active during the COVID-19 pandemic while following preventative protocols and measures [6–9]. Nursing education has evolved from a traditional face-to-face model to one based on virtual learning modes [10]. Virtual education has necessitated the rapid conversion of in-person content into an online format, resulting in a lack of clinical practice opportunities for students, as is usual for traditional nursing programs [6]. Students had to adjust quickly to the challenges associated with virtual classes and assessments as a result of innovative approaches to assessment in this mode of education.

It is therefore necessary for students to consider new methodologies for organizing, preparing, and interacting with their studies in this context. As a result, students became more independent and self-directed when it came to completing course requirements. In online environments, self-directed learning is one of the best predictors of better learning outcomes and academic achievement [11]. A significant amount of research has shown that locus of control (LOC) and self-directed learning (SDL) have significant effects on students' performance and readiness for online learning [11–14].

The locus of control refers to how one believes he or she can control oneself [13], while self-directed learning competency refers to the extent to which one accepts responsibility for learning. To be successful in the future, nursing students must develop their SDL to develop professionalism [15]. With distance learning, students manage a variety of circumstances to succeed academically while taking responsibility for their education [16]. Motivation to learn is derived from the LOC [17]. Global pandemics can negatively affect LOC and affect academic performance [18,19]. A lifelong learning process requires the acquisition of SDL and LOC, which enables individuals to critically evaluate the knowledge they have acquired [20,21]. COVID-19 presents similar challenges [6]. It has been found that integrating lifelong learning strategies into nursing education results in a higher level of education and professional competence [22], which in turn fosters the development of professional values and improves nursing outcomes [21,23]. There is a significant correlation between these traits and Saudi Vision 2030 [23–25]—a road map that seeks to transform health delivery systems, education, and nursing, among many other fields, in order to develop a globally competitive and prosperous country by 2030.

One of the major consequences of the COVID-19 pandemic has been psychological challenges [24]. Students of higher education have also been reported to experience stress and anxiety. During COVID-19, Saudi students were reported to experience moderate to extreme levels of anxiety, with stress levels perceived to be as high as 35% [25]. In addition, recent studies indicate that students' perceived stress is significantly correlated with their locus of control [26,27] and that the locus of control influences their learning outcomes [28,29]. Concomitantly, a high level of academic achievement depends on their internal locus of control [29–34].

Developing SDL skills is crucial in preparing college students for life after graduation [33,35,36]. A study by Cheng et al. indicates that the learner formulates learning objectives, selects appropriate learning strategies, diagnoses learning needs, identifies resources, and evaluates learning outcomes, with or without external support [37]. SDL is utilized in a wide variety of contexts, including problem-solving, contract negotiations, distance learning, and clinical documentation [36]. As a result of SDL, nursing students develop independent learning skills [38]. Moreover, SDL enhances students' self-confidence and motivation, which are vital to both their personal and professional success [39].

Furthermore, it fosters purposeful change, which is essential for effective personal and professional lives [22,40,41]. Lee et al. [22] found that SDL has an important direct impact on nursing students' professional values. Considering the proficiency of the new generation in using the Internet and other information sources, the findings of this study should encourage nursing educators to promote SDL among nursing students. Researchers have consistently observed a strong correlation between SDL use and positive educational outcomes in various countries, including Oman, Saudi Arabia, China, and Turkey [30,32,38,39,42].

Assessing nursing students' self-direction levels can be achieved through the measurement of their self-directed learning readiness (SDLR) [42]. A study conducted at Al-Jouf University in Saudi Arabia revealed that 77% of nursing students demonstrated high levels of SDLR [38], which positively correlated with academic performance in undergraduate nursing students [43]. Despite a study showing no significant gender-based differences in SDLR scores [44], Alsufyani et al. raised concerns about the involvement of factors such as gender, age, and clinical experience in SDLR scores [42].

The concept of LOC has been examined by Rotter in a psychological context [45], referring to individuals' beliefs about their ability to control causality, situations, and life experiences. Among educators, LOC refers to the way students interpret the factors contributing to their academic success. It has been classified by Rotter [45] as internal or external. Individuals with an external LOC attribute their behavior to external influences, while internally oriented individuals believe that their behavior is primarily shaped by their own decisions and efforts. Moreover, LOC plays a critical role in motivating learning [46,47]. It is significantly linked to academic achievement [18], a crucial aspect for students [46]. According to past research, students with high internal LOCs are more likely to persist in online education and achieve higher academic outcomes than students with low internal LOCs [48–50]. By contrast, Harrell and Bower found no significant relationship between LOC and student persistence in online learning [51]. Bahçekapılı and Karaman concluded that external LOC negatively and insignificantly influences students' academic achievement [52]. Even though students with high levels of internal LOC are better prepared for SDL in a traditional classroom setting than students with low levels of internal LOC, regardless of their year of study, Arkan et al. [15] analyzed the influence of internal LOC on nursing students.

Following numerous calls for an exploration of the impact of the COVID-19 pandemic across all sectors, particularly health and education, extensive research has been conducted to determine students' readiness to embrace SDL [30–32,42–44]. While nursing students in Saudi Arabia experienced the COVID-19 pandemic, the literature is unclear as to whether the locus of control affects their SDL readiness level [33,34]. The current study fills this literature gap by exploring nursing students' readiness for SDL and their locus of control. With many nursing schools using online learning platforms to guide student learning, this study's potential contribution is more valuable than ever. Our study is the first to link students' locus of control to their readiness to learn independently during COVID-19 outbreaks in Saudi Arabia. For nursing educators, academic leaders, educational psychologists, and policymakers, this study provides new insights into nursing students' learning.

1.1. Aim of the Study

The purpose of this study was to investigate the relationship between LOC and readiness for SDL among nursing students during the first wave of the COVID-19 pandemic contingency.

1.2. Research Questions

1. What is the nature of the nursing students' locus of control?
2. What is the level of readiness for self-directed learning among nursing students?
3. Is there a relationship between locus of control and readiness for self-directed learning among nursing students during the COVID-19 pandemic?

2. Methods

2.1. Study Design

For this study, a cross-sectional, descriptive, cross-sectional, correlational design was employed to examine relationships among the study variables, SDL and LOC. A cross-sectional study design involves the simultaneous collection and analysis of data for a given phenomenon. As well as describing a concept's status and examining relationships and connections between variables, descriptive correlational studies do not infer causality [53].

2.2. Setting

During the academic year 2020–2021, this study was conducted at the Nursing College, at one of the reputable universities in Saudi Arabia. Currently, this Bachelor of Science in the Nursing program has eight levels, including classroom as well as laboratory activities that are integrated with clinical experiences. The study commenced during the first and the second academic semesters to include students who attended the classrooms, the nursing simulation labs, and/or practiced extracurricular activities.

2.3. Participants

Nursing students enrolled in a bachelor's degree program at a Saudi Arabian university in the 2020–2021 academic year made up the study population (N = 967, 497 females and 470 males). To obtain a sufficient sample size, a convenience sampling methodology was used to select participants. Nursing students registered at the third through the eighth academic levels of their bachelor's program who were available to participate in the survey at the time of data collection were invited. The sample size was calculated using Raosoft website's sample calculator (http://www.raosoft.com/samplesize.html (accessed on 21 October 2023)). To achieve a medium effect size ($f^2 = 0.3$), assuming a significance level (α) of 0.05 and a power of 0.95, a minimum sample size of 276 participants was required to detect the associations among the study variables. In order to account for attrition and/or withdrawals, an additional 5% of participants were invited, leaving 290 participants eligible to participate.

2.4. Eligibility Criteria

Nursing students (both males and females) enrolled at the third through eighth academic levels who were available during data collection and willing to participate in the study were eligible to participate in the study.

2.5. Measurements

Data collection was done using a structured self-report questionnaire, which consisted of three parts. The first part assessed participants' demographic characteristics, including their age, marital status, academic level, permanent residence, and years of experience. The Self-Directed Learning Readiness Scale for Nursing Education, developed by Fisher et al. [36] and revised and validated by Fisher and King [54], was used in the second part of the study. The original version of this scale was created to help nursing educators diagnose the necessary attitudes, abilities, and personality characteristics for nursing students' self-directed learning. There are 40 items on the scale, divided into three categories: self-management (13), learning desire (12), and self-control (15). To measure students' responses, a Likert scale from 1 to 5 was used. For statements that were negatively stated, reverse scoring was implemented (e.g., strongly agree to strongly disagree). Overall scores ranged from 40 to 200, with higher scores reflecting stronger SDL readiness. Various nursing education studies [36,54–56] tested the validity and reliability of the scale, finding Cronbach's alpha values between 0.70 and 0.85. The third part of the questionnaire used the Locus of Control Scale, developed by Dag [57], which was adapted from Rotter's Internal-External Locus of Control Scale [45]. This scale aims to evaluate whether individuals believe that the consequences of their actions are internally or externally influenced. This scale includes 47 items, divided into five categories. They address a range of factors, namely personal control (18 items), belief in chance (11 items), meaninglessness of effort (10 items), fate (3 items), and an unjust world (5 items). The Likert scale was used to rank responses (1 = not at all suitable to 5 = fully suitable). Higher scores indicated a stronger belief in external LOC. Cronbach's alpha and Pearson's product-moment correlation test values of 0.88 and 0.92, respectively, were obtained for the original scale, indicating good internal consistency [57]. According to Beaton et al.'s guidelines for cross-cultural adaptation of self-report measures [58], the Locus of Control Scale was cross-culturally and linguistically adapted. Two bilingual nursing professionals independently translated the scale into English and conducted a blind back-translation into Turkish to determine construct validity. Three academics and two professionals proficient in both Turkish and English reviewed the scale, comparing the back-translations to the original. An online survey was conducted using Google Forms. Ten students participated in a pilot study to assess whether the scales were linguistically clear and culturally coherent in relation to the Saudi Nursing Academic culture and nursing practices. Since the students reported no problems with the clarity or relevance of the questionnaire, the pilot test responses were included in the main study. Cronbach's coefficients for both scales produced a Cronbach's ratio of 0.91 for the locus of control survey and 0.86 for the self-directed learning survey. The CHERRIES Checklist for electronic surveys was followed [59].

2.6. Data Collection Procedure

In accordance with COVID-19 restrictions and the university's epidemic prevention and control policies, and after obtaining approval from the Standing Committee for Scientific Research Ethics at the university, all students were approached online, as physical contact was not possible. Nursing students who consented to participate were emailed a link to the online questionnaire by the college's scientific research unit in coordination with researchers and the college's academic advising committee. Academic Coordinators were given e-survey links to share with students via their academic emails. Data collection took place over a 12-week period from January to March 2021.

2.7. Ethical Considerations

Study approval was obtained from the Institutional Review Board (bioethical committee of the researchers' university) (IRB log number KSU-HE-21-02. Furthermore, approval was obtained from the vice deanship for academic affairs, academic advisors, academic level coordinators, and faculty teaching nursing students. The authors gave their permission to translate the LOC scale and adapt both LOC and RSDL. As part of the consent process, participants were asked to click "agree" to confirm that they understood the purpose, nature, benefits, and uses of the data, as well as their voluntary acceptance of participation in the study. No names or personally identifiable information were collected in survey responses as a means of ensuring anonymity, indicating that the survey did not use the respondent's IP address, username, contact information (e.g., email address), or respondent tracking functionality, and anyone with access to the survey could not relate a response to a respondent [59].

2.8. Statistical Analysis

A statistical analysis was performed with SPSS version 24 (IBM Corp., Armonk, NY, USA). The Excel spreadsheet was screened for missing and incomplete responses using data-cleaning techniques before being declared valid. Continuous quantitative variables were described after assessing their normal distributions, which were assessed using the Shapiro–Wilk test. Means and standard deviations (SD) of normal distribution variables were calculated, while frequencies (f) and percentages (%) were used to describe nominal categorical variables.

A descriptive statistic was used to summarize participants' demographic characteristics and to assess their levels of RSDL and LOC to answer the first and the second research questions, including frequencies, percentages, means, standard deviations, minimums, and maximums. The Pearson product–moment correlation analysis was used to determine the relationship between students' LOC and their readiness for SDL to answer the third research question. The statistical significance threshold was set as ($p < 0.05$).

3. Results

3.1. Descriptive Analysis

Out of the 290 student participants, 277 completed the electronic survey, yielding a response rate of 95.5%. Table 1 presents an overview of the demographic characteristics of participants. Female students constituted 57% of the participants, whereas 43% were male. The mean reported age was 20.5 (±1.6) with the majority (98.6%) being single. Regarding academic level, 29.2% were at Level 6, 23.5% were at Level 7, 16.2% at Level 4, 14% at Level 3, and 10.8% at Level 5. Most participants were residents of Riyadh City and resided in their family homes (92.4%).

Table 1. Demographic characteristics of the study sample ($n = 277$).

Item		Number (%)
Gender		
Male		119 (43)
Female		158 (57)
Age	Mean	20.51 ± 1.6
Marital Status		
Single		273 (98.6)
Married		4 (1.4)
Academic level		
Level 3		39 (14.1)
Level 4		45 (16.2)
Level 5		30 (10.8)
Level 6		81 (29.2)
Level 7		65 (23.5)
Level 8		17 (6.1)
Residence		
Riyadh		255 (92.4)
Outside Riyadh		20 (7.2)

Research Question (1): What Is the Nature of the Nursing Students' Locus of Control?

The locus of control consists of five subscales: personal control, belief in chance, meaninglessness of effort, belief in fate, and belief in an unjust world. Table 2 shows that participants reported higher mean scores for external LOC (X = 86.2, SD = 19.7) than for internal LOC (X = 56.38, SD = 1.45), indicating that participants in this study believed that external factors or forces such as luck would determine their outcomes. The findings revealed that a higher mean score was reported for personal control (X = 56.38, SD = 1.45), followed by belief in chance (X = 32.21, SD = 7.97), belief in meaningless effort (X = 29.37, SD = 7.61), belief in an unjust world (X = 14.76, SD = 3.79), and belief in fate (X = 9.87, SD = 2.61).

Table 2. Results of Locus of Control subscale among the study sample.

Locus of Control Subscales	Minimum	Maximum	Mean (SD)
Personal control	18	90	56.38 (14.47)
Belief in chance	11	55	32.21 (7.97)
Meaningless of the effortfulness	10	50	29.37 (7.61)
Belief in fate	3	15	9.87 (2.61)
Belief in unjust world	5	25	14.76 (3.79)
Internal locus of control	18	90	56.37 (1.45)
External locus of control	29	235	86.2 (19.7)

Research Question (2): To What Extent Are Nursing Students Ready for Self-Directed Learning?

SDL was assessed using three subscales: self-management, desire for learning, and self-control. The results showed that almost 60% of participants reported a low level of readiness for SDL (144 ± 0.49), while 40% reported a high level. For the subscales, the highest mean score was for self-control (X = 52.36, SD = 12.45), followed by desire for learning (X = 45.02, SD = 10.38), and self-management (X = 39.52, SD = 9.04) (Table 3).

Table 3. Self-directed learning among the study participants (n = 277).

SDL Subscales	Minimum	Maximum	Mean (SD)	Level #	(%)
Self-management	13	65	39.52(9.04)	Low	227 (81.9)
				High	50 (18.1)
Desire for learning	12	60	45.02 (10.38)	Low	121 (43.6)
				High	156 (56.4)
Self-control	15	75	52.36 (12.45)	Low	157 (56.7)
				High	120 (43.3)
Total level of readiness for SDL	40	200	144.0 (0.49)	Low	166 (59.9)
				High	111 (40.1)

High level of readiness > 150, Low level of readiness < 150

3.2. Inferential Analysis

Research Question (3): Is There a Relationship between LOC and Readiness for Self-Directed Learning among Nursing Students during the COVID-19 Pandemic?

Correlation analysis demonstrated a significant association between the locus of control and level of readiness for SDL (r = 0.19 *, p = 0.001), with the internal locus of control showing a more substantial association with SDL (r = 0.22 *, p = 0.0001) than the external locus of control, which exhibited no statistically significant association (r = 0.10, p = 0.08). Moreover, the self-directed learning subscales displayed statistically significant correlations with all the locus of control subscales. Table 4 presents the results of the correlation analyses.

Table 4. Correlation analysis of the LOC subscales and SDL readiness subscales.

SDL Readiness Subscales	Locus of Control Subscales					
	Personal Control	Belief in Chance	Meaninglessness of the Effortfulness	Belief in Fate	Belief in Unjust World	Overall LoC
Self-management	r = 0.38 * p = (0.0001)	r = 0.26 * p = (0.0001)	r = 0.25 * p = (0.0001)	r = 0.37 * p = (0.0001)	r = 0.33 * p = (0.0001)	X
Desire for learning	r = 0.33 * p = (0.0001)	r = 0.20 * p = (0.003)	r = 0.21 * p = (0.002)	r = 0.36 * p = (0.0001)	r = 0.24 * p = (0.001)	X
Self-control	r = 0.40 * p = (0.0001)	r = 0.24 * p = (0.001)	r = 0.22 * p = (0.001)	r = 0.39 * p = (0.0001)	r = 0.26 * p = (0.0001)	X
Overall Level of readiness for self-directed learning	Internal LOC		External LOC			X
	r = 0.22 * p = 0.0001		r = 0.10 p = 0.08			r = 0.19 * p = 0.001

* $p \leq 0.05$.

4. Discussion

The study represents the first attempt to evaluate nursing students' LOC and RSDL in Saudi Arabia during the COVID-19 outbreak. As a critical component of problem-solving abilities, SDL significantly contributes to nursing students' clinical competence [60]. This study examined the nature of LOC and readiness for SDL among Saudi nursing students during the initial wave of the COVID-19 pandemic. The association between LOC and SDL readiness was also explored. A major strength of this study is its pioneering use of Dag's [57] English version of the Locus of Control Scale, which was cross-culturally adapted and validated for Saudi culture within the context of the COVID-19 pandemic contingency, resulting in its robustness.

The findings indicated that the study variables had a notable association. According to the current study, the student population's internal locus of control significantly decreased during the COVID-19 pandemic, whereas the external locus of control increased. In similar COVID-19 situations, previous studies found that the external locus of control was more prevalent among university students than the internal locus of control. Those findings are consistent with those of Misamer et al. [61], Wali et al. [62], and Hammoud [63], who observed that most of their studies' participants displayed a higher external LOC than internal LOC, and the LOC shifted substantially from internal to external during the initial COVID-19 outbreak. It is likely that students experienced heightened stress as a result of the challenging nature of the pandemic and the rapid changes associated with this. Those with an external LOC tend to react emotionally and withdraw from stressful situations (such as the COVID-19 pandemic) as compared to those with an internal LOC, who are better able to cope with stress and utilize problem-solving strategies to cope with its consequences [62].

According to the current study, approximately 60% of nursing students were not prepared for SDL. This finding is consistent with Ballad et al. [30], Nazarianpirdosti et al. [64], and Dogham et al. [65]. In contrast, Samarasooriya and colleagues [66] and Alsufyani et al. [42] concluded that students who completed bridging programs or who were registered nurses (RN) were significantly more likely to be ready for SDLs if they had prior clinical experience and self-reliance. Nazarianpirdosti et al. [64] concluded in a previous systematic review that SDL was insufficient in this context. Further, nursing students reported that they were prepared for SDL to a moderate extent.

In comparison to self-management and the desire to learn, self-control was the most influential subscale regarding SDLR readiness. Kaur et al. [67], Aljohani and Fadila [68], and Ballad et al. [30] also found that the majority of participating Indian, Saudi, and Omani students demonstrated high levels of self-control. In other words, nursing students are fully aware of and accountable for their learning processes. According to the current findings, nursing students are capable of managing their own conduct in pursuit of their ideals and goals, as well as effectively handling their learning within the online educational platform (LMS-Bb) available during the pandemic [69]. In contrast, students demonstrated fewer abilities, attitudes, and personality traits related to SDL.

A significant relationship was found between LOC and SDL readiness levels among student participants, particularly in regard to the internal locus of control, according to the current findings. It was found that this internal LOC is significantly related to SDLR and all its dimensions, including self-control, self-management, and learning desire. Several studies have identified the association between internal LOC and academic self-regulation (self-control), including those by Sidola et al. [70], Syahputra and Affandi [71], Javidkar et al. [72] and Arkan et al. [15].

Based on this study, students with external LOCs were found to be low or moderately ready for SDL, and their achievements were largely determined by external circumstances. According to this association, students with an external LOC lack control over their behaviors, emotions, and thoughts in pursuit of long-term goals. In particular, they have difficulty managing their emotions, thoughts, behaviors, and energy in ways conducive to their academic achievement, well-being, and learning [70].

Referring to the findings of this study, the internal LOC was significantly positively associated with self-management and the desire to learn subscales. According to Rafique et al. [73], students who were internally controlled had a greater desire to learn as compared to those with an external LOC in terms of readiness for SDL. Students with an internal LOC showed greater confidence in executing their study plans, requesting timely assistance, managing their time, and setting learning goals, as well as having higher learning expectations. They also demonstrated effective self-management and a genuine interest in learning, as well as demonstrating more innovation, motivation, and sharing their ideas with colleagues and teachers. Externally controlled students, however, did not possess these characteristics and relied more on external support to attain their goals [73].

4.1. Limitations

As the study was conducted at a single nursing college, convenience sampling was used, and the sample size was relatively small, the findings cannot be generalized. The data were collected using an e-questionnaire that measured independent and dependent variables simultaneously. Therefore, it could not provide sound information regarding the causal relationships among the investigated variables. Also, this study focused on the relationship between LOC and SDLR and did not consider external variables that could affect students' SDL, such as mood, health status, or gender. Therefore, further longitudinal studies are required. The findings also heavily depend on the COVID-19 crisis as the main precipitating factor and do not explore the causes of students' external control and lack of SDL readiness.

4.2. Recommendations

The SDL process can be used to improve nursing students' learning processes [22]. Nursing education has been shown to benefit from SDL as it has been significantly associated with academic achievement [74], professional competence, communication self-efficacy, assertiveness, accountability [64,75], and clinical competency [76]. The importance of SDL in nursing education should motivate nursing educators to encourage students to use SDL effectively.

Additionally, since SDL is a crucial component of nursing student clinical competence, it is necessary to encourage this form of education. Prior to incorporating SDL skills into their curriculum, nursing professors should train their students and impart these skills. Through the adoption of problem-based and student-centered curricula, nursing education and teaching methods can be improved. Considering that nursing students are not attaining the desired level of SDL, future studies should investigate factors influencing their readiness for SDL and evaluate the effectiveness of educational interventions. To understand the factors that facilitate and inhibit SDL, qualitative studies are necessary.

4.3. Further Studies

Future studies should replicate this study using different target settings and populations, including nursing and non-nursing health colleges. Although these findings are applicable at the target-setting (college) level, they can be replicated both nationally and internationally.

4.4. Conclusions

As indicated by the preceding findings, respondents had a tendency towards an external locus of control. Most respondents scored poorly across all dimensions of SDL readiness. Although the majority of respondents demonstrated low readiness levels for SDL, self-control is the most important dimension in comparison to self-management and desire to learn. According to this finding, nursing students can regulate their behavior and manage their learning effectively based on the available resources and their goals. A statistical analysis of the data indicated a significant positive correlation between internal locus of control and readiness for SDL. As a result, most student participants with an external LOC may benefit from educational administration and academic staff cultivating an environment where they feel confident that they will be able to execute their study plans, seek timely assistance, manage their time, set goals, and achieve higher learning expectations. They will be more innovative, motivated, inclined to share ideas with colleagues and teachers, skilled at self-management, and enthusiastic about learning.

Considering these findings, nursing students should be encouraged to develop a sense of self-direction so that they can become self-directed learners, a trait that is considered positive among nurses and known to enhance their ability to achieve their desired goals. In addition, the internal locus of control significantly contributes to all three dimensions of SDL readiness in nursing students. Nursing students' internal locus of control is crucial to their developing lifelong learning strategies, becoming more competent in clinical situations, and succeeding in academic life.

4.5. Relevance to Clinical Practice

When the COVID-19 pandemic hit, education methods and learning experiences were abruptly changed, resulting in conflicts among students and educators. A more optimistic view of the COVID-19 contingency is that it created new opportunities for university education. Several factors were taken into consideration when these improvements were implemented, including nursing education. By enhancing students' SDL skills, nursing educators were able to foster students' creativity, interaction, and innovative learning as they transitioned from the traditional in-class learning methods to self-directed learning. Moreover, curricula and academic policies should undergo annual reviews and development. This encourages students to augment their autonomy in learning by directing them to acquire knowledge in a relevant and meaningful manner. Further, students' awareness of their own SDL skills can be developed and enhanced through a variety of mechanisms, including the employment of learning contracts, promoting creative, innovative, critical thinking, and independent learning approaches, implementing contemporary teaching and assessment strategies that encourage SDL, and providing the necessary administrative and technical support systems.

Author Contributions: H.A.A. (Hanan A. Alkorashy) and H.A.A. (Hanan A. Alotaibi) contributed to the design and implementation of the study. H.A.A. (Hanan A. Alotaibi) collected the data and H.A.A. (Hanan A. Alkorashy) analyzed the data. Both researchers H.A.A. (Hanan A. Alkorashy) and H.A.A. (Hanan A. Alotaibi) wrote the final report and manuscript. Both the authors read and approved the version for submission. H.A.A. (Hanan A. Alkorashy) conceived and supervised the project. All authors have read and agreed to the published version of the manuscript.

Funding: This research project was funded by the Research Center of the Female Scientific and Medical Colleges, Deanship of Scientific Research, King Saud University.

Institutional Review Board Statement: The study was conducted in accordance with the Declaration of Helsinki and approved by the Bioethical Committee of the Institutional Review Board of the researchers' university (IRB log number: KSU-HE-21-02). Additional approval was obtained from the vice deanship for academic affairs, academic advisors, academic-level coordinators, and faculty members instructing undergraduate nursing students at academic levels 3rd through 8th.

Informed Consent Statement: Informed consent was obtained from all participants involved in the study.

Data Availability Statement: Data are available upon reasonable request.

Public Involvement Statement: No public involvement in any aspect of this research.

Guidelines and Standards Statement: This manuscript was drafted against the (STROBE) for a cross-sectional study.

Acknowledgments: The authors wish to thank the academic staff and students for their time and authentic participation in this study. The authors are thankful to the Deanship of Scientific Research, College of Nursing Research Center at King Saud University for funding this research. Moreover, the authors extend their appreciation to the Deanship of Scientific Research at King Saud University for the logistic support of this work through the Research Assistant Internship Program, Project number (RAIP-2-20-228). Moreover, the authors extend their acknowledgment to "Prince Naif Health Research Center, Investigator Support Unit" for the language editing service provided. The statistics of this research study were checked prior to submission by a professor of nursing and an expert statistician, Hanem Mohamed (dr.hfm7@gmail.com). Both authors extend their gratitude to her and affirm that the methods used in the data analyses are suitably applied to their data within their study design and context, and the statistical findings have been implemented and interpreted correctly.

Conflicts of Interest: The authors declare no conflict of interest.

References

1. Jack, A.; Smyth, J. Coronavirus: Universities face a harsh lesson. *Financial Times*, 2020. Available online: https://www.ft.com/content/0ae1c300-7fee-11ea-82f6-150830b3b99a(accessed on 21 October 2023).
2. Mustafa, N. Impact of the 2019-20 Coronavirus pandemic on education. *Int. J. Health Prefer. Res.* **2020**, *5*, 31–44.
3. Onyema, E.M.; Eucheria, N.C.; Obafemi, F.A.; Sen, S.; Atonye, F.G.; Sharma, A.; Alsayed, A.O. Impact of Coronavirus Pandemic on Education. *J. Educ. Pract.* **2020**, *11*, 108–121. [CrossRef]
4. Tran, T.; Hoang, A.-D.; Nguyen, Y.-C.; Nguyen, L.-C.; Ta, N.-T.; Pham, Q.-H.; Pham, C.-X.; Le, Q.-A.; Dinh, V.-H.; Nguyen, T.-T. Toward sustainable learning during school suspension: Socioeconomic, occupational aspirations, and learning behavior of vietnamese students during COVID-19. *Sustainability* **2020**, *12*, 4195. [CrossRef]
5. Plakhotnik, M.S.; Volkova, N.V.; Jiang, C.; Yahiaoui, D.; Pheiffer, G.; McKay, K.; Newman, S.; Reißig-Thust, S. The Perceived Impact of COVID-19 on Student Well-Being and the Mediating Role of the University Support: Evidence from France, Germany, Russia, and the UK. *Front. Psychol.* **2021**, *12*, 642689. [CrossRef]
6. Agu, C.F.; Stewart, J.; McFarlane-Stewart, N.; Rae, T. COVID-19 pandemic effects on nursing education: Looking through the lens of a developing country. *Int. Nurs. Rev.* **2021**, *68*, 153–158. [CrossRef]
7. Son, C.; Hegde, S.; Smith, A.; Wang, X.; Sasangohar, F. Effects of COVID-19 on college students' mental health in the United States: Interview survey study. *J. Med. Internet Res.* **2020**, *22*, e21279. [CrossRef]
8. Gadi, N.; Saleh, S.; Johnson, J.A.; Trinidade, A. The impact of the COVID-19 pandemic on the lifestyle and behaviours, mental health and education of students studying healthcare-related courses at a British university. *BMC Med. Educ.* **2022**, *22*, 115. [CrossRef]
9. XinhuaNet. Chinese Universities to Remain Closed until Effective Control of Epidemic. 2020. Available online: http://www.xinhuanet.com/anglad/2020-02/25/c_138814715.htm (accessed on 24 September 2023).
10. Lade, K.; Gaglani, H.; Khare, S.; Muley, S.; Jha, R. Perception of student's towards online learning during COVID-19 pandemic. *Int. J. Health Sci.* **2022**, *6*, 473–480. [CrossRef]
11. Torun, E.D. Online Distance Learning in Higher Education: E-Learning Readiness as a Predictor of Academic Achievement. *Open Prax.* **2019**, *12*, 191–208. [CrossRef]
12. Martin, F.; Stamper, B.; Flowers, C. Examining student perception of readiness for online learning: Importance and confidence. *Online Learn. J.* **2020**, *24*, 38–58. [CrossRef]
13. Boddu, V.K.; Rebello, A.; Chandrasekharan, S.V.; Rudrabhatla, P.K.; Chandran, A.; Ravi, S.; Unnithan, G.; Menon, R.N.; Cherian, A.; Radhakrishnan, A. How does "locus of control" affect persons with epilepsy? *Epilepsy Behav.* **2021**, *123*, 108257. [CrossRef]
14. Dwilestari, S.; Zamzam, A.; Susanti, N.W.M.; Syahrial, E. The Students' Self-Directed Learning in English Foreign Language Classes During The Covid-19 Pandemic. *J. Lisdaya* **2021**, *17*, 38–46. [CrossRef]
15. Arkan, B.; Ünsal Avdal, E.; Yildirim Sari, H. Locus of Control and Self Directed Learning Relation on Nursing Students. *Int. J. Caring Sci.* **2016**, *9*, 514–519.
16. Naseer, N.; Kanwal, S.; Habib, Z. Exploration of Distance Learners' Nature of Locus of Control: Qualitative Analysis. *Glob. Educ. Stud. Rev.* **2020**, *V*, 20–31. [CrossRef]
17. Sigurvinsdottir, R.; Thorisdottir, I.E.; Gylfason, H.F. The impact of COVID-19 on mental health: The role of locus on control and internet use. *Int. J Environ. Res. Public Health* **2020**, *17*, 6985. [CrossRef]
18. Alipio, M.M. Academic success as estimated by locus of control and motivation. *edArXiv* **2020**, 1–9. Available online: https://edarxiv.org/smf84/ (accessed on 21 October 2023).
19. Hosseini, S.N.; Mirzaei Alavijeh, M.; Matin, B.K.; Hamzeh, B.; Ashtarian, H.; Jalilian, F. Locus of control or self-esteem; Which one is the best predictor of academic achievement in Iranian college students. *Iran J. Psychiatry Behav. Sci.* **2016**, *10*, e2602. [CrossRef]
20. Cadorin, L.; Ghezzi, V.; Camillo, M.; Palese, A. The self-rating scale of self-directed learning tool: Findings from a confirmatory factor analysis. *J. Nurs. Educ. Pract.* **2016**, *7*, 31–37. [CrossRef]
21. Qalehsari, M.Q.; Khaghanizadeh, M.; Ebadi, A. Lifelong learning strategies in nursing: A systematic review. *Electron Physician* **2017**, *9*, 5545–5550. [CrossRef]
22. Lee, S.; Kim, D.H.; Chae, S.M. Self-directed learning and professional values of nursing students. *Nurse Educ. Pract.* **2020**, *42*, 102647. [CrossRef]
23. Mlambo, M.; Silén, C.; McGrath, C. Lifelong learning and nurses' continuing professional development, a metasynthesis of the literature. *BMC Nurs.* **2021**, *20*, 62. [CrossRef]
24. Hossain, S.F.A.; Nurunnabi, M.; Sundarasen, S.; Chinna, K.; Kamaludin, K.; Baloch, G.M.; Khoshaim, H.B.; Sukayt, A. Sociopsychological impact on angladeshi students during COVID-19. *J. Public Health Res.* **2020**, *9*, 1911. [CrossRef]
25. Khoshaim, H.B.; Al-Sukayt, A.; Chinna, K.; Nurunnabi, M.; Sundarasen, S.; Kamaludin, K.; Baloch, G.M.; Hossain, S.F.A. How students in the Kingdom of Saudi Arabia are coping with COVID-19 pandemic. *J Public Health Res.* **2020**, *9*, 1898. [CrossRef]

26. Ganjoo, M.; Farhadi, A.; Baghbani, R.; Daneshi, S.; Nemati, R. Association between health locus of control and perceived stress in college student during the COVID-19 outbreak: A cross-sectional study in Iran. *BMC Psychiatry* **2021**, *21*, 529. [CrossRef]
27. Mori, M.; Seko, T.; Ogawa, S. Association of Social Capital and Locus of Control with Perceived Health during the COVID-19 Pandemic in Japan. *Int. J. Environ. Res. Public Health* **2022**, *19*, 9415. [CrossRef]
28. Al Mulhim, E.N. Flipped Learning, Self-Regulated Learning and Learning Retention of Students with Internal/External Locus of Control. *Int. J. Instr.* **2020**, *14*, 827–846. [CrossRef]
29. Animba, I.E.; Ezema, E.O.; Chukwu, P.N.; Nwobodo, P. Locus of control, self-efficacy and academic performance of secondary school students in enugu state, Nigeria. *GPH-Int. J. Educ. Res.* **2022**, *5*, 45–52. Available online: http://www.gphjournal.org/index.php/er/article/view/707/471 (accessed on 21 October 2023).
30. Ballad, C.A.C.; Labrague, L.J.; Cayaban, A.R.R.; Turingan, O.M.; Al Balushi, S.M. Self-directed learning readiness and learning styles among Omani nursing students: Implications for online learning during the COVID-19 pandemic. *Nurs. Forum* **2022**, *57*, 94–103. [CrossRef]
31. Luu, T.M.V. Readiness for Online Learning: Learners' Comfort and Self-Directed Learning Ability. *Int. J. TESOL Educ.* **2022**, *2*, 213–224. [CrossRef]
32. Titiek Murniati, C.; Hartono, H.; Cahyo Nugroho, A. Self-directed Learning, Self-efficacy, and Technology Readiness in e-learning Among University Students. *KnE Soc. Sci.* **2022**, *7*, 213–224. [CrossRef]
33. Oktrivina, A.; Achmadi, A.; Hendryadi, H. Ethical Perceptions Of Accounting Students: The Role of The God Locus of Control, Moral Disengagement, and Love of Money. *J. Reviu Akunt. Dan Keuang.* **2022**, *12*, 144–158. [CrossRef]
34. Uysal, Ş.K.; Karadağ, H.; Tuncer, B.; Şahin, F. Locus of control, need for achievement, and entrepreneurial intention: A moderated mediation model. *Int. J. Manag. Educ.* **2022**, *20*, 100560. [CrossRef]
35. Almomani, L.M.; Halalsheh, N.; Al-Dreabi, H.; Al-Hyari, L.; Al-Quraan, R. Self-directed learning skills and motivation during distance learning in the COVID-19 pandemic (case study: The university of Jordan). *Heliyon* **2023**, *9*, e20018. [CrossRef]
36. Fisher, M.; King, J.; Tague, G. Development of a self-directed learning readiness scale for nursing education. *Nurse Educ. Today* **2001**, *21*, 516–525. [CrossRef]
37. Cheng, S.F.; Kuo, C.L.; Lin, K.C.; Lee-Hsieh, J. Development and preliminary testing of a self-rating instrument to measure self-directed learning ability of nursing students. *Int. J. Nurs. Stud.* **2010**, *47*, 1152–1158. [CrossRef]
38. El-Gilany, A.H.; Abusaad, F.E.S. Self-directed learning readiness and learning styles among Saudi undergraduate nursing students. *Nurse Educ. Today* **2013**, *33*, 1040–1044. [CrossRef]
39. Morris, T.H. Self-directed learning: A fundamental competence in a rapidly changing world. *Int. Rev. Educ.* **2019**, *65*, 633–653. [CrossRef]
40. Deacon, A.K.; Larson, N.; O'Neill, T.A.; Brennan, R.W.; Eggermont, M.; Rosehart, W. The self-directed learning readiness scale, conscientiousness, and the prediction of engineering student learning outcomes. In Proceedings of the Canadian Engineering Education Association (CEEA), University of Calgary, Canmore, AB, Canada, 8–11 June 2014. Available online: https://ojs.library.queensu.ca/index.php/PCEEA/article/view/5953 (accessed on 3 November 2023)
41. O'Shea, E. Self-directed learning in nurse education: A review of the literature. *J. Adv. Nurs.* **2003**, *43*, 62–70. [CrossRef]
42. Alsufyani, A.M.; Aboshaiqah, A.; Moussa, M.L.; Baker, O.G.; Aljuaid, D.A.; Alshehri, F.A. Self-Directed Learning Readiness of Students in Bridging Nursing Programs in Saudi Arabia—A Descriptive Study. *Midwifery Pract. Nurs. Stand* **2020**, *1*, 16–23. [CrossRef]
43. Alotaibi, K.N. The learning environment as a mediating variable between self-directed learning readiness and academic performance of a sample of saudi nursing and medical emergency students. *Nurse Educ. Today* **2016**, *36*, 249–254. [CrossRef]
44. Alharbi, H.A. Readiness for self-directed learning: How bridging and traditional nursing students differs? *Nurse Educ. Today* **2018**, *61*, 231–234. [CrossRef]
45. Rotter, J.B. Generalized expectancies for internal versus external control of reinforcement. *Psychol. Monogr.* **1966**, *80*, 1–28. [CrossRef] [PubMed]
46. Ozuome, C.C.; Oguzie, A.E.; Mokwelu, O.B.; Anyamene, A. Locus of Control as a Correlate of Secondary School Students' Academic Achievement in Imo State, Nigeria. *J. Guid. Couns. Stud.* **2020**, *4*, 374–385. [CrossRef]
47. Yang, J.C.; Lin, Y.L.; Liu, Y.C. Effects of locus of control on behavioral intention and learning performance of energy knowledge in game-based learning. *Environ. Educ. Res.* **2017**, *23*, 886–899. [CrossRef]
48. Lowes, S.; Lin, P. Learning to learn online: Using locus of control to help students become successful online learners. *J. Online Learn. Res.* **2015**, *1*, 17–48.
49. Association for the Advancement of Computing in Education (AACE): Waynesville, NC, USA Retrieved 2 October 2023. Available online: https://www.learntechlib.org/primary/p/149845/ (accessed on 3 November 2023).
50. Brammer, S.E.; Punyanunt-Carter, N.M. Getting the attention of online learners. *Commun. Educ.* **2022**, *71*, 155–157. [CrossRef]
51. Harrell, I.L.; Bower, B.L. Student characteristics that predict persistence in community college online courses. *Am. J. Distance Educ.* **2011**, *25*, 178–191. [CrossRef]
52. Bahçekapılı, E.; Karaman, S. A path analysis of five-factor personality traits, self-efficacy, academic locus of control and academic achievement among online students. *Knowl. Manag. E-Learn.* **2020**, *12*, 191–208. [CrossRef]
53. Polit, D.F.; Beck, C.T. *Nursing Research: Generating and Assessing Evidence for Nursing Practice*, 11th ed.; LWW: Philadelphia, PA, USA, 2021.

54. Fisher, M.J.; King, J. The self-directed learning readiness scale for nursing education revisited: A confirmatory factor analysis. *Nurse Educ. Today* **2010**, *30*, 44–48. [CrossRef]
55. Abdulghani, H.; Almndeel, N.; Almutawa, A.; Aldhahri, R.; Alzeheary, M.; Ahmad, T.; Alshahrani, A.; Hamza, A.; Khamis, N. The validity of the self-directed learning readiness instrument with the academic achievement among the Saudi medical students. *Int. J. Med. Sci. Public Health* **2019**, *9*, 44–50. [CrossRef]
56. Fooladvand, M.; Nadi, M. Validation of revisited self-directed learning readiness scale for nursing education among Iranian nursing and midwifery students. *J. Educ. Health Promot.* **2019**, *8*, 266. [CrossRef]
57. Dag, I. Locus of Control Scale: Scale Development, Reliability and Validity Study. *Turk Psikol. Derg.* **2002**, *17*, 77–90.
58. Beaton, D.E.; Bombardier, C.; Guillemin, F.; Ferraz, M.B. Guidelines for the process of cross-cultural adaptation of self-report measures. *Spine* **2000**, *25*, 3186–3191. [CrossRef] [PubMed]
59. Eysenbach, G. Improving the Quality of Web Surveys: The Checklist for Reporting Results of Internet E-Surveys (CHERRIES). *J. Med. Internet Res.* **2004**, *6*, e34. [CrossRef] [PubMed]
60. Manuaba, I.B.A.P.; No, Y.; Wu, C.C. The effectiveness of problem based learning in improving critical thinking, problem-solving and self-directed learning in first-year medical students: A meta-analysis. *PLoS ONE* **2022**, *17*, e0277339. [CrossRef]
61. Misamer, M.; Signerski-Krieger, J.; Bartels, C.; Belz, M. Internal Locus of Control and Sense of Coherence Decrease During the COVID-19 Pandemic: A Survey of Students and Professionals in Social Work. *Front. Sociol.* **2021**, *6*, 705809. [CrossRef] [PubMed]
62. Wali, O.; Vanka, S.; Vanka, A.; Alamoudi, N. Locus of Control—A Dental Student Perspective. *J. Evol. Med. Dent. Sci.* **2021**, *10*, 573+. Available online: https://link.gale.com/apps/doc/A654627503/AONE?u=anon~7d130064&sid=googleScholar&xid=83e38e55 (accessed on 2 October 2023). [CrossRef]
63. Hammoud, S. Achievement Motivation and Its Relationship to Locus of Control among Nursing Faculty Students in Tishreen University. *Tishreen Univ. J.-Med. Sci. Ser.* **2021**, *43*, 95–109. Available online: https://journal.tishreen.edu.sy/index.php/hlthscnc/article/view/10558 (accessed on 2 October 2023).
64. Nazarianpirdosti, M.; Janatolmakan, M.; Andayeshgar, B.; Khatony, A. Evaluation of Self-Directed Learning in Nursing Students: A Systematic Review and Meta-Analysis. *Educ. Res. Int.* **2021**, 2112108. [CrossRef]
65. Dogham, R.S.; Elcokany, N.M.; Ghaly, A.S.; Dawood, T.M.A.; Aldakheel, F.M.; Llaguno, M.B.B.; Mohsen, D.M. Self-directed learning readiness and online learning self-efficacy among undergraduate nursing students. *Int. J. Afr. Nurs. Sci.* **2022**, *17*, 100490. [CrossRef]
66. Samarasooriya, R.C.; Park, J.; Yoon, S.H.; Oh, J.; Baek, S. Self-directed learning among nurse learners in Sri Lanka. *J. Contin. Educ. Nurs.* **2019**, *50*, 41–48. [CrossRef]
67. Kaur, A.; Lakra, P.; Kumar, R. Self-directed Learning Readiness and Learning Styles among Nursing Undergraduates. *Nurs. Midwifery Res. J.* **2020**, *16*, 45–50. [CrossRef]
68. Aljohani, K.A.; Fadila, D.E.S. Self-directed learning readiness and learning styles among Taibah nursing students. *Saudi J. Health Sci.* **2018**, *7*, 153–158. [CrossRef]
69. Nwagu, E.N.; Enebechi, J.C.; Odo, A.N. Self-Control in Learning for Healthy Living Among Students in a Nigerian College of Education. *Sage Open* **2018**, *8*, 371. [CrossRef]
70. Sidola, S.; Saini, S.; Kang, T.K. Locus of control as correlate of self-regulation among college students. *Pharma Innov. J.* **2020**, *9*, 116–122.
71. Syahputra, I.A.; Affandi, G.R. The Relationship between Internal Locus of Control and Academic Self-Regulation in Class 11 Vocational High School Students in Sidoarjo. *Psikologia J. Psikol.* **2021**, *6*, 1–6. [CrossRef]
72. Javidkar, S.; Divsar, H.; Saeedi, M.; Hadavizadeh, A. A Path Analysis of Autonomy Supportive Teaching, EFL Learners' Willingness to Communicate, Self-Regulation, Academic Engagement, and Perceived Locus of Control. *J. Mod. Res. Engl. Lang. Stud.* **2022**, *9*, 25–49.
73. Rafique, G.M.; Mahmood, K.; Warraich, N.F.; Rehman, S.U. Readiness for Online Learning during COVID-19 pandemic: A survey of Pakistani LIS students. *J. Acad. Librariansh.* **2021**, *47*, 102346. [CrossRef] [PubMed]
74. Avdal, E.Ü. The effect of self-directed learning abilities of student nurses on success in Turkey. *Nurse Educ. Today* **2013**, *33*, 838–841. [CrossRef]
75. Song, Y.; Yun, S.Y.; Kim, S.A.; Ahn, E.K.; Jung, M.S. Role of self-directed learning in communication competence and self-efficacy. *J. Nurs. Educ.* **2015**, *54*, 559–564. [CrossRef]
76. Taylor, T.A.H.; Kemp, K.; Mi, M.; Lerchenfeldt, S. Self-directed learning assessment practices in undergraduate health professions education: A systematic review. *Med. Educ. Online* **2023**, *28*, 2189553. [CrossRef]

Disclaimer/Publisher's Note: The statements, opinions and data contained in all publications are solely those of the individual author(s) and contributor(s) and not of MDPI and/or the editor(s). MDPI and/or the editor(s) disclaim responsibility for any injury to people or property resulting from any ideas, methods, instructions or products referred to in the content.

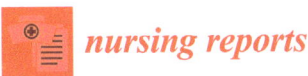

Article

Evaluation of the Use of Project-Based Learning in the Nursing Degree

Laura Parra-Anguita [1], María Dolores López-Franco [1,*], Juan Miguel Martínez-Galiano [1,2], Manuel González-Cabrera [1], Sara Moreno-Cámara [1] and Nani Granero-Moya [1]

[1] Department of Nursing, Faculty of Health Sciences, University of Jaén, 23071 Jaén, Spain; lparra@ujaen.es (L.P.-A.); jgaliano@ujaen.es (J.M.M.-G.); mgonzale@ujaen.es (M.G.-C.); smcamara@ujaen.es (S.M.-C.); jgranero@ujaen.es (N.G.-M.)

[2] Consortium for Biomedical Research in Epidemiology and Public Health (CIBERESP), 28029 Madrid, Spain

[*] Correspondence: mlfranco@ujaen.es; Tel.: +34-953213667

Abstract: Project-based learning (PBL) is a teaching methodology that allows students to acquire knowledge and competencies through the completion of projects that respond to real-life problems. The aims of this study were to evaluate the acquisition of knowledge of students of the Aging Nursing subject through a PBL-based intervention and determine the degree of student satisfaction with the use of this methodology. A mixed, quasi-experimental, pre–post study was conducted without a control group using an educational intervention based on PBL and descriptive phenomenology with content analysis of the experiences reported after it. A knowledge questionnaire about nursing homes was administered before the start of the intervention. After using PBL to carry out the subject project, the same knowledge questionnaire and an ad hoc questionnaire on satisfaction, assessment, and improvement aspects were administered. In total, 111 nursing students participated. The difference in knowledge after the educational intervention was significant. The mean pre-intervention score was 5.56, SD 1.50, and the mean post-intervention score was 7.14, SD 1.59, ($p = 0.001$). In total, 74% of the students stated that they were very satisfied with the use of this methodology. The students had a positive perspective on the process of acquiring knowledge that PBL allows. The students improved their knowledge about the planning and management of nursing homes with the use of the project-based learning teaching methodology. They were very satisfied with said activity. Teachers must be adequately trained for the correct implementation of this teaching methodology. This study was not registered.

Keywords: project-based learning; higher education; satisfaction; nursing; nursing homes

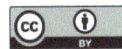

1. Introduction

Project-based learning (PBL) is a teaching methodology that allows students to acquire knowledge and competencies through the development of projects that respond to real-life problems. The PBL methodology is considered an innovation in higher education and facilitates the development of professional competencies in university students [1].

PBL can potentially increase students' sense of responsibility and control over their learning. PBL provides an environment in which students are engaged in a continuous hands-on activity in which they give and receive constructive feedback, guidance, and support from other students and teachers. Multiple interactions are also performed in addition to conflict resolution [2]. Likewise, the exploratory process involved in PBL can develop multiple cognitive abilities and problem-solving abilities, thus achieving effective learning [3]. The use of PBL in mixed learning environments, where different teaching methodologies centered on the student or the teacher are combined, allows nursing students to acquire practical skills that provide many benefits for nursing work in real-care settings.

PBL is associated with "students' ability to discover problems", while practical training based on experience is associated with "students' ability to sustain action". This didactic methodology focuses on the creation and development of specific projects that should not be confused with another similar methodology in terms of student participation and motivation, which is problem-based learning aimed at solving problems [4].

Research in nursing students through project-based learning is being used through different methodological designs. We found studies with a quasi-experimental study design using a pretest–posttest design of a non-equivalent control group [5] or accounts of experiences on the use of PBL in the course of educational actions in nursing practice [6]. PBL is also being used in professional-level training for quality-of-care improvement by using project-based learning to teach advanced practice nurses [7].

This methodology has been used in research at the university level with Nursing degree students [2,4], Early Childhood Education students [1,8], and Pedagogy degree students [9], as well as in different geographical areas, such as Japan [4], Taiwan [3], the United States [10], and Spain [8,9].

Project-based learning is perceived as more effective at increasing knowledge acquisition and problem-solving compared to other methodologies, such as conferences, flipped classrooms, or problem-based learning [10]. In addition, students are more satisfied with courses that use this student-centered learning pedagogy [10,11]. The effects of PBL are difficult to specify as they depend on the subject areas, the duration of the implementation in the classroom, and the circumstances of the institution or center where they are carried out [12], as well as the size of the group, the use of technological support, or the educational stage where it is implemented [13].

As a consequence of the aging population and social changes in family structures, many of the elderly are cared for in nursing homes. There is a great lack of knowledge about the functioning and organization of these institutions among nursing students. This aspect made us consider the organization of the Aging Nursing subject (this is the name given to Gerontological Nursing in our curriculum) to address issues such as the preparation and organization of nursing homes, their financing, and resources (professional and material) as well as the quality of care they should provide using this active learning methodology based on projects through the creation of a nursing home for the elderly. Therefore, the following objectives were proposed:

- Evaluate the acquisition of knowledge about nursing homes for older adults using the PBL methodology.
- To assess the experience and satisfaction with the use of the PBL teaching method in the Aging Nursing subject of the Nursing degree.

2. Materials and Methods

2.1. Design

This research used a mixed-methods approach combining a quantitative and a qualitative study. First, a quasi-experimental, pre–post study without a control group was developed through an educational intervention based on PBL with students of Nursing of Aging in the Nursing degree at the University of Jaén (Spain). This was followed by a descriptive phenomenological study of the experiences reported after the educational intervention.

2.2. Sample

The target population included all the students enrolled in the Aging Nursing course at the University of Jaén: a total of 133, of whom 106 were women and 27 were men, and their ages ranged from 20 to 52 years. This subject is taught in the third year of the nursing degree, which consists of 4 courses. It was decided to include all these students since the completion of the project was part of the overall evaluation of the course. The final sample consisted of students who voluntarily participated in the research.

2.3. Procedures

In the subject of Nursing Aging, topics related to physiological changes in the aging process, the most prevalent diseases in the elderly, or social and healthcare resources in the community are dealt with. In relation to this last aspect, the project is developed through the PBL methodology. The students were divided into 30 work groups. The students self-selected into groups of 4 to 5 students. The random selection of students was not possible; therefore, it is a non-probabilistic convenience sample. Each work group had to carry out a project that consisted of planning and managing a residential care facility for older adults where quality gerontological care would be provided. Every decision in the planning and management of the nursing home had to be based on the necessary gerontological care. This project was carried out during the course of the entire subject (one semester), and it was elaborated through PBL. The students received a document that provided general indications for the elaboration of the work. It included the structure to be presented, information on the requirements for the presentation, and the way in which the evaluation would be carried out. In order to ensure that all the members of the group participated equally, they were told that the final grade was individual. The calculation of the final grade was the result of the project grade (group work) and a personal grade (± 2 points on the group grade) obtained from the evaluation of the presentation and a defense made by each of the students in the group. The project should have contained the following sections: Section 1.—Opinions or previous knowledge about what a nursing home for the elderly is; Section 2.—Research and information search; and Section 3.—Development of the project of the nursing home (organization, operation, staff, programs, activities, etc.). A maximum length of 15 pages was required for the Word document. The main researcher and coordinator of the subject in question carried out two mandatory group tutorials with all the students, where both the purpose of the project and the indications to carry it out were explained as well as the possibility of participating in the research on a voluntary basis. The realization of the project was mandatory as it was part of the evaluation of the subject.

The 30 groups made the final presentation of the project, for which they had about 20 min to present their project and 10 min of debate and discussion with the rest of their classmates and teachers. On the first day of class, all the students filled out a self-administered multiple-choice questionnaire on knowledge related to nursing homes. At the end of the project (ten weeks later), and after their presentation, they all filled out the same knowledge questionnaire and a survey, which collected their degree of satisfaction, their perspectives on the most positive and negative aspects of carrying out the project, and improvements to be implemented. Both questionnaires were developed by the research team.

2.4. Instruments

The data were collected through self-administered questionnaires prepared ad hoc through an online tool (Google form) for subsequent analysis. The knowledge questionnaire consisted of 11 multiple-choice questions with 4 response options where only one was true. The content of the questionnaire was based on the main topics of the subject and, in particular, on the aspects relevant and necessary for the development of the project. The maximum achievable score was 11 points. The second questionnaire addressed the satisfaction of the students using a 5-point Likert scale (from "not at all satisfied" to "very satisfied") in relation to carrying out this training activity and their perception of the organization and planning of the information presented by the students themselves (from "very bad" to "very good" or "I would have liked the structure to be previously determined by the teacher"). Open questions were asked about the most positive and negative aspects of carrying out the training activity, the suggestions for the next PBL project, and the usefulness of the PBL methodology (Table 1).

Table 1. Questions from both questionnaires.

Pre–Post Questionnaire Elderly Nursing Homes
1. The minimum ratio of nurses required in a nursing home in a situation of dependency is:
2. Which of the following services is mandatory for a nursing home with more than 60 residents?
3. The following principles shall govern the operation of nursing homes for the elderly in a situation of dependency:
4. Which of the following protocols should be in the Junta de Andalucía's nursing homes?
5. What is the primary goal of active aging?
6. The "giants of geriatrics" are:
7. Regarding Comprehensive Geriatric Assessment, point out the WRONG statement.
8. How often should an ear canal examination be recommended for the elderly population?
9. Which of the following technical aids does the Junta de Andalucía provide subsidy for?
10. Which of the following is not an objective of preventive gerontology?
11. Abuse suffered due to abandonment or neglect of duties in the care of a person is referred to as:
Satisfaction Questionnaire. Nursing Homes Project
Indicate the degree of satisfaction with this training activity.
Indicate the most positive and negative aspects of this training activity (indicate at least 1 positive and 1 negative aspect).
What suggestions for improvement do you have for future calls?
How did you feel about deciding on the organization and planning of the information presented?
Doing this project as a group has seemed to me:
Working with this project-based learning methodology has helped you to... (you can check more than one option)

2.5. Data Analysis

The data normality was verified using the Kolmogorov–Smirnov test. Both univariate and bivariate analyses were performed. Descriptive analysis of each variable was performed by calculating the measures of frequency and percentage for the qualitative variables and the measures of central tendency and dispersion for the quantitative variables. To compare the means of knowledge before and after the intervention, the Student's t test or the Wilcoxon test was used, after checking for normality. Inadequately or incompletely completed questionnaires were excluded. The software package SPSS v.24 was used to perform the analyses. The significance level was set at 0.05.

The responses of the qualitative dimensions were analyzed by means of a content analysis based on the proposal of Taylor et al. [14]. The qualitative analysis of the speeches followed an iterative process in several stages: exhaustive reading of the texts, fragmentation of those considered significant into units of analysis, and subsequent coding. Finally, the codes were grouped into thematic categories taking the open questions asked in the questionnaire as a reference. To support the credibility of the study, triangulation was performed in the analysis by two different researchers [15].

2.6. Ethical Considerations

At the beginning of the project, the students were informed of the objectives, and their participation was voluntary at all times. By completing the questionnaires, they gave their consent to participate in the research. The students had the right to withdraw at any time without affecting their academic situation. The confidentiality of their personal data was maintained. The data collected was used for specific research purposes and is kept in the custody of the researchers. Ethical approval was granted by the Research Ethics Committee of the University of Jaen (SEPT.22/1.PRY).

3. Results

The final study sample consisted of 111 students enrolled in the Aging Nursing course (133 enrolled). The response rate was 83.4%.

Of these, 78.03% were women, while 21.97% were men. The age range was from 20 to 52 years. The mean age was 22.51 (SD 5.85).

3.1. Knowledge Acquisition

The mean pre-intervention score was 5.56 (SD 1.50), and the mean post-intervention score was 7.14 (SD 1.59). The distribution of the score difference variable had a different distribution than the normal KMO (0.095 p = 0.015), so the Wilcoxon non-parametric tests were performed, showing the existence of a significant difference between them ($Z = -6.018$ $p = 0.001$).

Regarding the questionnaire items, we can say that the item that showed the greatest learning was item 2 *"Which of the following services is mandatory for a residential care facility for older adults with more than 60 users"* (only 2 students answered it correctly in the pre-questionnaire and 54 in the post-questionnaire). The item that most students answered correctly in the pretest was item 5 *"What is the primary objective of active aging?"* (106 students answered it correctly in the pre-questionnaire and 111 in the post-questionnaire). The item with the least variation in terms of the number of correct answers was item 11 *"The mistreatment suffered due to abandonment or failure to fulfill the care obligations of a person is called"* (the number of correct answers only increased by two between the pre and post-questionnaires).

3.2. Student Satisfaction

Regarding the questionnaire on satisfaction with carrying out this learning activity, 74.4% indicated that they were *Very satisfied*, 24.8% were *Satisfied*, and 0.8% were *Somewhat satisfied*. When asked what they thought of deciding on the organization and planning of the information presented, 65.9% stated that it was *Very good*, 20.2% stated *Good*, 13.2% stated *I would have liked the structure to be previously determined by the teacher*, and 0.8% thought it was *Very bad*. Another aspect asked was their opinion about carrying out this group project. In total, 76% stated it was *Very useful*; 23.3% stated it was *Useful*, and 0.8% stated it was *Not at all useful*.

The open questions inquired about the students' experience in carrying out the proposed activity using PBL. The categories and subcategories emerged as shown below.

3.2.1. Positive Aspects/Strengths of Work Using PBL

The students had a positive perspective regarding the operation of nursing homes (protocols, organization, strengths, and weaknesses), the work carried out by different professionals within them, and the possibilities for improvement that they present or the real needs of older adults (Table 2). Carrying out the project contributed to modifying many students' perceptions about the reality of nursing homes/residential care facilities for older adults. The knowledge acquired allowed them to identify which organizational and care models are the most appropriate to implement in a residential facility for older adults, as well as the elements for improvement.

The following are some examples of student comments:

(A positive aspect has been) *"knowing the current situation regarding the nursing homes and knowing how they are organized, care and activities offered"*.

"Be aware that (nurses) must be the axis of care for older adults".

"A positive aspect is the change in mentality regarding nursing homes".

"Positively assess the function of a nursing home".

The students' positive remarks about the project include an emphasis on the acquisition of the predetermined competencies, the teamwork that allows sharing and discussing different experiences and opinions, and the joint exposition that facilitated hearing the proposals and reflections of their classmates. The promotion of critical thinking, the autonomy to carry out the activity or the construction of one's own learning, and the awareness of the evolution in their knowledge about the needs of older adults also emerged.

"Sharing our ideas generates a broader and more open knowledge about nursing homes".

"By getting involved, we learn so much more".

"The freedom for creativity has allowed us to really enjoy it".

Table 2. Positive aspects of work using PBL.

Related to Residential Care Facilities	
Knowledge Regarding	Functioning Professionals' work Needs of older adults Improvement possibilities in nursing homes
Recognizing The Value of Nursing Homes	
Project as a Facilitator of a Change in Perspective	
Regarding the Learning Method	
Group Work	Shared experiences Distribution of work
Active Role of Student	Development of own learning Awareness of learning evolution Autonomy Satisfaction Encouragement of critical thinking

3.2.2. Negative Aspects/Weaknesses of PBL Work Project

Regarding the weaknesses or negative aspects of the project, the students especially referred to the need to spend a lot of time carrying it out, as well as the little time allocated for presenting their project. In some cases, they alluded to the proposed page limit. For some, it was insufficient, while for others it was excessive. Also, they referred to a lack of specific instructions on the development of the project.

"The negative aspect is that it has taken me a considerable time of work".
"We didn't have the time to be able to present well what our ideal nursing home would be like".
"I would have liked a slightly longer page limit".

On the other hand, they found that similar ideas appeared during the presentation of the different groups, and this repetition was considered a negative point. In addition, some of the common drawbacks of joint work were pointed out, such as the difficulty in meeting or coordinating tasks.

"It gets a bit repetitive because the ideas are similar".
"It is difficult to meet to do group work".

Another issue the students reported was the frustration that appears when confronting their work with reality and verifying that it remains more on the plane of the ideal or utopian.

"We have proposed an ideal nursing home, and in reality, they really are not like we suggest".

Finally, there were those who thought that the information provided to carry out the activity was a negative aspect, as they considered that it was insufficient and inaccurate to develop the project.

"I didn't have much information on how to do the project".

3.2.3. Improvement Suggestions for Future Projects

The students considered that the following proposals could be interesting for future editions of the activity:

Regarding the development of the activity and to enrich the final work:

Many students considered it important to incorporate the opinions of different actors: relatives of the older adults or the workers. They stated that they would especially like to know what older people think. For this, they proposed a visit to a nursing home or requested guest speakers to explain their experiences. A conversation or interview with older adults could offer an important basis to help build the project from their preferences, desires, or real needs.

"Bring older people to talk about how they live in a nursing home".

"*Approach from different perspectives: students, parents, grandparents...*"

Likewise, they also mentioned that in order to have more points of view and reduce repetition, some students could carry out a negative residential care facility project, that is, pointing out those aspects that should never exist in a center. Along these lines, they suggested inverting the approach: by first identifying the negative aspects present in some residential care centers and proposing improvements from there. They also indicated that it would be interesting if specific aspects on which to focus the design of the nursing home were distributed among the different work groups. This would allow for deeper knowledge and better variation in the projects.

"*Create a nursing home to which we would not like to go*".

"*That each group do a different directed project, that is, an ideal residence for older adults, another depending on the workers, another how the families see it*".

In addition, they proposed carrying out research on residential facilities in other environments and on different centers, such as day centers. Delving further into the nursing care that is provided there was also suggested.

"*Propose that different residential facilities in different countries be investigated*".

"*Delve deeper into the work of the residential care nurses*".

In relation to the project, its structure, or programming:

The students suggested that the time devoted to carrying out the project should be greater, as well as the duration of its presentation. With respect to the length, linked to one of the negative aspects, some believed that the pages of the report should be limited while there are those who believed that, on the contrary, they should be expanded.

"*Provide more time for projects*".

"*Expand the extension and exposure time*".

Finally, and repeatedly, many students proposed greater exhaustiveness in the information offered to carry out the work: more instructions, more specificity, greater clarification of the content, carrying out a group tutorial before beginning, or even a guide on how to perform it.

"*Explain something else in the informative document and not only the sections that we have to follow*".

"*Explain more the contents that must be included*".

"*Put a clearer guide for what needs to be done*".

"*Put in the instructions what general sections we must include in the work*".

As one of the students explained, "We are used to being given very detailed guidelines, and the moment they leave us a little more to our devices, we get lost."

4. Discussion

After carrying out the intervention, a significant increase in the level of knowledge on the subject studied was observed. Therefore, project-based learning is ideal for increasing knowledge about essential aspects of institutions dedicated to caring for older adults.

Although the difference in knowledge after the educational intervention was statistically significant, the authors expected that the final mean knowledge would have been higher and, thus, that the students would have experienced significant learning. The students did not have previous experience in the use of this didactic methodology, so it is believed that the results were not influenced by this aspect. We recommend further research comparing different teaching methodologies in order to be able to demonstrate which one produces greater learning.

In Garnjost's study, which compared four different student-centered methodologies (problem-based, service-learning, flipped classroom, and project-based) with lectures (teacher-centered pedagogy), the students only perceived that project-based learning had a significant impact on problem-solving and knowledge acquisition compared to lectures and that the satisfaction was significantly higher than the other methodologies [10].

Research that has used this same teaching methodology but online affirms that the use of PBL promotes the development of teamwork skills and encourages autonomy, proactivity, commitment, respect for the opinion of others, and the exercise of creativity [6], coinciding with the findings of our research.

In the use of the PBL methodology, the supervisory role of the tutor becomes essential, involving students in the creation and execution of the project [6]; the tutor must be trained to effectively guide the teamwork of undergraduate nursing students throughout the PBL process so that they achieve their goal [16]. This aspect makes the use of this methodology difficult because it requires greater involvement of the tutor and adequate training to establish a connection with the real world and promote the transfer of knowledge to practical situations, as well as greater involvement of the students.

The majority (74.4%) stated they were very satisfied with this training activity. There are also other studies along the same lines, in which PBL has been used in the university setting. These studies conclude that PBL produces an increase in the motivation and commitment of the students and has a positive effect on the knowledge of fundamental content and the development of the so-called 21st-century skills, such as collaboration, critical thinking, autonomy, problem-solving, time planning, or the ability to express oneself adequately [1,3,9,17].

Although PBL is a difficult methodology to apply in higher education, the results show the advantages that this type of methodology provides and the high level of satisfaction of the participating students [1] (79.6%) [8]. When exploring the association between group work skills and satisfaction with PBL in the university setting, the results show that there is a significant and positive relationship between both [18].

Regarding the qualitative study of the experience in the nursing home project, the open questions allowed us to explore the students' experiences. On the one hand, the question about the positive and negative aspects of carrying out the activity gives us a subjective assessment of the task carried out, which is something that we consider important to reveal the perception that emerges from the speeches. On the other hand, the question about suggestions for improvement for future activities places us in the scenario of reflection on the work and the projection of ideas acquired both in the preparation of the project itself and in the presentation of the different groups. Some suggestions for improvement made by the students require commenting on ethical considerations, such as conducting a "negative" nursing home project or making visits to nursing homes to analyze them. If these proposals were to be carried out, it would have to be made clear that when bad examples of care were detected, they would be acted upon.

One of the aspects valued as positive has to do with group work. Collaborative learning work is dynamic, and the need for students to work together to achieve common goals favors the development of knowledge and skills and generates a profitable and positive interdependence for students [18].

In addition, our study, like that of Mora [19], found that the student feels satisfied with this methodology as they become an active subject within their training, and they appreciate the development of skills such as critical thinking. This methodology improved the critical thinking and autonomy of the students by encouraging their active participation and motivation to learn. Also, a greater emotional involvement was generated, since the students were involved in the creation and execution of a project that was relevant and interesting to them about the needs of older adults.

On the other hand, the use of this didactic methodology results in the achievement of different specific learning results regarding the subject of Aging Nursing, such as describing the structures and operation of the centers where care is provided to older adults. And, in achieving certain competencies, such as demonstrating the ability to gather and interpret the relevant data to make judgments that include a reflection on social, scientific, or ethical issues. In addition to this, other training is carried out in generic or transversal skills, such as resource management, public speaking skills, decision-making, or interpersonal relationships.

Although, in general, PBL turns out to be a positive experience in terms of the time allotted for carrying out the activity, it can lead to it being perceived as unsatisfactory, and, in this regard, our results coincide with what was stated by Hernando et al. [20].

Proposing a change in methodology, encouraging active learning [5], and offering the freedom to interpret the required content can generate some difficulty and restlessness in those who are used to greater precision. In addition, that which, in principle, we consider as an opportunity to expand the possibilities of intervention is considered a burden that generates insecurity and requires greater involvement of both teachers and students.

Among the limitations is the small size of the sample. The possibility of generalizing the results is limited because the study population was limited to the students of a single subject of the Nursing degree at the University of Jaen. Finally, it is important to consider the limitations of using ad hoc questionnaires as well as the use of a self-reported survey method as a data collection system for both quantitative variables and qualitative dimensions.

5. Conclusions

The students of the Aging Nursing subject of the Nursing degree at the University of Jaen improved their knowledge about the planning and management of nursing homes with the use of the project-based learning teaching methodology. The students who participated in the project were very satisfied with the activity. The students had a positive perspective on the process of acquiring knowledge with PBL, with in-depth learning of some aspects, such as the operation of nursing homes, the work carried out by different professionals within them, and the needs of older adults as well as the possibilities of the improvement of these institutions. In terms of the learning methodology, they considered group work and the active role of students to be positive. They assessed the need to spend a lot of time to carry it out or the lack of precise indications about the development of the work as negative aspects.

It is recommended that faculties should facilitate teacher training in this teaching methodology in order to be able to implement similar projects with guaranteed success.

More research is needed to compare project-based learning with other teaching methodologies in order to determine which one is more recommendable.

Author Contributions: Conceptualization, L.P.-A. and N.G.-M.; methodology, L.P.-A. and N.G.-M.; validation, S.M.-C. and M.G.-C.; formal analysis, N.G.-M. and J.M.M.-G.; investigation, L.P.-A., M.D.L.-F., M.G.-C., S.M.-C., N.G.-M. and J.M.M.-G.; resources, S.M.-C.; data curation L.P.-A. and N.G.-M.; writing—original draft preparation, L.P.-A. and N.G.-M.; writing—review and editing, L.P.-A., M.D.L.-F., M.G.-C., S.M.-C., N.G.-M. and J.M.M.-G.; visualization, M.D.L.-F.; supervision, N.G.-M.; project administration, L.P.-A.; funding acquisition, L.P.-A. All authors have read and agreed to the published version of the manuscript.

Funding: This research was funded by the University of Jaen through the Project-Based Learning Teaching Innovation Project in the Nursing degree (PIMED02_202022).

Institutional Review Board Statement: Ethical approval was granted by the Research Ethics Committee of the University of Jaen (SEPT.22/1.PRY).

Informed Consent Statement: Informed consent was obtained from all the subjects involved in the study.

Data Availability Statement: The datasets used and analyzed during the current study are available from the corresponding author on request.

Public Involvement Statement: There was no public involvement in any aspect of this research.

Guidelines and Standards Statement: This manuscript was drafted against the Strengthening the Reporting of Observational Studies in Epidemiology (STROBE) for the quantitative study and Consolidated Criteria for Reporting Qualitative Research (COREQ) for the qualitative study.

Acknowledgments: The authors wish to thank Ingrid de Ruiter for the English language support and translation and all the students that participated in this study.

Conflicts of Interest: The authors declare no conflict of interest. The funders had no role in the design of the study; in the collection, analyses, or interpretation of the data; in the writing of the manuscript; or in the decision to publish the results.

References

1. Toledo Morales, P.; Sánchez García, J.M. Aprendizaje basado en proyectos: Una experiencia universitaria. *Rev. Curric. Profess.* **2018**, *22*, 429–449. [CrossRef]
2. Chen, J. Problem-based learning: Developing resilience in nursing students. *Kaohsiung J. Med. Sci.* **2011**, *27*, 230–233. [CrossRef] [PubMed]
3. Sung, T.; Wu, T. Learning with e-books and project-based strategy in a community health nursing course. *CIN Comput. Inform. Nurs.* **2018**, *36*, 140–146. [CrossRef] [PubMed]
4. Lee, H.; Shimotakahara, R.; Fukada, A.; Shinbashi, S.; Ogata, S. Impact of differences in clinical training methods on generic skills development of nursing students: A text mining analysis study. *Heliyon* **2019**, *5*, e01285. [CrossRef] [PubMed]
5. Koo, H.; Gu, Y.; Lee, B. Development of a project-based learning program on high-risk newborn care for nursing students and its effects: A quasi-experimental study. *Int. J. Environ. Res. Public Health* **2022**, *19*, 5269. [CrossRef] [PubMed]
6. Pascon, D.M.; Vaz, D.R.; Peres, H.H.C.; Leonello, V.M. Profissional Aprendizagem baseada em projetos no ensino remoto para estudantes ingressantes da graduação em enfermagem. *Rev. Esc. Enferm. USP* **2022**, *56*, e20220058. [PubMed]
7. McDermott, J. Using Project-Based Learning to Teach Advanced Practice Nurses About Quality Improvement. *AACN Adv. Crit. Care* **2022**, *33*, 376–381. [CrossRef] [PubMed]
8. Ferreiro, A.A. Aprendizaje basado en proyectos para el desarrollo de la competencia digital docente en la formación inicial del profesorado. *Relatec. Rev. Latinoam. Tecnolog. Educ.* **2018**, *17*, 9–24.
9. Ausín, V.; Abella, V.; Delgado, V.; Hortigüela, D. Aprendizaje basado en proyectos a través de las TIC: Una experiencia de innovación docente desde las aulas universitarias. *Form. Univers.* **2016**, *9*, 31–38. [CrossRef]
10. Garnjost, P.; Lawter, L. Undergraduates' satisfaction and perceptions of learning outcomes across teacher-and learner-focused pedagogies. *Int. J. Manag. Educ.* **2019**, *17*, 267–275. [CrossRef]
11. Bilbao-Aiastui, E. Desarrollo de la competencia científica mediante el aprendizaje basado en proyectos y TIC en Educación Primaria. *Digit. Educ. Rev.* **2021**, *39*, 304–318. [CrossRef]
12. Hallermann, S.; Larmer, J.; Mergendoller, J.R. *PBL in the Elementary Grades: Step-by-Step Guidance, Tools and Tips for Standards-Focused K-5 Projects*, 2nd ed.; Buck Institute for Education: Novato, CA, USA, 2016.
13. Chen, C.; Yang, Y. Revisiting the effects of project-based learning on students' academic achievement: A meta-analysis investigating moderators. *Educ. Res. Rev.* **2019**, *26*, 71–81. [CrossRef]
14. Taylor, S.J.; Bogdan, R. *Introducción a los Métodos Cualitativos de Investigación*; Paidós: Barcelona, Spain, 1987.
15. Farmer, T.; Robinson, K.; Elliott, S.J.; Eyles, J. Developing and implementing a triangulation protocol for qualitative health research. *Qual. Health Res.* **2006**, *16*, 377–394. [CrossRef] [PubMed]
16. Wosinski, J.; Belcher, A.E.; Dürrenberger, Y.; Allin, A.; Stormacq, C.; Gerson, L. Facilitating problem-based learning among undergraduate nursing students: A qualitative systematic review. *Nurse Educ. Today* **2018**, *60*, 67–74. [CrossRef]
17. Sánchez, J. Qué dicen los estudios sobre el Aprendizaje Basado en Proyectos. *Actual. Pedagógica* **2013**, *1*, 1–4.
18. Melguizo-Garín, A.; Ruiz-Rodríguez, I.; Peláez-Fernández, M.A.; Salas-Rodríguez, J.; Serrano-Ibáñez, E.R. Relationship Between Group Work Competencies and Satisfaction with Project-Based Learning Among University Students. *Front. Psychol.* **2022**, *13*, 811864. [CrossRef] [PubMed]
19. Mora Escalante, E. El Aprendizaje Basado en Problemas para la Intervencion de la Enfermeria con la Persona Adulta Mayor. *Rev. Enferm. Act. Costa Rica* **2011**, *20*. Available online: https://revistas.ucr.ac.cr/index.php/enfermeria/article/view/3649 (accessed on 20 October 2023). [CrossRef]
20. Hernando, C.G.; Martín, M.Á.C.; Ortega, F.L.; Villamor, P.M. Aprendizaje Basado en Problemas y satisfacción de los estudiantes de Enfermería. *Enfermería Glob.* **2014**, *13*, 97–112.

Disclaimer/Publisher's Note: The statements, opinions and data contained in all publications are solely those of the individual author(s) and contributor(s) and not of MDPI and/or the editor(s). MDPI and/or the editor(s) disclaim responsibility for any injury to people or property resulting from any ideas, methods, instructions or products referred to in the content.

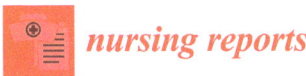

Article

Analysis of the Attitudes towards Sexuality in People with Intellectual Disabilities: A Cross-Sectional Study

José Carlos López-García [1,2], Azucena González-Sanz [2], Elena Sutil-Rodríguez [2], Carlos Saus-Ortega [3], Regina Ruiz de Viñaspre-Hernádez [4,*], Raúl Juárez-Vela [4,*], Vicente Gea-Caballero [5], Juan Luis Sánchez-González [6], Clara Isabel Tejada-Garrido [4], Ana Cobos-Rincón [4], José María Criado-Gutiérrez [7] and Consuelo Sancho-Sanchez [7]

[1] Doctoral Program in Health, Disability, Dependence, and Welfare, University of Salamanca, 37008 Salamanca, Spain; josecarlosdue@usal.es
[2] Adscript Center of Zamora, School of Nursing, University of Salamanca, 37008 Zamora, Spain; agonzalezsa@usal.es (A.G.-S.); esutil@usal.es (E.S.-R.)
[3] Adscript Center of La FE, School of Nursing, University of Valencia, 46003 Valencia, Spain; carles.saus-ortega@uv.es
[4] Faculty of Health Sciences, University of La Rioja, 26006 Logroño, Spain; clara-isabel.tejada@unirioja.es (C.I.T.-G.); ana.cobos@unirioja.es (A.C.-R.)
[5] Faculty of Health Sciences, International University of Valencia, 46003 Valencia, Spain; vagea@universidadviu.com
[6] Faculty of Nursing and Physiotherapy, University of Salamanca, 37008 Salamanca, Spain; juanluissanchez@usal.es
[7] Faculty of Medicine, University of Salamanca, 37008 Salamanca, Spain; jmcriado@usal.es (J.M.C.-G.); sanchoc@usal.es (C.S.-S.)
* Correspondence: reruizde@unirioja.es (R.R.d.V.-H.); raul.juarez@unirioja.es (R.J.-V.)

Abstract: The barriers faced by people with intellectual disabilities are many. One of the areas in which many problems have been identified is the sexual domain. This descriptive study aims to analyze the attitudes of the family environment, professional carers, and the general population toward their sexuality. A cross-sectional descriptive study was carried out between 2022 and 2023, using convenience sampling among family members and carers from different centers working with people with intellectual disabilities in Spain, and among the general population not related to people with intellectual disabilities. A total of 583 responses were received and significant differences were found for all variables, with the variables related to family or work proximity being those that provided the most significant and relevant results. It was observed that the male sex has a more paternalistic attitude and that in rural areas there is a more permissive attitude towards the sexuality of people with intellectual disabilities. People who work with people with disabilities have more positive attitudes towards this group, while direct relatives have more paternalistic attitudes. Nursing care in the community and specialized centers should be based on an adequate therapeutic relationship and personalized care.

Keywords: intellectual disability; sexuality; attitudes

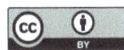

1. Introduction

Intellectual disability (ID) is a concept that has evolved over the last few decades. These changes have affected the way the condition itself is described, to avoid linguistic degradation, but also its defining characteristics, which include people with below-average IQ, but with the addition of adaptive limitations to the environment, and all this limited to a diagnosis before the age of 22 [1]. Limitations related to social skills and adaptation to family, work, and social environments are a fundamental pillar of diagnosis [1]. The types and causes of ID are diverse and it is necessary to use psychometric tools to make a correct diagnosis and identify the main needs for its management from a multidisciplinary approach [2].

The barriers faced by people with ID are numerous, ranging from limitations inherent in their diagnosis to social or work limitations [3,4]. One of the fields in which numerous problems have been demonstrated in people with ID has been the sexual domain. Sexuality is inherent in human beings from the moment of conception. It affects all developmental domains and every social facet of our everyday life [5]. The way of living and manifesting sexuality is multiple. It is influenced by culture, education, and multiple personal and social aspects [6].

Sexuality is often associated with genitality [7]. A comprehensive view of sexuality considers several dimensions of sexuality, such as the biological, psychological, and social domains [8]. This broad vision is reflected in the WHO definition of sexuality [9], which refers to the multiple ways of feeling and expressing it through thoughts, fantasies, desires, beliefs, attitudes, values, behaviors, practices, roles, and relationships. Despite the importance of sexuality, rights in this area are effected in all cultures and by any physical or psychological change in the individual. Acute and chronic illnesses, the need for hospitalization and surgery, the use of multiple medications [10], and mental health problems of all kinds, especially chronic ones [11], hurt sexuality. Globally, there are still problems affecting sexuality that are difficult to address due to their social, cultural, and economic roots, such as trafficking in women [12], clitoral cutting [13], gender-based violence, sexual abuse, and pornography and the inclusion of new issues such as sexting [14], which limit freedom in the area of sexuality.

Many specific problems have been described concerning the experience of sexuality in the population with ID, such as difficulties in education, higher rates of sexual abuse, and changes in affectivity or perception, among others [15]. Many attempts have been made to identify the causes of these problems, and the solution has focused on improving the sexual education of people with ID [16]. However, an increasing number of studies have investigated attitudes towards and around people with ID as a source of problems in sexual matters for people with ID [17–20]. To analyze this situation, several surveys have been developed to determine the influence of these attitudes.

The role of nursing with the ID collective is little addressed. There is little research that discusses the roles of nursing in the team of people in contact with this collective [21,22].

The present study aims to find and apply a validated scale and to analyze the attitudes of different population groups according to their proximity to people with ID. We will consider assessing the influence of being a family member of a person with ID, the influence of being a caregiver of a person with ID, or having no relationship with a person with ID. The influence of sociodemographic factors will also be considered to determine the influence on attitudes toward the sexuality of people with ID.

2. Material and Methods

A cross-sectional, descriptive, and analytical study was carried out.

2.1. Setting and Sample

A multicenter study was conducted in Spain and there were no exclusion criteria. The study was conducted between October 2022 and January 2023.

Professionals from centers working with people with intellectual disabilities, family members of people with intellectual disabilities, and the general population were invited to participate in the study. To select the sample, cluster sampling was carried out among the different associations working with groups of people with ID, asking them to disseminate the survey among their employees and family members. The sample of professionals and relatives of people with ID was recruited in different professional centers, preferably in Castilla-León, but also in other Autonomous Communities of Spain, which were contacted and informed about the study. To obtain the sample of the general population, non-probabilistic snowball sampling was performed, using different digital media to complete the questionnaire.

2.2. Tool

A literature search was conducted to find a suitable questionnaire on the attitudes of the population towards the sexuality of people with ID.

The search was conducted in the Web of Science and PubMed databases in September 2022. The search was limited to articles published in the last 20 years in Spanish, English, and Portuguese. The terms "intellectual disability", "scale", and "attitude" were used in the search, and the Boolean operators "AND" and "OR" were used. The initial reference search was performed by the first author of the manuscript and 526 articles were found. The selection and search for scales was carried out by the second and third authors of the manuscript, after reading the titles and abstracts. The scales should meet certain criteria such as "as up-to-date as possible, with a limited number of questions, easy to complete and disseminate, and covering all dimensions of sexuality, not only sexual relations". The literature search provided three scales, namely the Perception of Sexuality Scale (POS) [23], the questionnaire on attitudes towards sexuality in people with intellectual disabilities (ASQ-ID) [24], and the questionnaire Attitudes Towards Sexuality of Individuals with Intellectual Disability (ASEXID) [25].

To select the most appropriate questionnaire, five experts in ID were asked to analyze the questionnaires and give a score from 0 to 10 according to five criteria of the scale: appropriateness of the number of items, adaptability to the study population, breadth of topics addressed by the questionnaire about sexuality, comprehension of the questions, and speed of response. After analyzing the different questionnaires, the ASEXID questionnaire [25] (Assessment of attitudes towards the sexuality of people with intellectual disabilities) was selected. This questionnaire assesses attitudes towards sexuality in people with ID through 18 items with a Likert-type response format with five levels of frequency (from strongly disagree to strongly agree). This questionnaire has been validated in Spanish among professionals and family members of people with ID and the general population.

The 18 items are grouped into three factors: normalizing attitudes, expressing the similarity between people with and without ID; denying attitudes, expressing a lower sexual desire in people with ID; and paternalistic attitudes, expressing a perceived lack of impulse control in people with ID. This questionnaire is designed to be completed by people with family members with ID, caregivers of people with ID, and the general population. In addition to the ASEXID questionnaire, five short questions on some sociodemographic characteristics are requested for further analysis, which are:

1. Whether they have a direct family member with ID.
2. Whether they are a caregiver of a person with ID.
3. Their age, which is grouped into several intervals (0–20, 20–40, 40–60, and over 60).
4. Their sexual identity: male or female.
5. Whether they live in rural or urban areas.

2.3. Ethical Considerations

This study was approved by the Bioethics Committee of the University of La Rioja, which issued a favorable report with verification URL: https://sede.unirioja.es/csv/code/p2Cc6Wk1S6UT6lszlr3Gg9ukhS3Ey7ha (accessed on 5 July 2023).

Furthermore, the study was conducted following the principles of the Declaration of Helsinki and good clinical practice. Reporting was performed following the guidelines for strengthening the reporting of observational studies in epidemiology (STROBE) [26].

2.4. Procedure

After being fully informed about the purpose of the study and giving their informed consent, participants were asked to complete an anonymous questionnaire through the Google Forms ® platform. Contact with family members and workers was made through the directors of the centers working with people with ID, who facilitated access to the questionnaire online. The distribution of the questionnaire to the general population was carried out through the use of social networks.

2.5. Statistical Analysis

We established a 95% confidence interval by entering all the variables in the SPSS v.27 program and analyzing the characteristics of the responses given, as well as the relationship between the different variables. The Kolmogorov–Smirnov test [27] and visual inspection of the histograms were performed to evaluate the distribution of the data (p values < 0.05 were considered non-normal, a result obtained for some of our variables).

With the results of the Kolmogorov–Smirnov test and taking into account the characteristics of the variables to be analyzed, the Mann–Whitney U test [28] was used for the independent variables: the presence of a direct relative, the gender of the respondent, the caregiver of a relative with ID, or the place of residence. For the age analysis, Spearman's Rho [29] and Kendall's Tau c [30] were used, which were determined to be the most appropriate tests, since both variables are ordinal.

3. Results

The total number of responses was 583. Most of the people who accessed the survey agreed to answer it (99.1%). Despite the difficulty in finding direct relatives or caregivers of persons with ID, 7.4% and 13.9% of the responses were obtained from these groups of participants, respectively. The number of participants who had no professional or personal relationship with a person with ID was 459 (78.7%). The age of respondents varied, but the vast majority (85.4%) were between 20 and 60 years old. Most respondents lived in urban areas (81.4%). The number of women was higher at 67.7% compared to 27.4% who were men. The sociodemographic characteristics of the participants are shown in Table 1.

Table 1. Sociodemographic characteristics of the participants.

		N = 583	
		N	%
Gender	Male	160	27.4%
	Female	395	67.7%
	No answer	28	4.8%
Age	0–20 years old	46	7.9%
	20–40 years old	261	44.8%
	40–60 years old	219	37.6%
	+60 years old	36	6.2%
	No answer	21	3.63%
Residence	Urban	459	78.7%
	Rural	105	18%
	No answer	19	3.3%
Professional carers of people with intellectual disabilities	Yes	81	13.9%
	No	494	84.7%
	No answer	8	1.3%
A direct relative of a person with ID	Yes	43	7.4%
	No	532	91.2%
	No answer	8	1.4%

In general, the highest percentage of responses to the questionnaire were grouped in one of the extremes of the Likert scale ("Strongly disagree" or "Strongly agree"). If we add to the majority response the closest response on the Likert scale, the sum of both responses exceeds 75% of the total responses in most questions. However, there are several exceptions:

1. In question 7 questioning whether people with ID can control their sexual urges, the middle three responses reached 87.6%.
2. In question 11 on whether they agreed that people with ID can have sex without penetration, 71.6% of respondents disagreed ("Strongly disagree" or "Somewhat disagree").
3. In question 13 on whether people with ID need a guardian to decide their sexuality, the responses were almost equally distributed between "Strongly disagree", "Somewhat disagree", and "Neither agree nor disagree" answers.
4. Questions 15, 16, and 18 have the largest differences between their responses. The biggest difference between one response and another is seen in question 15 on whether people with ID see the danger of sexual abuse. In question 16 on whether they are okay with people with ID viewing pornography, the majority take a neutral stance, although they are more in favor of yes. The question with the greatest degree of dispersion is question 18 ("A woman with ID should be prevented from getting pregnant by using contraception"), with 1/3 of people in the neutral zone, 1/3 choosing "Agree" or "Strongly agree", and 1/3 selecting "Somewhat disagree" or "Strongly disagree" (Table 2).

Table 2. Analysis of ASEXID scale responses.

	Questions	Likert Scale Responses					
		1 Strongly Disagree	2 Somewhat Disagree	3 Neither Agree nor Disagree	4 Agree	5 Strongly Agree	No Answer
1.	People with ID have less interest in sexuality than people without [2]	306 52.5%	146 25%	98 16.8%	22 3.8%	4 0.7%	7 1.2%
2.	Sexual education should only be provided to people with ID when they demand it [2]	436 74.8%	107 18.4%	15 2.6%	10 1.7%	7 1.2%	8 1.4%
3.	Talking to people with ID about sex encourages them to practice it [2]	425 72.9%	92 15.8%	48 8.2%	8 1.4%	3 0.5%	7 1.2%
4.	Masturbation can harm people with ID [2]	498 85.4%	43 7.4%	22 3.8%	7 1.2%	3 0.5%	10 1.7%
5.	It seems good to me that people with ID masturbate [1]	12 2.1%	5 0.9%	95 16.3%	174 29.8%	289 49.6%	8 1.4%
6.	A person with ID can live their sexuality as anyone else [1]	14 2.4%	59 10.1%	38 6.5%	204 35%	260 44.6%	8 1.4%
7.	People with ID can control their sexual impulses [3]	10 1.7%	139 23.8%	225 38.6%	147 25.2%	52 8.9%	10 1.7%
8.	People with ID should have their privacy [1]	1 0.2%	4 0.7%	8 1.4%	147 25.2%	413 70.8%	10 1.7%
9.	People with ID can have a partner [1]	1 0.2%	5 0.9%	15 2.6%	165 28.3%	387 66.4%	10 1.7%
10.	It seems good to me that people with ID kiss or caress with another person [3]	2 0.3%	4 0.7%	25 4.3%	149 25.6%	393 67.4%	10 1.7%
11.	It seems good to me that people with ID have sex as long as there is no penetration [3]	289 49.6%	128 22%	123 21.1%	22 3.8%	11 3.9%	10 1.7%
12.	It seems good to me that people with ID have sexual intercourse even with penetration [1]	6 1%	9 1.5%	73 12.5%	210 36%	276 47.3%	9 1.5%
13.	People with ID need another adult guardian to decide about their sexuality [3]	183 31.4%	170 29.2%	142 24.4%	65 11.1%	13 2.2%	10 1.4%
14.	People with ID are always heterosexual [2]	406 69.6%	90 15.4%	40 6.9%	3 0.5%	3 0.5%	10 1.7%
15.	People with ID perceive the danger of sexual abuse [3]	81 13.9%	198 34%	165 28.3%	96 16.5%	34 5.8%	9 1.5%

Table 2. Cont.

	Questions	Likert Scale Responses					
		1 Strongly Disagree	2 Somewhat Disagree	3 Neither Agree nor Disagree	4 Agree	5 Strongly Agree	No Answer
16.	It is normal for people with ID to see pornography [1]	41 / 7%	50 / 8.6%	231 / 39.6%	167 / 28.6%	84 / 14.4%	10 / 1.7%
17.	People with ID can use condoms properly to prevent infections [3]	4 / 0.7%	23 / 3.9%	67 / 11.5%	195 / 33.4%	284 / 48.7%	10 / 1.7%
18.	We should prevent women with ID from becoming pregnant through the use of contraceptives [3]	86 / 14.8%	83 / 14.2%	201 / 34.5%	132 / 22.6%	74 / 12.7%	7 / 1.2%

[1] Normalizing attitude that expresses the similarity between people with and without ID. [2] Denying attitude that expresses a lower sexual desire in people with ID. [3] Paternalistic attitude that expresses a supposed lack of impulse control in people with ID.

If we analyze the relationship between the responses to the ASEXID scale and demographic characteristics, we find that highly significant differences are found in the variables "Direct family of people with ID", "Professional caregiver of people with ID", and in the different "Age groups". The analysis of the variables is shown in Table 3.

Table 3. Analysis of socio-demographic variables and ASEXID questionnaire.

	Question	Sex	Age	Place of Residence	Professional Carer	Immediate Family ID
		p				
1.	People with ID have less interest in sexuality than people without [2]	0.024 *	0.011 *	0.543	<0.001 *	0.531
2.	Sexual education should only be provided to people with ID when they demand it [2]	0.209	0.444	0.600	0.124	0.706
3.	Talking to people with ID about sex encourages them to practice it [2]	0.003 *	0.291	0.231	0.090	0.314
4.	Masturbation can harm people with ID [2]	0.335	0.354	0.334	0.115	0.305
5.	It seems good to me that people with ID masturbate [1]	0.577	<0.001 *	0.769	0.002 *	0.153
6.	A person with ID can live their sexuality as anyone else [1]	0.423	0.059	0.636	0.012 *	0.053
7.	People with ID can control their sexual impulses [3]	0.644	0.214	0.125	0.577	0.249
8.	People with ID should have their privacy [1]	0.456	<0.001 *	0.241	0.01 *	0.137
9.	People with ID can have a partner [1]	0.111	<0.001 *	0.445	0.022 *	0.017 *
10.	It seems good to me that people with ID kiss or caress with another person [3]	0.648	<0.001 *	1.000	0.26	0.002 *
11.	It seems good to me that people with ID have sex as long as there is no penetration [3]	0.070	0.177	0.192	0.458	0.635
12.	It seems good to me that people with ID have sexual intercourse even with penetration [1]	0.143	<0.001 *	0.616	0.047 *	0.007 *

Table 3. Cont.

	Sex	Age	Place of Residence	Professional Carer	Immediate Family ID
			p		
Question					
13. People with ID need another adult guardian to decide about their sexuality [3]	0.097	<0.001 *	0.036 *	0.076	0.505
14. People with ID are always heterosexual [2]	0.70	0.036 *	0.744	0.02 *	0.947
15. People with ID perceive the danger of sexual abuse [3]	0.118	<0.001 *	0.009 *	0.014 *	0.038 *
16. It is normal for people with ID to see pornography [1]	0.687	<0.001 *	0.998	0.008 *	0.452
17. People with ID can use condoms properly to prevent infections [3]	0.139	0.294	0.652	0.545	0.423
18. We should prevent women with ID from becoming pregnant through the use of contraceptives [3]	0.460	<0.001 *	0.333	0.314	0.728

[1] Normalizing attitude that expresses the similarity between people with and without ID. [2] Denying attitude that expresses a lower sexual desire in people with ID. [3] Paternalistic attitude that expresses a supposed lack of impulse control in people with ID. * $p < 0.05$ are considerate with statistical signitication U-Mann-Whitney and Rho Spearman test.

With the variable "gender", a high significant difference is obtained in question 1 (People with ID have less interest in sexuality than people without ID) with a p of 0.024 and in question 3 (Talking about sex with people with ID is to encourage them to practice it) with a p of 0.003. In both questions, it is men who consider that people with ID have less sexual desire.

The variable "age" had the highest number of significant differences in 11 of the 18 questions, with a high degree of significance in 9 of them, with values lower than $p < 0.01$. To evaluate the association between these ordinal variables, Spearman's Rho and Kendall's Tau c were used. In both tests, the results were similar, but when interpreting Spearman's correlation coefficient, it can be observed that it is very low or low in all cases. When analyzing the age groups, in the questions related to affective aspects, friendship, or courtship, it is the older groups that have a more permissive attitude towards IDs, while in the questions related to explicit sexual relations or parenting, the older groups have a more paternalistic attitude (which is defined as the tendency to apply the father's forms of authority and protection in the traditional family to other forms of social relations: political, labor, etc.).

In the variable "Place of residence", significant differences are obtained in questions 13 (People with ID need a guardian) and 15 (People with ID perceive sexual abuse) with degrees of significance of 0.036 and 0.009, respectively, and in which a more "paternalistic" attitude of people residing in urban versus rural areas is observed since they consider a higher percentage of people in urban areas do believe that they should have a guardian and that they do not perceive sexual abuse.

The variable "Professional caregiver of people with ID" shows a significant number of significant results in questions that include the three factors analyzed in the ASEXID scale (normalizing attitude, negative attitude, and paternalistic attitude), and all of them reflect a more favorable attitude of professional caregivers towards the sexuality of people with ID than the general population or family groups, except for question 15 where they think that people with ID do not perceive sexual abuse.

The variable "Direct relative of a person with ID" is highly significant in pre-questions 9, 10, and 12, which evaluate the factor "Normalizing attitude". In all of them, it is worse than in the group of caregivers and the general population. Question 15 increased with the group of caregivers and both thought that people with ID do not perceive the risk of sexual abuse in comparison with the general population.

4. Discussion

We present a novel study on the topic. Significant differences were found in all the variables analyzed: proximity to people with ID is a determining factor and what most determines the level of protection and attitudes towards this group is kinship.

The first analysis suggested by this study is the percentage of female respondents compared to male respondents. The sample search did not focus on predominantly female groups; however, the 3:1 response rate suggests that we should analyze whether this is a recurring circumstance in many surveys and why, or whether it is specific to this topic.

As with gender, there is a significant difference between caregivers and family members of people with ID. The survey was distributed in a significant number of organizations; if we take into account the number of workers caring for people with ID, which will always be lower than the number of people with ID, and the number of family members, which will always be much higher, we might think that the responses of family members would exceed those of caregivers. However, twice as many caregivers than family members responded.

The variable "gender" shows only two responses with significant differences in both cases: it is the male gender that shows a more conservative response to sexuality in ID, a result that coincides with other studies [18–20,29].

A study conducted in Australia in 2009 evaluated the same population groups (family members, caregivers, and the general population) and found that fathers were more conservative than workers about sexuality, and both were more conservative than the rest of society concerning parenting. Age also represented a difference in attitudes, with people over 60 also being more conservative. They relate this to the fact that in many cases the parents are older than 60 years and it is not specified whether this applies to all questions or only to some [18]. The same scale was used in a 2015 study in England to measure attitudes toward the sexuality of people with ID, but in this case, different cultural groups were compared, determining that people of Asian origin are less considerate and have greater social control vis-à-vis the sexual rights of people with ID [19].

Other scales, such as the ASQ-GD (for the general population) and the ASQ-ID (for people with ID) used in Australia in 2010, assessed the attitudes of leisure workers towards sexuality in people with ID. The results showed a generally positive attitude, although they noted that men had less self-control, thought that women with ID should have less sexual freedom, and were very cautious about their attitude toward parenting in this group [20]. Another study conducted in Australia in 2012 using the same scale suggests that sexuality training may benefit direct care workers with ID, especially older female workers [31]. A meta-analysis of articles using the ASQ-ID scale was conducted in 2022 [32].

The POS Sexuality Perception Scale in a 1996 study in Alaska showed that college students viewed the sexual behavior of people with ID as less acceptable than their own [33].

5. Nursing Clinical Implications

The role of the nurse in this group is little known. However, nurses care for this type of patient in the community setting for primary care and are present in most specialized centers working with people with ID. Two literature reviews [21,22] stand out in which the key role of the nurse in the multidisciplinary team that cares for these people is identified, focusing attention on establishing appropriate therapeutic communication and individualizing the care plan according to personal needs. Nursing is key to enabling people with ID to adapt to their environment holistically: facilitating the development of social skills, teaching new cognitive skills to enable information processing and problem-solving, and creating new tools to enhance learning in new situations of daily living.

6. Study Limitations

The main limitation found in the study is the lack of response from people who are part of the ID environment. About 100 organizations involved in the care of people with ID were contacted to disseminate the survey among workers and their families, but the number of responses was low to the number of organizations contacted, and this is even though the survey was completely anonymous, brief, and concrete. There are even organizations that have refused to disseminate the survey because it deals with a topic related to sexuality in ID on the part of the organizations or at the request of partners or family members. These data cannot be reflected in the study, as they have not been quantified or analyzed, but they suggest comprehensive analysis in the future to determine the importance of this refusal in this and other topics related to ID. In general, the samples in all the studies analyzed are not very large.

7. Conclusions

With the "gender" variable, a more paternalistic attitude can be observed in the male population compared to the female population.

Regarding the place of residence, there are no previous studies to compare and in this case, the data show a more paternalistic attitude in the urban population compared to the rural population.

The younger age groups have a more paternalistic attitude in matters of friendship or courtship; however, this attitude is reversed and it is the older population groups that have a more paternalistic attitude in matters of more explicit sex or in matters related to the upbringing of people with ID.

It can be affirmed that the group of caregivers is more concerned about this issue, responding to this survey in a higher percentage, and they present a more respectful attitude compared to the group of relatives, who have a more paternalistic attitude.

It is suggested that similar studies be carried out with a larger sample size to extrapolate the results and implement them in practice in the future to achieve a decrease in sexual complications in people with ID and improve their level of satisfaction in this area.

Most studies and actions focus on the people closest to the people with ID, but more actions should be carried out in the general population so as not to stigmatize the group. It would be interesting to assess whether these actions would have an impact on the attitudes of family members toward the sexuality of people with ID.

Author Contributions: Conceptualization, J.C.L.-G.; methodology, J.C.L.-G., A.G.-S. and R.J.-V.; software, E.S.-R.; validation, C.S.-O.; formal analysis, R.R.d.V.-H. and J.C.L.-G.; investigation, J.C.L.-G., A.G.-S. and E.S.-R.; resources, R.J.-V.; data curation, A.C.-R. and V.G.-C.; writing—original draft preparation, C.I.T.-G., J.C.L.-G., V.G.-C., J.M.C.-G. and C.S.-S.; writing—review and editing, V.G.-C., J.C.L.-G., C.S.-S. and J.M.C.-G.; visualization, J.L.S.-G.; supervision, C.S.-S. and R.J.-V.; project administration, R.R.d.V.-H.; funding acquisition, C.S.-S. and J.M.C.-G. All authors have read and agreed to the published version of the manuscript.

Funding: This research received no external funding.

Institutional Review Board Statement: This study was approved by the Bioethics Committee of the University of La Rioja which issued a favorable report with verification URL: https://sede.unirioja.es/csv/code/p2Cc6Wk1S6UT6lszlr3Gg9ukhS3Ey7ha (accessed on 1 July2023).

Informed Consent Statement: Informed consent was obtained from all subjects involved in the study.

Data Availability Statement: Data will be available by contacting the first author.

Public Involvement Statement: There has been no public involvement in any aspect of this research.

Guidelines and Standards Statement: This manuscript was drafted against the STROBE guidelines for Observational Studies.

Conflicts of Interest: The authors declare no conflict of interest.

References

1. Schalock, R.L.; Luckasson, R.; Tassé, M.J. *Intellectual Disability: Definition, Diagnosis, Classification, and Systems of Supports*, 12th ed.; AAIDD: Silver Spring, MD, USA, 2021.
2. Navas, P.; Verdugo, M.A.; Gómez, L.E. Diagnosis and classification on intellectual disability. *Psychosoc. Interv.* **2008**, *17*, 143–152. [CrossRef]
3. Barreras para las personas con discapacidades | Las discapacidades y la salud | NCBDDD | CDC'. 2020. Available online: https://www.cdc.gov/ncbddd/spanish/disabilityandhealth/disability-barriers.html (accessed on 16 September 2020).
4. Flores, N.; Jenaro, C.; Tomsa, R.; Lucas, J.L.; Beltrán, M. Actitudes, barreras y oportunidades para el empleo de personas con discapacidad intelectual. *Int. J. Dev. Educ. Psychol.* **2016**, *4*, 613. [CrossRef]
5. OPS. Salud Sexual para el Milenio: Declaración y documento técnico. 2009. Available online: https://www.paho.org/es/documentos/salud-sexual-para-milenio-declaracion-documento-tecnico-2009 (accessed on 20 May 2022).
6. WHO. Sexual Health and Its Linkages to Reproductive Health: An Operational Approach. Available online: http://old.aidsdatahub.org/sites/default/files/publication/WHO_Sexual_health_and_its_linkages_to_reproductive_health_2017.pdf (accessed on 26 July 2022).
7. Masters, W.; Johnson, V. *El Vínculo Del Placer*; Grijalbo: Barcelona, Spain, 1978.
8. Rathus; Spencer, A.; Nevid, J.S.; Fichner-Rathus, L.; Sánchez, F.L. *Sexualidad Humana*, 6th ed.; Pearson Educación: Madrid, Spain, 2005.
9. Development and Research Training in Human Reproduction UNDP/UNFPA/UNICEF/WHO/World Bank Special Programme of Research. *La Salud Sexual y su Relación con la Salud Reproductiva: Un Enfoque Operativo*; Organización Mundial de la Salud: Ginebra, Colombia, 2018. Available online: https://apps.who.int/iris/handle/10665/274656 (accessed on 7 July 2023).
10. Montejo, A. Frecuencia de Los Problemas Sexules Provocados Por Psicofármacos: Antidepresivos, Antipsicótcios, Benzodiazepinas y Eutimizantes. Impacto Cliínico y Propuestas de Actuación. *Actas Esp. De Psiquiatr.* **2002**, *1*, 54–65.
11. Fernández, V.; Alba; Bravo, M.Á.E. Sexualidad y Salud Sexual en Pacientes con Esquizofrenia: Revisión Bibliográfica. 2020, Volume 33. Available online: https://www.google.com.hk/url?sa=t&rct=j&q=&esrc=s&source=web&cd=&cad=rja&uact=8&ved=2ahUKEwjLv-Ke97qCAxUPsFYBHWz8AVcQFnoECBMQAQ&url=https%3A%2F%2Frepositori.udl.cat%2Fbitstreams%2Fa61a7205-f8ef-491b-9a08-b311fa314f8c%2Fdownload&usg=AOvVaw0q5JZiDn5pC_65j8ybZ2Ru&opi=89978449 (accessed on 7 July 2023).
12. Ministerio de Sanidad. *Poblaciones-Mercancía: Tráfico y Trata de Mujeres en España*; Ministerio de Sanidad, Política Social e Igualdad. Centro de Publicaciones: Madrid, Spain, 2011. Available online: https://violenciagenero.igualdad.gob.es/otrasFormas/trata/datosExplotacionSexual/estudios/DOC/PoblacionesMercancia.pdf (accessed on 3 July 2023).
13. Gallego, M.A.; López, M.I. Mutilación Genital Femenina: Revisión y Aspectos de Interés Médico Legal. *Cuad. De Med. Forense* **2010**, *16*, 145–151. [CrossRef]
14. Arta, D.; Sesar, K. Sexting Categories. *Mediterr. J. Clin. Psychol.* **2020**, *8*, 1–26. [CrossRef]
15. David, M.; Aunos, M.; Pacheco, L.; Hahn, L. Reconsidering Sexuality, Relationships, and Parenthood for Adults with Intellectual Disability. In *APA Handbook of Intellectual and Developmental Disabilities: Clinical and Educational Implications: Prevention, Intervention, and Treatment*; American Psychological Association: Washington, DC, USA, 2021; Volume 2, pp. 383–417. [CrossRef]
16. Yıldız, G.; Cavkaytar, A. Effectiveness of a Sexual Education Program for Mothers of Young Adults with Intellectual Disabilities on Mothers' Attitudes Toward Sexual Education and the Perception of Social Support. *Sex. Disabil.* **2017**, *35*, 3–19. [CrossRef]
17. Povilaitienė, N.; Radzevičienė, L. Teachers' and Parents' Attitude to Relevance of Sexuality Education of Adolescents with Mild Intellectual Disabilities. *Soc. Welf. Interdiscip. Approach* **2015**, *5*, 82–90. [CrossRef]
18. Cuskelly, M.; Bryde, R. Attitudes towards the Sexuality of Adults with an Intellectual Disability: Parents, Support Staff, and a Community Sample. *J. Intellect. Dev. Disabil.* 2009. [CrossRef]
19. Sankhla, D.; Theodore, K. British Attitudes Towards Sexuality in Men and Women with Intellectual Disabilities: A Comparison Between White Westerners and South Asians. *Sex. Disabil.* **2015**, *33*, 429–445. [CrossRef]
20. Gilmore, L.; Chambers, B. Intellectual Disability and Sexuality: Attitudes of Disability Support Staff and Leisure Industry Employees. *J. Intellect. Dev. Disabil.* **2010**, *35*, 22–28. [CrossRef]
21. Pridding, A.; Watkins, D.; Happell, B. Mental Health Nursing Roles and Functions in Acute Inpatient Units: Caring for People with Intellectual Disability and Mental Health Problems—A Literature Review. *Int. J. Psychiatr. Nurs. Res.* **2007**, *12*, 1459–1471. [PubMed]
22. Bakken, T.L.; Sageng, H. Mental Health Nursing of Adults With Intellectual Disabilities and Mental Illness: A Review of Empirical Studies 1994–2013. *Arch. Psychiatr. Nurs.* **2016**, *30*, 286–291. [CrossRef] [PubMed]
23. Scotti, J.R.; Slack, B.S.; Bowman, R.A.; Morris, T.L. College Student Attitudes Concerning the Sexuality of Persons with Mental Retardation: Development of the Perceptions of Sexuality Scale. *Sex. Disabil.* **1996**, *14*, 49–63. [CrossRef]
24. Cuskelly, M.; Gilmore, L. Attitudes to Sexuality Questionnaire (Individuals with an Intellectual Disability): Scale Development and Community Norms. *J. Intellect. Dev. Disabil.* **2007**, *32*, 214–221. [CrossRef]
25. Gil-Llario, M.D.; Fernández-García, O.; Castro-Calvo, J.; Caballero-Gascón, L.; Ballester-Arnal, R. Validation of a Tool to Assess Attitudes Towards Sexuality of Individuals with Intellectual Disability (ASEXID): A Preliminary Study. *Sex. Disabil.* **2021**, *39*, 147–165. [CrossRef]

26. Von Elm, E.; Altman, D.G.; Egger, M.; Pocock, S.J.; Gøtzsche, P.C.; Vandenbroucke, J.P. The Strengthening the Reporting of Observational Studies in Epidemiology (STROBE) Statement: Guidelines for Reporting Observational Studies. *Lancet* **2007**, *370*, 1453–1457. [CrossRef]
27. IBM Documentation. Available online: https://www.ibm.com/docs/es/spss-statistics/saas?topic=tests-one-sample-kolmogorov-smirnov-test (accessed on 5 October 2022).
28. IBM Documentation. Available online: https://www.ibm.com/docs/es/spss-statistics/beta?topic=tests-mann-whitney-u-test (accessed on 7 December 2021).
29. Martínez Ortega, R.M.; Tuya Pendás, L.C.; Martínez Ortega, M.; Pérez Abreu, A.; Cánovas, A.M. El coeficiente de correlacion de los rangos de spearman caracterizacion. *Rev. Habanera De Cienc. Médicas* **2009**, *8*.
30. Davis, M.K.; Chen, G. Grafing Kendall's @t. Computational Statistics and Data Analysis', Grafing Kendall's @t. *Comput. Stat. Data Anal.* **2007**, *51*, 2375–2378. [CrossRef]
31. Meaney-Tavares, R.; Gavidia-Payne, S. Staff Characteristics and Attitudes towards the Sexuality of People with Intellectual Disability. *J. Intellect. Dev. Disabil.* **2012**, *37*, 269–273. [CrossRef]
32. Correa, A.B.; Moreno, J.D.; Castro, A. A Meta-Analytic Review of Attitudes towards the Sexuality of Adults with Intellectual Disabilities as Measured by the ASQ-ID and Related Variables: Is Context the Key? *J. Intellect. Disabil. Res.* **2022**, *66*, 727–742. [CrossRef]
33. Swango-Wilson, A. Caregiver Perception of Sexual Behaviors of Individuals with Intellectual Disabilities. *Sex. Disabil.* **2008**, *26*, 75–81. [CrossRef]

Disclaimer/Publisher's Note: The statements, opinions and data contained in all publications are solely those of the individual author(s) and contributor(s) and not of MDPI and/or the editor(s). MDPI and/or the editor(s) disclaim responsibility for any injury to people or property resulting from any ideas, methods, instructions or products referred to in the content.

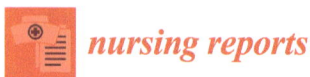 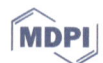

Systematic Review

Media Exposure of Suicidal Behaviour: An Umbrella Review

Teresa Sufrate-Sorzano [1,2], Marco Di Nitto [3], María Elena Garrote-Cámara [1,2], Fidel Molina-Luque [4,5,6], José Ignacio Recio-Rodríguez [7,8], Pilar Asión-Polo [9], Ángela Durante [10], Vicente Gea-Caballero [11], Raúl Juárez-Vela [1,2,12,*], Jesús Pérez [12,13,14] and Iván Santolalla-Arnedo [1,2]

[1] Care and Health Research Group, GRUPAC, Nursing Deparment, University of La Rioja, 26006 Logroño, Spain; teresa.sufrate@unirioja.es (T.S.-S.); maria-elena.garrote@unirioja.es (M.E.G.-C.); ivan.santolalla@unirioja.es (I.S.-A.)
[2] Biomedical Research Centre of La Rioja, CIBIR, 26006 Logroño, Spain
[3] Department of Health Sciences, University of Genoa, 16126 Genova, Italy; marco.dinitto@unige.it
[4] Faculty of Education, Psychology and Social Work, University of Lleida, 25001 Lleida, Spain; fidel.molinaluque@udl.cat
[5] Group for the Study of Society, Health, Education and Culture (GESEC), University of Lleida, 25001 Lleida, Spain
[6] Research Institute in Social and Territorial Development (INDEST), University of Lleida, 25001 Lleida, Spain
[7] Faculty of Nursing and Physiotherapy, University of Salamanca, 37008 Salamanca, Spain; donrecio@usal.es
[8] Primary Care Research Unit of Salamanca (APISAL), Institute of Biomedical Research of Salamanca (IBSAL), 37008 Salamanca, Spain
[9] Aragonese Health Service (SALUD), 50017 Zaragoza, Spain; piasion@unirioja.es
[10] Department of Translational Medicine, University of East Piedmonet, 13100 Vercelli, Italy; angela.durante@uniupo.it
[11] Faculty of Health Sciences, International University of Valencia, 46002 Valencia, Spain; vagea@universidadviu.com
[12] Prevention and Early Intervention in Mental Health (PRINT), Institute of Biomedical Research of Salamanca (IBSAL), 37008 Salamanca, Spain; jesusperez@usal.es
[13] Faculty of Medicine, University of Salamanca, 37008 Salamanca, Spain
[14] Department of Psychiatry, University of Cambridge, Cambridge CB2 1TN, UK
* Correspondence: raul.juarez@unirioja.es

Citation: Sufrate-Sorzano, T.; Di Nitto, M.; Garrote-Cámara, M.E.; Molina-Luque, F.; Recio-Rodríguez, J.I.; Asión-Polo, P.; Durante, Á.; Gea-Caballero, V.; Juárez-Vela, R.; Pérez, J.; et al. Media Exposure of Suicidal Behaviour: An Umbrella Review. *Nurs. Rep.* 2023, 13, 1486–1499. https://doi.org/10.3390/nursrep13040125

Academic Editor: Richard Gray

Received: 16 August 2023
Revised: 14 October 2023
Accepted: 19 October 2023
Published: 25 October 2023

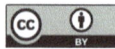

Copyright: © 2023 by the authors. Licensee MDPI, Basel, Switzerland. This article is an open access article distributed under the terms and conditions of the Creative Commons Attribution (CC BY) license (https://creativecommons.org/licenses/by/4.0/).

Abstract: Aim: To analyse recommended interventions for the safe and responsible dissemination of suicidal behaviour in the media for preventive purposes. Background: Suicide is a serious public health problem that leads to more than 700,000 deaths per year, which translates into one death every forty seconds. The media play a significant role in shaping public perceptions and reflecting societal issues. Because of its active role in the construction of reality, the way in which the media report and expose suicidal behaviour has the capacity to influence the population in either a preventive or harmful way. Design: An umbrella review was carried out and a report was written according to the Preferred Reporting Items for Overviews of Reviews. Methods: We systematically searched for reviews published from inception to February 2023 in MEDLINE (PubMed), CINAHL and PsycInfo (via EBSCOhost), Web of Science, Embase, Cochrane Library of Systematic Reviews, Scopus, and Google Scholar. A narrative synthesis of the results was conducted. Results: Six systematic reviews with a moderate to high quality level were selected. Among the recommended interventions were the inclusion of positive messages of hope, resilience, or of overcoming the event, narratives with information on available resources or the promotion of support-seeking attitudes as an effective prevention mechanism, as well as the avoidance of repetitive reporting of the same suicide. The appropriate and responsible dissemination of information on suicidal behaviour in the media with complete and up-to-date information on available centres, organisations, institutions, and resources has proven to be effective, especially in vulnerable populations. Conclusion: Educating and training the media in an appropriate approach to disseminating suicidal behaviour helps to reduce the number of suicidal behaviours. Knowing what information is advisable to include in the news item as well as what information to avoid is a strong point. Guidelines to promote responsible media reporting are a key component of suicide prevention strategies. This study was prospectively registered in the International Prospective Register of Systematic Reviews (PROSPERO) on 23 April 2022 with the registration number CRD42022320393.

Keywords: communications media; general literature review; Papageno effect; prevention; suicide; suicidal behaviours; suicidal ideation and Werther effect

1. Introduction

In 1976, the World Health Organization (WHO) defined the term suicide as *"an act with a lethal outcome, deliberately initiated and carried out by the subject, knowing or expecting its lethal outcome and through which they intend to obtain the desired changes"* [1]. It is known that the first suicidal behaviour dates to prehistoric times. The social conception of this universal phenomenon has changed according to the cultural, religious, and intellectual principles of history. Thus, the same lethal act has been accepted in some cultures as a transition to a new immortal stage, and in others, it has been punished and penalised as a crime [2]. Human beings have redefined what suicide represents in each historical context, and although the approaches have been disparate, no one has been indifferent to this phenomenon [3].

Suicide is now recognised as a serious public health problem due to the fact that there are more than 700,000 deaths per year, which translates into one death every forty seconds, and for every suicide, an estimated twenty attempts are made [4]. In addition, the psychological impact of suicidal behaviour (suicide ideation, attempt, and death by suicide) on close, personal circles, affecting, on average, six suicide loss survivors, is also highly significant [5]. Furthermore, it is currently estimated that an average of 100 community members may be affected after each suicide [6,7]. For these reasons, both the United Nations Sustainable Development Goals and the WHO's Comprehensive Mental Health Action Plan 2013–2030 have set a target of reducing these figures by one-third [8,9].

Suicidal behaviour is a complex phenomenon caused by a multitude of biological, psychological, social, cultural, and environmental factors which are associated with situations of crisis, stress, or traumatic moments that have not been dealt with, triggering suicide as an escape route [10]. Prevention is possible, and this requires the collaboration and coordination of different multidisciplinary teams that are committed to providing integrated and holistic care, as an individual approach is not effective in such a complex process [11].

Among the various health professionals needed to tackle the problem, the generalist nurse, and, specifically, the mental health specialist, play key roles in prevention. Their functions include treating underlying mental disorders and the identification and assessment of populations in situations of vulnerability, controlling environmental risk factors and stressful life events, identifying alcohol withdrawal, limiting access to the resources most frequently used for suicide, breaking the socio-cultural stigma that prevents access to mental health services, and promoting community health education as a highly vital method for the responsible, safe, and useful dissemination of information through the media [12].

The media play a significant role in shaping public perceptions and reflecting societal issues by allowing the transmission of information between sender and receiver; specifically, when the receiver is a social group, they are called Mass Media. Among the most prominent media are radio, internet, and television, whose news influences people's thoughts, values, and actions on political, economic, and social issues. Therefore, the media play an active role in society due to their direct influence on the way reality is perceived [13].

This approach is based on the theory of agenda-setting, which explains how the media are the most notable factor in the social construction of everyday reality so that the issues dealt with in the media will become the issues of greatest concern to society by directing attention and changing the way people think about them [14]. Therefore, the way in which the media report and expose suicidal behaviour can have a preventive or protective influence on suicidal behaviour or, conversely, a detrimental influence by causing an increase in numbers through contagion or imitation.

The origin of the Werther effect alludes to Goethe's novel "The Sorrows of Young Werther", where the protagonist takes his own life by shooting himself. After its publication, a wave of young people died by suicide using the same method, wearing the same clothes as the character, and making references to the work in their suicide notes [15–17]. Some authors propose that this effect may have originated earlier with William Shakespeare's Romeo and Juliet, as it caused a multitude of deaths among those unlucky in love. However, it was the sociologist Phillips in 1974 who framed this effect, stating that the more suicide was portrayed in the media, the higher the suicide figures were later on [15,16].

The basis of the protective effect, also called Papageno, aims to repeal the existing taboo on suicide by relying on responsible and truthful communication [16]. Such communication should meet established criteria such as the use of clear and understandable terminology, informing about the preventable nature of suicide, providing helpline numbers, informing about the link between suicide and depression, emphasising that it is a treatable condition, respecting the privacy of affected families, raising awareness among the general public so that they can be aware of risk indicators in the immediate environment, and providing information about support services and prevention programmes [17–19].

The Werther effect has repeated itself on several occasions throughout history; a recent media example is the broadcast of the series "13 Reasons Why" in March 2017 which explicitly and graphically showed the suicide of the teenage protagonist. Specifically, between March and April 2017, there were 1.5 million searches related to suicide on Google, with the most frequently searched phrases being *"how to slit your wrists"*, *"how to commit suicide"*, and *"how to kill yourself"* [20]. In 2019, research by Niederkrotenthaler et al. found an increase in suicides in the three months following the premiere of the series, higher than the general trend, among 10–19-year-olds and especially in females [21].

Frequently, media reports exaggerate the most tragic, lethal, and unusual methods, such as using a firearm or jumping onto railway tracks. These methods do not often correspond to the reality in most countries, where hanging is more common [22]. In this umbrella review, the concept of intervention is used to refer to the mode of media exposure and dissemination of suicidal behaviour. For that, we aimed to analyse the recommended interventions for the safe and responsible reporting of suicidal behaviour in the media for preventive purposes.

2. Materials and Method

This is an umbrella review conducted according to the Joanna Briggs Institute (JBI) methodological manual [23]. This systematic approach is guided by providing a comprehensive and objective synthesis through the use of rigorous and transparent methods. A preliminary search was conducted on PubMed to identify existing systematic reviews that met the inclusion criteria. From this preliminary search, several systematic reviews potentially falling within the inclusion criteria were found, which justified the use of an umbrella review for the purpose of the study. The report was written according to the Preferred Reporting Items for Overviews of Reviews (PRIOR) statement [24]. The protocol of this umbrella review was registered in the International Prospective Register of Systematic Reviews (PROSPERO) with registration code CRD42022320393.

Ethical considerations related to the review process: None of the data presented in this paper have been plagiarised, invented, manipulated, or distorted.

2.1. Search Strategy

A systematic search was conducted for systematic reviews published from inception to the 13 February 2023. Eight databases were consulted: MEDLINE (PubMed), CINAHL and PsycInfo (via EBSCOhost), Web of Science, Embase, Cochrane Library of Systematic Reviews, Scopus, and Google Scholar.

The search terms that guided the search were: suicide, "suicide, completed", "suicidal ideation", "suicide, attempted", "audiovisual aids", radio, television, telecommunications, and "systematic review". The search was first performed in PubMed, applying Mesh terms, free text terms, and using wildcards if deemed appropriate. Then, the final search was tailored for use in all the other databases considered. The complete search strategy can be found in Supplementary File S1.

2.2. Inclusion and Exclusion Criteria

We included all systematic reviews written in English, Spanish, or Italian regarding the dissemination of news in the communication media with the aim of reducing suicidal intentions. Primary studies, books, book sections, and grey literature (theses, conference proceedings, etc.) were excluded, as well as systematic reviews that did not focus on our topic.

2.3. Outcome Measures

The primary outcome of this umbrella review was suicide rate reduction following news dissemination. The secondary outcomes considered were the number of suicides and suicidal behaviour reduction.

2.4. Review Selection

All studies were retrieved from each database and were uploaded to a Microsoft Excel® (Version 16.66.1) spreadsheet and duplicates were removed. The Excel® tool was used to manage data collection, facilitating the organisation of information by title, journal, database, keywords, abstract, or year. Titles and abstracts were screened by two separate authors (Author 1 and Author 2) in accordance with the criteria for eligibility. After the preliminary phase, they separately evaluated the full texts of studies that might be pertinent for inclusion.

Any discrepancies were resolved by discussion between the authors, and when consensus was not reached, a third researcher (Author 3) was consulted.

2.5. Quality Assessment

The methodological quality of the selected papers was analysed independently by two reviewers (Author 1 and Author 2) (Table 1). When a consensus was not reached, a third researcher (Author 3) participated in the quality assessment. For this purpose, the Critical Appraisal Skills Programme Spanish (CASPe) tool was used in its version for systematic reviews [25]. The checklist consists of ten items designed to assess quality and considers three broad areas when evaluating a systematic review: are the results valid; what are the results; will the results help locally? The research team considered that if there was at least one response scored as "no" or "unclear" on one of the ten items, a moderate quality of the review would be inferred. If there were at least three "no" or "unclear" responses, it would be defined as a low-quality review. In the presentation of the results and the generalisation of the results, the reported quality was considered. The results obtained are shown in Table 1.

Table 1. Methodological quality analysis tool for systematic reviews using CASPe. Each criterion is scored as yes, no, or unclear.

	Authors					
Items	Niederkrotenthaler et al., 2022 [26]	Niederkrotenthaler et al., 2021 [27]	Niederkrotenthaler et al., 2020 [28]	Torok et al., 2017 [29]	Sisask et Värnik, 2012 [30]	Mann et al., 2005 [31]
Did the review address a clearly focused question?	Yes	Yes	Yes	Yes	Yes	Yes
Did the authors look for the right type of papers?	Yes	Yes	Yes	Yes	Yes	Yes
Do you think all the important, relevant studies were included?	Yes	Yes	Yes	Yes	No	No

Table 1. Cont.

	Authors					
Items	Niederkrotenthaler et al., 2022 [26]	Niederkrotenthaler et al., 2021 [27]	Niederkrotenthaler et al., 2020 [28]	Torok et al., 2017 [29]	Sisask et Värnik, 2012 [30]	Mann et al., 2005 [31]
Did the review authors do enough to assess the quality of the included studies?	Yes	Yes	Yes	Unclear	Unclear	Unclear
If the results of the review have been combined, was it reasonable to do so?	Yes	Yes	Yes	Yes	Yes	Yes
What are the overall results of the review?	Yes	Yes	Yes	Yes	Yes	Yes
How precise are the results?	Yes	Yes	Yes	Data was synthesised using a qualitative approach	Data was synthesised using a qualitative approach	Data was synthesised using a qualitative approach
Can the results be applied to the local population?	Yes	Yes	Yes	Yes	Yes	Yes
Were all important outcomes considered?	Yes	Yes	Yes	Yes	Yes	Yes
Are the benefits worth the harm and costs?	Yes	Yes	Yes	Yes	Yes	Yes

2.6. Data Extraction

Following the screening phase, two authors (Author 1 and Author 2) separately collected and extracted all data using a standard data collection form regarding systematic review characteristics: reference and year, general objective, review typology, databases, the period covered, and outcome data. Conflicts were resolved by consultation with a third reviewer (Author 3).

2.7. Data Synthesis

According to the JBI methodological manual [23], which emphasises that the results of an umbrella review are reported to provide existing research syntheses relevant to a particular topic, the data of the included systematic reviews were summarised in narrative form. The results were presented both in the form of a table and within the text.

3. Results

The search collected a total of 4520 articles (PubMed 204, CINAHL and PsycInfo 2981, Web of Science 212, Embase 936, Cochrane 115, Scopus 50, and Google Scholar 22). After the removal of duplicates, 4035 results were reviewed by title and abstract to assess relevance and eligibility criteria, eliminating 4010 records and including 25 papers. Finally, after eliminating 19 papers (n = 5 were not considered truly systematic reviews due to their methodology and n = 14 did not answer the research question posed for this umbrella review), 6 systematic reviews were analysed for the development of this research. Of the included reviews, three also included meta-analyses. The time range covered by the final reviews is from 2005 to 2022. The procedure followed in this umbrella review is described in Figure 1.

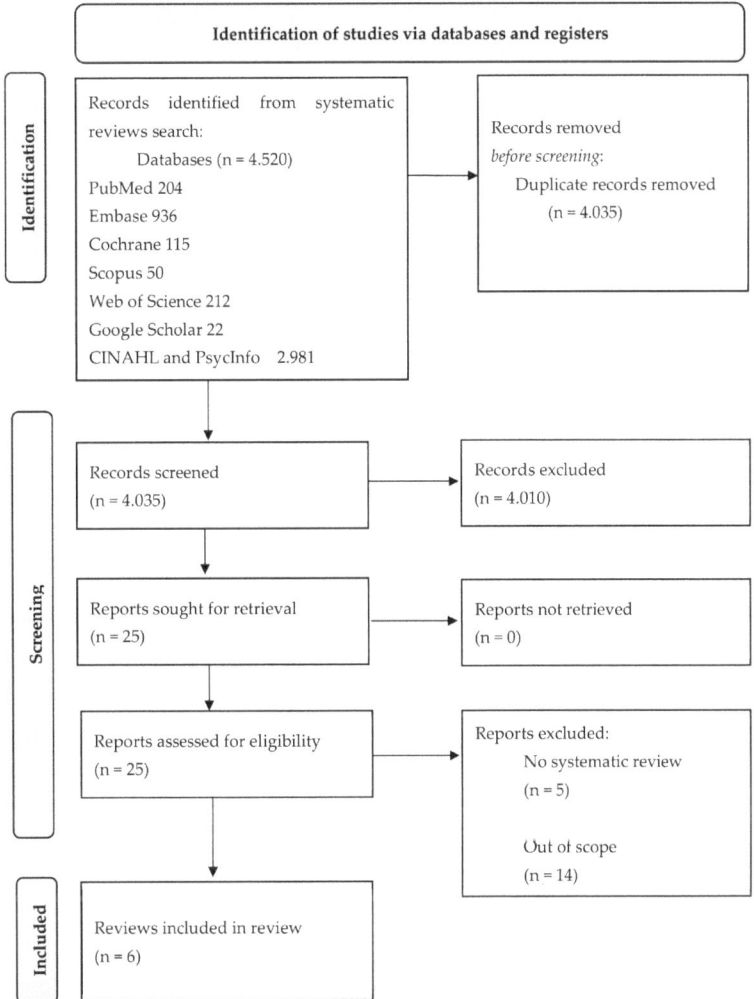

Figure 1. PRIOR flow diagram.

3.1. Methodological Quality Assessment

In relation to the assessment of methodological quality, three reviews were inferred to be of high quality [26–28] and three of moderate quality [29–31]. All reviews were included in the umbrella review as their results could be generalised and applied to the population. The main findings are presented as a narrative synthesis.

3.2. Characteristics of the Included Studies

The literature search dates of the included reviews ranged from the inception of the database to 2021. The reviews included a total of 195 unique primary studies. Descriptive observational designs were the most frequent primary study type (n = 136), followed by randomised controlled trials (n = 29), analytical observational studies (n = 25), and quasi-experimental studies (n = 5). A median of five primary studies (inter-quartile range 3–7) were included.

In the reviews included, the strategies or tools recommended being implemented by the media for the responsible and safe dissemination of suicidal behaviours to the population were considered as an intervention, either by adding certain aspects (n = 9) or by eliminating certain characteristics related to the suicidal behaviour described (n = 4).

A summary of the general characteristics of the included reviews is reported in Table 2.

Table 2. Data extraction form with the characteristics of the six systematic reviews included. Chronological order.

Reference and Year	General Objective	Review Typology	Database Included	Period Covered	Main Findings
Niederkrotenthaler et al., 2022 [26]	Summarise findings from randomised controlled trials on the effects of stories of hope and recovery on individuals with some degree of vulnerability to suicide.	Systematic review and meta-analysis.	PubMed, Scopus, Embase, PsycInfo, Web of Science, and Google Scholar	From inception until 6 September 2021	Exposure to narratives about hope and overcoming suicidal crises appears to have a beneficial effect on people with some vulnerability to suicidal ideation.
Niederkrotenthaler et al., 2021 [27]	Examine the association between portrayals of suicide and suicide attempts in entertainment media and suicidal behaviour in the population.	Systematic review and meta-analysis.	PubMed, Scopus, Embase, PsycInfo, Web of Science, and Google Scholar	From inception until 20 April 2021	The diffusion of suicidal behaviour in the media can increase suicides and suicide attempts among the population. Therefore, they should respect existing guidelines on their safe representation.
Niederkrotenthaler et al., 2020 [28]	Examine the association between reporting on suicides, especially deaths of celebrities by suicide, and subsequent suicides in the general population.	Systematic review and meta-analysis.	PubMed, Scopus, Embase, PsycInfo, Web of Science, and Google Scholar	From inception until 1 September 2019	Guidelines for responsible reporting of suicidal behaviour in the media are the best prevention intervention for the population. They should be more widely applied and promoted.
Torok et al., 2017 [29]	Address key knowledge gaps regarding how mass media campaigns can be optimised to prevent suicide by looking at their global efficacy and mechanisms related to successful outcomes.	Systematic review	PubMed, Scopus, Embase, PsycInfo, Web of Science, Cochrane Library, and Cochrane Central Register of Controlled Trials	From inception until 1 April 2016	Multilevel mass media outreach has positive effects on both suicide rates and suicide attempts. Repeated exposure and community involvement are key aspects of prevention campaigns.
Sisask et Värnik, 2012 [30]	Monitor and provide an overview of the research performed on the roles of the media in suicide prevention in order to find out the possible effects that the media reporting on suicidal behaviours might have on actual suicidality.	Systematic review	PubMed, PsycInfo, and Cochrane Library	From inception until 1 July 2011	Media reports are not representative of official data on suicides. They tend to sensationalise with the exposure of dramatic and very lethal methods which are infrequent in reality.
Mann et al., 2005 [31]	Examine the evidence for the effectiveness of specific suicide-preventive interventions and make recommendations for future prevention programmes and research.	Systematic review	PubMed, PsycInfo, and Cochrane Library	From 1966 to June 2005	Media exposure to suicide as a solution to problems may exacerbate the risk of developing these behaviours.

3.3. Overlap between Included Systematic Reviews and Studies

The primary studies included across the systematic reviews and relevant to the aim of this study were mapped and the overlap among all reviews was analysed. Only one primary study overlapped with another review. A total of thirty primary studies were cited thirty-one times across the six systematic reviews included in this overview, resulting in an overall corrected covered area (CCA) of 0.07, indicating almost no overlap across the included reviews. In Table 3, it can be seen that only one of these primary studies overlaps, i.e., it was analysed in two of the systematic reviews. This result is considered positive for the research as it infers that the included reviews did not analyse the same primary studies [32] (Table 3).

Table 3. Overlap between the systematic reviews and the studies included.

Studies	Niederkrotenthaler et al., 2022 [26]	Niederkrotenthaler et al., 2021 [27]	Niederkrotenthaler et al., 2020 [28]	Torok et al., 2017 [29]	Sisask et Värnik, 2012 [30]	Mann et al., 2005 [31]
Ftanou et al., 2021	x					
Niederkrotenthaler et al., 2020	x					
Till et al., 2020	x					
Niederkrotenthaler et al., 2019			x			
Till et al., 2019	x					
Handley et al., 2018		x				
King et al., 2018	x					
Sinyor et al., 2018			x			
Till et al., 2018			x			
Schmidt, 2017		x				
Till et al., 2017	x					
Arendt et al., 2016	x					
Kontopantelis et al., 2015		x				
Hawton et al., 2014		x				
Matsubayashi et al., 2014				x		
Niederkrotenthaler et al., 2014			x			
Robinson et al., 2014				x		
Robinson et al., 2013				x		
Till et al., 2013				x		
Chen et al., 2010					x	
Jenner et al., 2010				x		
Klimes-Dougan et al., 2010				x		
Niederkrotenthaler et al., 2010			x		x	
Niederkrotenthaler et al., 2009			x			
Klimes-Dougan et al., 2009				x		
Oliver et al., 2008				x		
Daigle et al., 2006				x		
Hegerl et al., 2006				x		
Sudak and Sudak, 2005					x	
Etzersdorfer et al., 1998						x

3.4. Summary of Evidence

For a better analysis and to facilitate understanding, the results are presented in terms of the aspects or characteristics that the media should include in the information dissemination related to suicidal behaviour and those that should be avoided, all with the ultimate aim of developing responsible dissemination based on prevention.

3.5. Recommended Strategies to Be Included in Responsible Dissemination

With regard to the strategies that are recommended to be included in the dissemination and found to be most widely represented in the reviews, the first is the inclusion in the narrative of positive messages of hope, resilience, and overcoming adversity [26–28,30,31], finding a protective effect of up to one month's duration in vulnerable populations [26]. Subsequently, the promotion and encouragement of the search attitude as an effective care tool for the general population are present in three studies [27,29,30]. In this line, the effectiveness of such an intervention when specifically focused on the male gender is worth highlighting [26,29]. With regard to the detrimental effect or Werther effect of developing suicidal behaviour following media reports, the work of Sisask et Värnik shows a strong association with age and gender, making young and old people more vulnerable to the imitation effect [30].

The inclusion in the narrative of complete and up-to-date information on available facilities, organisations, institutions, and resources has been shown to be effective [26,29,31]. This exposure includes providing the population with complete information, including contact telephone numbers or updated website addresses.

The media awareness of mental health and mental disorders [29,31] along with the dissemination of treatment availability, especially for depression, have also proven to be effective in the responsible and preventive dissemination of suicidal behaviour in the media [29]. Along these lines, there is a reference to awareness-raising as a method for literacy and public awareness in order to decrease the stigma of mental health in general and suicide in particular [29].

In the reviews analysed, some strategies focus on the contribution that health professionals and survivors of suicide can make to society, and community involvement has been shown to be critical to success [29]. Survivors are understood as those people negatively and significantly affected by the suicide of someone around them or those people who have faced a suicide attempt, highlighting, as a strategy in suicidal ideation, the dissemination of real personal stories and the sharing of stories that reflect overcoming or recovering from suicidal crises [26]. Regarding the specific role of healthcare professionals, the work of journalists or scriptwriters with experts in the field of mental health is effective for safe exposure [27]. Narratives that include the idea that suicide prevention is possible are also effective [29].

3.6. Strategies to Avoid Responsible Dissemination

In this section, as mentioned above, the strategies found in the included reviews that should be avoided for the dissemination and safe exposure of suicidal behaviour will be analysed. The omission of an explicit description of the method used and the location where the suicidal behaviour took place stands out in most of the works [27,28,30,31]. This strategy is based on the correspondence found between the subsequent increase in suicide rates following the media coverage of suicidal behaviour related to the explicit dissemination of the method used [29]. Along these lines, narratives that avoid a romantic, dramatic, or glorified depiction of suicidal behaviour have also been shown to be effective [28,30,31].

Not repeatedly reporting the same behaviour and not depicting suicide as an inevitable event with no option to intervene in prevention have also been shown to be effective interventions [28]. One response to these facts may lie in the bystander normalisation of suicidal behaviour as a quick escape route or solution to problems. In Table 4, the interventions found in the review are represented chronologically.

Table 4. Interventions found in the studies reviewed.

Interventions	Authors					
	Niederkrotenthaler et al., 2022 [26]	Niederkrotenthaler et al., 2021 [27]	Niederkrotenthaler et al., 2020 [28]	Torok et al., 2017 [29]	Sisask et Värnik, 2012 [30]	Mann et al., 2005 [31]
Positive messages of hope, resilience, and overcoming adversity.	x	x	x		x	x
Narratives with information on available centres, organisations, and resources.	x			x		x
Promote the attitude of seeking help as an effective mechanism.	x		x	x		

Table 4. Cont.

Interventions	Niederkrotenthaler et al., 2022 [26]	Niederkrotenthaler et al., 2021 [27]	Niederkrotenthaler et al., 2020 [28]	Torok et al., 2017 [29]	Sisask et Värnik, 2012 [30]	Mann et al., 2005 [31]
Personal narratives of overcoming suicidal crises.	x					
Specific information aimed at promoting support-seeking oriented towards the male gender.	x		x			
No explicit description of the method used or place/location.		x	x		x	x
No romantic, dramatic, or glorified description of suicide.			x		x	x
No repeated reporting of the same suicide.			x			
Narratives on the availability of treatment for mental disorders.					x	
No portrayal of suicide as inevitable.			x			
Narratives that suicide prevention is possible.				x		
Raise awareness of mental health in the media.				x		x
Work with mental health experts to ensure safe dissemination and exposure.		x				

4. Discussion

This is the first general review that explores the media as a key interpersonal and social factor. The media may function as a protective and/or risk factor for suicidal behaviour because it plays an active role in society by directly influencing the way reality is perceived. The way in which the media report and expose information related to suicidal behaviour is decisive. Well-managed information or exposure has a preventive influence in reducing suicide rates, while poor media reporting can lead to an increase in numbers through contagion or imitation. A broad search strategy has been used to ensure a comprehensive synthesis of the systematic reviews in this area, providing an integrated and comprehensive overview of a high level of evidence. The assessment of the methodological quality of the included systematic reviews, conducted by three independent reviewers, determined a high-quality rating for the majority of studies.

The results confirm that the inclusion in the narrative of positive messages of hope, resilience, and overcoming adversity is present as preventive and protective information in the most current systematic reviews published between 2020 and 2022 [26–28]. Establishing the adequate and responsible dissemination of suicidal behaviour in the media with complete and updated information on the centres, organisations, institutions, and resources available for dealing with suicidal behaviour has proven to be effective, especially in vulnerable populations and/or those with difficulties in accessing the health system [12,26,29,31]. The use of the media as a health literacy tool, reducing the stigma of mental illness in general and suicidal behaviour in particular, as well as the dissemination of available treatments, have been shown to be a preventive strategy in several studies [29,31]. Silencing suicide does not contribute to reducing the number of suicidal behaviours, but rather causes continuous stigmatisation of the event and its consequent consideration as a taboo subject by society [33]. The figure of the gatekeeper, understood as the person who acts as an information specialist, in the media is key to the prevention of suicidal behaviour, working in not only a *reactive* capacity, i.e., responding effectively to the demands for information that they receive, but also *proactively*, i.e., anticipating information needs before they are perceived [14]. Promoting the figure of the gatekeeper is a line of action to develop competencies for the prevention of suicidal behaviour in social agents who are in direct contact with the population [11]. The work of gatekeepers in the media for the protection of mental health and reduction in suicidal ideation and attempts can be carried out by health professionals, mental health nurses, psychologists, psychiatrists, etc., as well as by survivors or patients who tell personal stories of overcoming suicide; community participation has been shown to be fundamental for preventive success, with the key being to show suicide prevention as possible in the media [27,29]. The results of this umbrella review are in line with existing recommendations in the field and along the lines of providing well-managed information for suicide prevention. The WHO recommends providing accurate information on where to seek help; educating the community about the facts of suicide and suicide prevention, without spreading myths; and disseminating stories about how to cope with life stressors or suicidal thoughts, and how to obtain help [17]. The Action Alliance in its 2022 report suggests preventively working with mental health experts to ensure safe outreach and exposure; using non-judgmental language; and providing narratives with information on available facilities, organisations, and resources (including up-to-date contact numbers or websites) [34].

Following a review of the scientific literature, it can be determined that certain media interventions may become risk factors for suicidal behaviour. With regard to the placement of news about suicide, the Canadian Psychiatric Association and the Canadian Association for Suicide Prevention state that news about suicidal behaviour should not be displayed on the front or back page of newspapers, should avoid sensationalism, should not provide details about the site/location, should not explicitly describe the medium used, should not use photographs, video footage, or social media links, and should not repeat the news story unduly [35,36]. This is in line with the WHO, which has worked on several manuals to approach this issue, and their recommendations [17,37,38]. In 2017, an observational study by Acosta-Artiles et al. showed that the press publishes news in an unjustified manner, one-third of which is avoidable; it does not provide new information and it contains a high percentage of characteristics that are harmful to viewers, which may increase the risk of contagion. It should be taken into consideration that not only the quality of dissemination has an influence, but also the quantity [39]. In research by Armstrong et al., semi-structured interviews were conducted with media professionals in India who had previously published news about suicides, and several participants stated that violent and novel methods of suicide were of great interest to the press [40]; media education and intervention at this level is essential to prevent the dissemination of this type of sensationalist information which is a high-impact risk factor. The Action Alliance's 2022 report along these lines recommends not explicitly describing the method used and not reducing the multi-causality of suicidal behaviour to a single precipitating factor or a simple explanation [34].

In Spain, there is no suicide prevention plan at the national level on which to contrast results. In some autonomous communities, the Suicide Prevention Plan is included within a Strategic Mental Health Plan, a document that addresses the general objectives and interventions to be developed within mental health, but not expressly for suicide [41]. Specifically, in the community of La Rioja, there is a Suicide Prevention Plan. This document includes a specific section related to the prevention of suicidal behaviour and the media [42].

The results of this review are in line with this regional plan where the training of communication professionals and the development of style guides are indicated as effective interventions for the dissemination of suicidal behaviour.

5. Limitations

A possible limitation of the study is that if alternative search commands were used, additional studies might have been found. However, the authors believe that if the search procedure is modified, the conclusions may be largely the same, so this may not be such a serious limitation.

The focus of this umbrella review on suicidal behaviour and the media was on news descriptions and their dissemination. However, research on the specific representation of suicide in films, series, performing arts, or other forms of social dissemination could be of great interest.

Similarly, the number of studies included and the moderate quality in three of them can also be considered a limitation.

6. Implication for Practice

Although psychiatric disorders significantly increase the risk of suicide, interpersonal and social factors also play an important role. The media is a feature of the social environment in which suicidal behaviour can be learned; though the effect is probably smaller than that of other psychosocial risk factors for suicide, it is a significant agent in the social construction of reality, especially for vulnerable people [43].

7. Conclusions

Evidence confirms that suicide is preventable and that the comprehensive coordination of different multidisciplinary teams is necessary to be effective in suicide prevention. Educating and training the media in the appropriate approach for disseminating suicidal behaviour helps to reduce the number of suicidal behaviours. Knowing what information is advisable to include in the news item as well as what information to avoid is a strong starting point. Guidelines to encourage the responsible reporting of suicide in the media are a key component of suicide prevention strategies. Multidisciplinary health teams in collaboration with the media could be helpful in ensuring prevention-based outreach.

Supplementary Materials: The following supporting information can be downloaded at: https://www.mdpi.com/article/10.3390/nursrep13040125/s1, The complete search strategy can be found in Supplementary File S1. Supplementary File S2 contains the studies that met the inclusion criteria.

Author Contributions: Conceptualisation: T.S.-S., M.E.G.-C., M.D.N. and P.A.-P. Methodology: T.S.-S., M.D.N., M.E.G.-C. and P.A.-P. Software: R.J.-V., J.P., M.D.N. and F.M.-L. Validation: J.P., V.G.-C., M.E.G.-C., I.S.-A., J.I.R.-R. and R.J.-V. Formal analysis: T.S.-S., I.S.-A., J.I.R.-R. and M.D.N. Investigation: T.S.-S., M.E.G.-C. and P.A.-P. Resources: J.P., I.S.-A., R.J.-V., M.D.N., P.A.-P. and Á.D. Data curation: V.G.-C., I.S.-A., R.J.-V., F.M.-L., J.I.R.-R. and Á.D. Writing—original draft preparation: T.S.-S., M.D.N. and M.E.G.-C. Writing—review and editing: I.S.-A., R.J.-V., F.M.-L. and Á.D. Visualisation: T.S.-S. and M.E.G.-C. Supervision: J.P., I.S.-A., R.J.-V., F.M.-L., J.I.R.-R. and Á.D. Project Á.D. ministration: T.S.-S. All authors have read and agreed to the published version of the manuscript.

Funding: This research received no external funding.

Conflicts of Interest: The authors declare that they have no competing interests. The vision expressed in this paper is one of the authors and does not represent any involvement of the bodies or authorities of affiliation. M.D.N. has not received any fee or reimbursement for participating in the study and writing the article.

References

1. World Health Organization. The suicide. In *Notebooks on Public Health No. 59*; WHO: Geneva, Switzerland, 1977.
2. Guerrero-Díaz, M. Reflexiones sobre el suicidio desde la mirada histórica. *Boletín Psicoevidencias* **2019**, *25*, 1–6.
3. Amador Rivera, G.H. Suicidio: Consideraciones históricas. *Rev. Médica Paz* **2015**, *21*, 91–98.
4. Pan American Health Organization. Suicide Prevention. 2022. Available online: https://www.paho.org/en/topics/suicide-prevention (accessed on 26 December 2022).
5. Pompili, M.; Shrivastava, A.; Serafini, G.; Innamorati, M.; Milelli, M.; Erbuto, D.; Ricci, F.; Lamis, D.A.; Scocco, P.; Amore, M.; et al. Bereavment after the suicide of a significant other. *Indian J. Psychiatry* **2013**, *55*, 256–263. [CrossRef]
6. Cerel, J.; Brown, M.M.; Maple, M.; Singleton, M.; Van de Venne, J.; Moore, M.; Flaherty, C. How many people are exposed to suicide? Not six. *Suicide Life Threat. Behav.* **2019**, *49*, 529–534. [CrossRef] [PubMed]
7. Andriessen, K.; Rahman, B.; Draper, B.; Dudley, M.; Mitchell, P.B. Prevalence of exposure to suicide: A meta-analysis of population-based studies. *J. Psychiatr. Res.* **2017**, *88*, 113–120. [CrossRef]
8. Spanish Government. Sustainable Development Strategy 2030. Ministerio de Derechos Sociales. 2015. Available online: https://www.mdsocialesa2030.gob.es/agenda2030/documentos/eds-eng-acce.pdf (accessed on 24 January 2023).
9. World Health Organization. Comprehensive Mental Health Action Plan 2013–2030. World Health Organization. 2021. Available online: https://www.who.int/publications/i/item/9789240031029 (accessed on 15 February 2023).

10. Wasserman, D. A Stress–Vulnerability Model and the Development of the Suicidal Process: Danuta Wasserman Stress–Vulnerability Model. In *Suicide*; CRC Press: Boca Raton, FL, USA, 2001; pp. 38–53.
11. World Health Organization. Preventing Suicide: A Global Imperative. 2014. Available online: https://apps.who.int/iris/handle/10665/131056 (accessed on 17 February 2023).
12. Sufrate-Sorzano, T.; Pérez, J.; Juárez-Vela, R.; Garrote-Cámara, M.; de Viñaspre, R.R.; Molina-Luque, F.; Santolalla-Arnedo, I. Umbrella review of nursing interventions NIC for the treatment and prevention of suicidal behavior. *Int. J. Nurs. Knowl.* **2022**, *34*, 204–215. [CrossRef]
13. Diez, M.T.S.; Markina, I.C. La representación del suicidio en la prensa española. *Rev. Cienc. Soc.* **2020**, *2*, 168. [CrossRef]
14. Fong, Y.L. Reporting on suicide in Malaysia: Problem characterization and solution advocacy by media. *KOME* **2021**, *9*, 46–64. [CrossRef]
15. Phillips, D.P. The influence of suggestion on suicide: Substantive and theoretical implications of the Werther effect. *Am. Sociol. Rev.* **1974**, *39*, 340. [CrossRef]
16. Niederkrotenthaler, T.; Voracek, M.; Herberth, A.; Till, B.; Strauss, M.; Etzersdorfer, E.; Eisenwort, B.; Sonneck, G. Role of media reports in completed and prevented suicide: Werther v. Papageno effects. *Br. J. Psychiatry* **2010**, *197*, 234–243. [CrossRef]
17. World Health Organization. *Preventing Suicide: A Resource for Media Professionals*; World Health Organization: Geneva, Switzerland, 2017; Available online: https://apps.who.int/iris/handle/10665/258814 (accessed on 28 January 2023).
18. Durán, Á.; Fernández-Beltrán, F. Responsabilidad de los medios en la prevención del suicidio. Tratamiento informativo en los medios españoles. *Prof. Inf.* **2020**, *2*, 29. [CrossRef]
19. National Institute of Mental Health. Suicide Prevention. 2022. Available online: https://www.nimh.nih.gov/health/topics/suicide-prevention (accessed on 25 January 2023).
20. Ayers, J.W.; Althouse, B.M.; Leas, E.C.; Dredze, M.; Allem, J.P. Internet searches for suicide following the release of 13 reasons why. *JAMA Intern. Med.* **2017**, *177*, 1527. [CrossRef] [PubMed]
21. Niederkrotenthaler, T.; Stack, S.; Till, B.; Sinyor, M.; Pirkis, J.; Garcia, D.; Rockett, I.R.H.; Tran, U.S. Association of increased youth suicides in the United States with the release of 13 Reasons Why. *JAMA Psychiatry* **2019**, *76*, 933–940. [CrossRef] [PubMed]
22. Kõlves, K.; McDonough, M.; Crompton, D.; de Leo, D. Choice of a suicide method: Trends and characteristics. *Psychiatry Res.* **2018**, *260*, 67–74. [CrossRef]
23. Aromataris, E.; Fernandez, R.; Godfrey, C.; Holly, C.; Khalil, H. Methodology for jbi umbrella reviews. In *The Joanna Briggs Institute Reviewers Manual*; Aromataris, A.P.E., Ed.; Joanna Briggs Institute: Adelaide, Australia, 2014; pp. 5–34.
24. Gates, M.; Gates, A.; Pieper, D.; Fernandes, R.M.; Tricco, A.C.; Moher, D.; E Brennan, S.; Li, T.; Pollock, M.; Lunny, C.; et al. Reporting guideline for overviews of reviews of healthcare interventions: Development of the PRIOR statement. *BMJ* **2022**, *378*, e070849. [CrossRef]
25. CASP Checklists. Critical Appraisal Skills Programme. 2022. Available online: https://casp-uk.net/casp-tools-checklists/ (accessed on 5 June 2023).
26. Niederkrotenthaler, T.; Till, B.; Kirchner, S.; Sinyor, M.; Braun, M.; Pirkis, J.; Tran, U.S.; Voracek, M.; Arendt, F.; Ftanou, M.; et al. Effects of media stories of hope and recovery on suicidal ideation and help-seeking attitudes and intentions: Systematic review and meta-analysis. *Lancet Public Health* **2022**, *7*, e156–e168. [CrossRef] [PubMed]
27. Niederkrotenthaler, T.; Kirchner, S.; Till, B.; Sinyor, M.; Tran, U.S.; Pirkis, J.; Spittal, M.J. Systematic review and meta-analyses of suicidal outcomes following fictional portrayals of suicide and suicide attempt in entertainment media. *EClinicalMedicine* **2021**, *36*, 100922. [CrossRef]
28. Niederkrotenthaler, T.; Braun, M.; Pirkis, J.; Till, B.; Stack, S.; Sinyor, M.; Tran, U.S.; Voracek, M.; Cheng, Q.; Arendt, F.; et al. Association between suicide reporting in the media and suicide: Systematic review and meta-analysis. *BMJ* **2020**, *368*, m575. [CrossRef]
29. Torok, M.; Calear, A.; Shand, F.; Christensen, H. A systematic review of mass media campaigns for suicide prevention: Understanding their efficacy and the mechanisms needed for successful behavioral and literacy change. *Suicide Life Threat. Behav.* **2017**, *47*, 672–687. [CrossRef]
30. Sisask, M.; Värnik, A. Media roles in suicide prevention: A systematic review. *Int. J. Environ. Res. Public Health* **2012**, *9*, 123–138. [CrossRef]
31. Mann, J.J.; Apter, A.; Bertolote, J.; Beautrais, A.; Currier, D.; Haas, A.; Hegerl, U.; Lonnqvist, J.; Malone, K.; Marusic, A.; et al. Suicide prevention strategies: A systematic review: A systematic review. *JAMA* **2005**, *294*, 2064–2074. [CrossRef] [PubMed]
32. Hennessy, E.A.; Johnson, B.T. Examining overlap of included studies in meta-reviews: Guidance for using the corrected covered area index. *Res. Synth. Methods* **2020**, *11*, 134–145. [CrossRef] [PubMed]
33. Donovan, J.; Boyd, D. Stop the presses? Moving from strategic silence to strategic amplification in a networked media ecosystem. *Am. Behav. Sci.* **2021**, *65*, 333–350. [CrossRef]
34. Action Alliance. National Recommendations for Depicting Suicide. 2022. Available online: https://theactionalliance.org/messaging/entertainment-messaging/national-Recommendations (accessed on 14 February 2023).
35. Antebi, L.; Carmichael, V.; Whitley, R. Assessing Adherence to Responsible Reporting of Suicide Guidelines in the Canadian News Media: A 1-year Examination of Day-to-day. *Can. J. Psychiatry* **2020**, *65*, 621–629. [CrossRef]

36. Sinyor, M.; Schaffer, A.; Heisel, M.J.; Picard, A.; Adamson, G.; Cheung, C.P.; Katz, L.Y.; Jetly, R.; Sareen, J. Media guidelines for reporting on suicide: 2017 update of the Canadian psychiatric association policy paper. *Can. J. Psychiatry* **2018**, *63*, 182–196. [CrossRef]
37. World Health Organization. *Preventing Suicide: A Resource for Media Professionals*; World Health Organization: Geneva, Switzerland, 2008; Available online: https://apps.who.int/iris/bitstream/handle/10665/43954/9789241597074_nor.pdf (accessed on 14 August 2023).
38. Pan American Health Organization. *Suicide Prevention: A Resource for Media Professionals. Update*; Pan American Health Organization: Washington, DC, USA, 2018.
39. Acosta-Artiles, F.J.; Rodríguez-Caro, C.J.; Cejas-Méndez, M.R. Noticias sobre suicidio en los medios de comunicación. Recomendaciones de la OMS. *Rev. Española Salud Pública* **2017**, *91*, e201710040. Available online: http://scielo.isciii.es/scielo.php?script=sci_arttext&pid=S1135-57272017000100303&lng=es (accessed on 24 October 2017).
40. Armstrong, G.; Vijayakumar, L.; Cherian, A.; Krishnaswamy, K.; Pathare, S. Indian media professionals' perspectives regarding the role of media in suicide prevention and receptiveness to media guidelines: A qualitative study. *BMJ Open* **2021**, *11*, e047166. [CrossRef]
41. Sufrate-Sorzano, T.; Jiménez-Ramón, E.; Garrote-Cámara, M.E.; Gea-Caballero, V.; Durante, A.; Júarez-Vela, R.; Santolalla-Arnedo, I. Health plans for suicide prevention in Spain: A descriptive analysis of the published documents. *Nurs. Rep.* **2022**, *12*, 77–89. [CrossRef]
42. Working Group of the Suicide Prevention Plan in La Rioja. *Suicide Prevention Plan in La Rioja*, 1st ed.; Gobierno de La Rioja: Logroño, La Rioja, Spain, 2018.
43. Schmidtke, A.; Häfner, H. Public Attitudes towards and Effects of the Mass Media on Suicidal and Deliberate Self-Harm Behavior. In *Suicide and Its Prevention, The Role of Attitude and Imitation*; Diekstra, R.F.W., Maris, R., Platt, S., Schmidtke, A., Sonneck, G., Eds.; Brill: Leiden, The Netherlands, 1989; pp. 313–330.

Disclaimer/Publisher's Note: The statements, opinions and data contained in all publications are solely those of the individual author(s) and contributor(s) and not of MDPI and/or the editor(s). MDPI and/or the editor(s) disclaim responsibility for any injury to people or property resulting from any ideas, methods, instructions or products referred to in the content.

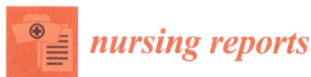

Article

Nursing Care for Stroke Patients: Current Practice and Future Needs

Lisa A. Babkair [1,*], Razan A. Safhi [1], Raghad Balshram [1], Rahaf Safhei [1], Atheer Almahamdy [1], Fatimah Hamad Hakami [2] and Ali Matouq Alsaleh [3]

[1] Faculty of Nursing, King AbdulAziz University, Jeddah 21589, Saudi Arabia; rsafhi0002@stu.kau.edu.sa (R.A.S.); rblsharm@stu.kau.edu.sa (R.B.); rsafhi0001@stu.kau.edu.sa (R.S.); aalmahamdy0001@stu.kau.edu.sa (A.A.)
[2] King Fahad General Hospital, Jeddah 23325, Saudi Arabia; fatimahhh@moh.gov.sa
[3] National Neuroscience Institute Nursing Administration, King Fahad Medical City, Riyadh 12231, Saudi Arabia; amalsaleh@kfmc.med.sa
* Correspondence: lbabkair@kau.edu.sa; Tel.: +966-506-509-985

Abstract: Background: Stroke is the second leading cause of death and the third leading cause of disability worldwide. Stroke nurses play an important role in the care of patients living with stroke by using best practices and adhering to stroke-management guidelines. This study aims at examining the current nursing practice for stroke patients in Saudi Arabia. Method: A cross-sectional descriptive design was used to collect data from nurses working in the stroke unit and intensive care unit between the period of February and June 2022 using electronic self-administered questionnaires. Results: A convenience sample of 131 nurses who provided care for stroke patients was enrolled. Significant differences in nursing practice were found between the stroke units and the intensive care units regarding the activation of the stroke code, X^2 (4, N = 131) = 48.34, $p < 0.001$; transferring stroke patients to a designated bed, X^2 (4, N = 131) = 48.74, $p = 0.002$; applying the NIHSS, X^2 (4, N = 131) = 70.11, $p < 0.001$; using the modified Rankin scale, X^2 (4, N = 131) = 61.24, $p < 0.001$; providing intervention for neglect syndrome, X^2 (4, N = 131) = 44.72, and hemianopsia, X^2 (4, N = 131) = 39.22; screening for poststroke depression, X^2 (4, N = 131) = 101.59, $p < 0.001$; assessing for psychosocial needs, X^2 (4, N = 131) = 74.44, $p < 0.001$, and encouraging patients to express their feelings, X^2 (4, N = 131) = 58.64, $p < 0.001$; educating patients and families about stroke prevention, X^2 (4, N = 131) = 40.51, $p < 0.001$. Conclusion: As per the results of the study, there is an urgent need for stroke units run by specialized stroke nurses to provide early stroke management and improve survivors' outcomes. Structured stroke-care programs are needed to improve nursing practice and meet the international standard of stroke care.

Keywords: critical care; nursing training; nursing practice; stroke; stroke patients; stroke unit

Citation: Babkair, L.A.; Safhi, R.A.; Balshram, R.; Safhei, R.; Almahamdy, A.; Hakami, F.H.; Alsaleh, A.M. Nursing Care for Stroke Patients: Current Practice and Future Needs. *Nurs. Rep.* **2023**, *13*, 1236–1250. https://doi.org/10.3390/nursrep13030106

Academic Editors: Antonio Martínez-Sabater, Elena Chover-Sierra and Carles Saus-Ortega

Received: 28 July 2023
Revised: 4 September 2023
Accepted: 8 September 2023
Published: 10 September 2023

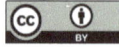

Copyright: © 2023 by the authors. Licensee MDPI, Basel, Switzerland. This article is an open access article distributed under the terms and conditions of the Creative Commons Attribution (CC BY) license (https://creativecommons.org/licenses/by/4.0/).

1. Introduction

Stroke is the second leading cause of death and the third leading cause of disability worldwide. Every year, 15 million individuals worldwide suffer from a stroke, with one-third dying and another one-third of survivors living with a permanent disability [1].

Incidences of stroke in Saudi Arabia have been increasing in recent decades because of its aging population. A recent systematic review reported that incidences of stroke in Saudi Arabia are 29 per 100,000 people annually [2]. Stroke is a devastating disease that affects stroke survivors' quality of life, causes severe physical disability, and increases mortality [3].

In Saudi Arabia, the Ministry of Health (MOH) is the major body supporting the medical services. Currently, Saudi Arabia has over 350 hospitals with a limited number of stroke centers [4]. In fact, just 5% of stroke patients in Saudi Arabia are admitted to acute stroke units and receive complete stroke care from specialists [5]. As a result, the present stroke services and staff numbers are insufficient to provide care to the increased number of expected stroke-incidence patients.

Because of the paucity of stroke centers in several Saudi Arabian regions, most stroke patients are commonly treated in the intensive care unit (ICU). Nurses in the ICU are currently providing care for stroke patients. Moreover, stroke nurses in Saudi Arabia generally gain their qualifications by the number of years of working experience with stroke patients.

Stroke nurses play a significant role in the care of stroke patients through appropriate practices, starting from following stroke-management guidelines in providing advanced care to stroke patients. Additionally, they focus on the patient's comprehensive care from the point the patient is admitted into the hospital until the patient is discharged to a rehabilitation department. Furthermore, stroke nurses provide a plan of care to ensure continuity of care for stroke patients after discharge. Therefore, implementing a stroke-care system will ensure advanced stroke management and provision of a high quality of care during acute and recovery care.

The focus in the acute phase appears to be on the "time is brain" principle. The principle emphasizes the time-sensitive necessity of early detection and management in patients with suspected strokes [6]. It is important that nurses be able to recognize stroke manifestations early and determine the onset of signs and symptoms to ensure that patients can receive appropriate treatment within a time window [7].

Furthermore, the use of several stroke scales can also be beneficial to detect stroke manifestations and assess the severity of a stroke [8]. Several studies have suggested that the National Institutes of Health Stroke Scale (NIHSS) is effective, and it is widely used, easy to learn, and rapidly completed on admission. It is considered the gold standard for determining the severity of a stroke. Based on the scale scores, nurses can determine the need for advanced stroke care for stroke patients [9].

According to previous studies on the early management of patients with stroke, one of the important members of the stroke-management team is the nursing staff [8]. Stroke nurses are well prepared to provide urgent care for stroke patients. According to the American Heart Association (AHA) and the European Consensus Group, patients with stroke need immediate medical attention. Early diagnosis of stroke and rapid hospitalization, primarily thrombolytic therapy, (tPA) tissue plasminogen activator and early rehabilitation, and early secondary prevention will reduce stroke mortality [10]. The purpose of all these practices is to address the diagnosis of the condition, achieve medical stability, and prevent early complications in the acute period of the stroke. Starting medical and nursing interventions as early as possible for stroke patients will enhance patient outcomes and minimize stroke complications.

Furthermore, nursing plays a vital role in the care of poststroke after the first 72 h of care [11] Poststroke nursing care focuses on rehabilitation services and secondary prevention measures to enhance stroke survivors' outcomes and avoid stroke recurrence. A study reported that appropriate nursing care and the provision of support from patients' families influences effective rehabilitation for stroke survivors [10]. Stroke has an impact on the patient's physical and psychological well-being, as well as their social and occupational integration [12]. The nurse's role is to follow up with the patient during the recovery phase to ensure continuity of care. However, stroke survivors might face care interruption during the transition from hospitals to rehabilitation or home. Therefore, nursing care practice should also focus on following up with stroke survivors to reduce the risk of readmission and improve the quality of survivors' lives [13].

Even today, the psychosocial health of a patient with a stroke remains under-recognized and undertreated [14]. According to the AHA and the American Stroke Association's (ASA) scientific statement, depression following a stroke is a dynamic phenomenon that affects up to one-third of stroke survivors [15]. Poststroke depression (PSD) among stroke survivors is associated with decreased functional independence and high stress levels, poor cognitive recovery, longer time to resume social activities, lower quality of life, and higher mortality rates. Nursing care guidelines are effective in guiding nursing practice to enhance the social integration of stroke survivors and screen survivors for PSD [16–19].

Furthermore, a study reported that years of experience of working with stroke patients improved nursing practice. A number of years of experience of acute stroke care increases stroke awareness and improves the actual practices associated with care [20]. In fact, obtaining a specialized certification, such as a stroke nursing certification, ensures a high quality of advanced care for patients with strokes. In some countries, working in specialized neuro-units requires that nurses must be certified to be competent to work in specialized clinical areas. However, as mentioned earlier, most of the stroke nurses in Saudi Arabia obtain their title from previous clinical experience with stroke patients.

A stroke is a medical emergency that needs immediate medical attention. Therefore, specialized stroke services, such as stroke units and specialized healthcare providers, will ensure that advanced stroke management is conducted during the periods of hyperacute, acute, and postacute care [21]. The continued lack of understanding of current nursing practices for the care of stroke patients has resulted in a lack of knowledge of the healthcare development needs, negatively affecting patient outcomes and quality of care. In Saudi Arabia, the number of stroke units is limited. Few studies have investigated nursing care for stroke patients in Saudi Arabia. This study aims at examining the current nursing practice for stroke patients in Saudi Arabia.

2. Materials and Methods

2.1. Research Design

This study employed a quantitative, descriptive, cross-sectional design to collect data about current nursing practice for stroke patients.

2.2. Setting and Sample

The study was conducted at three MOH hospitals: King Fahad Medical City (KFGH) is a nonprofit organization with a total capacity of 1200 beds, and it is one of the largest and fastest-growing medical complexes in the Middle East; King Fahad General Hospital (KFGH) in Jeddah is considered as one of the biggest MOH hospitals in the western region hospitals, with a 628-bed capacity; King Abdullah Medical Complex (KAMC) in Jeddah is a 500-bed hospital. The reason for selecting these hospitals was either that they had specialized stroke centers or were eligible to provide treatment for strokes.

A convenience sample of approximately 131 nurses was selected from the three hospitals. This study included head nurses, in-charge nurses, and registered nurses who provided direct care to stroke patients in the stroke unit or intensive care unit (ICU). New nursing staff in training or nursing interns were excluded from the study.

2.3. Recruitment and Data Collection

The participants were recruited after the researcher obtained the ethical permission for the study using the following procedure. The principal investigator sent an email to each hospital's nursing supervisor, along with a letter of invitation, an ethical approval form, and a document containing the study information. Then, the nursing supervisors sent the information to the heads of nursing at the selected units, including the link for the SurveyMonkey questionnaire. Finally, the heads of nursing emailed the questionnaire to the nursing staff.

The data in this study were collected using two questionnaires. The sociodemographic questionnaire consisted of eight items: nurses' age, gender, degree of education, working position, years of experience as a nurse, years of experience working with stroke patients, working sites, and working unit.

The second questionnaire focused on nursing practices with stroke patients and was composed of 71 items: prehospital care (7 items), acute care (30 items), and postacute care (34 items). The participants' responses were measured by using a 5-point Likert scale, as follows: (1) strongly disagree, (2) disagree, (3) neutral, (4) agree, and (5) strongly agree.

The researchers followed the following steps in developing the nursing practices for stroke patient questionnaire. The researchers developed the questionnaire after reviewing the literature and considering the most important practices in dealing with stroke patients according to the guidelines published by the AHA/ASA, European guidelines, and Saudi MOH guidelines. First, the researchers made the aim of the study a focal point of the questionnaire. Second, they selected a 5-point Likert scale to ascertain the degree of participant agreement with each nursing practice. Third, they determined the main dimensions of the questionnaire based on the available guidelines for stroke care. Last, each practice was selected carefully and placed under its associated dimension. All practices related to stroke-patient care were selected based on the authors' review of the literature and current stroke-care guidelines [19,22,23]. After completing the first draft of the questionnaire, the researchers submitted the questionnaire to an expert panel, which consisted of four nursing experts working in a stroke unit who had several years of experience in caring for stroke patients. The researchers revised the questionnaire three times according to the feedback from the expert panel. The approved version of the questionnaire consisted of three dimensions: prehospital care, acute care, and postacute care. The internal consistency of the questionnaire was calculated and found to be highly reliable. The prehospital-care subscale consisted of 7 items ($\alpha = 0.84$), the acute-care subscale consisted of 30 items ($\alpha = 0.88$), and the postacute-care subscale consisted of 34 items ($\alpha = 0.87$).

2.4. Data Analysis

Data were analyzed via SPSS version 26, with a descriptive analysis in the form of means, percentages, frequencies, and standard deviations. Further, an independent chi-square test was conducted to examine the differences in nursing practices between stroke units and the ICUs.

3. Results

3.1. Sociodemographic Characteristics

A sample of 131 nurses completed an online questionnaire. Table 1 shows the demographic characteristics of the sample. The nurses were relatively young (M = 33.27, SD = 5.82) and the ages ranged from 23 to 51 years. The majority of the sample (107; 81.7%) were females. The majority of nurses (107; 81.7%) had a bachelor's degree in nursing, whereas 105 (80.2%) nurses were staff nurses. Nearly half of the sample (47; 35.9%) had nursing experience of more than 10 years, and 64 (48.9%) nurses had five years of nursing experience with stroke patients. There were 52 (39.7%) nurses from KFMC, 35 (26.7%) from KFGH, and 44 (33.6%) from KAMC. More than half of the nurses, 73 (55.7%), were working in the ICU and 58 (44.3%) nurses were working in stroke units.

Table 1. Sociodemographic characteristics of the sample.

Characteristics		(N)	(%)
Gender	Male	24	18.3
	Female	107	81.7
Educational degree	Diploma	18	13.7
	Baccalaureate	107	81.7
	Master's	6	4.6
Current clinical position	Head nurse	7	5.3
	Charge nurse	19	14.5
	Staff nurse	105	80.2

Table 1. *Cont.*

Characteristics		(N)	(%)
Years of experience as a nurse	Less than one year	7	5.3
	1–5 years	41	31.3
	6–10 years	36	27.5
	More than 10 years	47	35.9
Years of experience with stroke patients	Less than one year	11	8.4
	1–5 years	64	48.9
	6–10 years	37	28.2
	More than 10 years	19	14.5
Working hospital	Hospital at Riyadh	52	39.7
	Hospital-1 at Jeddah	35	26.7
	Hospital-2 at Jeddah	44	33.6
Working unit	Stroke unit	58	44.3
	Intensive care unit	73	55.7

3.2. Survey of Nursing Practices for Stroke Patients

Table 2 presents the average score for nurses' responses to each nursing care practice for patients with stroke. Regarding the first dimension, prehospital care, the majority of the nurses agreed that nursing practices with stroke patients during the triaging phase, and nurses' ability to recognize associated medical histories, clinical signs and symptoms, and risk factors for stroke, are common practice. However, some participants were neutral about the activation of the stroke code practice ($M = 3.18$, $SD = 1.70$) and the rapid transfer of a stroke patient to a designated bed ($M = 3.23$, $SD = 1.66$).

Table 2. Nursing care practice for stroke patients.

Practices	Mean	Std. Deviation
Dimension 1: Prehospital care		
1.1. Triaging phase		
1.1.1. Identify stroke signs and symptoms (FAST)	4.21	1.162
1.1.2. Recognize the onset of stroke symptoms from the last time patient was seen as normal	4.10	1.073
1.1.3. Activate stroke code	3.18 *	1.703
1.1.4. Initiate rapid transfer to a designated bed	3.23 *	1.667
1.2. Recognize medical history and lifestyle risk factors for onset of stroke, including		
1.2.1. Medical/surgical history	4.14	1.080
1.2.2. Medication/anticoagulant history	4.21	1.065
1.2.3. Stroke risk factors	4.19	1.039
Dimension 2: Acute care		
2.1. Acute care		
2.1.1. Prepare for CT/CTA scan as soon as possible	4.55	0.825
2.1.2. Assess airway, breathing, and circulation	4.51	0.863

Table 2. Cont.

Practices	Mean	Std. Deviation
2.1.3. Connect patient on cardiac monitor/monitor vital signs	4.56	0.860
2.1.4. Assess stroke severity by applying the National Institutes of Health Stroke Scale (NIHSS)	3.19 *	1.763
2.1.5. Evaluate inclusion and exclusion eligibility criteria for tPA administration	4.07	1.242
2.1.6. Monitor blood glucose and provide treatment if <60 mg/dL according to physician's orders	4.43	0.912
2.1.7. Monitor and manage blood pressure appropriately and in accordance with physician's orders	4.52	0.862
2.1.8. Recognize targeted blood pressure needed for specific patient with stroke	4.48	0.906
2.1.9. Identify and differentiate stroke signs/symptoms and stroke mimics	4.44	0.870
2.1.10. Obtain 12 leads ECG and identify abnormal cardiac rhythm	4.43	0.895
2.1.11. Maintain oxygen saturation > 94%	4.44	0.896
2.1.12. Establish intravenous access, two eighteen-gauge cannula if possible	4.48	0.817
2.1.13. Administer appropriate fluids according to stroke type and following physician's orders	4.47	0.816
2.1.14. Assess need for NG/OG tube-insertion and catheterization-insertion before tPA administration	4.41	0.944
2.1.15. Perform initial bedside swallowing screening	4.25	1.018
2.1.16. Assess for transient ischemic attack (TIA) risk and recurrence using a proper tool	4.31	0.961
2.2. Post-tPA administration and considerations		
2.2.1. Monitor vital signs post-tPA	4.47	0.853
2.2.2. Transfer to the hyperacute stroke unit or ICU if needed, and attach to a cardiac monitor for 72 h post-tPA as per protocol	4.45	0.787
2.2.3. Perform neurological assessment post-tPA	4.53	0.835
2.2.4. Apply precautions post-tPA	4.48	0.862
2.2.5. Monitor for thrombolytic complications	4.52	0.798
2.2.6. Position patient appropriately post-tPA	4.46	0.834
2.2.7. Obtain the NIHSS score 24 h post-tPA administration	3.21 *	1.699
2.3. Pre- and postoperative management		
2.3.1. Obtain the NIHSS score before the procedure	3.18 *	1.659
2.3.2. Conduct preprocedural assessment, including vital signs, medical history, allergies, medications, and laboratory results	4.50	0.817

Table 2. *Cont.*

Practices	Mean	Std. Deviation
2.3.3. Discuss sedation with physician and document the blood-pressure plan	4.43	0.804
2.3.4. Monitor vital signs and conduct neurological assessment at least every 30–60 min preprocedure	4.51	0.768
2.3.5. Obtain the postprocedural NIHSS score	3.30 *	1.639
2.3.6. Check vital signs and conduct neurological assessment, check procedure site, and conduct postprocedural-circulation assessment	4.48	0.788
2.3.7. Monitor for postprocedural complications	4.53	0.778
Dimension 3: Postacute care		
3.1. Provide oxygen therapy and suctioning as needed	4.59	0.773
3.2. Monitor for signs of deterioration	4.59	0.793
3.3. Monitor for deep-vein-thrombosis (DVT) signs	4.58	0.784
3.4. Identify previous falls and assess risk for falls	4.60	0.751
3.5. Monitor for signs of infection	4.55	0.796
3.6. Conduct oral-hygiene assessment and oral care as needed	4.57	0.775
3.7. Manage nasogastric feeding tube safely	4.59	0.773
3.8. Assess for risk of aspiration	4.63	0.778
3.9. Assess nutritional need and nutritional deficiency	4.56	0.776
3.10. Assess for bowel constipation and urine retention and manage it by following physician's orders	4.60	0.752
3.11. Assess patient physical disability using the modified Rankin scale or other tools	3.41 *	1.650
3.12. Monitor gag reflex and ability to swallow	4.51	0.826
3.13. Assess for dysphasia due to injury in area of recognition of spoken language	4.34	0.918
3.14. Feed patient safely according to poststroke severity of dysphagia	4.46	0.888
3.15. Assess need for physical restraints and apply them safely	4.51	0.817
3.16. Conduct pain assessment and analgesic administration as needed following physician's orders	4.55	0.796
3.17. Conduct skin assessment using the Braden scale	4.52	0.826
3.18. Provide pressure relief mattress	4.55	0.787
3.19. Reposition patient every 2 h	4.50	0.826
3.20. Perform passive range-of-motion exercises to prevent contractures	4.47	0.816
3.21. Transfer patient from bed to chair or from bed to bed safely	4.48	0.854
3.22. Conduct appropriate management for patient with cognitive impairment	4.50	0.798

Table 2. Cont.

Practices	Mean	Std. Deviation
3.23. Neglect syndrome: teach patient to touch and use both sides of body	3.50 *	1.506
3.24. Hemianopsia: encourage patient to turn head to scan complete range of vision	3.64 *	1.468
3.25. Increase mobility as tolerated by patient and allowed by physiotherapist	4.44	0.833
3.26. Encourage independence in activities of daily living in safe manner	4.43	0.842
3.27. Refer patient to speech and language pathologist as prescribed	4.27	0.967
3.28. Screen for poststroke depression	2.76 *	1.724
3.29. Assess and report psychosocial needs	3.09 *	1.694
3.30. Encourage patient to express their feelings	3.39 *	1.567
3.31. Educate patient and family about stroke prevention and follow-up clinic after discharge	3.75 *	1.500
3.32. Refer family members to health educator to learn about how to provide home care	4.40	0.848
3.33. Provide end-of-life care for patient	4.41	0.803
3.34. Refer patient to physiatrist/rehabilitation team and assess need for rehabilitation program	4.41	0.822

* Participants disagreed or were neutral about application of the practices.

In the second dimension, acute care, the majority of the nurses agreed that most nursing practices with stroke patients during this phase were applicable. However, some nurses disagreed or were neutral about the need to assess stroke severity by applying the NIHSS ($M = 3.19$, $SD = 1.76$), obtaining NIHSS 24 h post-tPA administration ($M = 3.21$, $SD = 1.69$), obtaining NIHSS scores before conducting a procedure ($M = 3.18$, $SD = 1.65$), and obtaining NIHSS scores after conducting a procedure ($M = 3.30$, $SD = 1.63$).

Regarding the third dimension, postacute care, the majority of the nurses agreed that most nursing practices with stroke patients during this phase are applicable. However, some nurses disagreed or were neutral regarding nursing practices for the assessment of physical disability ($M = 3.41$, $SD = 1.65$), providing intervention for neglect syndrome ($M = 3.50$, $SD = 1.50$) and hemianopsia ($M = 3.64$, $SD = 1.46$), screening for PSD ($M = 2.76$, $SD = 1.72$), the assessment of psychosocial needs ($M = 3.09$, $SD = 1.69$), the encouragement of patient-feeling expression ($M = 3.39$, $SD = 1.56$), and educating patients and families about stroke prevention ($M = 3.75$, $SD = 1.50$).

3.3. Nursing Practices for Stroke Patients across Units

Further statistical analysis was conducted to determine whether there was a significant difference in nursing practices for stroke patients between the stroke units and the ICUs. We performed a chi-squared test of independence to examine the differences in each nursing practice and the two clinical units, stroke unit, and ICU. Table 3 shows the significant differences between nursing practices across units during prehospital care, including the activation of the stroke code, $X^2 (4, N = 131) = 48.34$, $p < 0.001$, and transferring stroke patients to designated beds, $X^2 (4, N = 131) = 48.74$, $p < 0.001$. Both nursing practices were more applicable in the stroke unit than in the ICU.

Table 3. Nursing practices for stroke patients during prehospital care across units.

Dimension 1: Prehospital Care	Practices	Stroke Unit N (%)	ICU N (%)	Chi-Square Tests of Independence
Activate stroke code	Strongly disagree	4 (3.1)	37 (28.2)	$X^2 (4) = 48.34$ $p < 0.001$
	Disagree	0 (0)	11 (8.4)	
	Neutral	4 (3.1)	4 (3.1)	
	Agree	18 (13.7)	8 (6.1)	
	Strongly agree	32 (24.4)	13 (9.9)	
Initiate rapid transfer to designated bed	Strongly disagree	4 (3.1)	33 (25.2)	$X^2 (4) = 48.74$ $p < 0.001$
	Disagree	0 (0)	14 (10.7)	
	Neutral	2 (1.5)	4 (3.1)	
	Agree	20 (15.3)	10 (7.6)	
	Strongly agree	32 (24.4)	12 (9.2)	

ICU = intensive care unit.

During the acute phase, we also found several significant differences in nursing practices across the two units. Table 4 shows that assessing stroke severity by applying the NIHSS was significant, $X^2 (4, N = 131) = 70.11, p < 0.001$; many nurses agreed that this scale was more commonly used by nurses in the stroke unit than in the ICU. Moreover, evaluating the inclusion and exclusion eligibility criteria for tPA administration was also significant, $X^2 (4, N = 131) = 20.14, p < 0.001$, between the two units. Furthermore, a similar significant difference was found with obtaining the NIHSS score 24 h post-tPA administration, $X^2 (4, N = 131) = 85.90, p < 0.001$, obtaining the NIHSS before the procedure, $X^2 (4, N = 131) = 84.61, p < 0.001$, and obtaining the NIHSS after the procedure, $X^2 (4, N = 131) = 78.08, p < 0.001$.

Table 4. Nursing practices for stroke patients during acute care across units.

Dimension 2: Acute Care	Practices	Stroke Unit N (%)	ICU N (%)	Chi-Square Tests of Independence
Assess stroke severity by applying the National Institution of Health Stroke Scale (NIHSS)	Strongly disagree	2 (1.5)	41 (31.3)	$X^2 (4) = 70.11$ $p < 0.001$
	Disagree	0 (0)	12 (9.2)	
	Neutral	1 (0.8)	3 (2.3)	
	Agree	13 (9.9)	8 (6.1)	
	Strongly agree	42 (32.1)	9 (6.9)	
Evaluate the inclusion and exclusion eligibility criteria for tPA administration	Strongly disagree	2 (1.5)	7 (5.3)	$X^2 (4) = 20.14$ $p < 0.001$
	Disagree	0 (0)	11 (8.4)	
	Neutral	3 (2.3)	6 (4.6)	
	Agree	12 (9.2)	23 (17.6)	
	Strongly agree	41 (31.3)	26 (19.8)	
Perform the NIHSS score 24 h post-tPA administration	Strongly disagree	1 (0.8)	35 (26.7)	$X^2 (4) = 85.90$ $p < 0.001$
	Disagree	0 (0)	19 (14.5)	
	Neutral	1 (0.8)	7 (5.3)	
	Agree	12 (9.2)	6 (4.6)	
	Strongly agree	44 (33.6)	6 (4.6)	

Table 4. Cont.

Dimension 2: Acute Care		Stroke Unit N (%)	ICU N (%)	Chi-Square Tests of Independence
Practices				
Obtain the NIHSS score before the procedure	Strongly disagree	1 (0.8)	32 (24.4)	$X^2 (4) = 84.61$ $p < 0.001$
	Disagree	0 (0)	23 (17.6)	
	Neutral	2 (1.5)	7 (5.3)	
	Agree	14 (10.7)	5 (3.8)	
	Strongly agree	41 (31.3)	6 (4.6)	
Obtain the postprocedural NIHSS score	Strongly disagree	1 (0.8)	30 (22.9)	$X^2 (4) = 78.08$ $p < 0.001$
	Disagree	0 (0)	20 (15.3)	
	Neutral	0 (0)	7 (5.3)	
	Agree	17 (13)	8 (6.1)	
	Strongly agree	40 (30.5)	8 (6.1)	

NIHSS = the National Institutes of Health Stroke Scale.

During the postacute phase, we detected some major differences in nursing practice across two units. Table 5 shows that assessing patient physical disability using the modified Rankin scale (mRS) or other tools was significant, $X^2 (4, N = 131) = 61.24, p < 0.001$. Many nurses reported that this scale was used more frequently in the stroke unit than in the ICU. Moreover, providing an intervention for neglect syndrome was significant, $X^2 (4, N = 131) = 44.72, p < 0.001$. This practice was more prevalent in the stroke unit than the ICU. We also found similarly significant values with providing intervention for hemianopsia, $X^2 (4, N = 131) = 39.22, p < 0.001$. There was a significant difference in screening for poststroke depression, $X^2 (4, N = 131) = 101.59, p < 0.001$. Assessment of psychosocial needs, $X^2 (4, N = 131) = 74.44, p < 0.001$, and the encouragement of patients to express their feelings was also significant, $X^2 (4, N = 131) = 58.64, p < 0.001$, between the two units. Furthermore, we found a significant difference in providing education to patients and families about stroke prevention and encouraging follow-up clinic after discharge, $X^2 (4, N = 131) = 40.51, p < 0.001$ between two units.

Table 5. Nursing practices for stroke patients during postacute care across units.

Dimension 3: Postacute Care		Stroke Unit N (%)	ICU N (%)	Chi-Square Tests of Independence
Practices				
Assess patient physical disability using the modified Rankin scale or other tools	Strongly disagree	1 (0.8)	27 (20.6)	$X^2 (4) = 61.24$ $p < 0.001$
	Disagree	0 (0)	22 (16.8)	
	Neutral	2 (1.5)	2 (1.5)	
	Agree	13 (9.9)	6 (6.9)	
	Strongly agree	42 (32.1)	13 (9.9)	
Neglect syndrome: teach the patient to touch and use both sides of the body	Strongly disagree	1 (0.8)	21 (16)	$X^2 (4) = 44.72$ $p < 0.001$
	Disagree	0 (0)	17 (13)	
	Neutral	5 (3.8)	9 (6.9)	
	Agree	18 (13.7)	12 (9.2)	
	Strongly agree	34 (26)	14 (10.7)	

Table 5. Cont.

Dimension 3: Postacute Care Practices		Stroke Unit N (%)	ICU N (%)	Chi-Square Tests of Independence
Hemianopsia: encourage the patient to turn the head to scan the complete range of vision	Strongly disagree	1 (0.8)	18 (13.7)	$X^2 (4) = 39.22$ $p < 0.001$
	Disagree	0 (0)	14 (10.7)	
	Neutral	5 (3.8)	11 (8.4)	
	Agree	14 (10.7)	14 (10.7)	
	Strongly agree	38 (29)	16 (12.2)	
Screen for poststroke depression	Strongly disagree	1 (0.8)	51 (38.9)	$X^2 (4) = 101.59$ $p < 0.001$
	Disagree	2 (1.5)	17 (13)	
	Neutral	6 (4.6)	1 (0.8)	
	Agree	13 (9.9)	2 (1.5)	
	Strongly agree	36 (27.5)	2 (1.5)	
Assess and report psychosocial needs	Strongly disagree	2 (1.5)	35 (26.7)	$X^2 (4) = 74.44$ $p < 0.001$
	Disagree	1 (0.8)	23 (17.6)	
	Neutral	3 (2.3)	3 (2.3)	
	Agree	16 (12.2)	2 (1.5)	
	Strongly agree	36 (27.5)	10 (7.6)	
Encourage the patient to express her or his feelings	Strongly disagree	1 (0.8)	21 (16)	$X^2 (4) = 58.64$ $p < 0.001$
	Disagree	1 (0.8)	27 (20.6)	
	Neutral	3 (2.3)	3 (2.3)	
	Agree	14 (10.7)	9 (6.9)	
	Strongly agree	39 (29.8)	11 (8.4)	
Educate patients and families about stroke prevention and follow-up clinic after discharge	Strongly disagree	2 (1.5)	14 (10.7)	$X^2 (4) = 40.51$ $p < 0.001$
	Disagree	0 (0)	22 (16.8)	
	Neutral	3 (2.3)	2 (1.5)	
	Agree	9 (6.9)	15 (11.5)	
	Strongly agree	44 (33.6)	20 (15.3)	

4. Discussion

This study examined current nursing practices for stroke patients in Saudi Arabia across three dimensions: pre-, acute, and poststroke care. Regarding the first dimension, prehospital care, our results showed that most nurses recognize stroke signs and symptoms. Consistent with previous studies, the identification and consistent use of a standardized assessment was found to provide reliable and consistent data. A possible explanation for this similarity is that the FAST test is easy to use and is a highly recommended screening tool when a patient presents with the signs and symptoms of a stroke [24].

Regarding prehospital care, the data revealed that 40% and 39%, respectively, of nurses disagreed with the application of activating the stroke code and the rapid transfer to designated bed practices. According to the AHA and ASA guidelines, the increased time taken from symptom onset to admission to an emergency department (ED) is the major cause of ineligibility for acute reperfusion treatments. This could be due to the lack of patients, and the public understanding of stroke signs and symptoms and of the necessity of immediate care. However, Saudi Arabia has provided a unified emergency number, as with 911, that might be used to create a faster medical and public response. The delay in the activation of the stroke code might be due to uncertainty with stroke onset and symptoms.

Regarding the second dimension, acute care, the data indicated that 40.5% of nurses disagreed about using the NIHSS in the ICU. Our study showed that most of those who did use it, 42%, were stroke-unit nurses. In line with another study, it was found that the use of the NIHSS is limited outside the stroke unit [25]. One explanation for this could be that nurses in other units, such as ICU nurses, are unfamiliar with this scale, or they do not use it frequently; therefore, nurses might need to be trained to use the NIHSS [25].

A total of 41% of ICU nurses reported they did not perform the NIHSS 24 h post-tPA administration, while 52% agreed to perform this practice. Nurses should frequently assess patients with the NIHSS after receiving tPA treatment to identify if there is a neurological deterioration [26]. Another study found that using the NIHSS can help manage and evaluate therapeutic effectiveness post-tPA administration and identify early complications [27]. It is well known that the patient's neurologic status changes within the first 24 h following intravenous thrombolysis therapy [28]. It is possible that this variation in NIHSS use is due to the fact that our nurses still need more training sessions on using stroke-tools assessment.

The analysis confirmed that the evaluation of inclusion and exclusion eligibility criteria for tPA administration was performed more in the stroke unit than in the ICU. This result is consistent with earlier findings. Treatments, including intravenous tPA, were used more frequently at primary stroke centers [29]. Moreover, stroke patients who were treated in stroke centers were more likely to receive tPA [30]. Although the stroke unit in Saudi Arabia is still being developed and improved, these findings are likely obtained because stroke nurses are more knowledgeable about stroke care than other nonspecialized nurses.

The current study found that, in stroke units, 42% of nurses reported applying the mRS or other measures to assess patient physical disability more frequently than in the ICU. Comparing the results with those of another study, they found that the mRS is the most widely used major outcome measure for acute stroke. Additionally, nurses use other assessment tools with the mRS to address the defects and provide a more comprehensive understanding of poststroke disability [31]. Healthcare agencies must grasp the importance of involving nurses in rehabilitation services. They should clarify the roles of nurses in stroke rehabilitation and develop systematic procedures to ensure adequate time is provided for rehabilitation nursing care. In fact, the mRS is widely used as a measure of long-term functional outcomes in community settings after a stroke [31].

There may be potential complications after a stroke according to the AHA scientific statement (2021). Nurses and other healthcare professionals should prevent and manage these complications. Neglect syndrome is one of the major complications associated with a stroke [32]. According to this study's findings, stroke nurses are willing to deal with neglect syndrome. Further, this practice is applied more in the stroke unit than in the ICU. This finding is consistent with a qualitative study that found most nurses adopt various behaviors to increase patient awareness of their left side. This includes verbally telling patients to pay attention to their left side or picking up something from their left side [33]. Moreover, it was mentioned in a prior study that nurses play a key role in hemianopsia management, as well as in educating the patients and their families [34]. The reason behind this might be that approximately half of the nurses in this study, 48.9%, had at least five years of experience working with stroke patients.

According to our survey, a significant percent, 52%, of participants disagreed about using the poststroke depression (PSD) screening. This finding is supported by a recent study conducted in Saudi Arabia. The study reported that the majority of stroke survivors are discharged from hospitals without receiving PSD screening [14]. Additionally, although nurses recognize the necessity of screening and detecting depression symptoms, they rarely utilize recommended depression-screening tools [19]. Furthermore, incidences of PSD increase when stroke survivors lack social support and experience social isolation. We found similar results regarding the lack of psychosocial support, which further validated our findings from the perspective of a lack of attention to psychosocial needs. As evidenced by previous studies, stroke survivors with PSD have reported a lack of perceived social support, restricted social involvement, and a poor quality of life [14]. In line with our findings, there is a lack of practices encouraging patients to express their feelings. A possible explanation for this could be that most of the practices are focused on acute-stage concerns, whereas postacute care, including consideration of the patient's psychosocial status, is mostly ignored. The literature has reported that healthcare providers pay little attention to the psychological state of stroke patients [14]. According to another study, clinical care practices for stroke patients are mainly focused on general care, regardless of the stage of the disease. This could be because the nurses focus on stroke priority outcomes rather than rehabilitation nursing care [35]. Furthermore, generally, most hospitals are lacking transition-of-care programs from the stroke unit to home care, in which patients get lost in the middle of the care [36].

Patient education after a stroke is an important element to prevent stroke recurrence. Family members require education sessions to learn skills to provide home care for stroke survivors. However, in this study, about 28% of the ICU nurses disagreed about patient-education practices in the ICU. The AHA/ASA highly recommend post-stroke patient education to prevent stroke recurrence [22]. One explanation for the study's finding is that stroke patients are usually admitted to the ICU during the acute stage and are discharged once they are medically stable, which means that the ICU nurse would not be able to provide education to the patient and their family members during the acute stage.

There are some limitations to consider in this study in using convenience sampling, which increases the risk for selection bias. In Saudi Arabia, there are no equivalent national studies on nursing practices with stroke patients. Moreover, the number of stroke-care units available is limited and has fewer nurses to participate in the study than the ICU. Therefore, the heterogeneity of the results of some nursing practice between the ICU and stroke unit was clearly identified in the analysis of the study. However, this is the first study in Saudi Arabia to examine evidence-based nursing practice in stroke care. The researchers compared stroke units to the ICUs in three hospitals, in which the gap in nursing practice across clinical areas should receive further attention to improve quality of stroke care. Further, the survey for this study was developed based on standardized stroke-care guidelines.

Based on the study findings, we recommend the development of a stroke unit for patient care in several Saudi Arabian regions. This will help in early stroke identification and allow advanced stroke management within the treatment window. It will also help improve the application of evidence-based practices and standardized guidelines in providing appropriate interventions for patients with strokes. Moreover, we recommend providing educational and training programs to critical nurses to increase their knowledge and skills to use the NIHSS. During the rehabilitation phase, we recommend nurses provide and pay adequate support and attention to stroke survivors. Psychosocial support plays an important role in stroke survivors' and their families' health. Based on current poststroke recommendations, early depression screening is one of the most critical screenings among stroke survivors. Hospitals should have a clear policy for screening stroke patients for depression. Nurses should be trained on using depression-screening tools for early-depression-symptom identification to improve patient outcomes. Further research is needed to examine how nurses can improve stroke outcomes in different care units, regardless of whether they are stroke units or ICUs. Moreover, stroke care should be provided with specialized competent stroke nurses. Further examination for obtaining stroke certification from an accredited body is highly recommended for nurses to work in specialized stroke areas. This will improve clinical outcomes for stroke patients and prevent long-term complications in stroke survivors.

5. Conclusions

In this study, we aimed to examine current nursing practices and determine the future nursing needs of patients with strokes in Saudi Arabia. We found a significant variation between several nursing practices across stroke units and ICUs regarding the activation of the stroke code, transferring stroke patients to a designated bed, applying the

NIHSS, using the modified Rankin scale, providing intervention for neglect syndrome and hemianopsia, screening for poststroke depression, assessing for psychosocial needs and encouraging patients to express their feelings, and educating patients and families about stroke prevention. These practices were more prevalent in the stroke unit than in the ICU. However, the majority of nurses agreed that most care practices for stroke patients were applicable. There is a variability of standards in some aspects of nursing stroke care, and, as a result, there is scope for their improvement. A stroke-care program and specialized certification is highly recommended for nurses who provide care for patients with strokes.

Author Contributions: Conceptualization, L.A.B., R.A.S., R.B., R.S., A.A., F.H.H. and A.M.A.; methodology, L.A.B., R.A.S., R.B., R.S. and A.A.; software, R.A.S., R.B., R.S. and A.A.; validation, L.A.B., F.H.H. and A.M.A.; formal analysis, L.A.B., R.A.S., R.B., R.S. and A.A.; investigation, L.A.B., R.A.S., R.B., R.S. and A.A.; resources, L.A.B., F.H.H. and A.M.A.; data curation, L.A.B., F.H.H. and A.M.A.; writing—original draft preparation, R.A.S., R.B., R.S. and A.A.; writing—review and editing, L.A.B.; visualization, L.A.B.; supervision, L.A.B.; project administration, L.A.B. All authors have read and agreed to the published version of the manuscript.

Funding: This research received no external funding.

Institutional Review Board Statement: The ethical permission was obtained from the Faculty of Nursing at King Abdulaziz University and the Ministry of Health hospitals in Saudi Arabia, NREC serial no: Ref No 2B. 06.

Informed Consent Statement: Informed consent was obtained from all subjects involved in the study.

Data Availability Statement: The data will be shared by the authors of this research paper upon request.

Public Involvement Statement: No public involvement in any aspect of this research.

Guidelines and Standards Statement: This manuscript was drafted against the STROBE (The Strengthening the Reporting of Observational Studies in Epidemiology) for cross-sectional studies.

Acknowledgments: The authors want to acknowledge the efforts of the research assistant who facilitated the data collection.

Conflicts of Interest: The authors declare no conflict of interest.

References

1. World Health Organization—Regional Office for the Eastern Mediterranean. Stroke, Cerebrovascular Accident. 2020. Available online: http://www.emro.who.int/health-topics/stroke-cerebrovascular-accident/index.html (accessed on 18 February 2022).
2. Alqahtani, B.A.; Alenazi, A.M.; Hoover, J.C.; Alshehri, M.M.; Alghamdi, M.S.; Osailan, A.M.; Khunti, K. Incidence of stroke among Saudi population: A systematic review and meta-analysis. *Neurol. Sci.* **2020**, *41*, 3099–3104. [CrossRef] [PubMed]
3. Al-Senani, F.; Al-Johani, M.; Salawati, M.; Alhazzani, A.; Morgenstern, L.B.; Ravest, V.S.; Cuche, M.; Eggington, S. An Epidemiological Model for First Stroke in Saudi Arabia. *J. Stroke Cerebrovasc. Dis.* **2020**, *29*, 104465. [CrossRef] [PubMed]
4. Basri, R.; Issrani, R.; Hua Gan, S.; Prabhu, N.; Khursheed Alam, M. Burden of stroke in the Kingdom of Saudi Arabia: A soaring epidemic. *Saudi Pharm. J.* **2021**, *29*, 264–268. [CrossRef] [PubMed]
5. Al-Senani, F.; Salawati, M.; AlJohani, M.; Cuche, M.; Seguel Ravest, V.; Eggington, S. Workforce requirements for comprehensive ischaemic stroke care in a developing country: The case of Saudi Arabia. *Hum. Resour. Health* **2019**, *17*, 90. [CrossRef]
6. Ashcraft, S.; Wilson, S.E.; Nyström, K.V.; Dusenbury, W.; Wira, C.R.; Burrus, T.M.; American Heart Association Council on Cardiovascular and Stroke Nursing and the Stroke Council. Care of the Patient with Acute Ischemic Stroke (Prehospital and Acute Phase of Care): Update to the 2009 Comprehensive Nursing Care Scientific Statement: A Scientific Statement from the American Heart Association. *Stroke* **2021**, *52*, e164–e178. [CrossRef] [PubMed]
7. Chauhdry, H. Understanding the importance of recognising, treating and preventing stroke. *Nurs. Stand.* **2022**, *37*, 77–82. [CrossRef] [PubMed]
8. Škodrić, A.; Marić, G.; Jovanović, D.; Beslać-Bumbaširević, L.; Kisić-Tepavčević, D.; Pekmezović, T. Assessment of nursing care-associated predictors of in-hospital mortality in the patients with acute ischemic stroke. *Vojnosanit. Pregl.* **2019**, *76*, 373–378. [CrossRef]
9. Lyden, P. Using the National Institutes of Health Stroke Scale: A Cautionary Tale. *Stroke* **2017**, *48*, 513–519. [CrossRef]
10. Jaromin, J.; Tomaszewska, A.; Waluś, A.; Pelan, M.; Śleziona, M.; Graf, L. Nurses' Opinion on Nursing Problems in the Care of Patients after Stroke. *J. Neurol. Neurosurg. Nurs.* **2017**, *6*, 73–80. [CrossRef]
11. Clare, C.S. Role of the nurse in acute stroke care. *Nurs. Stand.* **2020**, *35*, 68–75. [CrossRef]

12. Loft, M.I.; Poulsen, I.; Esbensen, B.A.; Iversen, H.K.; Mathiesen, L.L.; Martinsen, B. Nurses' and nurse assistants' beliefs, attitudes and actions related to role and function in an inpatient stroke rehabilitation unit-A qualitative study. *J. Clin. Nurs.* **2017**, *26*, 4905–4914. [CrossRef]
13. Ross, S.Y.; Roberts, S.; Taggart, H.; Patronas, C. Stroke Transitions of Care. *Medsurg. Nurs.* **2017**, *26*, 119–123.
14. Babkair, L.A. Risk Factors for Poststroke Depression: An Integrative Review. *J. Neurosci. Nurs.* **2017**, *49*, 73–84. [CrossRef] [PubMed]
15. Virani, S.S.; Alonso, A.; Benjamin, E.J.; Bittencourt, M.S.; Callaway, C.W.; Carson, A.P.; Chamberlain, A.M.; Chang, A.R.; Cheng, S.; Delling, F.N.; et al. Heart Disease and Stroke Statistics—2020 Update: A Report From the American Heart Association. *Circulation* **2020**, *141*, e139–e596. [CrossRef] [PubMed]
16. Babkair, L.A.; Chyun, D.; Dickson, V.V.; Almekhlafi, M.A. The Effect of Psychosocial Factors and Functional Independence on Poststroke Depressive Symptoms: A Cross-Sectional Study. *J. Nurs. Res.* **2021**, *30*, e189. [CrossRef] [PubMed]
17. Khedr, E.M.; Abdelrahman, A.A.; Desoky, T.; Zaki, A.F.; Gamea, A. Post-stroke depression: Frequency, risk factors, and impact on quality of life among 103 stroke patients—Hospital-based study. *Egypt. J. Neurol. Psychiatry Neurosurg.* **2020**, *56*, 66. [CrossRef]
18. Bartoli, F.; Di Brita, C.; Crocamo, C.; Clerici, M.; Carrà, G. Early Post-stroke Depression and Mortality: Meta-Analysis and Meta-Regression. *Front. Psychiatry* **2018**, *9*, 530. [CrossRef]
19. Bjartmarz, I.; Jónsdóttir, H.; Hafsteinsdóttir, T.B. Implementation and feasibility of the stroke nursing guideline in the care of patients with stroke: A mixed methods study. *BMC Nurs.* **2017**, *16*, 72. [CrossRef]
20. Hisaka, Y.; Ito, H.; Yasuhara, Y.; Takase, K.; Tanioka, T.; Locsin, R. Nurses' Awareness and Actual Nursing Practice Situation of Stroke Care in Acute Stroke Units: A Japanese Cross-Sectional Web-Based Questionnaire Survey. *Int. J. Environ. Res. Public. Health* **2021**, *18*, 12800. [CrossRef]
21. Harrison, M.; Ryan, T.; Gardiner, C.; Jones, A. Psychological and emotional needs, assessment, and support post-stroke: A multi-perspective qualitative study. *Top. Stroke Rehabil.* **2016**, *24*, 119–125. [CrossRef]
22. Winstein, C.J.; Stein, J.; Arena, R.; Bates, B.; Cherney, L.R.; Cramer, S.C.; Deruyter, F.; Eng, J.J.; Fisher, B.; Harvey, R.L.; et al. Guidelines for Adult Stroke Rehabilitation and Recovery: A Guideline for Healthcare Professionals From the American Heart Association/American Stroke Association. *Stroke* **2016**, *47*, e98–e169. [CrossRef] [PubMed]
23. Powers, W.J.; Rabinstein, A.A.; Ackerson, T.; Adeoye, O.M.; Bambakidis, N.C.; Becker, K.; Biller, J.; Brown, M.; Demaerschalk, B.M.; Hoh, B.; et al. Guidelines for the Early Management of Patients with Acute Ischemic Stroke: 2019 Update to the 2018 Guidelines for the Early Management of Acute Ischemic Stroke: A Guideline for Healthcare Professionals from the American Heart Association/American Stroke Association. *Stroke* **2019**, *50*, e344–e418. [PubMed]
24. Crause, K.G.; Stassen, W. The accuracy of the FAST stroke assessment in identifying stroke at initial ambulance call into a South African private emergency call centre. *S. Afr. J. Crit. Care.* **2020**, *36*, 35. [CrossRef] [PubMed]
25. Dancer, S.; Brown, A.J.; Yanase, L.R. National Institutes of Health Stroke Scale in Plain English Is Reliable for Novice Nurse Users with Minimal Training. *J. Emerg. Nurs.* **2017**, *43*, 221–227. [CrossRef] [PubMed]
26. Hinkle, J.L. Reliability and Validity of the National Institutes of Health Stroke Scale for Neuroscience Nurses. *Stroke* **2014**, *45*, e32–e34. [CrossRef] [PubMed]
27. Rangaraju, S.; Frankel, M.; Jovin, T.G. Prognostic Value of the 24-Hour Neurological Examination in Anterior Circulation Ischemic Stroke: A post hoc Analysis of Two Randomized Controlled Stroke Trials. *Interv. Neurol.* **2015**, *4*, 120–129. [CrossRef] [PubMed]
28. Wouters, A.; Nysten, C.; Thijs, V.; Lemmens, R. Prediction of Outcome in Patients with Acute Ischemic Stroke Based on Initial Severity and Improvement in the First 24 h. *Front. Neurol.* **2018**, *9*, 308. [CrossRef] [PubMed]
29. Higashida, R.; Alberts, M.J.; Alexander, D.N.; Crocco, T.J.; Demaerschalk, B.M.; Derdeyn, C.P.; Goldstein, L.B.; Jauch, E.C.; Mayer, S.A.; Meltzer, N.M.; et al. Interactions within Stroke Systems of Care: A Policy Statement from the American Heart Association/American Stroke Association. *Stroke* **2013**, *44*, 2961–2984. [CrossRef]
30. Johnson, M.; Bakas, T. A Review of Barriers to Thrombolytic Therapy: Implications for Nursing Care in the Emergency Department. *J. Neurosci. Nurs.* **2010**, *42*, 7. [CrossRef]
31. Zerna, C.; Burley, T.; Green, T.L.; Dukelow, S.P.; Demchuk, A.M.; Hill, M.D. Comprehensive assessment of disability post-stroke using the newly developed miFUNCTION scale. *Int. J. Stroke* **2020**, *15*, 167–174. [CrossRef]
32. Lui, S.K.; Nguyen, M.H. Elderly Stroke Rehabilitation: Overcoming the Complications and Its Associated Challenges. *Curr. Gerontol. Geriatr. Res.* **2018**, *2018*, 9853837. [CrossRef]
33. Someya, A.; Tanaka, M. The process by which patients become aware of unilateral spatial neglect: A qualitative study. *Neuropsychol. Rehabil.* **2021**, *32*, 2370–2391. [CrossRef]
34. Wolberg, A.; Kapoor, N. Homonymous Hemianopsia. In *StatPearls [Internet]*; StatPearls Publishing: Orlando, FL, USA, 2021.
35. Meng, X.; Chen, X.; Liu, Z.; Zhou, L. Nursing practice in stroke rehabilitation: Perspectives from multi-disciplinary healthcare professionals. *Nurs. Health Sci.* **2020**, *22*, 28–37. [CrossRef]
36. Camicia, M.; Lutz, B.; Summers, D.; Klassman, L.; Vaughn, S. Nursing's Role in Successful Stroke Care Transitions Across the Continuum: From Acute Care Into the Community. *Stroke* **2021**, *52*, e794–e805. [CrossRef]

Disclaimer/Publisher's Note: The statements, opinions and data contained in all publications are solely those of the individual author(s) and contributor(s) and not of MDPI and/or the editor(s). MDPI and/or the editor(s) disclaim responsibility for any injury to people or property resulting from any ideas, methods, instructions or products referred to in the content.

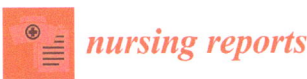

Article

Validity and Reliability of a Short Form of the Questionnaire for the Reflective Practice of Nursing Involving Invasive Mechanical Ventilation: A Cross-Sectional Study

Makoto Tsukuda [1,*], Atsuko Fukuda [2], Junko Shogaki [2] and Ikuko Miyawaki [2]

1. College of Nursing Art and Science, University of Hyogo, 13-71 Kitaoji-Cho, Akashi 673-0021, Hyogo, Japan
2. Graduate School of Health Sciences, Kobe University, 7-10-2 Tomogaoka, Suma-Ku, Kobe 654-0142, Hyogo, Japan
* Correspondence: makoto_tsukuda@cnas.u-hyogo.ac.jp; Tel./Fax: +81-78-925-9419

Abstract: The number of patients on ventilators is rapidly increasing owing to the coronavirus pandemic. The previously developed Questionnaire for the Reflective Practice of Nursing Involving Invasive Mechanical Ventilation (Q-RPN-IMV) for the care of patients on ventilators includes nurses' thought processes as items. This study aims to develop a short form of the Q-RPN-IMV for immediate use in practice and to test its reliability and validity. A convenience sample of 629 participants was used to explore the factor structure using factor analysis. The test–retest reliability was assessed using the intraclass correlation coefficient (ICC). The study was a cross-sectional design instrument development study and was reported according to GRRAS guidelines. Q-RPN-IMV short form was divided into ventilator management and patient management. The ventilator management comprised 31 items organized into six factors. Cronbach's alpha ranged from 0.82 to 0.91, and the ICC ranged from 0.82 to 0.89. The patient management comprised 27 items organized into five factors. Cronbach's alpha ranged from 0.75 to 0.97, and ICC ranged from 0.75 to 0.97. The Q-RPN-IMV short form is a reliable and validated instrument for assessing care for patients on ventilators. This study was not registered.

Keywords: invasive mechanical ventilation; validity; reliability; questionnaire; short form

Citation: Tsukuda, M.; Fukuda, A.; Shogaki, J.; Miyawaki, I. Validity and Reliability of a Short Form of the Questionnaire for the Reflective Practice of Nursing Involving Invasive Mechanical Ventilation: A Cross-Sectional Study. *Nurs. Rep.* **2023**, *13*, 1170–1184. https://doi.org/10.3390/nursrep13030101

Academic Editor: Richard Gray

Received: 28 July 2023
Revised: 24 August 2023
Accepted: 29 August 2023
Published: 1 September 2023

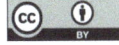

Copyright: © 2023 by the authors. Licensee MDPI, Basel, Switzerland. This article is an open access article distributed under the terms and conditions of the Creative Commons Attribution (CC BY) license (https://creativecommons.org/licenses/by/4.0/).

1. Introduction

The essential skills required for nursing practice for patients on ventilator support include knowledge of ventilators, invasive techniques for preventing complications, and risk prediction for safe management [1,2]. Therefore, management in the intensive care area is generally recommended for patients on ventilator support because it is well-equipped and has qualified experts to manage such patients [3]. Recently, the number of patients with respiratory diseases due to aging has increased worldwide. Moreover, the number of patients with severe respiratory symptoms due to the spread of coronavirus disease 2019 (COVID-19) is rapidly increasing [4–6]; thus, the number of patients on ventilators during treatment has inevitably increased. In the current scenario of the ongoing pandemic, intensive care units cannot exclusively manage patients on ventilators. Therefore, the general ward continues to serve as an urgent management site for such patients [7–10].

Respiratory therapists in Europe and the United States are coping with the pressures of a growing number of patients suffering from infectious diseases; however, in the event of a pandemic, there could be a worldwide shortage of ventilators and specially trained respiratory therapists [11,12]. General nurses from various backgrounds would therefore be forced to manage patients on ventilators and provide in-hospital and home care, including oxygen therapy, respiratory assistance, and ventilator therapy [13]. Furthermore, even if nurses have little experience caring for patients on ventilators, they are expected to have the minimum knowledge and skills necessary to safely manage these patients. Therefore, nurses in charge of patients requiring ventilators carry a heavy burden because of a substantial amount of responsibility and potential lack of experience, frequently leading to negative emotions, such as anxiety, stress, and lack of self-confidence [9].

Despite this situation, inexperienced nurses currently provide ventilator education to other nursing staff using the methods of the facility. Furthermore, most nursing education programs generally solely focus on imparting knowledge on the individual skills of ventilator care [14]. During the pandemic, it was difficult to ensure the quality and safety of nursing care for patients on ventilators because conducting group training in the hospital was impossible due to the increased number of patients. Therefore, with the rapid increase in the number of patients on ventilators, there is a need for an evaluation sheet that allows inexperienced nurses to provide safe nursing care to patients on ventilators and for nurses who practice on such patients to look back on their practice and self-evaluate it.

In a previous study, we developed the Questionnaire for the Reflective Practice of Nursing Involving Invasive Mechanical Ventilation (Q-RPN-IMV), a comprehensive, itemized measure of nursing practice of ventilator care by professional and certified nurses who are considered experts in fields related to ventilator care, including their thought processes [15]. This questionnaire differs from previous checklists because it is not simply a checklist to determine whether self-care has been practiced. However, because ventilator care is complex and includes advanced-level practice items practiced by specialized and certified nurses, the number of items is notably large, and the so-called "Q-RPN-IMV long form" could not be used routinely by inexperienced nurses. Even for inexperienced nurses to safely manage ventilator-implanted patients and to be able to use the questionnaire immediately in clinical practice, the number of items in the questionnaire must be carefully selected and consolidated. Therefore, we carefully selected suitable items from the Q-RPN-IMV developed in previous studies and created a short form that can be easily used by inexperienced nurses. This study aims to develop a short form of the Q-RPN-IMV, based on the Q-RPN-IMV, for immediate use in practice and to test its reliability and validity.

2. Materials and Methods

2.1. Study Design

Scale development was based on the guidelines described in Scale Development: Theory and Applications and the Consensus-based Standards for the Selection of Health Status Measurement [16]. Moreover, we followed the Guidelines for Reporting Reliability and Agreement Studies (GRRAS) [17].

2.2. Setting and Participants

Using convenience sampling, we selected clinical nurses who had experience caring for patients on ventilators. To meet the criteria for good methodology, a sample size of at least seven times the number of survey items and an absolute number of at least 100 are required [18]. The first version of the questionnaire contained 71 items; therefore, the minimum sample size was 497. The purpose of this study was explained in writing and orally to the facility director to be surveyed, and permission was obtained before the start of the study. A questionnaire on ventilator care was distributed to clinical nurses working in wards where ventilators were used. Criteria for participation were full-time employment in a general hospital with at least 500 beds that was considered to offer group training on ventilators. Certified nurses, nursing managers, licensed practical nurses/nursing assistants, and midwives were excluded from the study. Nurses' responses to the questionnaire were collected from April 2020 to December 2021. The nurses were asked to post their responses in a collection box set up in the ward within 1 week after distribution. Furthermore, the participants were asked to answer a questionnaire on ventilator care after 10–14 days for test–retest reliability to examine the stability of the study. A filled-in questionnaire implied the nurses' consent to participate in the study [19].

2.3. Instrument

Participants answered a questionnaire consisting of the following three sections: (1) demographic characteristics, (2) the Self-Evaluation Scale for Nursing Involving Invasive Mechanical Ventilation, and (3) the educational needs assessment tool for clinical nurses.

2.3.1. Participant Demographic Characteristics

From the participants, we collected data on age, clinical career (years of work experience), number of patients on ventilators received to date, hospital affiliation, and presence or absence of certified nurse support.

2.3.2. Self-Evaluation Scale for Nursing Involving Invasive Mechanical Ventilation

To investigate the participants' nursing practice with patients on ventilators, we utilized the nursing practice process items related to ventilator care required by clinical nurses from the Q-RPN-IMV. The Q-RPN-IMV is a questionnaire that was itemized by observing the respiratory care for patients on ventilators practiced by certified nurses in previous studies, including their thought processes. Furthermore, the Q-RPN-IMV comprises 136 items: 26 observation, 66 judgment, and 44 implementation items. These items were relevant to the respiratory care of patients on ventilators by certified nurses. From these 136 items, the most essential were selected for immediate use by inexperienced nurses.

Content validity refers to whether the content of the scale adequately captures the constructs and requires expert judgment. The content validity index (CVI) is the most widely reported content validity approach in instrument development and can be calculated using Item-CVI (I-CVI) and Scale-Level-CVI (S-CVI). To verify content validity, the Delphi method was performed three times by 20 certified nurses, and the items were selected by more than 80% of the experts on all three occasions [20]. Furthermore, those items were classified by an expert panel of certified nurses into two groups to make them easier to understand by less experienced nurses; items were classified into two groups, "ventilator management" and "patient management". After reviewing the items, they were classified into "ventilator management" and "patient management", and 71 items were adopted as proposal items. Thus, a ventilator evaluation scale consisting of 32 items for machine management and 39 for patient management was proposed for 71 items. Each item was rated on a 5-point Likert scale from 1 (not at all) to 5 (always) to determine the frequency of implementation. The resulting questionnaire was pretested on five nurses in a general ward, and the superficial validity of the proposed scale was examined by checking for unclear expressions and the time required for easy comprehension, even by inexperienced nurses.

2.4. Data Analysis

In the statistical analysis, questionnaires with missing items were excluded, and item analysis was performed first. Subsequently, exploratory factor analysis (EFA), confirmatory factor analysis (CFA), and criterion-related validity were performed to assess the scale's validity. Finally, internal consistency and reproducibility were examined to assess the reliability. All statistical analyses were performed using IBM SPSS version 28 and Amos 28 (IBM Corp., Armonk, NY, USA).

2.4.1. Item Analysis

Standard deviations and means for all items were estimated to detect ceiling and floor effects.

2.4.2. Validity Analysis

EFA was conducted to determine the factor structure supporting "ventilator management" and "patient management" of patients on ventilators. To assess the suitability of the data for factor analysis, the Kaiser–Meyer–Olkin (KMO) test for sampling adequacy and Bartlett's specificity test were performed [18]. The number of factors was visually inspected using scree plots to identify the ideal number of potential factors and to determine if the

KMO criterion of an eigenvalue ≥ 1 was met, and the proportion of variance explained by each factor [21]. Maximum likelihood methods with promax rotation were then performed [22]. Items with factor loadings < 0.4 were excluded [23]. As a rule, the sum of the variance explained should be greater than 50% [24]. EFA was conducted again with the removed items (Items with factor loadings < 0.4). The number of factors was determined to include all items with factor loadings of 0.40 or greater. For items with approximate factor loadings, a valid factor analysis was conducted using a covariance structure analysis, considering the item content included in that factor.

The CFA was performed to test the model fit. For the CFA, we used maximum-likelihood estimation and evaluated model fit. Model fit was tested based on the χ^2, normed χ^2 (χ^2/df), comparative fit index (CFI), and root mean square error of approximation (RMSEA) index used to assess the fit of the scale. A χ^2/df value of ≤ 3 is considered adequate. Furthermore, the fit was considered good if the CFI value was >0.90 and the RMSEA value was <0.08 [25,26].

2.4.3. Reliability Analysis

Reliability was verified using Cronbach's alpha coefficients for the entire scale and each factor. To examine stability and verify the test–retest reliability, we determined the intraclass correlation coefficient (ICC) of the response scores to the scale obtained at the two-time points [19]. ICCs were determined as <0.50 (poor), 0.50–0.80 (fair to good), and >0.80 (excellent) [27].

2.5. Ethical Consideration

Participants were informed of the purpose and methods of the study and the risks and benefits of participation. In addition, participants were informed that their participation was voluntary, that they were free to drop out at any time, and that their privacy would not be affected. Data were collected anonymously using assigned IDs and were strictly controlled. Data handling and disposal procedures were also explained. In the interest of transparency, it was further explained that some of the findings would be presented in a public forum. Researchers provided participants with contact information. Ethical approval was obtained from the Institutional Review Board (IRB) Ethics Committee of the author's university (No. 696). All methods were performed in accordance with relevant guidelines and regulations.

3. Results

3.1. Participant Characteristics

Table 1 presents the participant characteristics. Questionnaires were distributed to 945 clinical nurses working in general hospitals with more than 500 beds and with experience working with patients on ventilators, and 754 returned the questionnaires.

Table 1. Participant characteristics (n = 629).

		n	%
Sex			
	Men	49	(7.8)
	Women	580	(92.2)
Nursing experience			
	<3 years	60	(9.5)
	<3–5 years	152	(24.2)
	<6–10 years	145	(23.1)
	>10 years	272	(43.2)
Number of patients requiring IMV			
	1	16	(2.5)
	2–3	63	(10.0)

Table 1. Cont.

	n	%
4–5	237	(37.7)
6–10	61	(9.7)
>10	252	(40.1)
Support from professional		
Yes	516	(82.0)
No	113	(18.0)

Data are presented as n (%). IMV: invasive mechanical ventilation.

Of the 754 returned questionnaires, 125 with >20% missing data were excluded, and 629 questionnaires were included in the analysis. The questionnaire collection rate was 79.8%, and the effective response rate was 83.4%. For the stability study, 157 questionnaires were collected, and 122 were analyzed after excluding 35 with missing data. The number of nurses with less than 5 years of experience was 212 (33.7%), which is higher than the percentage of nurses in Japan, but this is because the survey excluded managers. Approximately half of the participants were responsible for more than six ventilators.

3.2. Item Analysis

Each of the 71 items was analyzed. The mean individual item scores ranged from 3.03 to 4.89 (standard deviation 0.44–1.53), with no ceiling or bottom effects.

3.3. Factor Analysis

EFA was performed on managing ventilator items (32 items) and patient items (39 items) using the main factor method and promax rotation.

The following results were obtained according to the conditions for factor selection.

3.3.1. Ventilator Management

The KMO measure of sampling adequacy was 0.90. There were six factors based on eigenvalues ≥ 1 and the scree criterion. Items with a loading value of ≥ 0.4 were retained, and item 12 was deleted because the factor loadings were <0.4. The six factors covered the following roles: initial confirmation, artificial airways, alarm management, humidification management, emergency management, and airway fixation. The contributions of factors 1–6 were 32.29%, 10.79%, 6.03%, 5.36%, 4.91%, and 3.75%, respectively, and the cumulative contribution was 63.13%. The model fit index for the scale was calculated using CFA, and the results showed that $\chi^2 = 2058.1$, $\chi^2/df = 4.91$, CFI = 0.844, and RMSEA = 0.079 (Table 2). The model fit was not optimal, although it was acceptable with respect to the factor contribution ratio.

3.3.2. Patient Management

The KMO measure of sampling adequacy was 0.90. There were five factors based on eigenvalues ≥ 1 and the scree criterion. Items with a loading value of ≥ 0.4 were retained, and item 12 was deleted because the factor loadings were <0.4. These five factors covered the following roles: prevention of complications, prevention of VAP, safe transfer, skin management, and post-transfer assessment. The contributions of factors 1–5 were 31.81%, 12.87%, 6.13%, 5.44%, and 4.18%, respectively, and the cumulative contribution was 60.43%. The model fit index for the scale was calculated using CFA, and the results showed that $\chi^2 = 1723.9$, $p < 0.01$, $\chi^2/df = 5.49$, CFI = 0.841, and RMSEA = 0.085 (Table 3). Factor contributions were acceptable. Model coefficients were not good, despite attempts to improve the model index as much as possible by removing items.

Table 2. Ventilator Management (Cronbach's α = 0.91).

Domain/Item Number and Content		Factor Loadings					
		Factor 1	Factor 2	Factor 3	Factor 4	Factor 5	Factor 6
Factor 1							
	Initial confirmation (Cronbach's α = 0.82)						
16	At the start of a shift, confirm the alarm settings for the artificial respirator together with another staff member.	0.76	−0.08	−0.18	−0.06	−0.01	−0.09
18	Confirm that the power is plugged into an outlet that is either red or brown.	0.71	−0.08	0.01	0.03	0.00	−0.03
19	Confirm the patient's respiratory data displayed on the artificial respirator (number of breaths, volume of air per breath, volume of air per minute, maximum respiratory tract internal pressure) every two hours.	0.69	−0.13	0.12	0.02	−0.07	−0.05
21	In case the artificial respirator alarm rings, confirm the alarm message displayed on the LCD screen.	0.68	0.22	−0.03	−0.02	0.03	0.02
17	When confirming the presence or absence of a circuit leak, confirm that each individual artificial airway connection and circuit component is connected properly by both sight and touch.	0.63	0.01	0.19	−0.06	−0.01	0.09
15	At the start of a shift, confirm the artificial respirator instructions and settings together with another staff member.	0.59	−0.05	0.10	0.04	−0.11	0.15
13	Confirm that a cannula of the same type and size as the one currently inserted in the tracheostomy tube, lubricant, and an 11 mL syringe are prepared on the patient's bedside table	0.50	0.09	−0.04	0.03	0.08	−0.16
11	Confirm cuff pressure at the start of each shift	0.48	−0.10	0.12	−0.01	0.06	0.07
64	Ensure no contamination or damage to the artificial respirator circuit	0.45	0.38	−0.08	0.08	−0.02	0.02
Factor 2							
	Artificial airway (Cronbach's α = 0.82)						
32	In a situation where a patient's sputum viscosity is low and a humidifier is in use, consider that to be a sign that the patient's artificial nose needs to be replaced.	−0.20	0.89	−0.03	−0.03	−0.03	0.02
33	In a situation where a patient's sputum viscosity is high and an artificial nose is in use, consider that to be a sign that the patient needs to be switched to a humidifier.	−0.04	0.86	−0.10	0.03	−0.12	0.08
26	Be aware that artificial noses and heated humidifiers must not be used at the same time.	0.25	0.56	−0.08	−0.03	0.11	−0.01
14	If an accidental removal of the tracheotomy tube occurs, one should call a doctor, ventilate with VBM from the mouth, and prepare a tracheostomy tube of the same size and an emergency cart (prepare for intubation).	0.05	0.55	0.06	−0.07	0.22	−0.12

Table 2. Cont.

Domain/Item Number and Content			Factor Loadings					
		Factor 1	Factor 2	Factor 3	Factor 4	Factor 5	Factor 6
	6	In the event of accidental removal of the intubation tube, one should ventilate with VBM, prepare an emergency cart (prepare for intubation), and call a doctor.	−0.12	0.55	0.18	0.12	−0.04	−0.01
	31	Confirm the volume and characteristics of sputum by observing surface viscosity and consistency.	0.18	0.49	0.00	−0.02	−0.05	−0.06
	4	If oral care causes the fixation of the tracheal tube to loosen, reaffix it.	−0.21	0.46	0.27	−0.02	0.00	0.01
Factor 3		Alarm management (Cronbach's α = 0.89)						
	23	If a "high pressure" alarm rings, confirm that there are no abnormal values for SpO$_2$, pulse, blood pressure, single breath volume, or breath volume per minute and check that there is no accumulated sputum or blockage in the circuit.	−0.01	−0.02	0.96	−0.01	−0.06	−0.06
	25	If the "low pressure" alarm rings, since this indicates a possibility of a leak in the circuit, check the circuit and cuff pressure	0.04	0.01	0.81	0.02	0.00	−0.08
	24	If the "apnea" alarm rings, confirm the number of breaths and consult with a doctor about changing the ventilation mode setting and alarm setting as and when necessary.	0.03	0.00	0.76	−0.02	0.01	−0.02
	22	If a "high pressure" alarm rings, confirm the presence or absence of fighting or bucking, respiratory tract blockage due to secretions, or bending of the circuit.	−0.08	0.17	0.70	0.00	0.04	0.01
	20	Consider the alarms related to the artificial respirator as having a possibility of being directly linked to the lives of patients.	0.12	0.12	0.51	0.00	0.01	0.11
	10	Use cuff pressure to assess whether there is a possibility of damage and ulceration of the respiratory tract mucosa.	0.19	−0.06	0.45	−0.01	0.06	0.08
Factor 4		Humidification management (Cronbach's α = 0.87)						
	28	Confirm that heated humidifiers are on.	−0.09	0.02	−0.05	0.98	0.07	−0.08
	27	Check and refill the water chambers of heated humidifiers to ensure the water does not run out.	−0.03	−0.11	0.02	0.90	−0.03	0.04
	30	Confirm that artificial noses are clean and free of contaminants and change them in case they are not.	0.11	0.13	0.00	0.61	−0.07	0.02
	29	Confirm that the water inside the water chambers of heated humidifiers is clean and free of contaminants.	0.17	0.01	0.04	0.59	0.06	0.04
Factor 5		Emergency management (Cronbach's α = 0.87)						
	7	Confirm that the tracheostomy tube is attached at the midline.	−0.12	0.00	0.00	0.01	0.95	−0.01
	8	Attach the tracheostomy tube using the pressure of one finger on each side.	0.15	−0.09	−0.01	0.01	0.84	−0.05

Table 2. Cont.

Domain/Item Number and Content			Factor Loadings					
			Factor 1	Factor 2	Factor 3	Factor 4	Factor 5	Factor 6
Factor 6	54	Confirm that the attachment band of the tracheal tube is not loose before and after adjusting a patient's body position. Airway fixation (Cronbach's $\alpha = 0.82$)	−0.03	0.05	0.02	0.01	0.54	0.25
	2	Confirm that the tape holding the tracheal tube in place is not likely to unstick due to wetness or peeling.	0.01	−0.04	−0.07	−0.02	0.02	0.99
	1	Confirm that the tracheal tube is fixed in place at the corners of the mouth or confirm the measurement (in cm) from the incisors specified in the instructions.	−0.09	0.02	0.01	0.01	0.02	0.78
Cumulative contribution ratio		Contribution ratio	32.29	10.79	6.03	5.36	4.91	3.75
				43.08	49.11	54.47	59.38	63.13
Factor correlations		Factor 1	-	0.20	0.54	0.49	0.46	0.47
		Factor 2		-	0.54	0.46	0.39	0.36
		Factor 3			-	0.47	0.48	0.55
		Factor 4				-	0.38	0.43
		Factor 5					-	0.46
		Factor 6						-

$\chi^2 = 2058.1$, $p < 0.01$, $\chi^2/df = 4.91$, CFI = 0.844, RMSEA = 0.079
Factor extraction method: main factor method, motation method: Promax method with Kaiser normalization.
Squared figures: factor loadings > 0.4.
31 items from 32 initial items.
The following items had low loadings and were excluded from the assessment:
12   Set cuff pressure to a range between 22 and 32 cmH$_2$O.

Table 3. Patient Management (Cronbach's α = 0.91).

Domain/Item Number and Content			Factor Loadings				
			Factor 1	Factor 2	Factor 3	Factor 4	Factor 5
Factor 1		Complication prevention (Cronbach's α = 0.88)					
	58	Make sure there is plenty of slack in the breathing circuit when adjusting a patient's body position.	0.85	−0.02	−0.14	0.01	−0.03
	63	Except when contraindicated, make sure the head is always at an angle of at least 30 degrees.	0.82	−0.05	0.06	−0.06	−0.09
	36	Carry out oral care at least once during each shift.	0.73	−0.05	−0.09	0.03	0.02
	70	When moving patients to beds, stretchers, inspection tables, or operating tables, one staff member holds the tracheal tube in place with their hands.	0.69	0.01	−0.03	0.01	0.02
	39	Before oral care, apply suction to the upper cuff area, oral cavity, nasal cavity, and trachea in that order.	0.66	−0.07	0.13	−0.02	−0.04
	48	Use a suction tube insertion length that reaches about 1 to 2 cm from the tip of the tracheal tube, inserting until just before the bifurcation of the trachea.	0.65	0.02	−0.14	0.03	0.05
	41	For patients who have teeth, brush the ir teeth with a toothbrush.	0.61	0.13	−0.08	0.02	0.06
	40	As a rinsing liquid, use 50 mL or more of tap water administered in 3–5 mL units while applying suction.	0.46	0.13	0.15	−0.07	0.03
	5	If there is drooling, carry out intraoral suction at intervals of once every 30 min to 1 h.	0.43	0.00	0.30	0.10	−0.15
	59	Adjust a patient's body position together with the help of another staff member.	0.41	0.13	0.30	−0.05	−0.03
Factor 2		Prevent ventilator-associated pneumonia (VAP) (Cronbach's α = 0.86)					
	52	Consider that body position is affected by the movements of the diaphragm and the chest.	−0.11	0.92	−0.06	−0.02	0.00
	34	Consider that the self-cleaning function of an intubated patient's oral cavity declines when the patient is intubated.	−0.14	0.69	0.21	0.11	−0.10
	44	Consider that accumulated secretions in the upper cuff area, oral cavity, and nasal cavity drop into the lungs as a result of coughing induced by tracheal suction.	0.10	0.68	−0.04	−0.08	−0.04
	62	Understand that there is a possibility of inducing VAP due to the backflow of stomach contents.	0.04	0.60	−0.01	0.02	0.12
	35	Understand that dental plaque contains a large amount of bacteria and cannot be removed without brushing.	0.04	0.60	0.09	−0.02	−0.11
	43	Consider it possible that pulmonary alveoli could collapse as a result of tracheal suction.	0.15	0.57	−0.09	−0.06	0.10
	51	Consider the possibility that changing body position can result in differences in the volume of air per breath.	0.01	0.56	−0.10	0.03	0.34

Table 3. *Cont.*

Domain/Item Number and Content			Factor Loadings				
			Factor 1	Factor 2	Factor 3	Factor 4	Factor 5
Factor 3		Transfer the patient safely from one location to the other (Cronbach's α = 0.75).					
	69	Prior to transport, attach a test lung to the artificial respirator and conduct a startup inspection.	−0.02	−0.07	0.74	−0.04	0.12
	67	Confirm that portable artificial respirator circuits are properly connected.	0.03	−0.03	0.64	0.05	0.18
	68	When patients are being transported, prepare a back valve mask, oxygen tank, spare tracheotomy cannula set, and a transport-use monitor (which can monitor ECG and SpO$_2$).	−0.08	−0.16	0.64	−0.05	0.15
	38	Adjust cuff pressure to between 22 and 32 cmH$_2$O before and after oral care.	0.14	0.28	0.46	0.00	−0.10
	46	Record the volume and characteristics of sputum recovered from tracheal suction once per shift.	−0.07	0.28	0.41	0.06	−0.07
Factor 4		Skin management (Cronbach's α = 0.97)					
	3	Confirm the presence or absence of redness and ulceration of the lips.	0.03	−0.06	0.06	0.98	0.00
	9	Confirm the presence or absence of maceration, redness, and ulceration in the skin surrounding the tracheostomy incision.	−0.03	0.01	−0.07	0.98	0.00
Factor 5		Assessment post transferred (Cronbach's α = 0.77)					
	71	After changing the transport-use respirator and artificial respirator, check the settings, number of breaths, volume of air per breath, maximum intratracheal pressure, volume of breaths per minute, breathing sounds, number of breaths, SpO$_2$, and subjective symptoms to confirm that they are as they were before the change.	0.13	−0.02	0.14	0.01	0.83
	66	Do not execute nursing care within 30 min before or after the transport of patients.	−0.23	0.03	0.20	−0.04	0.71
	65	Prior to moving a patient, assess whether they have stable breathing and circulation.	0.27	0.19	−0.08	0.05	0.46
Contribution ratio			31.81	12.87	6.13	5.44	4.18
Cumulative contribution ratio				44.68	50.81	56.25	60.43
Factor correlations		Factor 1	-				
		Factor 2	0.58	-			
		Factor 3	−0.01	0.36	-		
		Factor 4	0.40	0.48	0.25	-	
		Factor 5	0.36	0.61	0.29	0.26	-

Table 3. *Cont.*

Domain/Item Number and Content	Factor Loadings				
	Factor 1	Factor 2	Factor 3	Factor 4	Factor 5
37 For orally intubated patients, carry out oral care together with another staff member.					
42 Consider that tracheal secretions are affected by gravity.					
45 For patients without restrictions, perform sputum drainage and adjust their position to an angle of at least 40 to 60 degrees alternating between the left and right sides to prevent atelectasis.					
47 Record any changes in the volume or characteristics of sputum recovered from tracheal suction.					
49 Complete suction within 15 s after inserting the suction catheter.					
50 After tracheal suction, confirm breath sounds, number of breaths, SpO$_2$, and subjective symptoms to confirm that all sputum has been removed.					
53 Before adjusting a patient's body position, remove water from the circuit.					
55 Perform oral cavity suction prior to adjusting a patient's body position.					
56 When changing the orientation of the body or moving the neck, use hands to keep the tracheal tube base in place.					
57 When adjusting a patient's body position, position the breathing circuit lower than the tracheal tube to prevent water in the breathing circuit from flowing into the trachea.					
60 Adjust the position of the pillows to prevent the patient's neck from getting into an extended position.					
61 Before and after touching artificial respirators or patients, sterilize hands with quick-drying alcohol (if there is visible dirt, wash hands with soap and water).					

$\chi^2 = 1723.9$, $p < 0.01$, $\chi^2/df = 5.49$, CFI = 0.841, RMSEA = 0.085
Factor extraction method: main factor method, rotation method: Promax method with Kaiser normalization.
Squared figures: factor loadings above 0.4.
27 items from 39 initial items.
The following items had low loading and were excluded from the assessment

3.4. Reliability Testing

The Cronbach's alpha coefficient for "Ventilator Management" was 0.91 at the scale level and 0.82, 0.82, 0.89, 0.87, 0.87, and 0.82 for factors 1–6, respectively (Table 2). In contrast, for "Patient Management", the coefficients were 0.91 at the scale level and 0.88, 0.86, 0.75, 0.97, and 0.77 for factors 1–5, respectively (Table 3). For reproducibility, the ICC intraclass correlation coefficient for factors, calculated using data from the 152 participants who returned their test–retest responses, ranged from 0.75 to 0.97 (Table 4). All factors of ventilator management show high reliability. Patient management factors 1, 2, and 4 showed high reliability. Factors 3 and 5 showed acceptable reliability. A lower ICC was predicted because the frequency of practice increased as nurses reflected on ventilator care in their nursing practice through retesting.

Table 4. Intraclass correlation coefficient and 95% confidence intervals.

		ICC *	95%CI **	*p*-Value ***
Ventilator Management				
	Factor 1	0.816	0.794–0.837	<0.001
	Factor 2	0.823	0.800–0.843	<0.001
	Factor 3	0.886	0.871–0.899	<0.001
	Factor 4	0.869	0.852–0.885	<0.001
	Factor 5	0.868	0.849–0.885	<0.001
	Factor 6	0.823	0.793–0.849	<0.001
Patient Management				
	Factor 1	0.875	0.860–0.889	<0.001
	Factor 2	0.861	0.844–0.877	<0.001
	Factor 3	0.752	0.720–0.781	<0.001
	Factor 4	0.968	0.962–0.972	<0.001
	Factor 5	0.771	0.738–0.800	<0.001

ICC * = intra-class correlation coefficient; CI ** = confidence interval; *p*-value *** = the statistically significant reference.

4. Discussion

The basis for this study was the Q-IMV-RPN, developed from the existing literature and observations of actual skilled nursing practice, which include their thought processes concerning the nursing practices required for ventilator care. The rating scale was developed by selecting essential items that should be used immediately by nurses in general wards. However, the nursing skills to be provided to patients with respiratory distress are complex. Therefore, for each machine and patient management, essential nursing practices were consolidated according to the nursing process, and a scale was created.

Mechanical management of ventilator care in a general hospital ward comprises six factors. These included essential information, such as setting alarms and damaging the ventilator circuit, which should be checked at regular intervals and personnel shifts. Factor 1, "initial confirmation", included confirming the forced ventilation mode setting, volume of single breaths, and respiratory frequency. Factor 2, "artificial airway", included an assessment to prevent incidents related to artificial airways that occur most frequently in general wards [28] and an assessment related to humidification. Factor 3, "alarm management", included an assessment of the patient's situation when the alarm went off. This is a crucial factor because even if alarms are set, it is impossible to prevent or manage abnormalities in the patient without being able to assess what is happening during the alarm [29]. Factor 4 was related to the confirmation and implementation of "humidification management". Heating and humidification are essential assessment items for ventilator-associated pneumonia (VAP) prevention; however, they are also important factors, as inadequate management can lead to serious incidents, such as airway burns. Factors 5 and 6 included the confirmation and implementation items related to the artificial airway [30]. Therefore, it is obvious that machine management for ventilator care includes the management of machine settings and alarms and the nursing practice process related to the management of the artificial airway, including heating and humidification.

Management of patients in a general hospital ward essentially comprises five factors. Factor 1, "complication prevention", consists of items for implementing necessary care, such as intraperiod suctioning, repositioning, and oral care, to prevent pneumonia and unscheduled extubation. We believe that the essential care items that should be implemented for patients using ventilators are concentrated in this category. Factor 2, "prevent VAP", comprises a collection of items describing the perspectives and rationale for preventing VAP, such as repositioning, oral care, and endotracheal suctioning. Therefore, it should be practiced continuously in conjunction with factor 1. Factor 2, the perspective of assessment, and factor 1, the implementation of safe care, can be regarded as practices to prevent complications [31]. Factor 3, "transfer safely", includes items such as checking the connection and setting the ventilator. Many incidents related to ventilators in general wards involve unscheduled extubation during transfer, poor aftercare connection, and incorrect ventilator settings. Therefore, it is considered a crucial factor in safety management [28]. Factor 4, "skin management", concentrates on items related to skin damage caused by the fixation of the artificial airway. Generally, great emphasis should be placed on preventing the unscheduled removal of artificial airways. Therefore, there is a high likelihood of skin damage due to immobilization. Tracheal tube fixation is essential for safe breathing. However, skin damage from fixation can prevent stable fixation from being maintained, increase patient distress, and reduce the patient's quality of life after extubation. Therefore, we value this factor as a perspective for implementing care while maintaining safety. Factor 5, "assessment post-transfer", consolidates items related to the assessment and the rationale for factor 3. Factors 3 and 5 together can be considered to pertain to safety management practice. Patient management for ventilator care focuses on nursing practices to prevent VAP and the unscheduled removal of the artificial airway. This is also expected to occur during the transfer of the patient from one location to another before and after care. The content pertains to nursing care aiming to prevent skin damage and improve safety management.

In Japan, nurses control the use of ventilators. However, this is not covered in basic nursing education. Instead, nurses are trained in the field of practice while working in hospitals. However, during the pandemic, the number of patients on ventilators increased. Moreover, there was no time to train nurses who could care for patients on ventilators because they were faced with urgent life-and-death situations. Therefore, we believe that the scale developed in this study is highly beneficial for inexperienced nurses to manage ventilators safely. Furthermore, nurses' ability to practice ventilator care can be assessed using this scale, which can further help evaluate the ability of wards to manage ventilators. Moreover, managers can evaluate which wards can safely manage patients on ventilators removed from the intensive care unit during trying times. It can also be used for objective evaluation by a third party to assess ventilator management capabilities and to help in education. This scale itemizes the nursing practice process of ventilator care that should be practiced by nurses, including thought processes. Therefore, it can benefit nurses with limited experience to safely practice ventilator care. Simultaneously, it can be used to assess the practice and educational impact of group education on ventilator care and which items should be taught effectively. Therefore, it is possible to evaluate the developmental stages of nurses using this scale. Furthermore, this scale can help hospital administrators evaluate which nurses can practice ventilator management and to what extent it can be used as a material to consider which area to move patients with ventilators. As there has been a rising need for human resources to provide ventilator care, it is believed that safe care for patients on ventilation can be provided using this system with the currently used checklist.

Regarding the item content, the items were narrowed down to the minimum necessary while verbalizing the practice of professional nurses, including their thought processes. Furthermore, the scale was divided into ventilator management and patient management so that routine nurses and inexperienced nurses could safely practice ventilator care. Therefore, this scale can be used to self-evaluate one's nursing practice and as an evaluation tool for others for educational purposes. In particular, we believe that, in cases where actual practical exercises or group training could not be conducted, including pandemics, the scale created in this study will allow even novices to practice the minimum necessary ventilator care and to reflect on the content of their practice.

However, this study had several limitations. First, the scale was developed only for Japanese nurses. Therefore, whether this scale can be used in other countries needs to be examined. Second, this study included only generalists working in Japanese hospitals with 500 or more beds. Therefore, future studies investigating its applicability to nurses working in smaller hospitals are needed. Third, if pediatric patients had participated in this study, it is highly likely that their attitudes and methods toward ventilator management would have changed. Therefore, the model as a scale is not optimal and needs to be improved. In the future, the number of items for each target nurse should be considered, and the structure should be balanced. In addition, it is necessary to create a scale that can be adapted according to the target patients.

5. Conclusions

The short form developed in this study is based on the Q-RPN-IMV, and the items are carefully selected to provide the minimum necessary content for nursing practice professionals to care for patients on ventilators. Furthermore, to facilitate use by generalist nurses, the scale is divided into thirty-one items with six factors related to ventilator management and twenty-seven items with five factors related to patient management to ensure reliability and validity.

Author Contributions: Conceptualization, M.T. and I.M.; methodology, M.T.; software, J.S.; validation, M.T. and I.M.; formal analysis, M.T.; investigation, J.S.; resources, J.S.; data curation, M.T.; writing—original draft preparation, M.T.; writing—review and editing, M.T., A.F., J.S. and I.M.; visualization, M.T.; supervision, I.M.; project administration, M.T.; funding acquisition, M.T. All authors have read and agreed to the published version of the manuscript.

Funding: This research was funded by JSPS KAKENHI, grant number JP18K10347.

Institutional Review Board Statement: Informed consent was obtained from all participants involved in the study. This study was approved by the ethics committee of the university to which the authors are affiliated (approval number 696).

Informed Consent Statement: Not applicable.

Data Availability Statement: The datasets used during the current study are available from the corresponding author upon request.

Public Involvement Statement: No public involvement in any aspect of this research.

Guidelines and Standards Statement: This manuscript was drafted against the guidelines described in the *Scale Development: Theory and Applications* and the Consensus-based Standards for the Selection of Health Status Measurement. Moreover, we followed the Guidelines for Reporting Reliability and Agreement Studies (GRRAS).

Acknowledgments: The authors are grateful to all participants in the study.

Conflicts of Interest: The authors declare no conflict of interest.

References

1. Li, J.; Ni, Y.; Tu, M.; Ni, J.; Ge, H.; Shi, Y.; Ni, Z.; Chen, R.; Yao, R.; Liang, Z. Respiratory care education and clinical practice in Mainland China. *Respir. Care* **2018**, *63*, 1239–1245. [CrossRef]
2. Zisk-Rony, R.Y.; Weissman, C.; Weiss, Y.G. Mechanical ventilation patterns and trends over 20 years in an Israeli hospital system: Policy ramifications. *Isr. J. Health Policy Res.* **2019**, *8*, 20. [CrossRef]
3. Oakley, C.; Pascoe, C.; Balthazor, D.; Bennett, D.; Gautam, N.; Isaac, J.; Isherwood, P.; Matthews, T.; Murphy, N.; Oelofse, T.; et al. Assembly Line ICU: What the Long Shops taught us about managing surge capacity for COVID-19. *BMJ Open Qual.* **2020**, *9*, e001117. [CrossRef]
4. Boilève, A.; Stoclin, A.; Barlesi, F.; Varin, F.; Suria, S.; Rieutord, A.; Blot, F.; Netzer, F.; Scotté, F. COVID-19 management in a cancer center: The ICU storm. *Support. Care Cancer* **2020**, *28*, 5037–5044. [CrossRef] [PubMed]

5. Litton, E.; Bucci, T.; Chavan, S.; Ho, Y.Y.; Holley, A.; Howard, G.; Huckson, S.; Kwong, P.; Millar, J.; Nguyen, N.; et al. Surge capacity of intensive care units in case of acute increase in demand caused by COVID-19 in Australia. *Med. J. Aust.* **2020**, *212*, 463–467. [CrossRef]
6. Khan, M.; Adil, S.F.; Alkhathlan, H.Z.; Tahir, M.N.; Saif, S.; Khan, M.; Khan, S.T. COVID-19: A global challenge with old history, epidemiology and progress so far. *Molecules* **2020**, *26*, 39. [CrossRef]
7. Wahlster, S.; Sharma, M.; Lewis, A.K.; Patel, P.V.; Hartog, C.S.; Jannotta, G.; Blissitt, P.; Kross, E.K.; Kassebaum, N.J.; Greer, D.M.; et al. The coronavirus disease 2019 pandemic's effect on critical care resources and health-care providers: A global survey. *Chest* **2021**, *159*, 619–633. [CrossRef]
8. Wongsurakiat, P.; Sangsa, N.; Tangaroonsanti, A. Mechanical ventilation of patients hospitalized on general medical ward: Outcomes and prognostic factors. *J. Med. Assoc. Thail.* **2016**, *99*, 772–776.
9. Kamio, T.; Masamune, K. Mechanical ventilation-related safety incidents in general care wards and ICU settings. *Respir. Care* **2018**, *63*, 1246–1252. [CrossRef]
10. Pham, J.C.; Williams, T.L.; Sparnon, E.M.; Cillie, T.K.; Scharen, H.F.; Marella, W.M. Ventilator-related adverse events: A taxonomy and findings from 3 incident reporting systems. *Respir. Care* **2016**, *61*, 621–631. [CrossRef] [PubMed]
11. Gattinoni, L.; Marini, J.J.; Collino, F.; Maiolo, G.; Rapetti, F.; Tonetti, T.; Vasques, F.; Quintel, M. The future of mechanical ventilation: Lessons from the present and the past. *Crit. Care* **2017**, *21*, 183. [CrossRef]
12. Mantena, S.; Rogo, K.; Burke, T.F. Re-examining the race to send ventilators to low-resource settings. *Respir. Care* **2020**, *65*, 1378–1381. [CrossRef]
13. Goldsworthy, S. Mechanical ventilation education and transition of critical care nurses into practice. *Crit. Care Nurs. Clin. N. Am.* **2016**, *28*, 399–412. [CrossRef] [PubMed]
14. Guilhermino, M.C.; Inder, K.J.; Sundin, D. Education on invasive mechanical ventilation involving intensive care nurses: A systematic review. *Nurs. Crit. Care* **2018**, *23*, 245–255. [CrossRef]
15. Tsukuda, M.; Fukuda, A.; Taru, C.; Miyawaki, I. Development of a questionnaire for the reflective practice of nursing involving invasive mechanical ventilation: Assessment of validity and reliability. *Nurs. Open* **2019**, *6*, 330–347. [CrossRef]
16. DeVellis, R.F. *Scale Development: Theory and Applications*, 5th ed.; Sage Publications: Thousand Oaks, CA, USA, 2022.
17. Kottner, J.; Audigé, L.; Brorson, S.; Donner, A.; Gajewski, B.J.; Hróbjartsson, A.; Roberts, C.; Shoukri, M.; Streiner, D.L. Guidelines for Reporting Reliability and Agreement Studies (GRRAS) were proposed. *J. Clin. Epidemiol.* **2011**, *64*, 96–106. [CrossRef]
18. Tabachnick, B.G.; Fidell, L.S. *Using Multivariate Statistics*, 7th ed.; Pearson Education: London, UK, 2019.
19. Lee, P.; Lu, W.S.; Liu, C.H.; Lin, H.Y.; Hsieh, C.L. Test-retest reliability and minimal detectable change of the D2 test of attention in patients with schizophrenia. *Arch. Clin. Neuropsychol.* **2018**, *33*, 1060–1068. [CrossRef] [PubMed]
20. McPherson, S.; Reese, C.; Wendler, M.C. Methodology update: Delphi studies. *Nurs. Res.* **2018**, *67*, 404–410. [CrossRef] [PubMed]
21. Hair, J.F.; Black, W.C.; Babin, B.J.; Anderson, R.E. *Multivariate Data Analysis*; Pearson Education Limited: Essex, UK, 2014.
22. Costello, A.; Osborne, J.W. Best practices in exploratory factor analysis: Four recommendations for getting the most from your analysis. *Pract. Assess. Res. Eval.* **2005**, *10*, 1–9. [CrossRef]
23. Stevens, J.P. *Applied Multivariate Statistics for the Social Sciences*, 2nd ed.; Erlbaum: Hillsdale, NJ, USA, 1992.
24. Streiner, D.L. Figuring out factors: The use and misuse of factor analysis. *Can. J. Psychiatry* **1994**, *39*, 135–140. [CrossRef]
25. West, S.G.; Taylor, A.B.; Wu, W. Model fit and model selection in structural equation modeling. In *Handbook of Structural Equation Modeling*; Hoyle, R.H., Ed.; The Guilford Press: New York, NY, USA, 2012; Volume 1, pp. 209–231.
26. Bae, B.R. *Structural Equation Modeling with Amos 19: Principles and Practice*; Chungram Books: Seoul, Republic of Korea, 2011; pp. 1–668.
27. Fleiss, J.L. *The Design and Analysis of Clinical Experiments*; John Wiley Sons: New York, NJ, USA, 1986.
28. Lin, S.J.; Tsan, C.Y.; Su, M.Y.; Wu, C.L.; Chen, L.C.; Hsieh, H.J.; Hsiao, W.L.; Cheng, J.C.; Kuo, Y.W.; Jerng, J.S.; et al. Improving patient safety during intrahospital transportation of mechanically ventilated patients with critical illness. *BMJ Open Qual.* **2020**, *9*, e000698. [CrossRef]
29. Scott, J.B.; De Vaux, L.; Dills, C.; Strickland, S.L. Mechanical ventilation alarms and alarm fatigue. *Respir. Care* **2019**, *64*, 1308–1313. [CrossRef] [PubMed]
30. Lavoie-Bérard, C.A.; Lefebvre, J.C.; Bouchard, P.A.; Simon, M.; Lellouche, F. Impact of airway humidification strategy in mechanically ventilated COVID-19 patients. *Respir. Care* **2022**, *67*, 157–166. [CrossRef] [PubMed]
31. Dexter, A.M.; Scott, J.B. Airway management and ventilator-associated events. *Respir. Care* **2019**, *64*, 986–993. [CrossRef] [PubMed]

Disclaimer/Publisher's Note: The statements, opinions and data contained in all publications are solely those of the individual author(s) and contributor(s) and not of MDPI and/or the editor(s). MDPI and/or the editor(s) disclaim responsibility for any injury to people or property resulting from any ideas, methods, instructions or products referred to in the content.

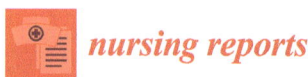

Article

A Modified Guideline for High-Fidelity Patient Simulation to Improve Student Satisfaction and Self-Confidence in Learning: A Mixed Study

Florence M. F. Wong [1,*] and David C. N. Wong [2]

1. School of Nursing, Tung Wah College, Kowloon, Hong Kong SAR 999078, China
2. Research Office, Tung Wah College, Kowloon, Hong Kong SAR 999078, China; shallwex@yahoo.com.hk
* Correspondence: florencewong@twc.edu.hk; Tel.: +(852)-34686838

Abstract: The coronaviral pandemic has led to a shift in traditional teaching methods to more innovative approaches, such as high-fidelity patient simulation (HFPS), which can improve students' clinical judgment and decision making for quality patient care. A modified guideline was introduced to enhance students' satisfaction and self-confidence in learning through HFPS. The study involved 189 baccalaureate nursing students, with 92 in the intervention group and 97 in the control group. The intervention group received the modified HFPS guideline, while the control group received standard treatment with basic instruction. After the HFPS debriefing session, students provided narrative feedback on their learning experiences. The quantitative results showed that students in the intervention group reported a significant improvement in satisfaction and self-confidence in learning compared to the control group. The modified HFPS guideline provided clear guidance for students to learn and apply knowledge and skills more effectively, leading to increased engagement during interactive simulation sessions. The results suggest that the HFPS guideline should be added to the curriculum to enhance students' satisfaction and self-confidence in learning, even for junior students. After the pandemic, innovative teaching methods, such as HFPS, can be necessary and beneficial for healthcare professional training.

Keywords: high-fidelity; simulation; satisfaction; confidence; learning; nursing education

Citation: Wong, F.M.F.; Wong, D.C.N. A Modified Guideline for High-Fidelity Patient Simulation to Improve Student Satisfaction and Self-Confidence in Learning: A Mixed Study. *Nurs. Rep.* **2023**, *13*, 1030–1039. https://doi.org/10.3390/nursrep13030090

Academic Editors: Antonio Martínez-Sabater, Elena Chover-Sierra and Carles Saus-Ortega

Received: 6 July 2023
Revised: 22 July 2023
Accepted: 25 July 2023
Published: 28 July 2023

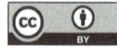

Copyright: © 2023 by the authors. Licensee MDPI, Basel, Switzerland. This article is an open access article distributed under the terms and conditions of the Creative Commons Attribution (CC BY) license (https://creativecommons.org/licenses/by/4.0/).

1. Introduction

The COVID-19 pandemic has had a significant impact on students' learning attitudes and behaviors, necessitating the use of innovative methods to encourage and enhance learning. It has presented new challenges for nurses, who now face more complex and immediate clinical situations. In addition to the advanced technology utilized in healthcare services, nurses are expected to take on greater accountability for managing complex clinical judgments and decisions. These higher expectations are necessary to ensure effective and appropriate patient care [1,2]. However, nurses often encounter challenges in making immediate clinical judgments and decisions [3]. As a result, there is a growing need for innovative, cost-effective, and high-quality training programs aimed at enhancing nursing competence and ultimately benefiting both patient care and healthcare services.

High-fidelity patient simulation (HFPS) is an advanced technology-based method widely used in professional training, including healthcare services. It has been shown to effectively improve knowledge acquisition and skill performance, enhancing clinical competence [4–6]. Nursing education includes theoretical knowledge, psychomotor skills training, and scenario-based nursing practice to improve competence in safe and appropriate practice [7,8]. Students can perform their learned knowledge and skills to foster clinical competence and ensure patient safety in a controlled and risk-free environment [9–12]. Students learn their roles and responsibilities in HFPS situations, discover their strengths and weaknesses [12,13], and develop motivation for lifelong learning and collaborative teamwork [13–16]. Students can interact and collaborate with their peers to exchange their learning experiences, enhancing their competence in nursing practice and teamwork skills in the HFPS. Therefore, HFPS acts as an important innovative teaching–learning method to foster students' ability in clinical judgment and decision making. However, students' satisfaction and confidence in learning through HFPS directly affect their motivation and engagement [17].

To address this, HFPS provides simulated patient training scenarios in clinical settings, allowing students to integrate their knowledge and psychomotor skills [18,19]. With the application of HFPS in the last decades, students have learned more effectively when they engage in this innovative learning activity [19–21]. Studies have shown that HFPS improves engagement, learning achievement, satisfaction, and confidence levels among students [22,23]. Therefore, it is important to increase their willingness and interest in learning. Students' satisfaction and their confidence in learning are essential elements, and they are intertwined. The more satisfaction students have, the more confidence they have to motivate themselves to undertake thinking and learning challenges [5,11]. HFPS is a multifaceted learning approach that necessitates students to engage in role playing and maximize their knowledge acquisition throughout the entire HFPS process [24]. With the growing popularity of simulations across various educational levels, different academic institutions have developed their unique simulation guidelines. HFPS is recognised as a motivating, secure, and cost-effective approach that not only provides students with hardware simulation devices but also incorporates engaging and instructive learning materials that are tailored to a specific learning environment. As a result, a well-designed HFPS is imperative in facilitating students' involvement in this high-expectation activity, delivering high-quality and cost-effective outcomes in student learning [24]. However, most of the studies were conducted in senior-year students. A guideline is useful to direct the HFPS and help students learn more effectively. In current nursing education, HFPS is employed in various courses to enhance students' understanding of patients' conditions and related treatment and care. Early application of HFPS in junior students may help them develop more personal and professional skills and better learning attitudes. To address this, a modified HFPS guideline was designed based on the Healthcare Simulation Standards of Best Practice (HSSOBP) by the International Nursing Association for Clinical Simulation and Learning [INACSL] [25] to provide systematic approaches to learning tasks and ensure students perform as expected throughout the learning process [22]. Four major sessions from HSSOBP, namely pre-briefing, simulation design, facilitation, and debriefing, were adopted to design a modified HFPS guideline for this study. This study aimed to examine the modified HFPS guidelines' impact on students' satisfaction and confidence in HFPS learning, and early application in junior students may develop personal and professional skills and better learning attitudes. The results could triangulate the findings with students' narratives after HFPS to understand how they achieved satisfaction and confidence in learning.

2. Materials and Methods

2.1. Study Design

A quasi-experimental with one intervention and one control group was conducted at a single tertiary institution in Hong Kong SAR, China between November 2021 and June 2022.

2.2. Study Objectives

The objective aims to investigate the impact of the modified HFPS guideline on student satisfaction and self-confidence in learning. By comparing the modified guideline with the standard HFPS, the study intends to evaluate whether the modified guideline leads to higher levels of SSSCL among first-year nursing students. The objectives align with the overall purpose of the study, which is to assess the effectiveness of the modified HFPS guideline in improving student satisfaction and self-confidence in learning.

2.3. Study Setting and Sampling

Students aged ≥ 18 years were recruited. Those who had received HFPS training before or had experienced clinical placement were excluded to avoid contamination. The sample size was calculated to reach a desired power of 0.95 and a type I error of 0.05 with an effect size of 0.5 based on a past study [26] using G*Power 3.1.9.4. The calculated minimum required number of participants was 176 students (88 in each group).

2.4. Modified Guideline for HFPS as the Study Framework

The modified HFPS guideline was based on the HSSOBP [25], which was developed to guide the integration, use, and advancement of simulation-based experiences in academia, clinical practice, and research. The HSSOBP is a comprehensive and evidenced-based tool that includes inputs from multiple healthcare professionals and experts in simulations [25]. It consists of nine standards, of which four were used to design the structured guideline for this study, as they were deemed most applicable. These four HSSOBP standards, namely pre-briefing, simulation design, facilitation, and debriefing, provided a systematic approach to direct students in engaging in their learning and simulated activities. The pre-briefing consists of preparation and briefing to ensure that students had the necessary learning materials, understood the ground rules, and were aware of their roles and responsibilities in the HFPS. Students are required to understand specific learning outcomes before HFPS. The simulation design provided a structural framework to develop effective logistics and strategies (including simulation case design) for promoting learning goals and improving the quality of care and patient safety. Facilitation aimed to provide guidance to students to meet their learning needs and achieve learning outcomes. The facilitator is assumed to be responsible for managing the entire HFPS and providing support to students to work cohesively during their simulation experience. Debriefing is a process that includes feedback, clarification, and guided reflection. The debriefing is essential to help students identify their strengths and weaknesses, gaps in knowledge, skills, personal attitudes, and emotional management in a simulation clinical situation. To evaluate the effects of the modified HFPS guideline, two groups were assigned either intervention or standard treatment. The differences in the four HFPS sessions between the two groups are illustrated in Table S1. Students in the intervention group were provided with the modified HFPS guideline as the intervention, which involved a more systematic approach to enable students to learn through the four sessions in a 2-h HFPS. Conversely, those in the control group received standard treatment with basic instructions for HFPS over the same period. This indicated that the standard treatment provided basic information and support from the facilitator in the four HSSOBP standards.

2.5. Instruments

The Student Satisfaction and Self-Confidence in Learning (SSSCL), which was developed by the National League of Nursing [27], would be used in this study. It consists of 13 items with a 5-point Likert scale (1 = strongly disagree and 5 = strongly agree) to measure students' perception of their satisfaction and self-confidence in learning. Five items are related to the subscale of students' satisfaction (SS) in simulation-based learning activities, and the remaining eight concern the subscale of self-confidence in learning (SCL). The Cronbach's alphas for the overall SSSCL and the subscales of SS and SCL were 0.95, 0.96, and 0.92, respectively, indicating excellent reliability in this study.

2.6. Study Procedure

Prospective participants were recruited via email and asked to select from three available timeslots for the HFPS. Students who agreed to participate were randomly assigned to either the intervention group, which received the HFPS following the new guidelines, or the control group, which received the standard guideline, according to their preference. Each laboratory group consisted of around eight to ten students, and the research assistant (RA) allocated students to the corresponding group. The RA was not involved in the implementation of HFPS. Once a group was filled, the RA contacted the students about the time and venue of the HFPS and emailed them the HFPS packages for preparation at an acceptable period, which was three days before HFPS for the students in the control group and one week for those in the intervention group. Two researchers were responsible for teaching the intervention and control groups, respectively, to ensure consistency. The tutorials were held at different campuses of the institution to avoid contamination. Students completed a baseline questionnaire before receiving the simulation on the study day and completed the same set of questionnaires immediately after the debriefing session.

On the day of HFPS, students were divided into three small groups and took turns in the role-play session to care for the simulated patient, with each group having 20 min in the simulation session. While one small group was assigned to the role-play session, the other two watched and provided feedback. In the debriefing session, students reflected on their learning throughout the HFPS, gave feedback to one another, and received feedback from the tutor. After the debriefing, students were asked to complete the post-intervention SSSCL survey and answer six open-ended questions about their learning in terms of satisfaction and confidence in learning through HFPS. The questions focused on the learning materials provided, the role-play session, the debriefing, and their effect on confidence in learning. The questions were: 'What do you think about the learning materials provided before the HFPS?', 'What do you think about the effect of learning materials on your confidence in learning through HFPS?', 'What do you think about the role-play you performed in the HFPS?', 'What do you think your role-play in the HFPS will affect your confidence in learning?', 'What do you think about the debriefing after the HFPS?', and 'What do you think about the effect on your confidence in learning after the HFPS?'.

2.7. Data Analysis

Statistical analyses were performed by a data analyst who was blinded to the students' allocation. Data were analysed using IBM SPSS version 26. Chi-square statistics were applied to compare the demographic characteristics (categorical data) between the intervention and control groups. Two-sample t-test statistics were applied to compare the student satisfaction and self-confidence in learning between the two groups. A two-sample independent t-test was used to examine the change of SSSCL between baseline and post-intervention (after debriefing) between the two groups. Secondary data analysis was conducted by ANOVA to examine the effect of HFPS on the change of SSSCL, adjusted for confounding factors. All statistical tests involved were two-sided, and p-values of <0.05 were considered statistically significant.

2.8. Ethical Consideration

Ethical approval was obtained from the research committee of the study institution (REC2021102). Informed consent was obtained from the students who agreed to participate. The participants were assigned by individual serial numbers, and the researchers would not be able to identify the participants during data analysis. All data with personal information were kept confidential.

3. Results

3.1. Students' Characteristics

A total of 189 students were recruited in this study without attrition, with 92 students (48.7%) in the intervention groups and 97 (51.3%) students in the control groups. Table 1 shows the demographic characteristics and students' satisfaction (SS) and self-confidence in learning (SCL) at baseline. Among the sampled participants, 73% participants were female, and the mean age was 20.56 (SD = 3.14). Around 71% of participants were studying for a bachelor's degree, and the remaining 29.1% were studying higher diploma. Over half of the participants were in the first year of study (54%), and the remaining 46% were in the second year of study. The baseline demographic characteristics were similar between the intervention and control groups, except that a higher proportion of participants studying for a bachelor's degree in the intervention group (79.3%) than in the control group (62.9%, $p = 0.013$). Both groups have similar levels of student satisfaction and self-confidence in learning at baseline.

Table 1. Students' characteristics, students' satisfaction, and self-confidence in learning.

	Overall (n = 189)		Intervention (n = 92)		Control (n = 97)		p-Value
	n	%	n	%	n	%	(between Groups)
Gender							0.210
Male	51	27	21	22.8	30	30.9	
Female	138	73	71	77.2	67	69.1	
Age							0.027 *
mean age (SD)	20.56 (3.14)		21.04 (3.65)		20.04 (2.41)		
18–24	170	89.9	85	92.3	85	87.6	
25 or older	19	10.1	7	7.7	12	12.4	
Program							0.013 *
Higher Diploma	55	29.1	19	20.7	36	37.1	
Bachelor of Science	134	70.9	73	79.3	61	62.9	
Study Year							0.919
1	102	54.0	50	54.3	52	53.6	
2	87	46.0	42	45.7	45	46.4	
Student satisfaction and self-confidence in learning	Mean	SD	Mean	SD	Mean	SD	p-value
SS	18.25	3.40	17.83	3.17	18.64	3.61	0.097
SCL	28.78	3.77	28.59	3.97	28.96	3.57	0.543
Overall SSSCL	47.03	6.98	46.41	6.57	47.61	7.35	0.239

SS: Student Satisfaction; SCL: Self-Confidence in Learning; SSSCL: Student Satisfaction and Self-Confidence in Learning. * $p < 0.05$.

3.2. Analysis of Outcomes

To assess the effectiveness of the intervention, the pre- and post-intervention scores of all subscales (SS and SCL), as well as the overall SSSCL, were compared between the intervention and control groups. The results showed a significant improvement in all subscales and overall SSSCL scores in both groups (<0.001). Table 2 illustrates the changes in subscales of SS and SCL and the overall SSSCL scores, which were observed to have improved in both intervention and control groups after the simulation.

Table 2. Comparison of the changes in students' satisfaction and self-confidence in learning before and after HFPS between intervention and control groups.

	Pre- and Post-Change			
	Mean	SD	p	95% CI
SS				
Intervention	5.14	3.27	0.004 **	−2.67 to −0.50
Control	3.56	4.18		
SCL				
Intervention	4.91	3.85	0.025 *	−2.81 to −0.19
Control	3.41	5.18		
Overall SSSCL				
Intervention	10.05	6.32	0.004 **	−5.18 to −0.99
Control	6.97	8.17		

SS: Student Satisfaction; SCL: Self-Confidence in Learning; SSSCL: Student Satisfaction and Self-Confidence in Learning. * $p < 0.05$; ** $p < 0.01$.

Compared with the control group, participants who were in the intervention group recorded a higher improvement in SSSCL (mean change in the intervention group = 10.05 vs. 6.97 in the control group, $p = 0.004$), as well as both the SS and SCL scores ($p = 0.004$ and 0.025 respectively) (Table 2); all subscales were found to have significant differences between the two groups. Consistent results were observed after accounting for the confounding variable (Table 3).

Table 3. Intervention effect on the changes of students' satisfaction and self-confidence in learning.

	Mean	SE	p
SS			
- Treatment (Intervention)	4.97	3.32	0.004 *
- Program (Bachelor)	9.73	6.20	0.312
SCL			
- Treatment (Intervention)	4.75	3.64	0.035 *
- Program (Bachelor)	4.75	3.64	0.304
Overall SSSCL			
- Treatment (Intervention)	9.73	6.20	0.005 *
- Program (Bachelor)	4.97	3.32	0.473

SS: Student Satisfaction, SCL: Self-Confidence in Learning, SSSCL: Student Satisfaction and Self-Confidence in Learning. * $p < 0.05$.

3.3. Effects of the Guideline on SSSCL through HFPS

Most students reported feeling satisfied and confident in their learning at each stage, according to the narrative feedback from the six open-ended questions. Students in the intervention group reported higher levels of satisfaction and confidence in learning than those in the control group. Some students in the intervention group mentioned that they had more satisfaction and confidence in learning due to the learning engagement at each stage. They found that when they had more satisfaction, they had better confidence in learning. During the preparatory stage, students in the intervention group followed the guideline and read the learning materials to manage the simulated patient. They reflected that the materials were useful in enhancing their understanding of the health problem and related management. In the role-play session, students in the intervention group were able to manage the scenario more efficiently. During the debriefing, all students learned from the educator and group feedback and their own self-evaluation. Table S2 summarizes students' feedback on their satisfaction and confidence in learning through three sessions of HFPS in the two groups.

4. Discussion

This study found significant improvement in the SSSCL in both groups, but there were more positive effects of the modified HFPS guideline on SSSCL through HFPS in the intervention group. All subscales of the SSSCL (SS and SCL) and the overall SSSCL showed significant differences ($p < 0.001$) between the pre- and post-intervention periods in both groups, indicating that HFPS itself improved student learning throughout the four-session HFPS [22]. HFPS uses advanced and innovative technology to foster student learning and learning motivation, providing a simulated clinical setting with a patient to allow students to actively participate in giving comfort care interventions, interacting with the patient, working with teammates, and receiving feedback from their facilitator [4]. Therefore, HFPS is an effective teaching method to allow students to practice patient care with learned knowledge and skills [18,21], aiming to enhance their clinical judgment and decision-making ability [8]. The modified guideline provided the necessary information and adequate support for students to be engaged in implementing care in a simulated patient situation during the process of HFPS, which informs more promising effects on student satisfaction and confidence in learning. Therefore, the HFPS guideline is a useful tool to enhance student learning and competence.

Comparing the changes in the subscales between the two groups, all subscales, particularly the subscales of SS ($p = 0.004$) and overall SSSCL ($p = 0.004$), showed significant differences before and after the intervention, with students in the intervention group reporting more changes in all SSSCL subscales. This suggests that the modified guideline greatly improved student learning, providing clearer direction and information for students to learn systematically, effectively, and sensibly [28]. The four sessions of HSSOBP were useful and effective in increasing students' SSSCL from their own self-directed study, group collaboration, self-reflection, and evaluation or feedback from peers and the tutor. Importantly, students need to engage in the entire four-session HFPS to obtain the benefits of SSSCL improvement [25]. Throughout this learning process in HFPS, students had the opportunity to increase their satisfaction and self-confidence by acquiring new knowledge and skills, ultimately enhancing their competence in clinical judgment and management [17,21,29]. Therefore, the modified HFPS guideline provides clear instruction and learning support that motivates students to engage in HFPS and improve their SSSCL.

The narratives of students in the intervention group substantiated the quantitative results, demonstrating more satisfaction and confidence in learning throughout the HFPS learning process. They found the learning material useful in making clinical judgments more confidently. Students can achieve a better sense of accomplishment when they are appropriately directed to learn and prepare. They also develop critical assessment and management skills to better understand the patient's experience and clinical practice in HFPS [30], ultimately enhancing their competence in clinical management [11,17]. During the role-playing session of the HFPS, students actively engaged in learning and practicing by interacting with the simulated patient and their teammates. They received opportunities to provide direct patient care and handle problem-based clinical situations, including sudden changes in health conditions, patient safety issues, and ethical concerns [21,31]. Working as a team in HFPS allowed students to collaborate with other team members for decision making and develop their personal and professional strengths together [14,15]. When students encountered difficult handling situations, they worked together for better clinical judgment and decision making [14,15,32]. Moreover, students in the intervention groups reported higher SSSCL through collaborative teamwork in the HFPS, which increased their competence in practicing safely and with appropriate intervention for the simulated patient. They also found that they learned from their educator, whose involvement as a facilitator enhanced their motivation and direction to learn more effectively during the role-play session of the HFPS [33].

In the debriefing session, all students appreciated the group and educator feedback, which allowed them to gain more learning and self-evaluate their performance for better practice and self-improvement [13–15,21]. Debriefing should be conducted as early as possible after the HFPS so that students can self-evaluate their performance for better practice and self-improvement [34]. In case immediate debriefing is not allowed, written self-debriefing is an alternative [34]. Despite a simulated situation, students are facing a range of emotions that profoundly stimulate students' learning and performance. Debriefing is, therefore, also beneficial to reduce psychological burden and distress when they have a similar situation in the real clinical setting [24,34]. Importantly, the HFPS environment tolerates errors and allows students to improve their professional development [35]. While students are allowed to make mistakes in the HFPS, they are also reminded to be more alert when practicing in similar clinical situations in future real settings. Therefore, debriefing informs the success of appropriate clinical decisions and increases teaching quality [36].

This study successfully demonstrated the benefits of the modified HFPS guideline for student learning by increasing SSSCL through HFPS. Despite only a part of HSSOBP [25] being adopted in this study, the modified guideline, comprising four HFPS sessions: pre-briefing, simulation design, facilitation, and debriefing, allowed students to learn step by step. Figure S1 shows a conceptual framework for the association of these four sessions with student learning and their satisfaction and confidence in learning and how students learned at each session of HFPS. It is important to note that students' self-study, their involvement, the tutor's facilitation, feedback from peers and tutor, and students' self-evaluation were also the key components to enhance their satisfaction and self-confidence in learning through HFPS. In general, the HFPS is usually employed in senior-year students to encourage them to practice their learned knowledge and skills. In this study, HFPS is also effective in stimulating students to learn individually and in a group, enhancing their learning attitudes, confidence, and satisfaction. Early development of confidence and satisfaction in learning ultimately allows students to enhance competence in practice, clinical judgment, and decision-making abilities. Thus, a structured guideline should be added to nursing courses with HFPS in the curriculum to facilitate students' learning. The results also promote the awareness of nurse educators in designing guidelines for HFPS-related activities to enhance SSSCL in learning, which is crucial for clinical judgment and decision making.

Strengths and Limitations

Strengths of this quasi-experimental with control study include providing reliable and accurate evidence of the effects of the modified guideline for HFPS. However, the generalizability of the results is limited due to the recruitment at a single professional training institution. Similar studies in multiple centers should be conducted to increase generalizability. The absence of randomization can limit the researcher's ability to make strong causal claims about the intervention's effectiveness and may introduce selection bias, as there may be systematic differences between the groups being compared.

5. Conclusions

HFPS has recently emerged as an effective teaching and learning method in professional training. The modified guideline in this study provides clear direction for students, including junior students, to learn step-by-step and apply specific knowledge and skills to a patient with specific health needs in a simulated clinical setting. The HFPS guideline improves students' ability to make informed clinical judgments and effective decisions, leading to enhanced patient care. The students' narratives supported the findings of the quantitative results on SSSCL through HFPS. A conceptual framework (Figure S1) was developed to understand student learning, their satisfaction, and confidence in learning, as well as the ultimate learning outcomes through HFPS. Throughout the learning process with the structured HFPS guideline, students can learn more effectively with higher satisfaction and confidence in learning. The results of this study increase educators' awareness of the application of an HFPS guideline in the training curriculum to achieve better teaching and learning outcomes.

Supplementary Materials: The following supporting information can be downloaded at: https://www.mdpi.com/article/10.3390/nursrep13030090/s1, Figure S1: A conceptual framework on the association of these four sessions with student learning and their satisfaction and confidence in learning; Table S1: Differences of the four sessions in HFPS between the two groups; Table S2: The summary of students' feedback on their satisfaction and confidence in learning through three sessions of HFPS in the two groups.

Author Contributions: Conceptualization, F.M.F.W.; methodology, F.M.F.W. and D.C.N.W.; validation, F.M.F.W. and D.C.N.W.; formal analysis, F.M.F.W.; investigation, F.M.F.W.; resources, F.M.F.W.; data curation, F.M.F.W. and D.C.N.W.; writing—original draft preparation, F.M.F.W.; writing—review and editing, F.M.F.W. and D.C.N.W.; visualization, F.M.F.W. and D.C.N.W.; supervision, WMF.; project administration, F.M.F.W.; funding acquisition, F.M.F.W. All authors have read and agreed to the published version of the manuscript.

Funding: This research was funded by Tung Wah College, grant number SRG210401.

Institutional Review Board Statement: The study was conducted in accordance with the Declaration of Helsinki and approved by the Research Ethics Committee of Tung Wah College (protocol code REC2021102 and 23 September 2021). This study was prospectively registered with ClinicalTrials.gov on 28 October 2021 with registration number NCT05111327 (Unique Protocol ID: REC2021102).

Informed Consent Statement: Informed consent was obtained from all subjects involved in the study. Written informed consent has been obtained from the subjects to publish this paper.

Data Availability Statement: The data presented in this study are available on request from the corresponding author. The data are not publicly available due to keep the confidentiality.

Public Involvement Statement: Guidance for Reporting Involvement of Patients and the Public Long Checklist was completed.

Guidelines and Standards Statement: This manuscript was drafted against the CONSORT Extension Checklist [37] for A mixed (a quasi-experimental and qualitative study) research.

Acknowledgments: We would like to show our appreciation for Alice ML Chan, Natalie PM Lee, and Kevin HK Luk for their assistance in data collection. We also acknowledge National League of Nursing for their kind generosity of their permission to use their instrument, Student Satisfaction and Self-Confidence in Learning.

Conflicts of Interest: The authors declare no conflict of interest.

References

1. Lee, J.; Lee, Y.; Lee, S.; Bae, J. Effects of high-fidelity patient simulation led clinical reasoning course: Focused on nursing core competencies, problem solving, and academic self-efficacy. *Jpn. J. Nurs. Sci.* **2016**, *13*, 20–28. [CrossRef]
2. Yang, G.F.; Jiang, X.Y. Self-directed learning readiness and nursing competency among undergraduate nursing students in Fujian province of China. *Int. J. Nurs. Sci.* **2014**, *1*, 255–259. [CrossRef]
3. Levett-Jones, T. *Clinical Reasoning: Learning to Think Like a Nurse*, 2nd ed.; Pearson: Sydney, Australia, 2018.
4. Aljohani, A.S.; Karim, Q.; George, P. Students' satisfaction with simulation learning environment in relation to self-confidence and learning achievement. *J. Health Sci.* **2016**, *4*, 228–235. [CrossRef]
5. Fuglsang, S.; Bloch, C.W.; Selberg, H. Simulation training and professional self-confidence: A large-scale study of third year nursing students. *Nurse Educ. Today* **2022**, *108*, 105175. [CrossRef]
6. Li, Z.; Huang, F.F.; Chen, S.S.; Wang, A.; Guo, Y. The learning effectiveness of high-fidelity simulation teaching among Chinese nursing students: A mixed-methods study. *J. Nurs. Res.* **2021**, *29*, e141. [CrossRef] [PubMed]
7. Dalton, L.; Gee, T.; Levett-Jones, T. Using clinical reasoning and simulation-based education to 'flip' the enrolled nurse curriculum. *AJAN* **2015**, *33*, 29–35. Available online: https://www.ajan.com.au/archive/Vol33/Issue2/4Dalton.pdf (accessed on 21 January 2023).
8. Gopalakrishnan, P.; Sethuraman, K.R.; Suresh, P. Efficacy of high-fidelity simulation in clinical problem-solving exercises - Feedback from teachers and learners. *SBV J. Basic. Clin. Appl. Health Sci.* **2018**, *2*, 14–22. [CrossRef]
9. Al Gharibi, K.A.; Arulappan, J. Repeated simulation experience on self-confidence, critical thinking, and competence of nurses and nursing students—An integrative review. *SAGE Open Nurs.* **2020**, *6*, 2377960820927377. [CrossRef]
10. Cura, S.Ü.; Kocatepe, V.; Yıldırım, D.; Küçükakgün, H.; Atay, S.; Ünver, V. Examining knowledge, skill, stress, satisfaction, and self-confidence levels of nursing students in three different simulation modalities. *Asian Nurs. Res.* **2020**, *14*, 158–164. [CrossRef]
11. Guerrero, J.G.; Ali, S.A.A.; Attallah, D.M. The acquired critical thinking skills, satisfaction, and self-confidence of nursing students and staff nurse through high-fidelity simulation experience. *Clin. Simul. Nurs.* **2022**, *64*, 24–30. [CrossRef]
12. Shirazi, F.; Kazemipoor, H.; Tavakkoli-Moghaddam, R. Fuzzy decision analysis for project scope change management. *Decis. Sci. Lett.* **2017**, *6*, 395–406. [CrossRef]
13. Kan, C.W.Y.; Wong, F.M.F. How students learn in small group through online mode during the coronavirus pandemic: Descriptive narratives. *Teach. Learn. Nurs.* **2023**, *18*, 281–285. [CrossRef]
14. Wong, F.M.F. A cross-sectional study: Collaborative learning approach enhances learning attitudes of undergraduate nursing students. *GSTF JNHC* **2018**, *5*. [CrossRef]
15. Wong, F.M.F. A phenomenological research study: Perspectives of student learning through small group work between undergraduate nursing students and educators. *Nurse Educ. Today* **2018**, *68*, 153–158. [CrossRef]
16. Wong, M.F.F. Development of higher-level intellectual skills through interactive group work: Perspectives between students and educators. *Med. Clin. Res.* **2020**, *5*, 164–169.
17. Kaliyaperumal, R.; Raman, V.; Kannan, L.; Ali, M.D. Satisfaction and self-confidence of nursing students with simulation teaching. *IJHSR* **2021**, *11*, 44–50.
18. Tawalbeh, L.I.; Tubaishat, A. Effect of simulation on knowledge of advanced cardiac life support, knowledge retention, and confidence of nursing students in Jordan. *J. Nurs. Educ.* **2014**, *53*, 38–44. [CrossRef]

19. Welman, A.; Spies, C. High-fidelity simulation in nursing education: Considerations for meaningful learning. *Trends Nurs.* **2016**, *3*, 1–16. [CrossRef]
20. Gates, M.G.; Parr, M.B.; Hughen, J.E. Enhancing nursing knowledge using high-fidelity simulation. *J. Nurs. Educ.* **2012**, *51*, 9–15. [CrossRef]
21. Powell, E.; Scrooby, B.; van Graan, A. Nurse educators' views on implementation and use of high-fidelity simulation in nursing programmes. *Afr. J. Health Prof. Educ.* **2020**, *12*, 215–219. [CrossRef]
22. Almasri, F. Simulations to teach science subjects: Connections among students' engagement, self-confidence, satisfaction, and learning style. *EAIT* **2022**, *27*, 7161–7181. [CrossRef]
23. Mahfouz, R.; Almutairi, A.; Eldesouky, E. Self-confidence of nursing students related to their simulation learning experience. *JEP* **2019**, *10*. [CrossRef]
24. Lesã, R.; Daniel, B.; Harland, T. Learning with simulation: The experience of nursing students. *CSN* **2021**, *56*, 57–65. [CrossRef]
25. The International Nursing Association for Clinical Simulation and Learning (INACSL). Onward and Upward: Introducing the Healthcare Simulation Standards of Best Standard. *CSN* **2021**, *58*, 1–4.
26. Reid, C.A.; Ralph, J.L.; El-Masri, M.; Ziefle, K. High-Fidelity Simulation and Clinical Judgment of Nursing Students in a Maternal-Newborn Course. *West. J. Nurs. Res.* **2020**, *42*, 829–837. [CrossRef]
27. Franklin, A.E.; Burns, P.; Lee, C.S. Psychometric testing on the NLN Student Satisfaction and Self-Confidence in Learning, Simulation Design Scale, and Educational Practices Questionnaire using a sample of prelicensure novice nurses. *Nurse Educ. Today* **2014**, *34*, 1298–1304. [CrossRef]
28. Kelleci, M.; Yilmaz, F.T.; Aldemir, K. The effects of high-fidelity simulation training on critical thinking and problem solving in nursing students in Turkey. *Educ. Res. Rev.* **2018**, *7*, e83966. [CrossRef]
29. Wong, F.M.F.; Tang, A.C.Y.; Cheng, W.L.S. Factors associated with self-directed learning among undergraduate nursing students: A systematic review. *Nurse Educ. Today* **2021**, *104*, 104998. [CrossRef]
30. Sarmasoglu, S.; Dinc, L.; Elcin, M. Using standardized patients in nursing education effects on students' psychomotor skill development. *Nurse Educ.* **2016**, *41*, E1–E5. [CrossRef] [PubMed]
31. Kim, J.; Park, J.H.; Shin, S. Effectiveness of simulation-based nursing education depending on fidelity: A meta-analysis. *BMC Med. Educ.* **2016**, *16*, 152. [CrossRef]
32. Carson, P.P.; Harder, N. Simulation use within the classroom: Recommendations from the literature. *CSN* **2016**, *12*, 429–437. [CrossRef]
33. Hustad, J.; Johannesen, B.; Fossum, M.; Hovland, O.J. Nursing students' transfer of learning outcomes from simulation-based training to clinical practice: A focus-group study. *BMC Nurs.* **2019**, *18*, 53. [CrossRef] [PubMed]
34. Miller, S.; Miller, M. Mind the gap! A strategy to bridge the time between simulation and debriefing. *CSN* **2021**, *51*, 10–13. [CrossRef]
35. Negri, E.C.; Mazzo, A.; Martins, J.C.A.; Pereira, G.A., Jr.; Almeida, R.G.D.S.; Pedersoli, C.E. Clinical simulation with dramatization: Gains perceived by students and health professionals. *Rev. Lat. Am. Enfermagem* **2017**, *3*, e2916. [CrossRef]
36. Silva, J.L.G.; Oliveira-Kumakura, A.R.S. Clinical simulation to teach nursing care for wounded patients. *Rev. Lat. Am. Enfermagem* **2018**, *71* (Suppl. S4), 1785–1790. [CrossRef]
37. Kwakkenbos, L.; Imran, M.; McCall, S.J.; McCord, K.A.; Fröbert, O.; Hemkens, L.G.; Zwarenstein, M.; Relton, C.; Rice, D.B.; Langan, S.M.; et al. CONSORT extension for the reporting of randomised controlled trials conducted using cohorts and routinely collected data (CONSORT-ROUTINE): Checklist with explanation and elaboration. *BMJ* **2021**, *373*, n857. [CrossRef]

Disclaimer/Publisher's Note: The statements, opinions and data contained in all publications are solely those of the individual author(s) and contributor(s) and not of MDPI and/or the editor(s). MDPI and/or the editor(s) disclaim responsibility for any injury to people or property resulting from any ideas, methods, instructions or products referred to in the content.

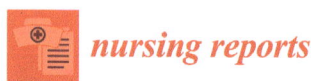

Article

Degree of Alarm Fatigue and Mental Workload of Hospital Nurses in Intensive Care Units

Yoonhee Seok [1], Yoomi Cho [2], Nayoung Kim [2] and Eunyoung E. Suh [3,*]

1. Department of Nursing, Kyungil University, Gyeongsan 38428, Republic of Korea; uri303@kiu.ac.kr
2. College of Nursing, Seoul National University, Seoul 03080, Republic of Korea
3. Center for Human-Caring Nurse Leaders for the Future by Brain Korea 21 (BK 21) Four Project, Research Institute of Nursing Science, College of Nursing, Seoul National University, Seoul 03080, Republic of Korea
* Correspondence: esuh@snu.ac.kr

Abstract: This study aimed to determine the degree of alarm fatigue and mental workload of ICU nurses, and to clarify the relationship between these two variables. A cross-sectional, descriptive research design was used. Data were collected from 90 nurses working in four ICUs in Seoul, Republic of Korea, using a questionnaire determining their degree of alarm fatigue and mental workload. Data were collected from 6 March to 26 April 2021 and were analyzed using a *t*-test, ANOVA, and Pearson's correlation coefficient. The average alarm-fatigue score was 28.59 out of 44. The item with the highest score was "I often hear a certain amount of noise in the ward", with a score of 3.59 out of 4. The average of the mental workload scores was 75.21 out of 100. The highest mental workload item was effort, which scored 78.72 out of 100. No significant correlation was found between alarm fatigue and mental workload. Although nurses were consistently exposed to alarm fatigue, this was not directly related to their mental workloads, perhaps owing to their professional consciousness as they strived to accomplish tasks despite alarm fatigue. However, since alarm fatigue can affect efficiency, investigations to reduce it and develop appropriate guidelines are necessary. This study was not registered.

Keywords: alarm fatigue; mental workload; intensive care units; patient safety; nursing

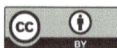

1. Introduction

The alarm sound generated by a medical device was listed as one of the top 10 health technology hazards in a report by the Emergency Treatment Research Institute in 2020 [1], with alarm fatigue being deemed a predominant medical-device-related technology risk in 2012. It is recognized as a national problem in many countries, and numerous studies are conducted on this topic annually [2]. The alarm was designed to monitor the patient's condition in real time and to rapidly identify and manage the patient if it is out of the appropriate range [3]. The intensive care units (ICUs) of hospitals are well-equipped with a range of medical devices to extensively observe and monitor critically ill patients, and high noise and alarm sounds are induced by such devices [4]. ICU nurses are the key personnel who manage various monitoring medical devices and respond to the alarm sounds. Thus, they are the ones most directly affected by medical-device alarm sounds.

Alarm fatigue is defined as the sensory overload and desensitization that make nurses unable to respond to real threats. [5]. An inadequate situational awareness of alarm sounds is one of the main factors causing safety accidents, which can lead to serious risks [6]. In ICUs, 72–99% of the alarm sounds generated are false-positive alarms. Excessive exposure to false-positive alarms that occur without accurate physiological data violations causes sensory overload in nurses, lowering their sensitivity to alarms. Therefore, they may fail to check these alarms, putting their patients at risk [7]. When these unnecessary alarms go off, if they are not resolved correctly, the cognitive response of the brain decreases and the alarm is ignored [8]. When a patient's crisis-related alarm is repeatedly rung, nurses' mental workload increases as a stress response, resulting in decreased situational awareness and job performance [9]. Inadequate measures against such alarm fatigue may cause medical personnel to become insensitive to the alerts, rendering them unable to differentiate between false-positive and actual alarms in real life-threatening situations. This may further lead to their inability to recognize alarms as serious and requiring immediate action [10]. Alarm fatigue is acknowledged as a contributor to staffs' environmental distractions and interferes with the ability of staff to perform critical patient care responsibilities resulting in patient safety issues. The Joint Commission (TJC) reported 98 alarm-related sentinel events between 2009 and 2012, of which 80 resulted in death, 13 in permanent loss of function, and five in unexpected prolonged care conditions. Of these incidences, the majority were associated with alarm malfunction, alarm misuse, or inadequate alarm settings, leading to the most common contributing factor—alarm fatigue [11].

Several studies demonstrated that continuous alarm fatigue can cause stress in nurses, with mental workload reported to be an additional cause [12]. Some studies reported that alarm-fatigue-related situations do not affect performance [9]. However, increased mental load owing to alarm fatigue affects prefrontal activity, which reduces coping strategies and increases psychophysiological demand [13]. It is thus important to clarify the degree of alarm fatigue and mental workload experienced by nurses to guarantee the quality and safety of patient care [14].

Globally, studies are actively being conducted on the effects of excessive alarm sounds on employees, nurses' responses to alarm sounds, technology to reduce false alarm sounds, and innovations to improve alarm systems [5]. However, in Republic of Korea, there are only four studies on the topic so far. One study addressed alarm-fatigue perception, management performance, and alarm-fatigue interference factors, while another verified the effectiveness of alarm-management education [15–18]. Studies on the mental workload that affects work performance are still lacking. In addition, previous studies show a limitation in accurately measuring the alarm fatigue of nurses by using the alarm-fatigue tool developed for industrial workers. Thus, it is impossible to be completely sure of the tool's sensitivity to alarm fatigue. Therefore, in this study, the alarm-fatigue measurement tool developed for nurses was used to understand their alarm fatigue in the ICU. This study aimed to investigate the relationship between alarm fatigue and nurses' mental workload to provide basic data for patient safety management.

Noise, Mental Workload, and Inhibitory Mechanism

Mental workload has a long association with human-factors research into safety-critical performance [19]. The prefrontal cortex (PFC) is a brain structure often identified as the neurophysiological source of limited resources. The PFC serves a control function during routine cognitive operations, such as action selection, retrieval/updating in working memory, monitoring, and inhibition [13]. In stressful situations, such as noise (alarm), the brain uses inhibitory mechanisms. Inhibitory mechanisms reduce neural activity associated with work or stimulation of high-level cortical areas (prefrontal cortex) to alleviate the activation of distracting neural assemblies. As a result, inhibitory mechanisms reduce the brain's ability to take into account new information or cope [20]. Excessive and repeated alarms result in noise-induced hearing impairment, interfere with speech interpretation, negatively impact psychophysiological and mental health, diminish overall performance, and interfere with intended activities [21].

2. Materials and Methods
2.1. Design, Setting, and Participants

This study used a cross-sectional, descriptive research design to not only understand the degree of alarm fatigue and mental workload experienced by ICU nurses but also to identify the relationship between these variables. Participants were nurses working in the ICU of Seoul National University Hospital in Republic of Korea. The nurses voluntarily agreed to participate in the study based on their understanding of the study's purpose.

The study was conducted in four ICUs belonging to one hospital. Nurses in the general ward, delivery room, recovery room, and operating room were excluded from the study because the frequency of exposure to the alarm sound differed significantly from that of the ICU nurses.

2.2. Target Number of Participants and Calculation Basis

The G*Power 3.1.9.4 program was used to calculate the number of samples required for the study, with a significance level of 0.05, the median effect size of 0.03, and power of 80%. The correlation between alarm fatigue and mental workload was calculated and the appropriate sample size involved 82 persons. Therefore, 90 Google form questionnaires were distributed, allowing for a 10% attrition rate. However, all 90 questionnaires were returned.

2.3. Instruments

2.3.1. Alarm Fatigue

The tool for alarm-fatigue measurement in ICU nurses was developed by Torabizadeh et al. [14]. This tool was approved for use and translation by the original author. It comprises 13 questions, rated on a five-point Likert scale ranging from 0 ("absolutely not") to 4 ("always"). Items 1 and 9 are reverse-scored. Possible scores range from 8–44, with higher scores indicating greater influence on nurses' performance owing to alarm fatigue. For example, in item 1, if the nurse selects "never," it means that he/she never readjusts the limits of alarms based on the clinical symptoms of patients and always sets them in a routine range, which is wrong, so it will be scored 4 meaning a greater impact of alarm fatigue on his/her performance. At the time of development, the reliability of these 13 questions was confirmed with a Cronbach's alpha of 0.91. The Cronbach's alpha in this study was 0.66.

The translation was performed in three steps. First, the English tool was translated into Korean by two researchers. Next, the translated Korean tool was retranslated into English by two professional translators, who are proficient in both English and Korean. Finally, a professor who majored in nursing was commissioned to evaluate the structural similarity of the language and meaning between the original text and reverse translation.

2.3.2. National Aeronautics and Space Administration Task Load Index (NASA-TLX)

The NASA-TLX is a subjective job difficulty assessment tool that was developed by NASA in the early 1980s. It is an openly accessible tool that can be used without a separate approval process [22]. The most effective way to evaluate a job's difficulty level is to directly assess the workers with relevant experience in that job. Various survey methods have thus been developed to evaluate the cognitive load of jobs. The NASA-TLX and subjective workload assessment technique (SWAT) are well-known assessments [23]. However, the NASA-TLX has been recognized as the most stable subjective task difficulty evaluation method [24]. It can quantify the overall workload based on the average score of six questionnaire items—mental demand, physical demand, temporal demand, effort, performance, and frustration level—with scores ranging between 0 and 100 in five-point increments. The higher the score, the higher the mental workload. NASA-TLX, both the split-half reliability and Cronbach's alpha coefficient were more than 0.80 [25]. The Cronbach's alpha in this study was 0.80.

2.4. Data Collection

Data were collected from nurses working in the ICU of a tertiary general hospital in Seoul from 6 March to 26 April 2021. Nurses who expressed their intention to participate in the study received an explanation about its purpose and procedure; written consent was then obtained from the nurses who wished to participate. Participants were then sent a survey questionnaire via email or Kakao Talk, a Korean chat app. The time required to complete the questionnaire was 10–15 min. There were no missing data in the responses among the 90 participants; thus, 90 questionnaires were used for statistical analysis.

2.5. Ethical Considerations

This study was approved by the Research Ethics Deliberation Committee of S Hospital for the conduct of research to ethically protect the study participants in the planning stage (no. 2102-158-1199; 22 March 2021). After obtaining consent from the hospital nursing department for data collection, the researcher directly posted an announcement of the study on the bulletin board of each department. The researcher personally interviewed the nurses who made contact after reading the notice. After asking and answering questions, if they agreed to participate in the study, a written consent form was provided to them. The nurses were assured that all data would be used for research purposes only, confidentiality would be maintained, and they could withdraw their participation at any time during the study. After data collection, a predetermined gift (mobile coupon of USD 3.0) was provided to all participants.

2.6. Data Analysis

Data were analyzed using SPSS 25.0 (IBM, Armonk, NY, USA). The distribution of participants' general characteristics was analyzed based on frequency and percentage. The degree of alarm fatigue and mental workload in ICU nurses was evaluated based on the mean and standard deviation. Differences in alarm fatigue and mental workload related to the general characteristics of nurses were assessed using *t*-tests and a one-way analysis of variance (ANOVA). The relationship between alarm fatigue and the mental workload of nurses was tested using Pearson's correlation coefficient.

3. Results

3.1. Participants' General Characteristics

The participants' mean age was 30.46 (5.30) years, with most participants being in their 20s (56.7%). There were 81 (90%) women, and 81 (90%) nurses with a bachelor's degree educational qualification. Of the participants, 83 (92.2%) were registered nurses, while 7 (7.8%) were charged nurses. Of the participants, 37 (41.1%) worked in the medical intensive care unit (MICU). Nurses' total ICU experience was 5.02 (4.95) years, with 52 (57.8%) having 1–5 years of experience. Meanwhile, 76 (84.4%) nurses stated that they oversaw care for two patients while on duty. Sixty-five (72.2%) nurses received education on alarm-sound management. Regarding ICU medical-device training within the past two years, 80 participants (88.9%) received training on the defibrillator the most, followed by 63 (70%) on the infusion pump, and 60 (66.7%) each for ventilators and physiological monitors, respectively. The number of nurses who did not experience an error related to the alarm sound was low at 16 (17.8%). Moreover, the number of nurses with direct or indirect experience of alarm-related event errors was high at 74 (82.2%). Finally, when asked whether they knew about the concept of alarm fatigue, 60 nurses (66.7%) answered that they did not (Table 1).

3.2. Nurses' Alarm Fatigue and Mental Workload

The average alarm-fatigue score was 28.59 (5.79) out of 44. The item with the highest score was "I often hear a certain amount of noise in the ward," with a score of 3.59 (0.58) out of 4. The item with the lowest score was "I regularly readjust the limits of alarms based on the clinical symptoms of patients," with a score of 1.05 (0.89) points. The average of the mental workload scores was 75.21 (14.70) out of 100. The performance and frustration level scores were low at 70.89 (21.58) and 70.50 (22.22) points, respectively. The highest mental load item was effort, with 78.72 (20.16) points (Table 2).

Table 1. Participants' General Characteristics (*n* = 90).

Characteristics	Category	n (%)	Mean (SD)
Age(years)	24~29	51 (56.7)	30.46 (5.30)
	30~49	39 (43.3)	
Gender	Male	9 (10.0)	
	Female	81 (90.0)	
Education	BSN	81 (90.0)	
	MSN	9 (10.0)	
Position	RN	83 (92.2)	
	CN	7 (7.8)	
ICU type	SICU	23 (25.6)	
	MICU	37 (41.1)	
	CCU	12 (13.3)	
	CPICU	18 (20.0)	
Total clinical experience (years)	1~5	51 (56.7)	5.52 (5.39)
	5~10	18 (20.0)	
	>10	21 (23.3)	
ICU clinical experience (years)	1~5	52 (57.8)	5.02 (4.95)
	5~10	20 (22.2)	
	>10	18 (20.0)	
Number of patients	2 patients	76 (84.4)	
	>3 patients	14 (15.6)	
Alarm-management education	Yes	65 (72.2)	
	No	25 (27.8)	
Trained medical equipment (within 2 years) (Multiple answers)	Ventilator	60 (66.7)	
	physiological monitor	60 (66.7)	
	Infusion pump	63 (70.0)	
	Defibrillator	80 (88.9)	
	Others (ECMO, CRRT, IABP, EV100, NO gas, servo-I, Masimo)	19 (21.1)	
Experience of alarm related accident	Yes	26 (28.9)	
	Indirected	48 (53.3)	
	No	16 (17.8)	
Insight of Concept	Yes	30 (33.3)	
	No	60 (66.7)	

SD, standard deviation; BSN, bachelor science of nursing; MSN, master science of nursing; RN, registered nurse; CN, charged nurse; SICU, surgical intensive care unit; MICU, medical intensive care unit; CCU, coronary care unit; CPICU, cardiopulmonary intensive care unit; ECMO, extracorporeal membrane oxygenation; CCRT, continuous renal replacement therapy; IABP, intra-aortic balloon pump; NO gas, nitric oxide gas.

3.3. Alarm Fatigue and Mental Workload According to General Characteristics

A *t*-test and one-way ANOVA were performed to verify the differences between nurses' general characteristics and alarm fatigue. Alarm fatigue showed no significant difference according to the nurses' age, sex, education level, position, ICU type, total ICU experience, number of patients overseen per person, presence or absence of alarm sound management training, or experience of safety accidents related to alarm sounds (Table 3).

However, alarm fatigue was significantly higher among those who were aware (vs. not) of its concept (t = 2.438, p = 0.017). The difference in the degree of mental workload according to general characteristics was also tested. The mental workload was higher when the number of patients cared for per person was >3, versus when there were 2 (t = 2.001, p = 0.048; Table 3).

Table 2. Nurse' Alarm Fatigue and Mental Workload (n = 90).

Domain	Possible Range	Min~Max	Mean (SD)
Alarm Fatigue	8~44	11~39	28.59 (5.79)
1. I regularly readjust the limits of alarms based on the clinical symptoms of patients			1.05 (0.89)
2. I turn off the alarms at the beginning of every shift.			1.48 (1.37)
3. Generally, I hear a certain amount of noise in the ward.			3.59 (0.58)
4. I believe much of the noise in the ward is from the alarms of the monitoring equipment			3.25 (0.63)
5. I pay more attention to the alarms in certain shifts			2.42 (1.21)
6. In some shifts the heavy workload in the ward prevents my quick response to alarms			2.88 (0.89)
7. When alarms go off repeatedly, I become indifferent to them.			1.80 (1.10)
8. Alarm sounds make me nervous.			3.38 (0.70)
9. I react differently to the low-volume (yellow) and high-volume (red) alarms of the ventilator.			1.11 (0.99)
10. When I'm upset and nervous, I'm more responsive to alarm sounds			2.15 (1.19)
11. When alarms go off repeatedly and continuously, I lose my patience.			2.43 (1.10)
12. Alarm sounds prevent me from focusing on my professional duties.			2.64 (0.97)
13. At visiting hours, I pay less attention to the alarms of the equipment.			1.15 (0.97)
Mental Workload	0~100	5~100	75.21 (14.70)
Mental demand	0~100	25~100	76.78 (20.00)
Physical demand	0~100	25~100	76.39 (20.00)
Temporal demand	0~100	25~100	78.00 (20.39)
Performance	0~100	20~100	70.89 (21.58)
Effort	0~100	25~100	78.72 (20.16)
Frustration level	0~100	10~100	70.50 (22.22)

SD, standard deviation.

Table 3. Alarm Fatigue and Mental Workload according to General Characteristics (n = 90).

Characteristics	Category	Alarm Fatigue Mean (SD)	Alarm Fatigue t/F	Alarm Fatigue p	Mental Workload Mean (SD)	Mental Workload t/F	Mental Workload p
Age (years)	24–29	28.53 (6.32)	−0.935	0.352	74.08 (12.29)	−0.612	0.542
	30–49	29.69 (5.15)			76.30 (17.31)		
Gender	Male	29.22 (7.41)	0.102	0.919	72.59 (14.92)	−0.522	0.603
	Female	29.01 (5.70)			75.29 (14.69)		
Education	BSN	28.73 (5.82)	−1.496	0.138	75.43 (14.82)	0.803	0.424
	MSN	31.78 (5.57)			72.28 (13.23)		
Position	RN	28.98 (5.93)	−3.200	0.750	75.44 (14.39)	0.946	0.347
	CN	29.71 (4.96)			69.99 (17.89)		
ICU type	SICU	28.91 (5.17)	2.551	0.061	73.84 (17.72)	1.092	0.357
	MICU	30.43 (5.61)			73.17 (13.42)		
	CCU	29.58 (5.88)			81.67 (14.27)		
	CPICU	25.94 (6.36)			75.88 (12.78)		
Total ICU clinical Experience (years)	1~5	28.73 (6.14)	0.169	0.845	75.30 (12.70)	2.298	0.107
	5~10	29.55 (5.84)			70.32 (19.84)		
	>10	29.33 (5.17)			80.42 (13.75)		
Number of patients	2 patients	28.93 (5.92)	−0.373	0.710	73.90 (14.67)	−2.001	0.048 *
	>3 patients	29.57 (5.58)			82.32 (13.14)		
Alarm management education	Yes	28.68 (6.04)	−0.933	0.354	74.41 (15.18)	−0.627	0.522
	No	29.96 (5.30)			76.59 (13.34)		
Experience of alarm related accident	Yes	30.23 (6.46)	1.810	0.170	75.68 (14.41)	0.096	0.909
	No	26.75 (5.53)			73.64 (19.29)		
	Heard that	29.14 (5.48)			75.12 (13.29)		
Insight of Concept	Yes	31.10 (5.09)	2.438	0.017 *	73.91 (13.75)	0.504	0.615
	No	28.00 (5.96)			75.57 (15.17)		

SD, standard deviation; BSN, bachelor science of nursing; MSN, master science of nursing; RN, registered nurse; CN, charged nurse; SICU, surgical intensive care unit; MICU, medical intensive care unit; CCU, coronary care unit; CPICU, cardiopulmonary intensive care unit; ECMO, extracorporeal membrane oxygenation; CCRT, continuous renal replacement therapy; IABP, intra-aortic balloon pump; NO gas, nitric oxide gas. * $p < 0.05$

3.4. The Relationship between Alarm Fatigue and Mental Workload

There was no significant correlation between alarm fatigue and the mental workload of ICU nurses ($r = 0.127$, $p = 0.232$; Table 4).

Table 4. The Relationship between Alarm Fatigue and Mental Workload ($n = 90$).

	Alarm Fatigue	Mental Workload
Alarm Fatigue	1	0.127 (0.232)
Mental Workload	0.127 (0.232)	1

4. Discussion

This study was conducted to identify the relationship between alarm fatigue and the mental workload of ICU nurses. In the detailed item evaluating alarm fatigue, nurses reported that they experienced a significant amount of alarm noise in their working environment and that this noise was mostly generated by medical monitoring devices. The items of the alarm-fatigue questionnaire included, "I regularly readjust the limits of alarms based on the clinical symptoms of patients" and "I react differently to the low-volume (yellow) and high-volume (red) alarms of the ventilator." This question should indicate a high score when the alarm-fatigue score is high. The participants in this study had a high overall alarm-fatigue score; however, they showed low scores for these two items. That is, if the alarm-fatigue score is high, nurses may not immediately respond to the alarm. Conversely, this study's participants reported that they responded immediately. This finding contradicts a study showing that 81% of nurses had a delayed response to the alarm sound or deactivated the alarm sound when they experienced alarm fatigue [26]. However, this is consistent with the current finding that alarm fatigue interferes with nurses' performance but does not affect response time [12,18]. These results show that the nurses have a sense of responsibility and alertness toward the patient. In fact, many nurses in Korea often sound an alarm when the patient's condition is constantly unstable around the target value but nurses tolerate the alarm sound and respond sensitively to changes in the patient's condition. Therefore, alarm fatigue may not directly affect job performance because the nurses remained alert to the alarm sound through previous patient safety accident experiences. On the other hand, we cannot rule out a bias in which the items in the survey lead nurses to choose the correct one as the type of question about moral conduct that they feel. This is because, in Korean hospital alarm management, nurses have to adjust the range of alarm sounds according to the patient's symptoms and respond according to the red and yellow alarm sounds [15].

In addition, previous studies showed that higher alarm fatigue caused stress and increased the mental workload among nurses but there was no significant correlation in this study [9,18].

In this study, the number of nurses who directly or indirectly experienced an alarm-related event error accounted for 82.2% of the total participants, which was higher than that of 66.7% in a previous study targeting tertiary hospitals [27]. It is, therefore, necessary to investigate the causes and influencing factors of medical-device-related patient safety accidents in the future. Moreover, it is necessary to establish strategies annually to reduce alarm fatigue by analyzing technology-related factors regarding patient safety at the organizational level.

Previous difficulties related to alarm fatigue that were experienced by nurses included the absence of documented data on alarm settings (75.8%) and a lack of education concerning these settings (47.8%) [28]. In this study, more nurses (72.2%) had received training on alarm management as compared to a previous study (50.3%) [29]. However, in this study, within the previous two years, less than 70% of nurses had received training on medical devices, such as ventilators, physiological monitors, and infusion pumps, and only 80% had received training on using a defibrillator. This suggests that medical-device education occurs only once and continuous and periodic education is necessary for alarm management in the field. In addition, it was confirmed that nurses with less than three years of experience lacked knowledge regarding how to control the alarm management according to the patient's situation and received unstructured and irregular education on alarm adjustment from the senior nurses when the alarm went off [15]. This suggests that it is necessary to develop a protocol for situational alarm management, in addition to providing training and a manual for alarm settings. In previous studies, it was found that improving education, customization of the alarm-sound parameters, and existing threshold algorithm improvement strategies were effective in reducing false positives to improve alarm fatigue [30,31].

There was no difference in alarm fatigue and mental workload between junior and senior nurses. Rather, there was a difference in nurses' mental workload according to the number of patients per nurse. Concerning senior nurses, their workload was immense owing to the task of managing the causes of alarms, which junior nurses could not resolve. For junior nurses, it was difficult to determine which alarms were associated with which patient and what problem caused them. When the number of managed patients is small, the number of alarm sounds to be managed also decreases; thus, it is suggested that there is a difference in the mental workload for alarms according to the number of patients [12,13].

Alarm fatigue is a nursing intervention item that requires continuous management and monitoring. In this study, alert fatigue did not affect the mental workload of nurses. Since alarm-sound fatigue is at a high level, it is a factor that affects patient safety; therefore, further research is needed in the future. Efforts to effectively manage medical-device alarms and reduce alarm fatigue can prevent potentially hazardous events [32].

Limitations

To determine the effect of alarm fatigue and mental workload, it would be more appropriate to record or observe nurses' reactions at the time the alarm sounds. This can be considered a supplement to this study. The Cronbach's alpha of the alarm-fatigue questionnaire used in this study was 0.66, which was a low value (more than an acceptable value of 0.7). This is in contradiction to the value of 0.91 obtained in the developed alarm-fatigue questionnaire. This is considered to be related to Korean culture or the hospital environment in Korea. In particular, in the case of questions 1 and 9, the alarm should never be turned off according to hospital rules and it should act according to the order of the alarm. In addition, in the case of Korea, they respond more sensitively to monitor alarms for a quiet environment during visits and to explain and focus more on the caregiver. To clarify this tool's reliability, it is necessary to repeat the study with different target hospitals and target nurses. We propose to identify the reality of alarm fatigue by applying a mixed method with the addition of a qualitative method for alarm fatigue. It also suggests the consideration of alert fatigue as a health risk for nurses.

5. Conclusions

A nurse's work environment directly or indirectly affects the safety and wellbeing of patients. Therefore, improving the working environment of nurses is directly related to patient safety and wellbeing. Alarm management is a nursing intervention that requires strategies to manage alarm fatigue while ensuring the delivery of safe patient care. This study was conducted to identify the degree of alarm fatigue and mental workload among nurses regarding the safety of patients and to investigate the relationship between them. However, there was no direct correlation between alarm fatigue and mental workload. This contradicts previous studies, which showed that alarm sounds cause stress and an increased mental workload among nurses. However, medical devices used in ICUs are continuously increasing and louder alarms are implemented in a noisier environment, causing psychological problems for nurses. Thus, a hospital-level alarm sound protocol and research on the reduction of alarm fatigue are necessary.

Author Contributions: Conceptualization, E.E.S. and Y.S.; methodology E.E.S., Y.S., Y.C. and N.K.; software, Y.S.; validation, E.E.S., Y.S. and Y.C.; formal analysis, Y.S. and Y.C.; investigation, Y.S. and N.K.; resources, Y.S. and Y.C.; data curation, Y.S., N.K. and Y.C.; writing—original draft, Y.S., N.K. and Y.C.; writing—review and editing, E.E.S. and Y.S.; visualization, Y.S.; supervision, E.E.S. All authors have read and agreed to the published version of the manuscript.

Funding: This research received no external funding.

Institutional Review Board Statement: This study was approved by the Research Ethics Deliberation Committee of S Hospital (2102-158-1199).

Informed Consent Statement: Written informed consent was obtained from all participants.

Data Availability Statement: Not applicable.

Public Involvement Statement: No public involvement in any aspect of this research.

Guidelines and Standards Statement: This manuscript was drafted against the (STROBE) for a cross-sectional study, descriptive research.

Acknowledgments: This work was supported by the Research Institute of Nursing Science, College of Nursing, Seoul National University Research Grant in 2021.

Conflicts of Interest: The authors declare that there are no conflict of interest.

References

1. ERCI. Top Ten Health Technology Hazards for 2020. Available online: https://elautoclave.files.wordpress.com/2019/10/ecri-top-10-technology-hazards-2020.pdf (accessed on 21 March 2021).
2. ECRI. Top 10 Health Technology Hazards for 2013. Available online: https://www.ecri.org/Resources/Whitepapers_and_reports/2013_Health_Devices_Top_10_Hazards.pdf (accessed on 21 March 2021).
3. Borowski, M.; Gorges, M.; Fried, R.; Such, O.; Wrede, C.; Imhoff, M. Medical device alarms. *Biomed. Tech.* **2011**, *56*, 73–83. [CrossRef]
4. Lee, M.H.; Sakong, J.; Kang, P.S. Effects of noise in hospital on patients and employees. *J. Yeungnam Med. Sci.* **2007**, *24*, S352–S364. [CrossRef]
5. Cvach, M. Monitor alarm fatigue: An integrative review. *Biomed. Instrum. Technol.* **2012**, *46*, 268–277. [CrossRef]
6. Kim, S.W.; Go, E.K.; Lee, B.H. Design to integrated display and caution function for KHP. *J. Korean Soc. Aeronaut.* **2017**, *45*, 481–489. [CrossRef]
7. Kenny, P.E. Alarm fatigue and patient safety. *Pa. Nurse.* **2011**, *66*, 3–22. [PubMed]
8. Sowan, A.K.; Tarriela, A.F.; Gomez, T.M.; Reed, C.C.; Rapp, K.M. Nurses' perceptions and practices toward clinical alarms in a transplant cardiac intensive care unit: Exploring key issues leading to alarm fatigue. *JMIR Hum. Factors* **2015**, *2*, e3. [CrossRef]
9. Mandrick, K.; Peysakhovich, V.; Rémy, F.; Lepron, E.; Causse, M. Neural and psychophysiological correlates of human performance under stress and high mental workload. *Biol. Psychol.* **2016**, *121*, 62–73. [CrossRef] [PubMed]
10. Hravnak, M.; Pellathy, T.; Chen, L.; Dubrawski, A.; Wertz, A.; Clermont, G.; Pinsky, M.R. A call to alarms: Current state and future directions in the battle against alarm fatigue. *J. Electrocardiol.* **2018**, *51*, S44–S48. [CrossRef]
11. Patricia, W.; Abbott, P. Alarm fatigue: A concept analysis. *OJNI* **2014**, *18*, 2.
12. Deb, S.; Claudio, D. Alarm fatigue and its influence on staff performance. *IISE Trans. Healthc. Syst. Eng.* **2015**, *5*, 183–196. [CrossRef]
13. Dehais, F.; Lafont, A.; Roy, R.; Fairclough, S. A neuroergonomics approach to mental workload, engagement and human performance. *Front. Neurosci.* **2020**, *14*, 268. [CrossRef] [PubMed]
14. Torabizadeh, C.; Yousefinya, A.; Zand, F.; Rakhshan, M.; Fararooei, M. A Nurses' alarm fatigue questionnaire: Development and psychometric properties. *J. Clin. Monit. Comput.* **2017**, *31*, 1305–1312. [CrossRef] [PubMed]
15. Kim, E.; Kim, M. Intensive care unit nurse's reaction experience to patient monitoring medical device alarms. *J. Korean Acad. Nurs. Adm.* **2021**, *27*, 215–226. [CrossRef]
16. Jeong, Y.J.; Kim, H. Evaluation of clinical alarms and alarm management in intensive care units. *J. Korean Biol. Nurs. Sci.* **2018**, *20*, 228–235. [CrossRef]
17. Hong, J.S. Effects of Patient Monitor Alarm Management Education for Intensive Care Unit Nurses. Master's Thesis, Jeju National University, Jeju, Republic of Korea, 2019.
18. Cho, O.M.; Kim, H.; Lee, Y.W.; Cho, I. Clinical alarms in intensive care units: Perceived obstacles of alarm management and alarm fatigue in nurses. *Healthc. Inform. Res.* **2016**, *22*, 46–53. [CrossRef]
19. Young, M.S.; Brookhuis, K.A.; Wickens, C.D.; Hancock, P.A. State of science: Mental workload in ergonomics. *Ergonomics* **2015**, *58*, 1–17. [CrossRef]
20. Munakata, Y.; Herd, S.A.; Chatham, C.H.; Depue, B.E.; Banich, M.T.; O'Reilly, R.C. A unified framework for inhibitory control. *Trends Cognit. Sci.* **2011**, *15*, 453–459. [CrossRef]

21. Oleksy, A.J.; Schlesinger, J.J. What's all that noise-Improving the hospital soundscape. *J. Clin. Monit. Comput.* **2019**, *33*, 557–562. [CrossRef]
22. Hart, S.G.; Staveland, L.E. Development of NASA-TLX (task load index): Results of empirical and theoretical research. *Adv. Psychol.* **1988**, *52*, 139–183. [CrossRef]
23. Rubio, S.; Diaz, E.; Martin, J.; Puente, J.M. Evaluation of subjective mental workload: A comparison of SWAT, NASA-TLX, and workload profile methods. *Appl. Psychol.* **2004**, *53*, 61–86. [CrossRef]
24. Hill, S.G.; Iavecchia, H.P.; Byers, J.C.; Bittner, A.C., Jr.; Zaklade, A.L.; Christ, R.E. Comparison of four subjective workload rating scales. *Human. Factors* **1992**, *34*, 429–439. [CrossRef]
25. Xiao, Y.M.; Wang, Z.M.; Wang, M.Z.; Lan, Y.J. The Appraisal of Reliability and Validity of Subjective Workload Assessment Technique and NASA-task Load Index. *Zhonghua Lao Dong Wei Sheng Zhi Ye Bing Za Zhi* **2005**, *23*, 178–181.
26. Casey, S.; Avalos, G.; Dowling, M. Critical Care Nurses' Knowledge of Alarm Fatigue and Practices Towards Alarms: A Multicentre Study. *Intensive Crit. Care Nurs.* **2018**, *48*, 36–41. [CrossRef]
27. Jeong, Y.J. Status of Clinical Alarms and Nurses' Attitudes, Fatigue and Practices toward the Alarms in Intensive Care Unit. Master's Thesis, Hallym University, Chuncheon, Republic of Korea, 2017.
28. Ramlaul, A.; Chironda, G.; Brysiewicz, P. Alarms in the ICU: A study investigating how ICU nurses respond to clinical alarms for patient safety in a selected hospital in Kwazulu-Natal province, South Africa. *J. Crit. Care* **2021**, *37*, 57–62. [CrossRef]
29. Mirhafez, S.R.; Movahedi, A.; Moghadam-Pasha, A.; Mohammadi, G.; Moeini, V.; Moradi, Z.; Kavosi, A.; Aryayi Far, M. Perceptions and practices related to clinical alarms. *Nurs. Forum.* **2019**, *54*, 369–375. [CrossRef] [PubMed]
30. Sendelbach, S.; Funk, M. Alarm fatigue: A patient safety concern. *AACN Adv. Crit. Care* **2013**, *24*, 378–386. [CrossRef] [PubMed]
31. Schmid, F.; Goepfert, M.S.; Franz, F.; Laule, D.; Reiter, B.; Goetz, A.E.; Reuter, D.A. Reduction of clinically irrelevant alarms in patient monitoring by adaptive time delays. *J. Clin. Monit. Comput.* **2017**, *31*, 213–219. [CrossRef] [PubMed]
32. Xie, H.; Kang, J.; Mills, G.H. Clinical review: The impact of noise on patients' sleep and the effectiveness of noise reduction strategies in intensive care units. *Crit. Care* **2009**, *13*, 208. [CrossRef]

Disclaimer/Publisher's Note: The statements, opinions and data contained in all publications are solely those of the individual author(s) and contributor(s) and not of MDPI and/or the editor(s). MDPI and/or the editor(s) disclaim responsibility for any injury to people or property resulting from any ideas, methods, instructions or products referred to in the content.

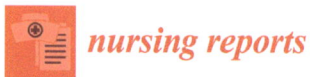

Systematic Review

The Influence of Smartphones on Adolescent Sleep: A Systematic Literature Review

Sofia de Sá [1,2,*], Ana Baião [1], Helena Marques [1], Maria do Céu Marques [3,4], Maria José Reis [5], Sandra Dias [1] and Marta Catarino [2,6,7]

1. Baixo Alentejo Local Health Unit, Public Business Entity, 7800-309 Beja, Portugal
2. Health Department, Polytechnic Institute of Beja, 7800-111 Beja, Portugal
3. Nursing Department, University of Évora, 7000-869 Évora, Portugal
4. Comprehensive Health Research Centre, 1150-082 Lisboa, Portugal
5. Algarve University Hospital Center, 8000-386 Faro, Portugal
6. Institute of Health Sciences (ICS), Universidade Católica Portuguesa, 1649-023 Lisboa, Portugal
7. Center for Interdisciplinary Research in Health (CIIS), Institute of Health Sciences (ICS), Universidade Católica Portuguesa, 1649-023 Lisboa, Portugal
* Correspondence: sofia.sa@ipbeja.pt

Abstract: (1) Background: Sleep is considered to be a complex condition for human beings, with the aim of ensuring physical and psychological recovery. Technology, including the cell phone, is a tool for teenagers that ensures they are always available to interact, even at night. This study aims to understand the influence of the use of smartphones on adolescent sleep quality. (2) Methods: The guidelines proposed by the Joanna Briggs Institute were followed. The search was conducted in October 2022 through the EBSCOhost platform, with access to the CINAHL Complete and Medline databases and through the b-On database. (3) Results: The use of electronic equipment plays an important role in adolescents' lives. There is a negative relationship between the use of electronic equipment, such as smartphones, and sleep, for reducing both the quality and quantity of sleep. There is also a relationship between nighttime smartphone use, insufficient sleep, and mental health problems. (4) Conclusions: The use of new technologies at night causes a change in the behavior of adolescents with repercussions in terms of the quality of sleep and sleep duration and consequent well-being and performance during the day.

Keywords: smartphone; children; well-being; sleep; teenagers; media

Citation: de Sá, S.; Baião, A.; Marques, H.; Marques, M.d.C.; Reis, M.J.; Dias, S.; Catarino, M. The Influence of Smartphones on Adolescent Sleep: A Systematic Literature Review. *Nurs. Rep.* 2023, 13, 612–621. https://doi.org/10.3390/nursrep13020054

Academic Editors: Antonio Martínez-Sabater, Elena Chover-Sierra and Carles Saus-Ortega

Received: 1 February 2023
Revised: 27 February 2023
Accepted: 4 March 2023
Published: 7 April 2023

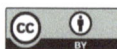

Copyright: © 2023 by the authors. Licensee MDPI, Basel, Switzerland. This article is an open access article distributed under the terms and conditions of the Creative Commons Attribution (CC BY) license (https://creativecommons.org/licenses/by/4.0/).

1. Introduction

Sleep is considered to be a very complex condition that serves to restructure all functions of an organism and to ensure the physical and psychic recovery of human beings. It is believed that during the sleep period, cell renewal, production of hormones and antibodies, protein synthesis, and metabolic regulation take place, which contribute in a very significant way to the physical growth of children [1].

In a questionnaire conducted in 2018 in Portugal regarding the sleep of Portuguese adolescents, it was concluded that 86.3% (N = 3894) reported difficulty in waking up in the morning and 59.7% (N = 3899) believed they sleep poorly [2]. Throughout growth, the sleep pattern undergoes changes, given that in adolescence, there is a shift in sleep patterns associated with deep changes that occur at a biological, psychological, and sociocultural level. As Bartel affirms: "The decline in adolescent sleep quantity and quality is multifactorial, and is influenced by biological, environmental, societal, and behavioral facts" [2] (p. 498).

The circadian rhythm of adolescents is bound to the inherent alterations in this growth stage. The sleep–wake cycle is regulated by melatonin, the hormone responsible for the onset of sleep, beginning its production at dusk. In adolescence, the production of this hormone occurs later, which implies that the adolescent will feel sleepy later and this sensation will last until later, coinciding with the waking hour [3].

As it is expected that changes inherent to this stage of growth will occur in adolescents' sleep patterns, it is important to take into consideration that "Adolescence is a sensitive age period for changes in sleep-wake patterns" [4] (p. 277) and that the National Sleep Foundation [5] recommends that an adolescent should sleep between 8 and 10 h. It is also proven that the quantity of sleep hours is not always associated with quality sleep.

The World Sleep Society [6] refers to the existence of studies suggesting that the quality of sleep holds a bigger impact than its quantity, both in terms of quality of life and daily period, such that poor-quality sleep combined with precarious health are closely related to a decrease in quality of life and happiness. The World Sleep Society highlights, in turn, that sleep centers around the world invite the teaching of good "sleep hygiene," advocating for the conservation of high-quality sleep in sufficient quantity. It also emphasizes that sleep is a basic human necessity as important as eating and drinking and indispensable for health and well-being. Good sleep along with a balanced diet and adequate physical exercise are important factors and some of the pillars of health. Finally, it states that sleep problems represent a global pandemic that puts at risk the health and quality of life of approximately 45% of the world's population, and in this sense, an adequate understanding of this problem will help to reduce the impact of sleep disturbances on society.

For good-quality sleep, three elements are considered: duration, continuity, and depth [6]. The World Sleep Society [6], through the document "Ten commandments for better sleep", which was released in the 2016 to celebrate the World Sleep Day, reveals the essential rules of proper sleep hygiene to maintain or restore deep, healthy, restful, and natural sleep, and underlines environmental conditions and the usage of electronic devices as a set of factors that influence the quantity and quality of sleep and, consequently, general well-being, which depends on high-quality sleep.

Nowadays, technology is constantly present in our life, and smartphones provide constant opportunities to connect with others [3], creating the need to be frequently connectable and connected to various social and sharing networks. This need is also felt among adolescents, who have, in technology, a tool that makes them always available for interaction [3]. This leads to a delay in the onset of sleep, as well as its frequent interruption through new technologies, namely the smartphone, as they coexist with the presence of noise and several standby lights, which disturb sleep [7].

This permanent connectivity that technological devices allow for increasingly presents itself as a risk factor for good-quality sleep among adolescents. Various studies confirm that "Sleep disturbance and adverse health outcomes related to screen media practices are on the rise affecting physical, cognitive, and behavioral health out-comes" [8] (p. 292).

The Portuguese Association of Sleep [7] demonstrates that, in Portugal, children and adolescents sleep, in general, for less time than is recommended, linking changes in the lifestyles of parents and children with alterations in sleep habit patterns.

Considering this topic as a current issue, since the quality of sleep is of extreme importance for good physical and intellectual development of adolescents, it was determined that this topic is of the utmost importance. The following question was formulated: "Does the use of smartphones affect adolescents' sleep?" Therefore, the objective of this review is to understand how the use of smartphones interferes with the quality of adolescents' sleep.

2. Materials and Methods

A Systematic Literature Review was performed, based on the methodological procedures defined by the Joanna Briggs Institute, and it was registered on PROSPERO platform (registration number CRD42023395696).

Using the PICO method (P—problem/population/participants (adolescents); I—intervention (use of smartphones); C—comparison/context (society); O—outcomes, results (influence in sleep)), the question for this review was formulated: "Does the use of smartphones affect adolescents' sleep?"

The search of articles was carried out on the platform EBSCOhost, with access to the databases CINAHL Complete and Medline, also on the database b-ON, following the Health Sciences Descriptors (DeCS) [9]. As keywords, the words "smartphone", "children", "well-being", "sleep", "teenagers", and "media" were selected, using the operator Boolean "AND" to combine the search terms. The research was conducted in October 2022 by two researchers simultaneously, applying the inclusion and exclusion criteria. A third researcher participated in the selection of studies for final review, confirming the selection and exclusion criteria, after individual reviews and researchers' meetings. For this review, inclusion criteria were defined: randomized controlled studies, experimental studies without randomization, cohort studies and controlled cases, observational studies without group control, case series and clinical trials, with published full text, with relevance to the identified problem, written in Portuguese, English or Spanish, and with publication date between 2014 and 2022. The review considered studies that included adolescents, according to the definitions of American Academy of Pediatrics, which considers all individuals from 11 to 21 years old.

The articles whose topic was not relevant for the review in question were excluded, and those that did not address the previously defined population and Systematic Literature Reviews.

Among the databases used, in total, 140 were obtained. The relevance of these articles was analyzed by reading the title, summary, and, whenever necessary, full-text reading. After applying the inclusion and exclusion criteria, 6 articles were selected, as illustrated in Figure 1.

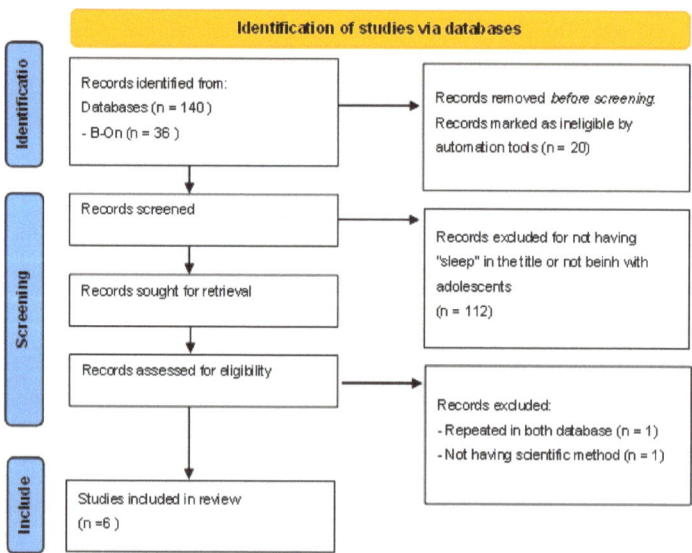

Figure 1. PRISMA of study selection and inclusion process [10].

After the selection of studies, they were evaluated critically by applying assessment grids of the level of evidence, reliability, and relevance, which allowed us to classify the studies found (Table 1).

To assess the level of evidence, the evaluation tools of Joanna Briggs Institute (JBI) were chosen [10], and to assess the methodological quality of the studies, the norms of Effective Public Health Practice Project (EPHPP) were chosen (Table 2).

Table 1. Critical evaluation of the results of the included studies according to the critical evaluation verification list by Joanna Briggs Institute [11].

Articles	Q1	Q2	Q3	Q4	Q5	Q6	Q7	Q8	Q9	Q10	Result
Tavernier et al. [4]	✓	✓	✓	✓	✓	✗	✓	✓	-	-	87.5%
Johansson et al. [3]	✓	✓	✓	✓	✓	✓	✓	✓	-	-	100%
Schweizer et al. [12]	✓	✓	✓	✓	✓	✓	✓	✓		-	100%
Garmy & Warde [13]	✓	✓	✓	✓	✓	✓	✓	✓	-	-	100%
Vernon et al. [14]	✓	✓	✓	✓	✓	✓	✗	✓	✓	✓	90%
Lemola et al. [15]	✓	✓	✓	✓	✓	✗	✓	✓	-		87.5%

Table 2. Classification of the selected studies according to evidence and methodological recommendation level.

Article	Level of Evidence JBI [11]	Methodological Recommendation (EPHPP)
Tavernier et al. [4]	4.b	87.5%
Johansson et al. [3]	4.b	100%
Schweizer et al. [12]	2.a	100%
Garmy and Warde [13]	4.b	100%
Vernon et al. [14]	4.c	90%
Lemola et al. [15]	4.b	87.5%

3. Results

The data collected on the characteristics of the studies were synthesized in a table (Table 3), facilitating mapping. The information in the table is complemented with a narrative summary, in which the findings of the studies included are clarified with the discussion of the results and the description of their correlation with the objective of the review and research question.

All articles selected in this Systematic Literature Review are studies published between 2014 and 2018, as journal articles, with five of these articles being observational descriptive studies and one article being a quasi-experimental study. They carefully present their aims, where they took place, the methods used, and their participants.

Regarding the place where the studies were performed, two were performed in the United States of America (USA), two in Switzerland, one in Sweden, and one in Australia.

All studies considered participants who were attending high school, so the results of different articles were obtained through self-report analysis of the adolescents, namely through interview. One of the articles analyzed [4] associated this method with an evaluation of sleep behavior using a motor activity recording device during sleep.

The analyzed studies evaluate, in general, the relation between the use of electronic devices and adolescents' sleep, with special emphasis on the use of smartphones in five of these articles [3,12–15].

Johansson et al. [3] reported that about 47% of the respondents used three or four devices before going to bed, and 97% used some type of technology in the hour before bedtime, in particular, the mobile phone (used by nearly 74% of respondents). They also concluded that the number of devices used before bedtime would be associated with reports of waking up too early and restless sleep, with repercussions in daytime sleepiness.

In fact, the use of mobile phones, specifically smartphones, is highlighted by several authors. Schweizer et al. [12] verified that smartphone owners were more likely to experience sleep problems than non-smartphone owners, who usually sleep the number of hours recommended by the National Sleep Foundation. They observed that as soon as the adolescents owned a smartphone, they would start to sleep less than what is recommended, increasing the prevalence of sleep problems to achieve the prevalence observed among owners.

Table 3. Extraction data.

Study Identification	Country	Method	Study Objective	Total of Participants	Intervention
Tavernier et al., (2017) [4]	USA	Analytical Cross-Sectional Study	To analyze the influence of use of time by the adolescents (in a technological, and face-to-face interactions with friends and family, activity base) in three sleep behaviors: time to fall asleep, duration and sleep efficiency.	71 students of 3 High School, from 11 to 18 years old	The participants used a device, in the non-dominant wrist, that registered the motor activity, for three nights, after a night of "familiarization" as a software and its algorithm were used to register data. The participants filled out a questionnaire about the time spent with eight activities of technological, and face to face interaction with friends and family, activity base.
			To understand the impact of technology use before bedtime on the sleep of adolescents and its repercussion the following day.	255 adolescents between 13 and 21 years old	Data obtained from a conducted study (National Sleep Foundation's 2011 Sleep in America Poll) with American population between 13 and 64 years old. A subsample was selected that answered a questionnaire developed by a group of experts in the field of sleep. The questionnaire had four categories: demographic data, sleep habits, quality of sleep and the use of technology one hour before bedtime and throughout the night.
Schweizer et al., (2017) [12]	Switzerland	Quasi-Experimental Study	To evaluate the influence of acquiring a smartphone in the sleep duration of adolescents.	591 students of 35 High Schools with an average age of 14.2 years old	The sample was grouped into owners of a smartphone, new owners, and non-owners. The initial collection was done through a questionnaire in classroom. The remaining data were collected through an online questionnaire.
Garmy & Ward, (2018) [13]	Sweden	Analytical Cross-Sectional Study	To understand the relation between the use of the mobile phone in the pre-sleep period and the sleep habits of adolescents.	278 students of 3 High Schools, with ages between 15 and 17 years old	A pre-test was applied to the students, following a session on health education about sleep and usage of social networks after which the test was repeated.
Vernon et al., (2018) [14]	Australia	Case Serie Study	Analyze the relation between the use of a mobile phone in night-time and the quality of sleep and well-being of adolescents.	1101 students, of 29 schools, who began Year 8 in high school	The data were extracted through a longitudinal study; Study based on data of self-report for four consecutive years (2010–2013), beginning in Year 8; All students were submitted to a data collection for at least 2 times.
Lemola et al., (2014) [15]	Switzerland	Analytical Cross-Sectional Study	To evaluate the relation between the use of electronic devices before bedtime and the possession of a smartphone; To understand the relation between sleep, depressive symptoms, and the use of electronic devices at night.	362 students at High School with ages between 12 and 17 years old.	The participants filled out a questionnaire about sleep, media consumption before sleep and psychological health. After completing the questionnaire, the students received information about sleep hygiene or general information about the topics related to sleep. One month after, the students were visited a second time and completed the same questionnaire.

Lemola et al. [15] also concluded that having a smartphone would be related to a greater use of electronic devices and, in particular, their use in bed, before sleep, by watching videos, phone calling, and texting with friends. The use of these electronic devices in bed before sleep was associated with less sleep time and difficulty in sleeping, such as being online in bed and with the phone turned on at night, which would intensify these changes.

Tavernier et al. [4] verified that adolescents sleep less when they spend more time than usual texting and working on the computer, and even that more time using the computer was associated with less sleep efficiency. On the contrary, they verified a positive association between the time spent in direct social contact (with friends and family) and the efficiency and latency of sleep; that is, when adolescents spend more time interacting directly with friends/family, they fall asleep faster.

Likewise, Garmy and Ward [13] highlighted the nighttime use of mobile phones, associating sending and receiving messages at night with much later hours to fall asleep, less regular hours to fall asleep, shorter times in bed, and irregular sleep habits. The authors also verified that tiredness during the day was frequently associated with this. Like these authors, Vernon et al. [14] also established a significative correlation between the nighttime use of phones, bad sleep behavior, and a decline in adolescents' well-being. The authors verified that the nighttime use of the phone would is also associated with depressive humor, low self-esteem, externalizing behavior, and low coping ability.

4. Discussion

Adolescence is a period of great physical, emotional, and social changes, in which sleep is susceptible to modification inherent to these changes. Variations in bedtime hour, waking hour, and sleep habits are very common among adolescents, with sleep disorders considered a public health problem in the United States of America, Europe, and Asian countries [13].

Technological development has been growing exponentially in the last few decades and, consequently, the use of electronic devices now plays an important role in adolescents' lives [13,14]. With the current systematic literature review, it was intended to understand the relation between the use of new technologies, particularly smartphones, and the sleep of adolescents. The studies analyzed corroborate the existing literature, reinforcing the fact that the use of technological gadgets influences the sleep of adolescents [3,4,12–15]. Among electronic devices, the smartphone stands out for its use, disseminated especially among adolescents, its ease of access, and its functionalities [12,14].

Schweizer et al. [11] verified that the owners of a smartphone were more prone to having sleep problems than non-owners, who slept, on average, for the number of hours recommended by the National Sleep Foundation. They observed that as soon as the adolescents owned a smartphone, they would start to sleep less than recommended, increasing the prevalence of sleep problems to achieve the prevalence observed among owners. The authors state that smartphones enable Internet access anywhere at any time, in addition to allowing communication through texts messages and free phone calls, which justifies the increase in possession of smartphones among adolescents.

Tavernier et al. [4] verified that adolescents sleep less when they spend more time than usual using electronic-based devices, such as texting and working on a computer, and, furthermore, more time using a computer was associated with reduced sleep efficiency. On the contrary, they verified a positive association between the time spent in direct social contact (with friends and family) and the efficiency and latency of sleep, meaning when adolescents spend more time than usual interacting directly with friends/family, they fall asleep faster.

The constant connectivity in technological devices has been a risk factor for good-quality adolescent sleep, as already confirmed in the literature [16]. The elevated quantity of time spent by adolescents with technological-based activities is undeniable, usage that is also verified at nighttime, namely the hour before bedtime, so several studies have focused on its use in this period. Lemola et al. [15] concluded that the possession of a smartphone would be related to a generally greater use of electronic devices, and, in particular, the use in bed, before sleep, watching videos, for phone calls, or texting friends.

If, on the one hand, the screen time stands out, on the other hand, there seems to be an association between owning a smartphone and the use of electronic devices at night.

The high amount of time spent by adolescents on technology-based activities is undeniable, with studies suggesting that this directly influences sleep time and efficiency.

In fact, Johansson et al. [3] verified that 97% of adolescents used some type of technology in the hour before bedtime (especially the mobile phone, used by nearly 74% of respondents). Further, 47% of the respondents used three or four devices in this time period. Vernon et al. [14] also corroborated this idea by concluding that there were few adolescents that did not use the mobile phone during nighttime after switching off the lights to sleep.

The studies reviewed suggest that there is a relationship between screen time and sleep, especially when used at night. Johansson et al. [3] verified the existence of a direct relation between the use of electronic devices and the sleep changes in adolescents, with its use before bedtime being associated with reports of waking up too early, restless sleep, and daytime sleepiness. This association was also verified by Vernon et al. [14] and by Lemola et al. [15], who highlighted that being online in bed and with the phone turned on at night would exacerbate these changes. Likewise, Garmy and Ward [13] highlighted the nighttime use of mobile phones, associating the sending and receiving of messages at night with much later hours to fall asleep, less regular hours to fall asleep, shorter times in bed, and irregular sleep habits. The authors also verified that frequently associated with this, there would be tiredness during the day.

Like these authors, Vernon et al. [14] also established a significative correlation between the nighttime use of phones and bad sleep behavior.

According to the literature, this influence can be explained, on the one hand, by the cognitive, emotional, and physiological excitement associated with social interactions and videogaming at night and, on the other, by the light exposure emitted by screens, which can suppress the secretions of melatonin, contributing equally to difficulties in falling asleep [3,13,14].

Many authors established the relation between sleep problems associated with the use of new technologies and the well-being and psychosocial behavior of adolescents. Vernon et al. [14] established a significative correlation among nighttime use of phones, bad sleep behavior, and the decline in adolescents' well-being. The authors verified that nighttime use of the phone would also be associated with depressive humor, low self-esteem, externalizing behavior, and low coping ability.

Lemola et al. [15] also concluded that the use of smartphones may be a partial mediator of the relation between the use of these electronic devices at night and depressive symptoms. They also established a relation regarding sleep, depressive symptoms, and the use of electronic devices before sleep, which meets the existing literature on the subject: "Recent studies show a link between insufficient sleep and mental health problems, including anxiety depression, low self-esteem and suicidality"; at the same time, it has negative effects on academic performance and overall performance during the day [13] (p.123). This phenomenon seems to occur, according to the author, because adolescents manifest feelings of concern and disconnection when unable to access technology, fearing the loss of information or important messages.

In Portugal, in 2017, a study was conducted about epidemiology of internet use in a population of adolescents and its relationship with sleep habits, published in Portuguese Medical minutes [17], in which 722 adolescents were inquired for establishing a parallel between use of the internet and, consequentially, the associated technology (mobile phones, online gaming devices, computers, tablets) and sleep habits. The study was based on the premise that the adolescents' use of internet and its excessive use were associated with dysfunctional coping strategies and worsen interpersonal relationships, negative impact on psychosocial development of adolescents, its association with suicidal behaviors (suicidal ideation and suicide attempts), depression, and anxiety. Therefore, the authors intended to "measure and characterize the use of internet in adolescence; determine the internet dependence on adolescence; evaluate the association between internet dependency and sleep changes/excessive daytime tiredness" [17] (p. 52).

Meeting the results of the findings in the present review, the study revealed that the internet dependence and its problematic use could have a significant influence on the sleep–wake cycle associated with intermediate insomnia, irregular sleep patterns, and excessive daytime tiredness, which was mentioned by Garmy and Ward [13]. It also tried to explain that the "negative impact of excessive internet use and sleep habits could be due to the use of devices (computer/mobile phone/tablet) while falling asleep, which conditions a state of excitement, therefore, interfering with the necessary procedures of a normal sleep-wake cycle" [17] (p. 531).

This study was the only one found about this topic for this age group in Portugal; it supports the analyzed studies of the present systematic literature review.

Therefore, although the mobile phone is a tool for social interaction that cultivates self-esteem, autonomy, and identity in adolescents, its excessive use, notably at nighttime, constitutes a problem, with an impact on the health of adolescents [14]. Thus, the parents/caregivers and the current policies have a preponderant role in the sensibilization of adolescents regarding the disadvantages of nighttime use of technologies/use of mobile phones in the sleep quality of adolescents.

Nursing has a privileged position in the contact with adolescents and families in their daily practice. Therefore, according to Garmy and Ward [13], nurses are in an ideal position to educate adolescents about the importance of healthy and consistent sleep habits and to alert them to the hazards of bad or insufficient sleep habits. According to the same authors, more than the adolescents, "School nurses are also in a unique position to discuss sleep health and educate not only students but also teachers and parents." (p. 124).

Johansson et al. [3] also considered that the results of the study have implications for nursing care practices: "Nurses are in the ideal position to address their goal by educating adolescents, their families, and the broader community about good sleep hygiene" (p. 502). The author also reinforces the importance of nurses in primary health care, as "Nurses in primary care or outpatient clinics should inquire about an adolescent's sleep habits, sleep quality, and technology use before bed. In addition, nurses should take the opportunity to counsel families in healthy sleep habits." (p. 502), meeting what was previously stated by Garmy and Ward [13].

In this sense, measures were suggested that are focused on the healthy use of technology in the beginning of adolescence, informing the adolescents and their parents that the acquisition of smartphone or other electronic devices can bring consequences regarding sleep quality, which repercuss in the adolescent's quality of life [3,13].

It is urgent to alert and study, alongside parents, strategies that limit the use of electronic devices, mainly during the nighttime period as a way of promoting quality sleep.

5. Conclusions

It was possible to find evidence that confirms the influence of technological devices, such as smartphones, computers, and tablets, in the sleep of adolescents. The results of the present systematic literature review suggest that this influence may be mainly associated with screen time. More studies are needed that explore the relation between adolescent sleep and screen time, even during the day.

The influence of technology, highlighting the use of smartphones, repercusses both in terms of quality and sleep duration, with manifestations in the performance of adolescents during the day and their well-being.

It becomes urgent to promote the implementation of measures that encourage a healthy use of new technologies, specifically at night.

Based on scientific assumptions, the nurse, in collaboration with other members of the multidisciplinary team, alongside adolescents, parents, and educators, could develop interventions that promote the thoughtful use of these resources, as this approach should be developed in the follow-up appointments of infant and juvenile health. Despite the present systematic literature review focusing on adolescents, the approach towards a healthy education for the use of this resource should be initiated as soon as possible.

6. Limitations/Future Prospects

Limitations were identified in some of the studies found, especially regarding the age of the study participants, which is not consensual, and it is not always identified for the authors to present only the year of schooling. Some of the results were also based on adolescents' self-report and, in some cases, obtained through questionnaires conducted in class, which may condition the adolescents' answers and their veracity. In the future, research will be needed that considers all these factors.

Author Contributions: Conceptualization, M.d.C.M. and M.C.; methodology, S.d.S., A.B. and M.C.; software, M.J.R. and H.M.; validation, H.M., S.D. and M.J.R.; formal analysis, S.d.S.; investigation, M.J.R. and S.D.; resources, S.d.S. and A.B.; data curation, M.d.C.M.; writing—original draft preparation, S.d.S. and A.B.; writing—review and editing, M.J.R.; visualization, S.D.; supervision, M.C.; project administration, S.d.S. and M.d.C.M. All authors have read and agreed to the published version of the manuscript.

Funding: This research received no external funding.

Institutional Review Board Statement: Not applicable.

Informed Consent Statement: Not applicable.

Data Availability Statement: Not applicable.

Conflicts of Interest: The authors declare no conflict of interest.

References

1. Sociedade Portuguesa de Pediatria [SPP]. *Recomendações sps-spp: Prática da Sesta da Criança*; Sociedade Portuguesa de Pediatria: Lisboa, Portugal, 2017. Available online: http://www.spp.pt/UserFiles/file/Noticias_2017/VERSAO%20PROFISSIONAIS%20DE%20SAUDE_RECOMENDACOES%20SPS-SPP%20SESTA%20NA%20CRIANCA.pdf (accessed on 3 October 2022).
2. Health Behaviour In School [HBS]—Aged Children, Dados Nacionais. *A Saúde dos Adolescentes Portugueses Após a Recessão. 2018 (1ª Edição)*; Equipa Aventura Social: Lisboa, Portugal, 2018.
3. Johansson, A.E.E.; Petrisko, M.A.; Chasens, E.R. Adolescent Sleep and the Impact of Technology Use Before Sleep on Daytime Function. *J. Pediatr. Nurs.* **2016**, *31*, 498–504. [CrossRef] [PubMed]
4. Tavernier, R.; Heissel, J.A.; Sladek, M.R.; Grant, K.E.; Adam, E.K. Adolescents' technology and face-to-face time use predict objective sleep outcomes. *Sleep Health* **2017**, *3*, 276–283. [CrossRef] [PubMed]
5. National Sleep Foundation [NSF]. *Sleep in America Poll. Communications Technology in the Bedroom*; Estados Unidos da América, National Sleep Foundation: Washington, DC, USA, 2011. Available online: https://teensneedsleep.files.wordpress.com/2011/05/national-sleep-foundation-2011-sleep-in-america-poll-communications-technology-in-the-bedroom.pdf (accessed on 6 October 2022).
6. World Sleep Society [WSS]. World Sleep Day. Portugal 2016: Eulália Semedo. 2019. Available online: http://worldsleepday.org/portugal-2016-translated-wsd-materials (accessed on 6 October 2022).
7. Associação Portuguesa do Sono [APS] (s.d). *Dormir Bem dá Saúde e Faz Crescer*; Associação Portuguesa do Sono: Lisbon, Portugal. Available online: https://www.apsono.com/index.php/pt/noticias/noticias-do-sono/69-dormir-bem-da-saude-faz-crescer (accessed on 8 October 2022).
8. Riesch, S.K.; Liu, J.; Kaufmann, P.G.; Doswell, W.M.; Cohen, S.; Vessey, J. Preventing adverse health outcomes among children and adolescents by addressing screen media practices concomitant to sleep disturbance. *Nurs. Outlook* **2019**, *67*, 492–496. [CrossRef] [PubMed]
9. Health Sciences Descriptors: DeCS São Paulo (SP): BIREME/PAHO/WHO. 2017. [updated 2017 May 18]. Available online: http://decs.bvsalud.org/I/homepagei.htm (accessed on 2 October 2022).
10. Tricco, A.C.; Lillie, E.; Zarin, W.; O'Brien, K.K.; Colquhoun, H.; Levac, D.; Moher, D.; Peters, M.D.J.; Horsley, T.; Weeks, L.; et al. PRISMA extension for scoping reviews (PRISMA-ScR): Checklist and explanation. *Ann. Int. Med.* **2018**, *7*, 467–473. [CrossRef] [PubMed]
11. JBI Global Wiki. Chapter 11: Scoping Reviews—JBI Manual for Evidence Synthesis. Available online: https://wiki.jbi.global/display/MANUAL/Chapter+11%3A+Scoping+reviews (accessed on 12 March 2021).
12. Schweizer, A.; Berchtold, A.; Barrense-Dias, Y.; Akre, C.; Suris, J.C. Adolescents with a smartphone sleep less than their peers. *Eur. J. Pediatr.* **2017**, *176*, 131–136. [CrossRef] [PubMed]
13. Garmy, P.; Ward, T.M. Sleep Habits and Nighttime Texting Among Adolescents. *J. Sch. Nurs.* **2018**, *34*, 121–127. [CrossRef] [PubMed]

14. Vernon, L.; Modecki, K.L.; Barber, B.L. Mobile Phones in the Bedroom: Trajectories of Sleep Habits and Subsequent Adolescent Psychosocial Development. *Child Dev.* **2018**, *89*, 66–77. [CrossRef] [PubMed]
15. Lemola, S.; Perkinson-Gloor, N.; Brand, S.; Dewald-Kaufmann, J.F.; Grob, A. Adolescents' Electronic Media Use at Night, Sleep Disturbance, and Depressive Symptoms in the Smartphone Age. *J. Youth Adolesc.* **2014**, *44*, 405–418. [CrossRef] [PubMed]
16. Hale, L.; Guan, S. Screen time and sleep among school-aged children and adolescents: A systematic literature review. *Sleep Med. Rev.* **2014**, *21*, 50–58. [CrossRef] [PubMed]
17. Ferreira, C.; Ferreira, H.; Vieira, M.J.; Costeira, M.; Branco, L.; Dias, N.; Macedo, L. Epidemiology of internet use by an adolescent population and its relation with sleep habits. *Acta Med. Port.* **2017**, *30*, 524–533. [CrossRef] [PubMed]

Disclaimer/Publisher's Note: The statements, opinions and data contained in all publications are solely those of the individual author(s) and contributor(s) and not of MDPI and/or the editor(s). MDPI and/or the editor(s) disclaim responsibility for any injury to people or property resulting from any ideas, methods, instructions or products referred to in the content.

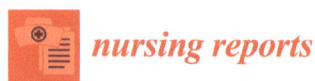

Article

Nursing Students' Preferences for Learning Medical and Bioscience Subjects: A Qualitative Study

Lars Kyte [1,*], Ingrid Lindaas [2], Hellen Dahl [2], Irene Valaker [1], Ole T. Kleiven [1] and Solveig Sægrov [1]

[1] Department of Health and Caring Sciences, Faculty of Health and Social Sciences, Western Norway University of Applied Sciences, Campus Førde, Svanehaugvegen 1, 6812 Førde, Norway; irene.valaker@hvl.no (I.V.); ole.kleiven@hvl.no (O.T.K.); solveig.nelly.segrov@hvl.no (S.S.)

[2] Department of Health and Caring Sciences, Faculty of Health and Social Sciences, Western Norway University of Applied Sciences, Campus Haugesund, Bjørnsonsgate 45, 5528 Haugesund, Norway; ingrid.lindaas@hvl.no (I.L.); hellen.dahl@hvl.no (H.D.)

* Correspondence: lars.kyte@hvl.no

Abstract: (1) Background: There are considerable challenges and concerns related to learning medical and bioscience subjects (MBS) in nursing education and integrating this knowledge into nursing. The aim of this study was to explore what learning methods nursing students prefer when studying MBS, and how this learning may be enhanced to facilitate the integration of these subjects into nursing. (2) Methods: Individual interviews with 10 nursing students. Transcripts from the interviews were analysed by systematic text condensation and the COREQ checklist for qualitative studies was completed. (3) Results: Students prefer varied and active learning methods in MBS. The participants in the study highlighted both organised tutorials in groups and working with fellow students outside of organised teaching. All participants used educational videos. Learning MBS by drawing was appreciated both during lectures and in student-initiated colloquia. Strategies that favour in-depth learning were appreciated, and it was found that lectures did not have to cover the entire curriculum. Teachers' attitudes toward students also were seen to have a considerable impact on students' motivation for learning. (4) Conclusion: Applying active learning methods and focusing on the most relevant topics in MBS appears to improve students' ability to integrate this knowledge into nursing; teachers should also be aware of their role as a motivator.

Keywords: in-depth interviews; learning methods; medical and bioscience subjects; nursing education; qualitative method

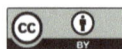

1. Introduction

Medical and bioscience subjects (MBS) are regarded as an important base for practising nursing and providing safe patient care [1–3]. Knowledge from MBS is necessary to ensure that the decisions nurses make in practice maximise the health impact and avoid harm to patients [4]. Furthermore, the ability to integrate theories from MBS when practising nursing correlates with improved patient outcomes [5]. In Norwegian nursing education, MBS include anatomy, physiology, biochemistry, microbiology, pathophysiology, and pharmacology. Many of these subjects are taught early in the nursing education programme. This forms a knowledge base that students need to apply in clinical practice later in their studies [6].

There are considerable challenges and concerns related to learning MBS in nursing education and integrating this knowledge into nursing practice [5,7]. Challenges include the large curriculum content, large class sizes, structuring MBS in the curriculum, course organisation and learning environment, student motivation and concentration, the integration of bioscience in clinical practice, and high failure rates at exams [3,7–9].

Many new nursing students are anxious about studying bioscience, and there is a need for improved support to facilitate their learning [1]. Students' prior competence in mathematics, chemistry, and biology is related to their achievements in bioscience [9] and pre-entry qualifications in science for nursing students have been proposed [7]. However, measures regarding entry qualifications will not solve the problem alone, and the focus must also be on higher education institutions and their responsibility to promote an organised learning environment that enhances learning in these subjects [7].

It can be a major challenge to teach MBS in a way that suits students of different ages and with varying learning styles [10]. Moreover, different studies show diverging results regarding what learning methods are preferable in facilitating students' learning process. One study showed that most students learned best kinaesthetically and that social learning was beneficial [11]. In a recent study, students following a flipped classroom model were both more satisfied and obtained better exam results than students following traditional lectures. This model was particularly effective for low-achieving students [12]. Another study found that most nursing students regarded classroom lectures as the most efficient approach when teaching anatomy and physiology. Group seminars were felt to be a waste of time for one-third of the students, while small group tutorials contributed well to the learning process [10]. However, although many students appreciate small group learning, this does not suit everyone, and there are challenges regarding time spent and tutors' competence [13]. A literature review revealed that there is a lack of knowledge on how to best support students' learning in bioscience subjects. New ways of teaching using digital tools, simulation, and different kinds of games enhance students' engagement and increase student satisfaction. However, the students' satisfaction with the teaching offered does not appear to correlate with their exam results [8].

The challenge regarding MBS in the nursing curriculum is also more complicated and involves more than simply considering students' achievement in exams in these subjects. Exam results probably do not tell the whole story about the benefits of this knowledge, as the reason for nursing students learning MBS is not to acquire this knowledge itself, but to apply this knowledge in nursing. Successful integration of MBS theory in nursing practice may be of great importance for patients; the appropriate application of bioscience in practice is vital in order to be able to offer safe and competent patient care [4,5].

This is the second article from a study exploring different aspects regarding the integration of MBS in nursing. The purpose of the first article was to describe how students experience the integration of medical and bioscience knowledge in nursing education. The findings presented in that article showed that students highlighted the importance of linking theory to practice [6]. Based on this, the aim of this study is to explore what learning methods nursing students prefer when studying MBS, and how the learning may be enhanced to facilitate the integration of these subjects into nursing.

2. Materials and Methods

2.1. Design

In this study, we applied a qualitative approach. The chosen design follows a hermeneutic-phenomenological tradition, as the aim was to explore students' own experiences and thoughts and capture their opinions about MBS in nursing education [14,15]. To achieve this, an interview guide for individual in-depth interviews with open-ended questions was constructed. The interview guide covered different aspects related to MBS in nursing education. The interview guide was partly semi-structured, as the interviewer was given the option to ask supplementary questions if necessary.

2.2. Recruitment of Participants

A total of 10 nursing students, two male and eight female, in the second or third year of their undergraduate studies, from two campuses at a university college in Norway, participated in this study (Table 1).

Table 1. Study participants.

Campus	Participant and Gender (f/m)
A	1 f
	2 f
	3 m
	4 m
	5 f
B	1 f
	2 f
	3 f
	4 f
	5 f

None of the participants dropped out of the study. A criterium for inclusion in the study was that the participants had completed their clinical placements in both surgical and medical wards in a hospital. The reason for this criterium was that during these placements students have to use medical and bioscience knowledge acquired earlier in their studies. To obtain permission to recruit participants for the study, we contacted the administration of the faculty responsible for nursing education at the students' university college. Students were subsequently recruited through information about the study in class. Of those who registered as participants, five students were randomly selected from each campus to participate in the study.

2.3. Data Collection

The COREQ checklist for qualitative studies [16] was completed. The research team consisted of four registered nurses (RN), one biologist, and one medical doctor (MD). At the time of the study, all researchers were employed as associate professors. All researchers (four women and two men) had experience from earlier research. Some of the researchers had been lecturers to some of the participants, but they had no personal relationship with them.

All interviews were performed face-to-face during 2019 and lasted approximately 30–60 min. The interviews took place on the campuses where the participants were studying. All participants on both campuses provided extensive information about how they perceived learning bioscience in their education, and how this knowledge base was integrated into nursing practice during their studies. When the data collection was completed, interviewers noted that saturation was obtained. Each interview was conducted by one of the researchers (I.V., I.L., or H.D.), audio-recorded, and subsequently transcribed. Some field notes were also made in connection with the interviews.

2.4. Data Analysis

After reading through the transcripts to gain an overall impression, all researchers discussed the content and agreed on the major themes of the interviews [14,17,18]. These themes covered content relevant to both this article and the first article in the project. The themes relevant to this article were chosen, and further analysis of this article was performed in accordance with the description of systematic text condensation by Malterud (2012, 2017) [14,18]. This part of the analysis was mainly performed by three of the researchers. The chosen themes formed the basis for code groups. Then, the meaning units from the transcripts were sorted into these code groups. Code groups were divided into subgroups, and during the analysis process code groups evolved and changed, in accordance with the description of the method [14,18]. Table 2 shows the code groups and subgroups that evolved through the analysis process with examples of meaning units corresponding to the different codes.

Table 2. Code groups and subgroups with examples of corresponding meaning units.

Examples of Meaning Units	Subgroups	Code Groups
"There has been a good variation in everything. Mostly, it has been teaching, but the fact that one . . . draws, shows drawings, some videos and then explanation again" (B5) "The seminars, I think these were useful, because then you have to kind of use both hemispheres of the brain" (A2)	Use of diverse learning methods	Active and varied learning methods
" . . . we actively listened to the others, we discussed and changed a little bit and discussed, so it was certainly helpful." (A3)	Collaborative learning	
"Yes, because if they manage to link the material to stories and their own experiences . . . , then we get a little more insight into what awaits us in working life" (B1)	Learning by understanding connections	In-depth learning
" . . . lecturers wanted to say as much as possible in the shortest possible time" (B1)	Knowledge must be manageable	
" . . . it's about showing commitment, . . . entering a classroom and wanting to teach [students] something" (B5) "A good lecturer for me is someone who doesn't rush through what we're going to learn in the curriculum, but actually takes time if there's something you don't understand to go through it a bit more, and include the students, not just stand and lecture, but actively actually ask." (B4)	During organised learning activities	The lecturer as a motivator for students' learning
"the most important thing when it comes to the lecturer is that you have someone who cares . . . and say hello when you meet them in the hallway. It makes it much more personal, especially when it becomes more personal for my own learning" (A1)	Outside of organised learning activities	

In the next step of the analysis, the meaning units of each subgroup were reduced to condensates. These condensates consisted of content from several meaning units given by different participants and were written as first-person statements ("artificial quotes"), according to the method [14,18]. Then, an analytic text for each subgroup was synthesized based on these first-person statements and quotes from the interviews. This analytic text formed the basis for the presentation of the results. No software was used in the analysis.

2.5. Ethical Considerations

The study was approved by the Data Protection Officer for Research at the Norwegian Centre for Research Data (NSD, no 287137). All participants were given written information about the project and signed consent forms prior to participation. To protect anonymity, participants' names were not used either in audio recordings or in transcripts. The recorded data and transcripts from the interviews were saved on a protected data server for research purposes belonging to the Western Norway University of Applied Sciences.

3. Results

The major themes revealed by the analysis were active and varied learning methods, in-depth learning, and the teacher as a motivator for students' learning. This corresponds to the code groups presented in Table 2.

3.1. Active and Varied Learning Methods

Many of the participants emphasised the importance of applying varied teaching methods during MBS lectures. It was stated that using PowerPoint alone is too monotonous, and that visual resources such as images, films, or animations can make it easier to understand and remember the material. Some highlighted "Kahoot!", a student response system (SRS), which encourages student activity by allowing students to answer questions in class by using a device. Several also pointed out that drawing during lectures enables better learning. It was emphasised that when students draw together with the lecturer, it makes it easier to understand the connections being taught in the subject. One of the participants put it this way:

> *If you sit and are taught [by the lecturer] all the time, then it becomes boring, but if you draw a bit or gets out some sheets of paper . . . , you learn with all your senses, so it is about using different methods* (B5).

Several participants said that they benefited greatly from digital resources as a supplement to other learning methods. All participants used educational videos, and several emphasised that this is useful, both because one can watch the videos when one has free time and because one can watch them several times in order to understand something better.

> *But it's when it is the physiological . . . what happens in the lungs, what happens in the kidneys, why the heart works that way, the chemical stuff. Then you may need to have it explained in different ways . . . it needs to mature, so you may have to listen to it several times* (B1).

It is also helpful to draw and take notes when hearing and watching videos because then you learn by using motor skills and several senses at the same time.

Several participants highlighted the benefits of seminars and other learning methods that required students to be active themselves and "do something". "And you remember in another way when you do it yourself than if you are only told it in a lecture" (A2). An example of this, which some of the participants remembered "very well", was running up and down a staircase while breathing through straws, in connection with learning about nursing for patients with chronic obstructive pulmonary disorders (COPD). Other examples were the use of anatomy models where students could pick up and look at the organs, dissection of the heart and kidneys (from pigs), and the cultivation of bacteria (from the hands). "It's nice to have visual resources like that; they're useful—it creates interest. We get to do it ourselves and can see with our own eyes . . . what is actually in the body" (A3).

The participants in the study appreciated organised tutorials in groups in MBS, where students can ask and students can answer, supervised by the teacher. In smaller groups the threshold for asking is lower; this makes you talk and discuss together. " . . . it brings out that discussion, that conversation, and you can learn in a different way . . . " (A1).

Many of the participants also preferred to work with fellow students outside of organised teaching. Quizzes, drawing on boards, and videos were used as learning methods in student-initiated colloquia. Some also pointed out that by explaining something to others, you remember things better: "I acquire a lot of knowledge by talking and explaining . . . and if you can explain it to someone, you've understood it so well that you know it" (A1).

However, most people do not want to work in groups all the time, and some students expressed a greater need to work on their own than others:

> *I prefer to work alone when I am reading. I think it's very nice to have groups, and to sit and discuss, but when I'm really going to work, I have to be alone. I can't concentrate if there's noise. So we work in different ways* (B1).

Some mentioned challenges regarding group work, as some group members contribute more than others. This may be frustrating when the group has to deliver a joint product.

3.2. In-Depth Learning

It was argued that lecturers prioritising the most important elements within each topic and not rushing through everything in the curriculum during the lectures may have an impact on students' sense of mastery.

> *. . . all the advanced diagnoses, we do not have to go through them during lectures. We can read about that ourselves . . . it is much better to know a lot about a little than a little*

about a lot when it comes to lectures. Then I think we could have left the classroom with a greater sense of mastery . . . (A4).

Discussing patient cases in class when learning MBS was also suggested, as discussion provides opportunities to hear other people's thoughts on a problem. It was argued that hearing others may widen the horizon and have an impact on clinical thinking: " . . . if you hear how other students think, and how they come up with a solution, it widens the horizon a little bit, and I think you eventually get a broader clinical view from hearing others" (B3).

One of the participants particularly highlighted the importance of not delaying reading until just before the exam, as that forces students to learn a lot in a short time. " . . . to some extent, when you cram something, you can achieve a good grade, but that way you don't retain it" (A1). It was argued that you need to understand something to be able to simplify it when explaining it to patients or relatives (in clinical practice later in the studies), i.e., if you cram everything, you are only able to reproduce what you have crammed.

Simulation-based learning was also highlighted as a learning method that enhanced students' understanding of clinical practice; as one of the students put it: " . . . in the simulation we have the opportunity to make mistakes and learn from them . . . " (A3).

3.3. The Teacher as a Motivator for Students' Learning

Regardless of the choice of learning methods, it was emphasised that teachers' attitudes towards students are important for students' learning and that it means a lot for students' motivation that the teacher cares about them. Several participants explained how teachers' ways of meeting students, both in organised learning activities and elsewhere, influenced learning.

In organised learning activities, it was emphasised that a good lecturer is someone who knows the subject matter, has good pedagogical abilities, shows commitment, and wants to teach students something. Several mentioned the importance of the lecturer including the students and creating dialogue in the classroom by both questioning the class and creating a safe framework that allows students to ask questions. " . . . he uses the board and is very engaged, and we have learned a lot from him . . . and that's also because he was so good at having dialogue with the class" (A5).

Several pointed out that what teachers do outside of organised learning activities is also important. The teacher's availability both at college and via e-mail was highlighted, and it was expressed how important it is for learning that the teacher cares about the students and treats them as individuals. It becomes more personal, even for students' learning, if the teachers say hello to students when they meet them in the hallway. It is also motivating when students find that the results of exams mean something not only to students but also to the teachers. One participant described what it means for motivation when the teacher cares, outside organised learning activities as well:

There was one thing we absolutely did not understand, and then we went to talk to the lecturer, and then he spent an hour getting our group of five people to understand this before the exam . . . it's the lecturers who do such things who make me want to do well too (B4).

4. Discussion

The aim of this study was to explore what learning methods nursing students prefer when studying MBS, and how that learning may be enhanced to facilitate the integration of these subjects into nursing.

4.1. Encourage Active Learning

Participants highly appreciated learning activities in MBS that forced them to be active learners. The term "active learning" is defined in several ways, and the definition has evolved over time, but it often means learning through activities or discussions that make students reflect on their understanding, by keeping them both mentally and physically active [19]. Freeman et al., 2014 constructed the following consensus definition: "Active learning engages students in the process of learning through activities and/or discussions in class, as opposed to passively listening to an expert. It emphasizes higher-order thinking and often involves group work" [20] (pp. 8413–8414). Following this definition, traditional lectures with a lecturer speaking to an audience are not viewed as active learning, and achieving active learning for students in lectures is challenging [21].

4.2. Variation during Lectures Is Needed

Lectures were widely used at both campuses, and the participants had various experiences regarding how lectures were delivered. A key result, highlighted by all participants, was the need for variation and student activity during lectures. In line with the definition of active learning [20] and the recommendations from Biggs (1999) [21], participants wanted lecturers to encourage students to participate in dialogue and discussions, something that may be challenging in large classes. They also highlighted the importance of creating a safe learning environment where students dare to speak up.

Two ways of promoting activity in class that were appreciated by participants in the study were the use of drawing and the use of "Kahoot!", a student response system (SRS). Several studies support the benefit of drawing, especially in anatomy [22–24]. Drawing makes lectures less boring, as students have to work actively [23]. When students draw simultaneously with the lecturer, it requires them to watch, reflect upon what they see, and draw themselves. This combination of visual stimuli, cognitive reflection, and motor activity may contribute to the learning process, and, in our study, it was mentioned that drawing enhanced the understanding of connections. This is in accordance with Fernandes et al., 2018 who proposed that drawing has an impact on a memory trace consisting of elaborative, motoric, and pictorial components [25]. There is also evidence that drawing may help students better retain knowledge [22,24], something that is important in being able to apply knowledge from MBS when practicing nursing later in their education.

"Kahoot!", an SRS that can deliver questions to students in a quiz format, was mentioned in our study as something that promotes variation. A large meta-analysis showed that "Kahoot!" has a positive effect on students' motivation and learning, and improves teacher-student interaction [26]. However, the extent to which it helps students retain information may vary [27]. On the other hand, this kind of tool may be used to promote discussions in class on topics in biology [28].

Nevertheless, the potential for discussion and dialogue in large classes is often limited, and learning methods other than lectures may be more suitable for achieving this, as several participants in our study clearly indicated. Learning methods that forced students to "do something" were appreciated, and various examples of these kinds of learning methods were given; many students learn best kinaesthetically and benefit from social learning [11].

4.3. Learning Together

Participants in our study appreciated the group tutorials led by teachers. They also highlighted the benefit of discussing bioscience with peer students in groups organised by the students themselves. According to Freeman (2014), active learning often involves group work [20]. Working together in groups also includes more than discussing topics verbally. Participants in our study used quizzes, watched online resources together, and made drawings together. Thus, working together implies a variety of learning methods, something that may help students to understand connections in the subject [10].

Data from a survey based on a national exam in anatomy, physiology, and biochemistry for nursing students showed that students working in groups obtained significantly higher grades than students who did not work together in groups [9]. When students discuss subjects they do not understand with fellow students, it motivates further learning [29]. Some of the participants in our study expressed that explaining difficult subjects to others strongly enhanced their own learning and facilitated the retention of knowledge. If students better retain knowledge from MBS, it will probably promote the integration of this knowledge into their nursing practice later in their education. When students try to explain something to fellow students, it generates valuable learning and also makes them aware of what they need to learn more about [29]. The combination of preparing to teach and explaining to others enhances learning [30]. The benefit of explaining to others was mentioned in our study in regard to the context of learning difficult material, and collaborative learning seems to be especially important when tasks are complex [31]. When students work together, they not only learn the subject studied but also experience that they need each other to achieve their goals [31]. Biggs (1999) argues that learning is a way of interacting with others, changing our conceptions so that we see something in a different way [21]. This is what one of the participants in our study highlighted when she stated that you can get a broader clinical view by listening to others.

However, participants also highlighted challenges regarding group work, for instance when the group has to deliver a joint product. This indicates that preparing students for group work and what it demands is important. Peer assessment of other group members' contributions has been found to enhance students' engagement in group work and make them take responsibility for their learning [32]. However, students learn in various ways, and their different perceptions regarding group work must be accepted. Teachers and fellow students may contribute to creating a positive learning atmosphere for students who feel insecure when working in groups [33]. Trust among group members is vital in order for a group to function, as students who rely on each other demonstrate stronger cognitive engagement and contribute more actively to group work [34]. Working together as students may also be advantageous regarding future work, as most nurses work in teams either in hospitals or in primary health care.

4.4. Videos Should Be Combined with Other Learning Methods

Most participants in our study highly appreciated the use of teaching videos when studying MBS. A meta-analysis covering more than 100 trials from various areas of higher education revealed that the use of videos led to improved learning outcomes [35]. Participants in our study particularly appreciated the opportunity to watch videos on difficult topics over and over again, something that may reduce cognitive overload [35].

Most participants preferred to use videos as a supplement to lectures or other learning methods. A recent report showed no clear connection between students' exam results and their use of an online video resource in bioscience, used by most students pursuing nursing education in Norway [9]. Several studies, including two major meta-analyses, support the idea that videos work best when combined with learning in face-to-face classes. This kind of blended approach also seems to be more efficient than classroom teaching alone [9,35,36]. Therefore, when the students in our study expressed that videos enhanced learning in MBS, it may be due to the effect of combining this kind of resource with other learning methods, such as lectures and discussions with peers.

4.5. Promoting In-Depth-Learning May Facilitate the Use of MBS Theory in Nursing Practice

Nursing students perceive bioscience as important for providing safe patient care [2,3], and it is essential for students to learn the fundamental principles of bioscience during their first year in order to facilitate the use of this knowledge later in their studies [7]. When teachers succeed in demonstrating the clinical relevance of bioscience for nursing, it motivates students to learn and may contribute both to a better understanding of the subjects taught and better exam results [9,37]. If teaching MBS focuses solely on theoretical aspects without linking to clinical practice, it may be reasonable to ask to what extent students' grades in these subjects reflect the usefulness of this kind of knowledge in clinical practice.

Our study highlights that rushing through all the curriculum during lectures may reduce students' experience of coping. Coping is important to promote students' interest and motivation for learning, thereby promoting deeper learning [38]. When students perceive an overload of tasks, it is demotivating for their learning [39]. This implies that teachers in MBS should help students to focus on the important and most relevant topics in the subject, rather than every detail in the curriculum, in order to better prepare them for the complexity of patient care. In patient care, knowledge from MBS must be used in connection with other kinds of knowledge such as nursing skills, ethics, and social sciences. This is far more complex than answering exam questions on anatomy and physiology during the first year of a nursing degree. This complexity should be made clear to students during their studies [3]. Simulation-based learning (SBE) may be a way of introducing this complexity [40]. In our study, SBE was highlighted as a safe way of training. When using SBE, different kinds of knowledge must be combined; this makes SBE an appropriate area for in-depth learning.

4.6. A Supportive Learning Environment

Several participants in the study clearly stated that teachers' concern for their students and their engagement and involvement in the student learning process are important for students' motivation. This is not primarily about the teacher giving a brilliant performance in class, but rather about the teacher's values and how these values can create an engaging learning environment that supports students [41]. The importance of this should not be underestimated, as the teacher is central to the students' learning environment. A supportive learning environment is important when students are to learn the basic principles of bioscience, and if this fails it may reduce their understanding of the importance of bioscience later in their studies [7]. This may counteract the integration of MBS in nursing practice. A recent systematic review showed that integrating bioscience in nursing by using clinical scenarios in the first year of the education program was associated with an increased understanding of bioscience and that supporting students with this integration is needed [42].

Nursing students are demotivated by negative comments from the teacher, or if they feel that the teacher is not interested in the students' learning [39]. A study among students in various kinds of higher education showed that the teachers' involvement in the student learning process and students' feeling of competence have an impact on students' achievement [43]. Thus, teachers' attitudes towards students are of great importance for students' motivation and learning. This is important throughout the education programme, and probably no less important at the beginning of the programme when students are not familiar with the demands and routines of higher education. As MBS is usually taught early in the nursing curriculum, teachers in these subjects should be aware of the importance of caring and involvement in students' learning process for students' motivation.

5. Study Limitations

One limitation of this study is the size of the study, as it was conducted at just two different campuses. Although students at these campuses had experienced several different learning methods, the results may not be directly transferable to other institutions with other educational approaches and learning methods. In addition, the students who registered as participants in the study may have been particularly interested in the topic and are not necessarily representative of all students.

Another limitation is the gender distribution of the participants, as only two of the participants were men. However, this reflects the gender distribution in Norwegian nursing education.

The interviews were conducted by three different researchers. Although all interviews followed the same interview guide, there may have been differences in how the interviews were carried out, and to what extent supplementary questions were asked during interviews.

6. Conclusions

In order to provide high-quality care for patients, nursing students need to learn MBS and be able to integrate this knowledge into nursing. This requires that education programmes focus on learning methods that support in-depth learning in these subjects. The knowledge must be manageable, and students need to understand how MBS theory relates to nursing practice. To achieve this, teachers must help students to focus on the most relevant topics in the subjects to better prepare them for the integration of this knowledge into patient care.

Nursing students prefer varied learning methods that actively engage them when studying MBS. These include drawing, watching videos, and teachers interacting with students during lectures. In addition, students appreciate working together and discussing, actively listening to others, and explaining professional issues to fellow students. This enhances learning and facilitates the retention of knowledge, thereby supporting the integration of this knowledge into their nursing practice later in their education.

A good teacher-student relationship has a considerable impact on students' motivation for learning. In class, the lecturer must involve students and contribute to a safe and supportive learning environment that allows students to ask questions. What teachers do outside of organised learning activities is also important, and students are motivated when they perceive that their teachers care about them and their learning process.

This study did not look at students' grades. Further studies are needed to investigate whether students' grades in MBS are related to their ability to retain this knowledge and integrate it into clinical practice.

Author Contributions: Conceptualisation: S.S., L.K., I.L., H.D., I.V. and O.T.K. Formal analysis: L.K., I.L., H.D., I.V., O.T.K. and S.S. Investigation: I.V., O.T.K. and H.D. Methodology: L.K., I.L., H.D., I.V., O.T.K. and S.S. Project administration: S.S. Supervision: S.S. and L.K. Writing—original draft: L.K. Writing—review and editing: L.K., I.L., H.D., I.V., O.T.K. and S.S. All authors have read and agreed to the published version of the manuscript.

Funding: This research received no external funding.

Institutional Review Board Statement: The study was conducted according to the guidelines of the Declaration of Helsinki and approved by the Data Protection Officer for Research at the Norwegian Centre for Research Data (NSD, no 287137).

Informed Consent Statement: Written informed consent was obtained from all subjects involved in the study.

Data Availability Statement: The data presented in this study are not publicly available due to ethical reasons. The participant consent and approval from the Norwegian Centre for Research Data (NSD, no 287137) prevents us from sharing data in public repositories. However, the data will be available from the corresponding author upon reasonable request. Transcripts from the interviews are saved on a protected data server for research purposes belonging to the Western Norway University of Applied Sciences. According to the informed consent signed by the participants, the data will be deleted two years after the project was finished (the project was finished on 31 July 2022).

Acknowledgments: We are grateful to the students who participated in this study.

Conflicts of Interest: The authors declare no conflict of interest.

References

1. Craft, J.; Hudson, P.; Plenderleith, M.; Wirihana, L.; Gordon, C. Commencing nursing students' perceptions and anxiety of bioscience. *Nurse Educ. Today* **2013**, *33*, 1399–1405. [CrossRef] [PubMed]
2. Molesworth, M.; Lewitt, M. Preregistration nursing students' perspectives on the learning, teaching and application of bioscience knowledge within practice. *J. Clin. Nurs.* **2016**, *25*, 725–732. [CrossRef]
3. Barton, M.J.; Bentley, S.; Craft, J.; Dupen, O.; Gordon, C.; Cayanan, E.A.; Kunst, E.; Connors, A.; Todorovic, M.; Johnston, A.N. Nursing students' perceptions of clinical relevance and engagement with bioscience education: A cross-sectional study of undergraduate and postgraduate nursing students. *Nurse Educ. Today* **2021**, *99*, 104767. [CrossRef]
4. Perkins, C. Enhanced bioscience content is urgently needed in UK pre-registration nursing curricula. *Nurse Educ. Pract.* **2019**, *34*, 7–11. [CrossRef]
5. Bakon, S.; Craft, J.; Christensen, M.; Wirihana, L. Can active learning principles be applied to the bioscience assessments of nursing students? A review of the literature. *Nurse Educ. Today* **2016**, *37*, 123–127. [CrossRef]

6. Sægrov, S.; Kyte, L.; Kleiven, O.T.; Dahl, H.; Lindaas, I.; Valaker, I. Medisinsk og naturvitskapleg kunnskap som grunnlag for utøving av sjukepleie [Medical and bioscience knowledge as a basis for practicing nursing]. *Nord. Sygeplejeforskning* **2022**, *12*, 1–10. [CrossRef]
7. McVicar, A.; Andrew, S.; Kemble, R. The 'bioscience problem' for nursing students: An integrative review of published evaluations of Year 1 bioscience, and proposed directions for curriculum development. *Nurse Educ. Today* **2015**, *35*, 500–509. [CrossRef] [PubMed]
8. Jensen, K.T.; Knutstad, U.; Fawcett, T.N. The challenge of the biosciences in nurse education: A literature review. *J. Clin. Nurs.* **2018**, *27*, 1793–1802. [CrossRef]
9. Haakens, M.; Karlsen, H.; Bråten, H. *Resultater på Nasjonal Deleksamen i Anatomi, Fysiologi og Biokjemi: Gode Resultater Eller Gode Studieprogrammer? [Results on the National Exam in Anatomy, Physiology and Biochemistry: Good Students or Good Study Programs?]*; NOKUT: Lysaker, Norway, 2021.
10. Evensen, A.E.; Brataas, H.V.; Cui, G. Bioscience learning in nursing: A cross-sectional survey of beginning nursing students in Norway. *BMC Nurs.* **2020**, *19*, 2. [CrossRef] [PubMed]
11. Johnston, A.N.; Hamill, J.; Barton, M.J.; Baldwin, S.; Percival, J.; Williams-Pritchard, G.; Salvage-Jones, J.; Todorovic, M. Student learning styles in anatomy and physiology courses: Meeting the needs of nursing students. *Nurse Educ. Pract.* **2015**, *15*, 415–420. [CrossRef]
12. Joseph, M.A.; Roach, E.J.; Natarajan, J.; Karkada, S.; Cayaban, A.R.R. Flipped classroom improves Omani nursing students performance and satisfaction in anatomy and physiology. *BMC Nurs.* **2021**, *20*, 1. [CrossRef]
13. Cui, G.; Laugsand, J.-B.; Zheng, W. A Survey of Norwegian Nursing Students' Responses to Student-Centered Small Group Learning in the Study of Human Anatomy and Physiology. *SAGE Open Nurs.* **2021**, *7*, 1–8. [CrossRef]
14. Malterud, K. *Kvalitative Forskningsmetoder for Medisin og Helsefag. En Innføring [Qualitative Research Methods for Medicine and Health Sciences: An Introduction]*, 4th ed.; Universitetsforlaget: Oslo, Norway, 2017.
15. Kvale, S.; Brinkmann, S.; Anderssen, T.M.; Rygge, J. *Det Kvalitative Forskningsintervju [The Qualitative Research Interview]*, 3rd ed.; Gyldendal Akademisk: Oslo, Norway, 2015.
16. Tong, A.; Sainsbury, P.; Craig, J. Consolidated criteria for reporting qualitative research (COREQ): A 32-item checklist for interviews and focus groups. *Int. J. Qual. Health Care J. Int. Soc. Qual. Health Care ISQua* **2007**, *19*, 349–357. [CrossRef] [PubMed]
17. Brinkmann, S.; Kvale, S. *InterViews: Learning the Craft of Qualitative Research Interviewing*, 3rd ed.; Sage: Thousand Oaks, CA, USA, 2015.
18. Malterud, K. Systematic text condensation: A strategy for qualitative analysis. *Scand. J. Public Health* **2012**, *40*, 795–805. [CrossRef]
19. Idsardi, R. Evidence-Based Practices for the Active Learning Classroom. In *Active Learning in College Science. The Case for Evidence-Based Practice*; Mintzes, J., Walter, E.M., Eds.; Springer: Cham, Switzerland, 2020; pp. 13–25.
20. Freeman, S.; Eddy, S.L.; McDonough, M.; Smith, M.K.; Okoroafor, N.; Jordt, H.; Wenderoth, M.P. Active learning increases student performance in science, engineering, and mathematics. *Proc. Natl. Acad. Sci. USA* **2014**, *111*, 8410–8415. [CrossRef] [PubMed]
21. Biggs, J.B. What the Student Does: Teaching for enhanced learning. *High. Educ. Res. Dev.* **1999**, *18*, 57–75. [CrossRef]
22. Amin, A. 'Drawing' to learn Anatomy: Exploring the theoretical underpinning and conditions favouring drawing based learning. *J. Pak. Med. Assoc.* **2020**, *70*, 2017–2022. [CrossRef] [PubMed]
23. Noorafshan, A.; Hoseini, L.; Amini, M.; Dehghani, M.R.; Kojuri, J.; Bazrafkan, L. Simultaneous anatomical sketching as learning by doing method of teaching human anatomy. *J. Educ. Health Promot.* **2014**, *3*, 50. [CrossRef] [PubMed]
24. Borrelli, M.; Leung, B.; Morgan, M.; Saxena, A.; Hunter, A. Should drawing be incorporated into the teaching of anatomy? *J. Contemp. Med. Educ.* **2018**, *6*, 34–48. [CrossRef]
25. Fernandes, M.A.; Wammes, J.D.; Meade, M.E. The Surprisingly Powerful Influence of Drawing on Memory. *Curr. Dir. Psychol. Sci.* **2018**, *27*, 302–308. [CrossRef]
26. Wang, A.I.; Tahir, R. The effect of using Kahoot! for learning—A literature review. *Comput. Educ.* **2020**, *149*, 103818. [CrossRef]
27. Holbrey, C.E. Kahoot! Using a game-based approach to blended learning to support effective learning environments and student engagement in traditional lecture theatres. *Technol. Pedagog. Educ.* **2020**, *29*, 191–202. [CrossRef]
28. Smith, M.K.; Knight, J.K. Clickers in the Biology Classroom: Strategies for Writing and Effectively Implementing Clicker Questions That Maximize Student Learning. In *Active Learning in College Science*; Springer: Cham, Switzerland, 2020; pp. 141–158.
29. Onshuus, K.; Jacobsen, T.-I. Å snakke med andre om sykepleie gjør at det sitter bedre. Medstudentsamarbeid som motivasjon til å lære mer i sykepleiestudiet [Talking to others about nursing makes you remember it better. Co-student collaboration as motivation to learn more in nursing education]. *Klin. Sygepleje* **2020**, *34*, 110–121. [CrossRef]
30. Kobayashi, K. Learning by Preparing-to-Teach and Teaching: A Meta-Analysis. *Jpn. Psychol. Res.* **2018**, *61*, 192–203. [CrossRef]
31. Scager, K.; Boonstra, J.; Peeters, T.; Vulperhorst, J.; Wiegant, F.; Knight, J. Collaborative Learning in Higher Education: Evoking Positive Interdependence. *CBE—Life Sci. Educ.* **2016**, *15*, ar69. [CrossRef]
32. Adesina, O.O.; Adesina, O.A.; Adelopo, I.; Afrifa, G.A. Managing group work: The impact of peer assessment on student engagement. *Account. Educ.* **2022**, *32*, 90–113. [CrossRef]
33. Lavy, S. Who benefits from group work in higher education? An attachment theory perspective. *High. Educ.* **2017**, *73*, 175–187. [CrossRef]
34. Poort, I.; Jansen, E.; Hofman, A. Does the group matter? Effects of trust, cultural diversity, and group formation on engagement in group work in higher education. *High. Educ. Res. Dev.* **2022**, *41*, 511–526. [CrossRef]

35. Noetel, M.; Griffith, S.; Delaney, O.; Sanders, T.; Parker, P.; del Pozo Cruz, B.; Lonsdale, C. Video Improves Learning in Higher Education: A Systematic Review. *Rev. Educ. Res.* **2021**, *91*, 204–236. [CrossRef]
36. Means, B.; Toyama, Y.; Murphy, R.; Baki, M. The Effectiveness of Online and Blended Learning: A Meta-Analysis of the Empirical Literature. *Teach. Coll. Rec. Voice Scholarsh. Educ.* **2013**, *115*, 1–47. [CrossRef]
37. Skavern, H.; Høye, S.; Ødbehr, L.S. Hvordan lærer sykepleierstudenter med lave opptakskarakterer anatomi, fysiologi og biokjemi (AFB)? [How do nursing students with low admission grades acquire knowledge in anatomy, physiology and biochemistry (AFB)?]. *Uniped* **2020**, *43*, 33–44. [CrossRef]
38. Damsgaard, H.L. *Studielivskvalitet. Studenters Erfaringer Med og Opplevelse av Kvalitet i Høyere Utdanning [Quality of Study Life. Students' Experiences with and Perception of Quality in Higher Education]*; Universitetsforlaget: Oslo, Norway, 2019.
39. Takase, M.; Niitani, M.; Imai, T.; Okada, M. Students' perceptions of teaching factors that demotivate their learning in lectures and laboratory-based skills practice. *Int. J. Nurs. Sci.* **2019**, *6*, 414–420. [CrossRef] [PubMed]
40. Chernikova, O.; Heitzmann, N.; Stadler, M.; Holzberger, D.; Seidel, T.; Fischer, F. Simulation-Based Learning in Higher Education: A Meta-Analysis. *Rev. Educ. Res.* **2020**, *90*, 499–541. [CrossRef]
41. Gibbs, G. Teacher engagement. *Uniped* **2016**, *39*, 184–187. [CrossRef]
42. Madhuvu, A.; Gao, W.; Rogers, R.; O'Halloran, M.; Bennett, N.; Morphet, J. Horizontal integration of bioscience and nursing in first-year nursing curricula: A systematic review. *Nurse Educ. Today* **2022**, *118*, 105519. [CrossRef] [PubMed]
43. Ayllon, S.; Alsina, A.; Colomer, J. Teachers' involvement and students' self-efficacy: Keys to achievement in higher education. *PLoS ONE* **2019**, *14*, e0216865. [CrossRef]

Disclaimer/Publisher's Note: The statements, opinions and data contained in all publications are solely those of the individual author(s) and contributor(s) and not of MDPI and/or the editor(s). MDPI and/or the editor(s) disclaim responsibility for any injury to people or property resulting from any ideas, methods, instructions or products referred to in the content.

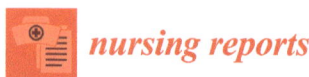

Article

Development and Validity of the Japanese Version of the Questionnaire on Factors That Influence Family Engagement in Acute Care Settings

Makoto Tsukuda [1,*], Yoshiyasu Ito [1], Shota Kakazu [2], Katsuko Sakamoto [3] and Junko Honda [1]

[1] College of Nursing Art and Science, University of Hyogo, 13-71 Kitaoji-cho, Akashi 673-0021, Japan; yoshiyasu_ito@cnas.u-hyogo.ac.jp (Y.I.); junko_honda@cnas.u-hyogo.ac.jp (J.H.)
[2] Graduate School of Nursing Sciences, St. Luke's International University, 10-1 Akashi-cho, Chuo-ku, Tokyo 104-0044, Japan; shota@slcn.ac.jp
[3] Nursing Department, Hyogo Prefectural KOBE Children's Hospital, 1-6-7 Minatojima Minamimachi, Chuo-ku, Kobe 650-0047, Japan; kachi.o.o.dolphin@gmail.com
* Correspondence: makoto_tsukuda@cnas.u-hyogo.ac.jp; Tel./Fax: +81-78-925-9419

Abstract: There exists an international consensus on the importance of family-centered care (FCC) in intensive care settings and the evaluation of collaboration between nurses and families; however, FCC is currently practiced blindly in Japan. In this study, we developed a Japanese version of the questionnaire, Factors that Influence Family Engagement (QFIFE-J) and examined its reliability and validity. A web-based survey was conducted with 250 nurses working in the intensive care unit (ICU). Exploratory and validatory factor analyses were used to ascertain factor validity. Criterion-related validity was tested using correlation analysis with the ICU Nurses' Family Assistance Practice Scale. Internal consistency and reproducibility were verified for reliability. Following exploratory and confirmatory factor analyses, a 15-item measure emerged comprising four factors: "ICU environment", "nurses' attitudes", "nurses' workflow", and "patient acuity". Confirmatory factor analyses showed a generally good fit. Cronbach's α for the overall scale was 0.78, indicating acceptable internal consistency. The intraclass coefficient for test–retest reliability was 0.80. It was found that the QFIFE-J was reliable and valid and may help determine the factors that promote or inhibit FCC. Additionally, this study has also clarified the current status and family support related issues in ICUs in Japan.

Keywords: QFIFE; ICU nurses' family assistance practice scale; exploratory and validatory factor analyses; family-centered care; Japanese version

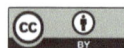

1. Introduction

Of late, intensive care technology has made dramatic progress, and various efforts have been made worldwide to focus on long-term goals such as daily life and social reintegration after discharge from the intensive care unit (ICU)—rather than short-term goals such as saving lives in the ICU. The background of this increased focus on long-term goals is the recognition of the fact that not only physical problems, but also mental disorders, including cognitive and emotional problems, may worsen long-term prognosis after discharge of critically ill patients from the ICU. Currently, this is termed Post-intensive Care Syndrome (PICS) [1].

The ICU provides advanced medical care, and patients admitted are often in life-threatening situations, causing sudden physical and mental stress, anxiety, confusion, and fatigue among their family members [2]. Uncertainty about such life crises, an unfamiliar hospitalization environment, and inadequate communication with healthcare providers can significantly affect families' interest in patient care and their coping abilities [3].

Mental disorders such as anxiety, depression, and complicated grief in the family that occur after the patient's admission to the ICU have gradually started gaining focus and are now recognized as PICS-Family (PICS-F). It is an urgent issue to consider both the patient and the family after ICU admission as objects of care as in PICS.

Recently, academic focus on PICS and the PICS-F for intensively treated patients and their families has been driven by improved life-saving rates and ICU outcomes. It is largely because, in the ICU setting, the emphasis is on the patient and their family, rather than on the physician and disease, which leads to better outcomes. International guidelines supporting family-centered care (FCC) have been developed, and advanced practices are required to improve care and outcomes for patients and their families [4]. However, studies have established that many of these practices do not adequately identify nurses' perceptions of care for patients' families [4,5]. Moreover, research concerning both patient's families and nurses have reported various barriers to patient care, including the presence of patients' families in the ICU [6–8]. However, studies have demonstrated the benefits of the patient's family's involvement in patient care in the ICU; and the current trend requires the promotion of family care participation in critical areas in Japan [9,10]. Nurses must consider the facilitators and barriers that they face regarding family participation in patient care to promote collaborative partnerships among patients, families, and critical care nurses.

In Japan, an assessment tool for PICS was developed by Harumi et al. [11], which focused on assessing patients' PICS. A new scale is thus needed to assess factors related to collaboration between the nurses and patients' families. Hetland et al. [10] developed the Questionnaire on Factors that Influence Family Engagement (QFIFE)—a reliable questionnaire to investigate the facilitators and barriers faced by nurses working in the ICUs in the United States regarding family involvement in patient care and their associations [12]. This study developed and tested the reliability and validity of the Japanese version of the QFIFE (QFIFE-J).

2. Materials and Methods

2.1. Design

A cross-sectional design was employed, and a psychometric validation study was conducted using a web-based questionnaire.

2.2. Materials

2.2.1. Questionnaire on Factors That Influence Family Engagement

The QFIFE was developed in the United States as an acute care family nursing instrument to assess nurses' perceptions for involving families in the care of the critically ill [7]. The degree of barriers to FCC can then be assessed by the nurses' perceptions. This is because nurses' attitudes are important in promoting FCC. The QFIFE has 15 items comprising four subscales: (1) ICU environment (items 1–5), (2) Patient acuity (items 6–7), (3) Nurses' workflow (items 8–10), and (4) Nurses' attitudes (items 11–15). Each item can be rated on a six-point Likert scale. Higher item scores indicate a factor that facilitates patient-family involvement, while lower scoring items suggest a potential barrier factor for patient-family involvement. The internal consistency reliability of the QFIFE total scores and subscales is well-established with Cronbach's alpha of 0.73, 0.77, 0.74, and 0.83 for the ICU environment, Patient acuity, nurses' workflow, and Nurses' attitudes, respectively.

2.2.2. The Japanese Version of the Questionnaire on Factors That Influence Family Engagement

Intensive care nurses and quantitative research specialists were involved in the development of the Japanese version of the QFIFE. Discussions were also held with the original authors, as translations of individual items needed to be semantic rather than literal to ensure conceptual and linguistic equivalence. Thereafter, the Japanese version was retranslated into the English version. At this time, the first person in charge of the translation compared the back-translation with each other and with the English version. The wording of the item was then revised to consider the differences between the back-translation and the English version, and the revised Japanese was then retranslated to English by two independent translators. After back-translation, the translated and back-translated scales were evaluated for semantic and conceptual aspects of the scales by bilingual translators and members of the re-study group. Finally, surface validity was confirmed by several nurses. The respondents were asked to ensure that all 15 questions were written in a clear, concise, and understandable manner. After checking the appropriateness of terminology and correcting spelling errors, a final version of the Japanese scale was created, which was named QFIFE-J.

2.3. Measures

2.3.1. Participants

This survey, which was conducted via an Internet-based questionnaire, was com-missioned by Rakuten Insight, Inc. (https://insight.rakuten.co.jp/en/, accessed on 9 June 2022). Approximately 6200 nurses working in ICUs are registered with Rakuten Insight, Inc. Survey requests were sent to ICU nurses who were registered with Rakuten Insight and who met the eligibility criteria of working full-time in the hospital ICUs. Associate nurses/nursing assistants and midwives were excluded. To validate a survey, a sample size that is at least seven times larger than the number of items it contains and an absolute number of at least 100 are required [13]. Of the nurses to whom the survey request was sent, those willing to participate were selected; the sampling continued until 250 nurses were recruited. To verify data collection, including reproducibility, two surveys were conducted to examine test–retest reliability. Two weeks after the first survey, a second survey was administered to all participants of the first survey. Data were collected between February to March 2022 in Japan.

2.3.2. Data Collection Procedures and Instruments

The questionnaire (the first survey) comprised (1) demographic characteristics, (2) the QFIFE-J, and (3) the Family Assistance Practice Scale for ICU Nurses [14].

1. Participants' demographic characteristics. Data on participants' age, sex, educational background, years of clinical experience, years of critical care experience, certification, job position, number of beds in the hospital where the participant works, and type of unit were collected.
2. The QFIFE-J. The QFIFE, developed by Hetland et al. [12], was used in the research survey by double-back-translation into Japanese, with the permission of the original creator. The six-question method, in which the answers to each question ranged from "strongly agree" to "completely disagree", was used to investigate the experiences and thoughts of the research collaborators.
3. Family Assistance Practice Scale for ICU Nurses [15]. The Family Assistance Practice Scale for ICU Nurses was used to validate the criterion-related validity. This scale comprises four factors and 24 items, including "emotional support", "informational support", "environmental adjustment support", and "evaluative support", and was developed to visualize the family support practices of ICU nurses and be used as a reflective evaluation by the nurses themselves. The model fit indices for the scale were comparative fit index (CFI) = 0.96 and root mean square error of approximation (RMSEA) = 0.07, and McDonald's ω coefficient for internal consistency was 0.92. Therefore, its reliability and validity have been confirmed in Japan. With the permission of the creator, this scale was used in a study to evaluate its criterion-related validity. The respondents' answers to each question were used on a six-point scale ranging from "strongly agree" to "completely disagree", to investigate their experiences and thoughts.

2.4. Data Analysis

For statistical analysis, an item analysis was performed. Items 6–10 were reverse coded before calculating the means of the total and subscales scores. Exploratory factor analysis (EFA), confirmatory factor analysis (CFA), and criterion-related validity were performed to assess the scale's validity. To assess the reliability, internal consistency and reproducibility were examined. For all analyses, a p-value of <0.05 was considered to be significant. All statistical analyses were performed using SPSS 28.0 software (IBM Japan, Tokyo, Japan).

2.5. Item Analysis

In the item analysis, ceiling and floor effects were identified from the standard deviations and means to see the bias in the distribution of the data. The good–poor (G-P) analysis and item–total (I-T) correlations were also detected to examine the validity of each item against the scale.

2.6. Validity Analysis

An EFA was conducted to examine the factor structure of QFIFE. The Kaiser–Meyer–Olkin (KMO) test and Bartlett's specificity test were performed to assess sampling adequacy and fit of the data to the factor analysis [16]. Scree plots were utilized to estimate the ideal number of potential factors. Thereafter, we assessed whether the variance explained by each factor had an eigenvalue ≥ 1 and a KMO > 0.5 [17]. Then, an EFA with maximum likelihood (ML) and Promax rotation was performed. [18]. Items with factor loadings <0.35 were excluded. In general, the total variance explained was >50% [19]. The CFA was used to evaluate the goodness-of-fit of the factor structure of the QFIFE-J. Hoyle [20] and Kline [21] recommend using at least four adjustment indices. Thus, in this study, the chi-square test, CFI, Tucker and Lewis's incremental index (TLI), and RMSEA were used to assess data fitness. The goodness-of-fit of the model was good with CFI > 0.90, TLI $\geq$ 0.90, and RMSEA < 0.08. Moreover, the ratio of chi-squares concerning degrees of freedom ($\chi^2/\text{df} < 2.00$) was evaluated. For criterion validity, Pearson's correlation coefficient was used to assess the correlation between the proposed scale scores and the Family Assistance Practice Scale for ICU Nurses' scores.

2.7. Reliability Analysis

To check the reliability of the scale, Cronbach's α coefficients were calculated for the entire scale and each subscale. To check for reproducibility, test–retests were conducted at two-week intervals, and intraclass correlation coefficients for the QFIFE-J response scores were calculated [13].

2.8. Ethical Considerations

It was explained in writing that research cooperation was based on free will, that no disadvantages would be incurred by the participants in the event of refusal, and that protection of personal information and privacy would be observed in the publication of the results. The questionnaire was answered only by those who agreed to participate in the study. Data were collected anonymously using serial IDs, and data confidentiality was maintained. Approval for the above was obtained from the Ethics Committee of the author's university (No. 2021F19).

3. Results

3.1. Participants' Demographic Characteristics

Participants of this study were 250 nurses in the critical care area; 67.2% were older than 30-years-old, 83.2% were women, 54% had a technical college degree, and 44% had a college degree (Table 1). More than half had more than six years of clinical nursing experience; however, more than half had less than five years of experience in the critical care area. Of the nurses, 15.6% held administrative positions in their departments and only a few were certified nurse specialist (CNS) or had certified nurse licenses. More than two-thirds of participants belonged to hospitals with more than 200 beds.

Table 1. Participants' characteristics (N = 250).

Characteristic	Category	n (%)
Age (in years)	<25	20 (8.0)
	25–29	62 (24.8)
	30–49	152 (60.8)
	>49	16 (6.4)
Sex	Male	42 (16.8)
	Female	208 (83.2)
Educational background	Vocational school	135 (54.0)
	University	110 (44.0)
	Graduate school	5 (2.0)
Clinical experience (in years)	<1	9 (3.6)
	1–5	67 (26.8)
	6–15	120 (48.0)
	>15	54 (21.6)
ICU experience (in years)	<1	44 (17.6)
	1–5	117 (46.8)
	6–15	82 (32.8)
	>15	7 (2.8)
Certification	Certified nurse specialist	5 (2.0)
	Certified nurse	6 (2.4)
	Registered nurse	239 (95.6)
Position	Nurse manager	8 (3.2)
	Assistant nurse manager	31 (12.4)
	General nurse	211 (84.4)
Number of hospital beds	<200	23 (9.2)
	200–300	34 (13.6)
	301–500	80 (32.0)
	501–800	57 (22.8)
	>800	56 (22.4)
Type of unit	Adult ICU	202 (80.8)
	Neonatal ICU	48 (19.2)

Abbreviation: ICU, intensive care unit.

3.2. Validity and Reliability of the QFIFE-J

Answer Distribution and Item Analysis

Data from 250 critical care nurses were used for item analysis (Table 2). Most items had the highest frequency of "4-point" responses, while Item 9 had the highest frequency of "1-point" responses. No ceiling or floor effects were found as the maximum value of the sum of the means and standard deviations for each item was 5.56 and the minimum value was 1.06. In the G-P analysis, a significant difference between the means of the high- and low-scoring groups was found for each item. The I-T correlations were significantly correlated with the overall scores for all items. Thus, no items were removed as a result of the item analysis.

3.3. Validity Testing

To determine the construct validity, item analysis was performed on the 15 items of the proposed scale, and no items were deleted. Therefore, EFA was performed using the ML method and Promax rotation on all 15 items. The KMO index for sampling adequacy was 0.799. Based on eigenvalues ≥ 1.0 and scree plots, four factors were identified. Items with loading values ≥ 0.35 were retained. Finally, a 15-item scale with a four-factor structure was used. To interpret and name each factor, the theoretical characteristics derived from the four-factor structure employed in the EFA were compared with the constructs identified in a previous study. Factor 1 comprised five items (Items 1–5) and was named "ICU environment". Factor 2 comprised five items (Items 11–15) and was named "nurses' attitudes". Factor 3 had three items (Items 8–10) and was named "nurses' workflow". Factor 4 comprised two items (6 and 7) and was named "patient acuity".

Table 2. The QFIFE-J item analysis (N = 250).

	Item	Mean (SD)	Good–Poor Analysis		Item–Total Correlation Analysis
			High Mean (SD)	Low Mean (SD)	
1	My unit is physically set up in a way that makes it possible to involve family caregivers in patient care.	3.32 (1.33)	3.98 (1.18)	2.70 (1.16)	0.58 **
2	My unit is adequately staffed to allow me time to involve family caregivers in patient care.	2.94 (1.32)	3.60 (1.26)	2.33 (1.07)	0.55 **
3	My unit has established written policies for involving family caregivers in patient care.	2.88 (1.26)	3.51 (1.20)	2.28 (0.99)	0.54 **
4	My unit supports family caregivers' presence during procedures (e.g., resuscitation, line placement).	2.41 (1.35)	2.79 (1.48)	2.05 (1.10)	0.32 **
5	There is a designated space and resources for families who wish to remain with their loved ones in the ICU.	3.23 (1.25)	3.78 (1.11)	2.71 (1.14)	0.52 **
6	Family caregivers of patients who are hemodynamically unstable should be excluded from participating in patient care.	3.86 (1.23)	4.14 (1.22)	3.60 (1.18)	0.31 **
7	Patients on life-sustaining treatments should not have family caregivers involved in patient care.	4.36 (1.20)	4.73 (1.14)	4.01 (1.14)	0.39 **
8	Allowing family caregivers to assist in patient care interrupts my work.	3.60 (1.13)	3.93 (1.10)	3.30 (1.08)	0.38 **
9	My clinical performance will be affected by the presence of family caregivers in the room while I am providing patient care.	3.60 (1.12)	3.90 (1.15)	3.31 (1.01)	0.35 **
10	I am too busy to incorporate family caregivers in patient care.	3.80 (1.19)	4.17 (1.17)	3.45 (1.10)	0.42 **
11	Allowing family caregivers to assist in patient care could help me more accurately assess distressing symptoms in my patients.	3.76 (0.99)	4.19 (0.88)	3.36 (0.93)	0.54 **
12	Allowing family caregivers to assist in daily patient care could improve the caregivers' levels of stress, anxiety, and fear.	4.20 (0.96)	4.59 (0.79)	3.84 (0.97)	0.47 **
13	I think that family caregivers who engage in patient care are better able to make care decisions for their loved ones.	4.06 (0.92)	4.50 (0.73)	3.64 (0.89)	0.57 **
14	I think involving family caregivers in patient care improves patient safety.	3.51 (1.03)	3.92 (0.98)	3.12 (0.93)	0.51 **
15	I think involving family caregivers in patient care improves overall quality of care.	4.17 (1.05)	4.76 (0.79)	3.62 (0.97)	0.65 **

Abbreviation: ICU, intensive care unit. ** $p < 0.01$.

Factors 1–4 explained 26.533%, 18.308%, 11.689%, and 6.357% of the total variance, respectively, with a cumulative contribution rate of 62.886%. The CFA for this 15-item model yielded the following indices: $\chi^2(84) = 153.535$, $\chi^2/df = 1.828$, CFI = 0.942, TLI = 0.917, and RMSEA = 0.057 (Table 3). The results of the criterion-related validity assessment are presented in Table 4. In this assessment, the extent that the total score on the QFIFE-J and each factor correlated with the total score on the Family Assistance Practice Scale for ICU Nurses was examined.

Table 3. Results of the exploratory factor analysis and Cronbach's α coefficients (N = 250).

	Item	Factor Loading				Mean (SD)
		1	2	3	4	
	Factor 1: ICU environment (α = 0.813)					2.96 (0.98)
3	My unit has established written policies for involving family caregivers in patient care.	**0.852**	−0.052	−0.104	0.045	
2	My unit is adequately staffed to allow me time to involve family caregivers in patient care.	**0.838**	−0.071	0.046	−0.002	
1	My unit is physically set up in a way that makes it possible to involve family caregivers in patient care.	**0.724**	0.059	−0.065	0.076	
5	There is a designated space and resources for families who wish to remain with their loved ones in the ICU.	**0.562**	0.132	0.109	−0.189	
4	My unit supports family caregivers' presence during procedures (e.g., resuscitation, line placement).	**0.387**	0.045	0.060	−0.146	
	Factor 2: Nurses' attitudes (α = 0.794)					3.94 (0.73)
12	Allowing family caregivers to assist in daily patient care could improve the caregivers' levels of stress, anxiety, and fear.	−0.152	**0.855**	−0.102	−0.018	
13	I think that family caregivers, involved in patient care, are better able to make care decisions for their loved ones.	0.035	**0.781**	−0.032	−0.005	
15	I think involving family caregivers in patient care improves overall quality of care.	0.164	**0.585**	−0.015	0.155	
11	Allowing family caregivers to assist in patient care could help me more accurately assess distressing symptoms in my patients.	0.069	**0.566**	0.099	−0.106	
14	I think involving family caregivers in patient care improves patient safety.	0.065	**0.400**	0.135	0.101	
	Factor 3: Nurses' workflow (α = 0.687)					3.67 (0.90)
8	Allowing family caregivers to assist in patient care interrupts my work.	−0.026	0.010	**0.882**	−0.048	
9	My clinical performance will be affected by the presence of family caregivers in the room while I am providing patient care.	−0.052	0.021	**0.598**	0.057	
10	I am too busy to incorporate family caregivers in patient care.	0.205	−0.066	**0.374**	0.202	
	Factor 4: Patient acuity (α = 0.780)					4.11 (1.10)
7	Patients on life-sustaining treatments should not have family caregivers involved in patient care.	−0.034	0.018	0.010	**0.867**	
6	Family caregivers of patients who are hemodynamically unstable should be excluded from participating in patient care.	−0.142	0.027	0.134	**0.638**	
	Factor loading (%)	26.533	18.308	11.689	6.357	
	Cumulative loading (%)		44.840	56.529	62.886	
	Cronbach's α (full scale) = 0.779					
Inter-factor correlations	Factor 1	1.000	0.387	0.093	−0.051	
	Factor 2		1.000	0.135	0.331	
	Factor 3			1.000	0.482	
	Factor 4				1.000	

Note. Factor loadings for each item in the factor are shown in bold.

Table 4. Relationship between the QFIFE-J and Family Assistance Practice Scale for ICU Nurses (N = 250).

		QFIFE-J			
	Total Score	Factor 1: ICU Environment	Factor 2: Nurses' Attitude	Factor 3: Nurses' Workflow	Factor 4: Patient Acuity
The Family Assistance Practice Scale for ICU Nurses					
Total score	−0.047	0.292 **	0.598 **	−0.848 **	−0.730 **
Emotional support	−0.157 *	0.131 *	0.594 **	−0.628 **	−0.648 **
Information provision support	−0.198 **	0.262 **	0.540 **	−0.911 **	−0.814 **
Environmental coordination support	0.043	0.363 **	0.511 **	−0774 **	−0.563 **
Family support behavior	0.045	0.275 **	0.542 **	−0.665 **	−0.558 **

Note. Pearson's rank correlation coefficient for the total score between QFIFE-J and Family Assistance Practice Scale for ICU Nurses. ** $p < 0.01$, * $p < 0.05$.

Pearson's rank correlation coefficient for the total scores was −0.047; the values for factors 1–4 ranged from −0.848 to 0.598 ($p < 0.01$).

3.4. Reliability Testing

The internal consistency analysis of the final four-factor, 15-item scale showed high reliability for all factors, with the Cronbach's α coefficient for the overall scale being 0.779.

The coefficients for the subscales "ICU environment", "nurses' attitudes", "nurses' workflows", and "patient acuity" were 0.813, 0.794, 0.687, and 0.780, respectively. Of the 250 respondents who completed the first survey, 160 (64.0%) participated in the second survey. The intraclass coefficient for test–retest reliability was 0.804 ($p < 0.01$) for the overall scale. The coefficients for the subscales "ICU environment", "nurses' attitudes", "nurses' workflow", and "patient acuity" were 0.762 ($p < 0.01$), 0.567 ($p < 0.01$), 0.587 ($p < 0.01$) and 0.560 ($p < 0.01$), respectively.

4. Discussion

In this study, the QFIFE-J was developed using a comprehensive approach. The initial scale items were developed incorporating ICU nurses' values and perspectives on cultural norms, which serve as the bias for tool development in psychometrics [22]. Moreover, the conceptual factor structure (construct validity) was assessed using an EFA. No floor or ceiling effects were found. The results indicated that family support in Japanese ICUs is best explained by a four-factor, 15-item model. Cronbach's alpha was 0.779 for the entire scale, indicating an acceptable internal consistency [23]. For test–retest reliability, the total score of the QFIFE-J showed high reliability. However, some factors did not show high reliability values on the subscales. This is expected because Factor 1, "ICU environment", varied a little; while Factor 2, "Nurses' attitudes", Factor 3, "Nurses' Workflow", and Factor 4, "patient acuity", were those that varied with changes in patient conditions, especially in ICUs. In ICUs, these factors fluctuate with changes in the patient's situation, and it was expected that the content would have changed over the two weeks measured [24]. Regarding construct validity, the EFA results revealed a four-factor construct, as defined in a previous study. Thus, this scale had good reliability and validity and can be considered a useful tool for measuring the barriers and facilitators of family support in the ICU.

Furthermore, the item analysis suggested that the mean scores for items related to nurses' attitudes were generally high, while those for the departmental environment were generally low, thus indicating that, although many nurses have a positive attitude toward involving family members in patient care, they lack organizational support to implement it, and the departmental environment is a challenge for promoting FCC in ICUs in Japan. Thus, it can be said that engaging families in the care of critically ill patients in the ICU requires a more focused team effort based on a shared culture and defined framework of FCC [25], which will require organizational support in the form of hospital and ICU policies and nurse education designed to promote FCC [4]. However, organizational support to facilitate such FCC in ICUs is lacking and has now become an international hindrance to FCC [26]. The current results show lower ratings for the departmental environment compared to the results in the U.S. [7], thereby highlighting the lack of organizational support as an issue for family care in Japanese ICUs.

The QFIFE-J can measure the perceived barriers and facilitators that affect critical care through nurses' attitudes toward family engagement, during care of critically ill patients. It contains only 15 items that are easy to use in practice. The QFIFE-J can also be used to assess four areas: ICU environment, nurses' attitudes, nurses' workflow and patient acuity, and attitude toward family caregiver engagement in care.

Involving the family in ICU care requires consideration of a variety of influencing factors; therefore, using a scale that takes a broad view may accurately capture the disincentive. In fact, the ability to clarify the facilitating and inhibiting factors in nurses' collaboration with families using this scale may help to accurately describe the current situation in ICUs and effectively collaborate with families. We believe that low scores for each factor of this scale will allow us to consider various measures to improve the factors that hinder collaboration with families.

Regarding the "ICU environment" factor, we should consider relaxing the restrictions on visiting hours and improving the environment for family members to enter the ICU. Regarding the "Nurses' attitudes" factor, we should consider the need for in-hospital family nursing education, i.e., education that enables positive recognition of collaboration with families or education on structured specific communication methods [25]. Regarding the "Nurses' workflow" factor, we should consider staffing, i.e., increasing the number of nurses or making consultation with professionals such as CNS seamless. Regarding the "Patient acuity" factor, we should always try to provide the best possible care to stabilize the patient's condition and carefully give feedback regarding the patient's progress to their family [27]. The recent COVID-19 pandemic has restricted family visits to patients during hospitalization, making it difficult for FCC to take root. It is thus necessary to promote qualitative improvement of nursing care in ICUs in Japan. By utilizing this scale, we believe that it is possible to evaluate what situations and patient attributes make it possible to practice FCC in ICUs in Japan. We also believe that this scale can be used to evaluate nursing education, and it also has implications for family involvement.

The ICU visiting policies vary widely depending on regional factors, cultural differences, laws, and hospital policies [28,29]. As the four subscales of the QFIFE may differ among institutions, systems, and countries, we believe that various comparative studies can provide suggestions for effective collaboration with families.

Study Limitations

As this study was conducted online and participants were limited to Rakuten Insight registrants, there was a possibility of selection bias. As the items comprising this scale are Japanese translations of the QFIFE, some items were not necessarily adapted depending on the ICU environment and standards in Japan. Therefore, to assess the facilitators of family care in ICUs in Japan, it is necessary to examine the details of ICU standards and family care practices in Japan, and the findings of nurses and physicians in particular.

5. Conclusions

The QFIFE-J is a reliable and valid instrument to quantitatively assess the facilitators and inhibitors of family entry into ICU patient care. Thus, using this scale to identify the facilitating and inhibiting factors in nurses' collaboration with families, it may be possible to accurately understand the current situation in ICUs and effectively collaborate with families.

Author Contributions: Conceptualization, M.T. and J.H.; methodology, M.T.; software, Y.I.; validation, M.T. and S.K.; formal analysis, M.T.; investigation, Y.I.; resources, Y.I.; data curation, Y.I.; writing—original draft preparation, M.T. and S.K.; writing—review and editing, M.T., S.K., Y.I., K.S. and J.H.; visualization, S.K.; supervision, J.H.; project administration, M.T.; funding acquisition, M.T. All authors have read and agreed to the published version of the manuscript.

Funding: The Foundation of Kinoshita Memorial Enterprise funded this research.

Institutional Review Board Statement: This study was approved by the ethics committee of the university to which the authors are affiliated (no. 2021F19).

Informed Consent Statement: Informed consent was obtained from all participants involved in the study.

Data Availability Statement: All data generated or analyzed during this study are included in this published article.

Acknowledgments: The authors are grateful to all study participants.

Conflicts of Interest: The authors declare no conflict of interest.

References

1. Inoue, S.; Hatakeyama, J.; Kondo, Y.; Hifumi, T.; Sakuramoto, H.; Kawasaki, T.; Taito, S.; Nakamura, K.; Unoki, T.; Kawai, Y.; et al. Post-intensive care syndrome: Its pathophysiology, prevention, and future directions. *Acute Med. Surg.* **2019**, *6*, 233–246. [CrossRef]
2. Nolen, K.B.; Warren, N.A. Meeting the needs of family members of ICU patients. *Crit. Care Nurs. Q.* **2014**, *37*, 393–406. [CrossRef] [PubMed]
3. Wong, P.; Liamputtong, P.; Koch, S.; Rawson, H. Barriers to regaining control within a constructivist grounded theory of family resilience in ICU: Living with uncertainty. *J. Clin. Nurs.* **2017**, *26*, 4390–4403. [CrossRef] [PubMed]
4. Davidson, J.E.; Aslakson, R.A.; Long, A.C.; Puntillo, K.A.; Kross, E.K.; Hart, J.; Cox, C.E.; Wunsch, H.; Wickline, M.A.; Nunnally, M.E.; et al. Guidelines for family-centered care in the neonatal, pediatric, and adult ICU. *Crit. Care Med.* **2017**, *45*, 103–128. [CrossRef] [PubMed]
5. Mitchell, M.; Gill, F.J.; Greenwood, M. *Partnering with Families in Critical Care*; ACCCN: Surrey Hills, Australia, 2015.
6. Wetzig, K.; Mitchell, M. The needs of families of ICU trauma patients: An integrative review. *Intensive Crit. Care Nurs.* **2017**, *41*, 63–70. [CrossRef]
7. Hetland, B.; McAndrew, N.; Perazzo, J.; Hickman, R. A qualitative study of factors that influence active family involvement with patient care in the ICU: Survey of critical care nurses. *Intensive Crit. Care Nurs.* **2018**, *44*, 67–75. [CrossRef]
8. Gwaza, E.; Msiska, G. Family involvement in caring for inpatients in acute care hospital settings: A systematic review of literature. *SAGE Open Nurs.* **2022**, *8*, 1–15. [CrossRef] [PubMed]
9. Burns, K.E.A.; Devlin, J.W.; Hill, N.S. Patient and family engagement in designing and implementing a weaning trial: A novel research paradigm in critical care. *Chest* **2017**, *152*, 707–711. [CrossRef]
10. Burns, K.E.A.; Misak, C.; Herridge, M.; Meade, M.O.; Oczkowski, S.; Patient and Family Partnership Committee of the Canadian Critical Care Trials Group. Patient and family engagement in the ICU. Untapped opportunities and underrecognized challenges. *Am. J. Respir. Crit. Care Med.* **2018**, *198*, 310–319. [CrossRef]
11. Harumi, E.; Emiko, S. Reliability and validity of assessment tool for early detection of post intensive care syndrome in Japan. *J. Jpn. Acad. Crit. Care Nurs.* **2021**, *17*, 11–20. (In Japanese) [CrossRef]
12. Hetland, B.; Hickman, R.; McAndrew, N.; Daly, B. Factors influencing active family engagement in care among critical care nurses. *AACN Adv. Crit. Care* **2017**, *28*, 160–170. [CrossRef]
13. Lee, P.; Lu, W.-S.; Liu, C.-H.; Lin, H.-Y.; Hsieh, C.-L. Test–retest reliability and minimal detectable change of the D2 test of attention in patients with schizophrenia. *Arch. Clin. Neuropsychol.* **2017**, *33*, 1060–1068. [CrossRef]
14. Berry, J.W. Introduction to methodology. In *Handbook of Cross-Cultural Psychology*; Triandis, H., Berry, J.W., Eds.; Allyn & Bacon: Boston, MA, USA, 1989; pp. 1–28.
15. Nishimura, N.; Yamaguchi, M. Development of a family assistance practice scale for ICU nurses. *Bull. Soc. Med.* **2020**, *37*, 138–149.
16. Tabachnick, B.; Fidell, L. *Using Multivariate Statistics*, 7th ed.; Pearson Education: London, UK, 2019.
17. Hair, J.F.; Black, W.C.; Babin, B.J.; Anderson, R.E. *Multivariate Data Analysis*; Pearson Education: Harlow, UK, 2014.
18. Costello, A.B.; Osborne, J.W. Best practices in exploratory factor analysis: Four recommendations for getting the most from your analysis. *Pract. Assess. Res. Eval.* **2005**, *10*, 7. [CrossRef]
19. Streiner, D.L. Figuring out factors: The use and misuse of factor analysis. *Can. J. Psychiatry* **1994**, *39*, 135–140. [CrossRef] [PubMed]
20. Hoyle, R.H.; Isherwood, J.C. Reporting results from structural equation modeling analyses in Archives of Scientific Psychology. *Arch. Sci. Psychol.* **2013**, *1*, 14–22. [CrossRef] [PubMed]
21. Kline, R.B. *Principles and Practice of Structural Equation Modeling*; Guilford: New York, NY, USA, 2010.

22. Streiner, D.L.; Norman, G.R. *Health Measurement Scales: A Practical Guide to Their Development and Use*, 5th ed.; Oxford University Press: New York, NY, USA, 2014.
23. Cronbach, L.J. Coefficient alpha and the internal structure of tests. *Psychometrika* **1951**, *16*, 297–334. [CrossRef]
24. Landis, J.R.; Koch, G.G. The measurement of observer agreement for categorical data. *Biometrics* **1977**, *33*, 159–174. [CrossRef] [PubMed]
25. Naef, R.; Brysiewicz, P.; McAndrew, N.S.; Beierwaltes, P.; Chiang, V.; Clisbee, D.; de Beer, J.; Honda, J.; Kakazu, S.; Nagl-Cupal, M.; et al. Intensive care nurse-family engagement from a global perspective: A qualitative multi-site exploration. *Intensive Crit. Care Nurs.* **2021**, *66*, 103081. [CrossRef] [PubMed]
26. Kiwanuka, F.; Shayan, S.J.; Tolulope, A.A. Barriers to patient and family-centred care in adult intensive care units: A systematic review. *Nurs. Open* **2019**, *6*, 676–684. [CrossRef]
27. Reifarth, E.; Garcia Borrega, J.; Kochanek, M. How to communicate with family members of the critically ill in the intensive care unit: A scoping review. *Intensive Crit. Care Nurs.* **2022**, *2022*, 103328. [CrossRef]
28. Cappellini, E.; Bambi, S.; Lucchini, A.; Milanesio, E. Open intensive care units: A global challenge for patients, relatives, and critical care teams. *Dimens. Crit. Care Nurs.* **2014**, *33*, 181–193. [CrossRef] [PubMed]
29. Milner, K.A.; Marmo, S.; Goncalves, S. Implementation and sustainment strategies for open visitation in the intensive care unit: A multicentre qualitative study. *Intensive Crit. Care Nurs.* **2021**, *62*, 102927. [CrossRef] [PubMed]

Disclaimer/Publisher's Note: The statements, opinions and data contained in all publications are solely those of the individual author(s) and contributor(s) and not of MDPI and/or the editor(s). MDPI and/or the editor(s) disclaim responsibility for any injury to people or property resulting from any ideas, methods, instructions or products referred to in the content.

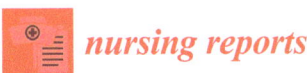

Article

Challenges Regarding Transition from Case-Based Learning to Problem-Based Learning: A Qualitative Study with Student Nurses

Ramoipei J. Phage *, Boitumelo J. Molato and Molekodi J. Matsipane

NuMIQ Research Focus Area, School of Nursing, Faculty of Health Sciences, North-West University, Ngaka Modiri Molema 2735, South Africa
* Correspondence: msg.paghe@gmail.com

Abstract: Background: The transition from case-based learning to problem-based learning can be challenging and may have negative effects on the academic, psychological, emotional, or social well-being of student nurses. As a result, this exposes student nurses to high failure rates, anxiety disorders, a loss of uniqueness, and fear of the unknown. However, student nurses employ different strategies aimed at overcoming challenges faced during this transition period. Methods: An exploratory, and descriptive research approach was used. A purposive non-probability sampling technique was used to select participants. Focus group discussions via Zoom video communication were used to collect data, which were analysed using Braun and Clarke's six steps of thematic analysis. Results: The following three themes emerged: challenges regarding facilitation, challenges regarding assessment, and strategies to overcome challenges. Conclusions: The study established that student nurses are faced with different challenges during the transition from one teaching strategy to another. Student nurses suggested strategies that could be used to overcome these challenges. However, these strategies are not enough and therefore more needs to be done to support and empower student nurses.

Keywords: case-based learning; challenges; problem-based learning; student nurses; transition

Citation: Phage, R.J.; Molato, B.J.; Matsipane, M.J. Challenges Regarding Transition from Case-Based Learning to Problem-Based Learning: A Qualitative Study with Student Nurses. *Nurs. Rep.* **2023**, *13*, 389–403. https://doi.org/10.3390/nursrep13010036

Academic Editors: Antonio Martínez-Sabater, Elena Chover-Sierra and Carles Saus-Ortega

Received: 10 January 2023
Revised: 8 February 2023
Accepted: 20 February 2023
Published: 2 March 2023

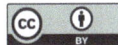

Copyright: © 2023 by the authors. Licensee MDPI, Basel, Switzerland. This article is an open access article distributed under the terms and conditions of the Creative Commons Attribution (CC BY) license (https://creativecommons.org/licenses/by/4.0/).

1. Introduction

Various active learning methods are used in the teaching and learning process in order to produce students who are creative, adaptive to team work and are able to find solutions to the problems of daily life by using the knowledge and skills gained [1]. Case-based learning (CBL) and problem-based learning (PBL) are among these methods of teaching and learning [1]. Keeping in view all the aforementioned facts, Liu et al (2019) asserted that CBL and PBL are long established pedagogic teaching strategies that have been widely implemented throughout various higher institutions of learning globally [2]. In a study conducted in China by Bi et al., (2019), CBL is an active teaching and learning strategy that focuses on student nurses as the centre of the learning environment [3].

Moreover, CBL encourages a student-centred and patient-oriented exploration of realistic and specific situations [3]. The authors also mention that student nurses focus on the patient's case, engage in self-directed learning, scientific inquiry, and collaboration with others in integrating theory and practice [1,3]. Furthermore, Hassoulas et al. (2017) state that CBL provides a practical model for students to relate content learning to professional practice and helps them improve the ability to collaborate when studying, thinking critically, and solving clinical problems [4]. Despite these benefits of CBL, there are also related challenges that student nurses may encounter which include: students feeling that CBL activities in the classroom take a lot of time, and other students finding it uncomfortable to engage in group learning activities since they prefer working independently [5].

Historically, CBL was invented in the United States of America (USA) in 1870 at Harvard University Law School, more than a century before PBL [6]. As a result, this endorses the fact that institutions of higher learning have indeed been using these two teaching methods for a very long time. According to literature, PBL was used initially in nursing education in the year 1969 at McMaster University Medical School in Canada [6]. PBL is a student-centred pedagogical approach in which students learn a subject through the experience of solving an open-ended problem found in trigger material [7]. PBL is known to increases student motivation and desire to learn, and strengthens cooperative learning skills [8]. Therefore, students are more likely to become active in their learning. Despite all these advantages, PBL has inherent limitations and disadvantages that cannot be overlooked. For example, PBL requires a significant amount of time, there is lack of training on PBL facilitation, and it is expensive to implement, to mention but a few [8].

In the South African (SA) context, Rakhudu et al. (2016) reported that five higher institutions of learning have adopted PBL as their teaching strategy [9]. Amongst five institutions that have adopted PBL in South Africa, there is one institution of higher learning in the North West Province (NWP) that has adopted both CBL and PBL as its teaching strategies in the undergraduate programme since 2002. This particular institution applies CBL in the first two years of study. During the third and fourth years, the same student nurses are expected to transition from CBL to PBL, which may cause anxiety to the student nurses due to a fear of anticipated challenges that may accompany a transition from one teaching strategy to another.

Since the implementation of both CBL and PBL in 2002 at a particular institution of higher learning in the NWP, South Africa, there has been no research study that has been conducted to explore and describe the challenges that student nurses may encounter during the transition period, thus resulting in a dearth of literature regarding their challenges. Therefore, the researchers deemed it necessary to explore and describe challenges faced by student nurses who transition from CBL to PBL in order to have a deep understanding from the student nurses' perspective with the aim of improving the teaching and learning process.

Transition is described as an internal, psychological process that results from a change. The actual change may occur quickly, but the transition process occurs much more slowly and is different for everyone [10]. The study conducted by Jindal-Snape et al. (2019) acknowledges that transition may have negative impact on the well-being of students, either psychological, emotional, or social [11]. Moreover, a transition from one teaching strategy to another exposes students to increased failure rates, anxiety disorder, a loss of uniqueness, and fear of the unknown [10]. The researchers are of the view that there might be challenges if the student nurses are to transition from the CBL to PBL teaching strategy. The researchers garner this view from the understanding that CBL and PBL as teaching strategies have their own challenges that may be compounded by the process of transitioning which on its own is a challenge to most students. Furthermore, the researchers believe that a profound understanding about the challenges faced by student nurses during transition from CBL to PBL in the NWP of South Africa is necessary in a sense that if they are successfully explored, this may assist in finding efficient and effective solutions to mitigate the challenges.

2. Material and Methods

2.1. Aim

The aim of this study was to explore and describe challenges faced by student nurses during transition from case-based learning (CBL) to problem-based learning (PBL) at one of the institutions of higher learning in the North West Province (NWP).

2.2. Research Design

An exploratory, and descriptive qualitative research approach was used to explore, describe, and contextualize challenges faced by student nurses during transition from CBL to PBL at one of the institutions of higher learning in the NWP, South Africa. An exploratory, descriptive, and contextual research approach was conducted to gain a new insight, and discover new ideas, thus increasing the knowledge about the phenomenon at hand.

2.3. Study Setting

The study was conducted at one of the institutions of higher learning in the NWP, South Africa, at which case-based learning and problem-based learning are used to facilitate teaching and learning. The study was conducted only in the Ngaka Modiri Molema (NMM) district in the NWP, because that is where the institution is situated. This institution has a capacity to accommodate four hundred student nurses on average. The higher institution is presently offering the undergraduate program Bachelor of Nursing Science (BNSc), whereby English is used as a medium of instruction. The BNSc program takes a minimum of four years to complete, from the first to fourth year level. Currently, the institution of higher learning has a total number of three hundred and nine student nurses.

2.4. Population and Sampling

The population of this study included student nurses in their third year of study who used CBL and are currently using PBL as their teaching and learning strategy. Although both the third and fourth-year student nurses have been exposed to CBL and PBL, the third-year student nurses were the only population of this study because they were recently exposed to PBL, which is new to them. As a result, the researcher believed that the third-year students were in a more vulnerable position than the fourth years as far as the transition from CBL to PBL was concerned. Furthermore, the researchers were of the opinion that the fourth-year students might have already grown used to PBL; hence, they were excluded from the population. A purposive non-probability sampling technique was used to sample the participants. Informed consent forms with additional important information about the study was emailed to the participants to read and sign. Each participant brought the signed consent form on the day of focus group. The sample size of the study was determined by data saturation.

2.5. Data Collection Method

Data were collected using semi-structured focus group discussions. Since there was the coronavirus (COVID-19) pandemic and mass gathering was prohibited, the researchers conducted the focus groups via Zoom video communication to avoid physical contact with participants, with the aim of minimizing the possible exposure to COVID-19.

Open-ended questions were asked and follow-up questions using probing, clarifying, and other communication techniques were used to improve communication dynamics. Based on Krishnasamy et al (2023), an example of a focus group questions is shown below in the form of Table 1 [12].

Table 1. Example of focus group questions.

Exploratory Questions
• What are the challenges you faced during transition from Case-based to Problem-based learning?
• What helps you to overcome the challenges?
• What else do you think other people can do to overcome the challenges?

Focus group sessions were audio-recorded with the permission of participants and transcribed verbatim into transcription data. The transcribed data were de-identified to maintain a principle of anonymity. Furthermore, all data was kept in a lockable safe place to promote privacy and confidentiality.

2.6. Data Analysis

The researchers and co-coder analysed data independently using Braun and Clarke's six steps of thematic analysis. The researchers prepared and organised data from all Zoom video communications. The researchers transcribed data from all Zooms and sent the transcribed data to the independent co-coder for coding. Data was coded using inductive process. Themes and subthemes were generated and can be viewed in Table 2 under results. Both the researchers and the co-coder held a meeting via Zoom video communication to discuss the themes and subthemes and agreed upon the themes and subthemes. Subsequently, the researchers narrated those themes and subthemes, quoted the participants, and supported them with the literature under discussions.

Table 2. Themes and subthemes.

Theme	Sub-Themes
1.1 Challenges regarding facilitation	1.1.1. Adaptation challenge 1.1.2. Group work 1.1.3. Information search 1.1.4. Workload and insufficient time for PBL content 1.1.5. Lack of proper guidance from lecturers 1.1.6. Learning issues 1.1.7. Online problem-based learning 1.1.8. Lack of student instructors (SI)
1.2 Challenges regarding assessment	1.2.1 Lack of revision 1.2.2. Lack of feedback
1.3 Strategies to overcome challenges	1.3.1 Collaborating with classmates/Peer learning 1.3.2. Use of relevant articles, prescribed books, and previous question papers 1.3.3. Plan study time 1.3.4. Consultation with lecturers

2.7. Ethical Considerations

The researchers submitted the research proposal to the North West University's scientific committee, Research Data Gatekeeper Committee (RDGC), and Health Research Ethics Committee (Ethics reference number: NWU-00218-21-s1), respectively, for ethical approval. Before the recruitment of participants and data collection, the study received unanimous approval from all the aforementioned committees. Participants were recruited via a wide range of methods, and all their rights were explained to them before signing consent forms. Participants signed consent forms before data collection and were addressed by alphabet rather than their names to maintain anonymity throughout the study. Furthermore, participants were also informed that they were free to withdraw from the study without consequences.

3. Results

A total of six focus group interviews consisting of six to eight participants via Zoom communication video were conducted and data saturation was reached with the sixth focus group. The results of the research study are discussed in to Table 2, which provides themes and subthemes. There are three themes and thirteen subthemes that emerged from the results of the study.

Student nurses expressed their challenges regarding the transition from case-based learning to problem-based learning in different ways. These challenges include facilitation challenges, assessment challenges, and strategies to overcome challenges. Each form of challenge faced by student nurses as a result of the transition were grouped into subthemes and discussed independently as follows:

3.1. Theme 1.1: Challenges Regarding Facilitation

The first theme focuses on the challenges regarding facilitation. This theme consists of seven sub-themes and are as follows: adaptation challenges, group work, information search, increased workload and insufficient time for problem-based learning content, lack of guidance from lecturers, learning issues, and online problem-based learning.

3.1.1. Subtheme 1.1.1: Adaptation Challenges

Adaptation challenges regarding the transition from CBL to PBL was identified as one of the subthemes. Participants revealed that it is challenging to adapt from one teaching strategy to the other. For instance, learning with PBL as a teaching strategy in third year while being used to a CBL teaching strategy from the first to second year of study. Participants expressed their views as follows:

"The challenge that I faced during transition was to adapt from case-based to problem-based learning."(**Participant U**).

Another participant supported the statement made by participant U and added:

"Well, my point supports the statement of student U. The main problem is that we struggled to adapt."(**Participant Y**).

Another participant described why they had a challenge regarding adaptation and said:

"With case-based learning, we were face to face with the lecturers. Lecturers guided us that is why we adapted very easily into case-based learning unlike in problem based learning." (**Participant W**).

3.1.2. Subtheme 1.1.2: Group Work

Working in groups emerged as a challenge student nurses faced the during transition period. Additionally, student nurses added that the poor participation of some of the group members, and changing of group members on a yearly basis are some of the reasons leading to group work challenges. Participants talked about the issue of group work versus poor participation and articulated the following:

"When we transit to problem-based learning, we were given problems to solve and we were working in groups. Some of the students did not want to participate, end up having to go to class unprepared, not being able to solve the given problems. So, the biggest problem was working in groups." (**Participant W**).

Another participant concurred with the statement made by participant W and said:

"The only issue that we had is poor participation from some group members. You gather your own information and end up doing the other member's part of the job delegated to him/her." (**Participant D**).

One of the participants explained how the issue of changing group members impact on group related work and added:

"The groups are changing every year. In the beginning of the year, we expect to have challenges because we are not used to each other as we are all new in the group and it is a big challenge. But as time goes on it becomes better since we get used to each other as group members. We get to know strengths and weaknesses of each other and we are delegating task based on strength and weaknesses. It becomes much easier to work together in that way. But now next year is the same routine again where I will get a new group and have to start the process all over again." (**Participant A1**).

3.1.3. Subthemes 1.1.3: Information Search

Searching for and finding relevant information on databases or search engines was another aspect that emerged as a subtheme. On top of that, student nurses added that there is lack of judgment from the lecturers as to whether the acquired information is relevant or not. Below are some of the views the participants mentioned:

"You have to go and look for information and sometimes you don't even know the sites (database) to get information from. You find out that sometimes you didn't get enough information and feedback from the lecturer and you don't know if you are right or wrong." **(Participant N)**.

Another participant described looking for information as a challenge and said:

"Problem-based learning was a whole new experience on its own as we look for information ourselves which is a challenge." **(Participant A5)**.

3.1.4. Subtheme 1.1.4: Workload and Insufficient Time for PBL Content

Student nurses reported that an increased workload accompanied by insufficient time for PBL content was a challenge aroused during transition from CBL to PBL. Most of the participants indicated that:

"It (PBL) needs you to be very flexible of which it comes with a lot of work and we don't have much of time because we are doing practicals as well as theory." **(Participant K)**.

The views shared by other participants were:

"With PBL we do a lot of different topics in a short period of time and we end up struggling remembering all the condition, we lose concentration." **(Participant Q)**.

"Another challenge is that the PBL workload is too much, as a student the work load is always a challenge but in this case it was too much to a point that we ended up doing the work for the sake of just submitting." **(Participant S)**.

"I don't know if it comes with problem-based learning but I feel like our lecturers gives us less time to do the work. They will give us work on Friday and say we must submit on Tuesday." **(Participant H)**.

3.1.5. Subtheme 1.1.5: Lack of Proper Guidance from Lecturers

A lack of proper guidance from lecturers emerged as one of the subthemes. Students raised concerns to say, since the transition from CBL to PBL, they are often not guided by lecturers when given homework. As a result, this poses a challenge. Some of the comments made by participants are as follows:

"Most of the work is being done by the student without the guidance of the lecturers, it's more like you are your own lecturer." **(Participant P)**.

"Sometimes we do not get clarity in class, we are usually given a topic or condition and we go and prepare when we come back to present, there is usually no clarity as to say what you did there was wrong and what you did there was right, you should go fix here and there." **(Participant A2)**.

"Personally the challenges that I face with transiting to problem-based learning (PBL) is that, we are given a problem and we have to go and find solutions ourselves, then we present it to the lecturers after that we are not being corrected or told that this and this is wrong, they are a learning issue if we ask questions." **(Participant Q)**.

3.1.6. Subtheme 1.1.6: Learning Issues

Learning issues emerged as one of the subtheme. A "learning issue" in this context is homework given to student nurses in class if students do not reach a consensus about certain information presented. The majority of the participants raised the concern about the challenge regarding learning issues and commented as follows:

"In problem-based learning, we facilitate everything ourselves. So we end up having learning issues, then we go research about them then come back the next day and present the same thing. We are not facilitated properly or corrected by the module facilitator in most cases actually hence we end up having learning issues." **(Participant U)**.

Other participants also commented on the problem of learning issues and said:

"Regarding transition to problem-based learning, during our classes there can be something new that is raised and if we do not the answer in class, it becomes a learning issue for a very long time." (**Participant A3**).

"If we can't find the correct information or answer for that learning issue it becomes a learning issue for about three weeks." (**Participant H**).

"It can become a learning issue forever because none of us comes up with a direct answer or if we come up with the wrong answer during presentations then it's going to be a learning issue until we come up with the right answer." (**Participant A6**).

Subsequently, another participant added and commented to say:

"Adding on the learning issues, yes my colleagues are correct with this process of us getting learning issues every week instead of the lecturers correcting us-It is a problem because if we were supposed to finish one module in 10 weeks we end up taking longer to finish the module because of those learning issues." (**Participant A1**).

3.1.7. Subtheme 1.1.7: Online Problem-Based Learning

Online problem-based learning facilitation was raised as one of the subthemes. Student nurses expressed their challenges relating to the conveyance of PBL via online platforms. As a result, this affected their transition to PBL. The majority of the participants raised a serious concern about PBL that was conducted online. The majority of participants have articulated that:

"I feel like it is the online learning that is challenging so I think since we are going back to contact learning I think it is going to be much better." (**Participant P**).

"The online learning also contributed in us not really understanding the problem-based learning. Even now, we don't fully understand problem-based learning, because we have been doing it online." (**Participant W**).

"Sometimes you will find that we attend class while we are in our beds and you will fall asleep and when you wake up you did not hear anything that's the problem. Because we are attending online in our own space, we will be sleeping and the lecturers are not even aware of that." (**Participant J**).

Other participants also raised their views and mentioned that:

"We are using online platforms such as google meetings and some people have connectivity problems. They will be having the correct answer but due to connectivity problem, they cannot give that answer then it becomes a learning issue." (**Participant A1**).

"Remember most of the lessons are conducted online and we have network issues, so sometimes when there is an assistance we experience connectivity issues and end up missing that segment of the lesson." (**Participant A5**).

"Most classes are online and there are connectivity issue sometimes. This makes it hard to voice out your opinion, so we can't express ourselves like in a contact classes." (**Participant P**).

One participant highlighted that she did not have a problem with the transition from CBL to PBL. However, the main challenge with PBL was that it was conducted online and they said:

"I did not have problems or challenges with transition from case-based learning to problem-based learning, so for me the issue was more of the online problem-based learning." (**Participant S**).

3.1.8. Subtheme 1.1.8: Lack of Student Instructors (SI)

A lack of student instructors (SI) also emerged as one of the subthemes. Student nurses expressed their concern relating to a lack of student instructors in their third year of study, where they need them the most. In this context, a student instructor (SI) is any senior student that will help junior students with their studies by facilitating extra classes during their spare time. Students mentioned that in their first and second year, when they were using case-based learning, they used to have student instructors and that helped them a lot. For this reason, they believe if the same principle can be applied in third year, in which they use problem-based learning, it can help them adapt well to the PBL teaching strategy. Participants expressed their own view regarding the lack of student instructors (SI) and said:

"it is not advise perse to the students but it's a suggestion on what the lecturers maybe can do or what the school of nursing can implement, like for our ancillary modules we used to have SI. So maybe if they can introduce SI's for third and fourth years whereby other students can actually conduct classes to explain further for those who needs further explanations. Like they are senior students so they are able to explain better to the junior students." (**Participant G**).

Another participant added:

"Sometimes I just wish like we had SI for certain modules, like other student who are doing different courses have SI to help them. So in this course we don't have SI who can help us with studying like other programs in the university." (**Participant A4**).

3.2. Theme 1.2: Challenges Regarding Assessment

The second theme focused of the challenges regarding the assessment of student nurses and produced two sub-themes, namely a lack of feedback and revision. The sub-themes were discussed as follows:

3.2.1. Subtheme 1.2.1: Lack of Feedback

A lack of feedback from lecturers is another subtheme that emerged. Student nurses raised their concern to say in PBL, lecturers usually do not give feedback or correct them when they are wrong, or when they do, it is not sufficient. As a result, this impacts their assessment negatively. One participant uttered:

"With lecturers in PBL we do not get correction or feedback." (**Participant Q**).

Another participant added to say:

"Sometimes you didn't get enough feedback from the lecturer and you don't know if you are right or wrong." (**Participant N**).

3.2.2. Subtheme 1.2.2: Lack of Revision

A lack of revision was raised as one of the subthemes. Student nurses reported that there is sometimes less time to revise, which somehow results in a challenge during assessments. One participant mentioned that:

"When we are busy with the learning issues, we can't move to other topics, that way we have less time to finish that module for that semester. In that way, we don't have enough revision time for exam." (**Participant H**).

Another participants added:

"Adding on the learning issues, yes my colleagues are correct with this process of us getting learning issues every week instead of the lecturers correcting us. It is a problem because if we were supposed to finish one module in 10 weeks we end up taking longer to finish the module because of those learning issues. The duration of a module becomes longer, it can take up to 16 weeks or 17 weeks and we end up finishing late and it waste the time we should be using revising the content of that module in preparation to the upcoming tests or exams." (**Participant A1**).

3.3. Theme 1.3: Strategies to Overcome Challenges

The third theme focuses on the strategies used by student nurses to overcome challenges faced during the transition from CBL to PBL. This theme consists of four sub-themes, namely collaboration with classmates/peer-assisted learning, the use of relevant study materials such as articles, prescribed books and past question papers, the planning of study time, and consultation with lecturers. The subthemes are discussed as follows:

3.3.1. Subtheme 1.3.1: Collaboration with Classmates/Peer-Assisted Learning

Collaboration with classmates, also referred to as peer-assisted learning, emerged as one of the subthemes. Students expressed the use of peer-assisted learning as one of the strategies they used to overcome the challenges faced during the transition from case-based to problem-based learning. Different participants explained:

"I will also ask the presentations of different groups and compile and study with it together with my own work because I can not only rely on my work to help me so that's how I manage to cope." **(Participant N)**.

"Studying as a group also helps because discussing amongst ourselves also makes it easier."
(Participant Q).

"We as student decided to share the presentations and slides that we have with each other and we would discuss with each other or go into other platform like YouTube to watch videos that would give more information. It made it much better." **(Participant S)**.

Further participants added:

"What helped was to consult with each other because you may find that some else understands the problem better than I do, then we would help each other that way." **(Participant A6)**.

"Collaborated team work will assist in getting information that the lecturer will, accept at the end of the day." **(Participant Y)**.

"I will advise student to utilize good communication it helps a lot to communicate with others especially when you approaching exams it happens that there are some things that you don't understand and my friend explains to me it is easy to remember what you friend said than remembering what the lecturer said because is intimidating." **(Participant L)**.

Subsequently, other participants mentioned that:

"What I did I studied was I put more effort and I also ask my fellow class mates to explain some things better to me, because sometimes it's a bit difficult to approach the lectures so I prefer to ask my colleagues to help me where they understand." **(Participant N)**.

"Studying as a group also helps because discussing amongst ourselves also makes it easier." **(Participant Q)**.

"To add on what student M was saying I think what also help to overcome the challenges is to get different presentation from different groups as some conditions have similar symptoms so by gathering all that information you will know what makes them different."
(Participant K).

3.3.2. Subtheme 1.3.2: Use of Relevant Study Materials Such as Articles, Prescribed Books, and Past Question Papers

The use of relevant study materials such as articles, prescribed books, and past question papers emerged as one of the subthemes. Student nurses reported the use of relevant study materials such as articles, prescribed books, and previous question papers as strategy to overcome the challenges faced during the transition from CBL to PBL. Participants stated that:

"The right prescribes text books and also relying on online books for more information helped me to improve on my second semester." (**Participant K**).

"So firstly, I will start with either google scholar and find information and after I will go to the library for additional information and more sources." (**Participant W**).

Another participant added that:

"What helped me was going through past question papers to see how the lecturers are setting- that's my other coping mechanism. So that one helped a lot." (**Participant Q**).

3.3.3. Subtheme 1.3.3: Plan Study Time

The planning of study time also emerged as a subtheme. Student nurses described the proper planning of study time as one of the strategies used to overcome the challenges faced during the transition from CBL to PBL. One of the participants articulated:

"I did what all the other students did basically. I put more effort and also practice time management. I look on the dates for tests, placement and exams. It is also helps to note them down so that you plan study time for yourself thus give you time to prepare." (**Participant M**).

Another participant said:

"Prepare before time like before going to class, so to know the topics that will be done." (**Participant P**).

3.3.4. Subtheme 1.3.4: Consultation with Lecturers

Consultation with lecturers emerged as one of the subthemes. Student nurses reported consultation with lecturers as a strategy to overcome the challenges faced during the transition from CBL to PBL. Participants expressed their views and mentioned that:

"If I feel like I have questions I usually go and consult with the module facilitator or the relevant person which we are referred to by the module facilitator to consult." (**Participant U**).

"Well what I can advise others is that they should consult with the lectures because some of us failed to consult that is where we encounter problems they should consult more and also use the library they can use the scenarios on the question papers." (**Participant N**).

Another participants added:

"I also forget to add consultation the lectures give you feedback and show you what to do." (**Participant P**).

"The consultations with the lecturers were helpful because they helped us identify the areas that were troubling us too much and we would try to work on them." (**Participant A5**).

"Attending class wholeheartedly, make notes and revise after each class in order to identify the areas where challenges are. After that consult with the lecturers with informed information because some lecturers like to ask what is it that you really don't understand and you can't say everything you have to be specific on what you don't understand." (**Participant M**).

4. Discussion

The study explored and described challenges faced by student nurses during the transition from case-based learning to problem-based learning at one of the institutions of higher learning in the North West Province (NWP). The data's findings particularly identified three themes: challenges regarding facilitation, challenges regarding assessment, and strategies to overcome challenges.

4.1. Challenges Regarding Facilitation

The transition from case-based learning (CBL) to problem-based learning (PBL) has presented several challenges to student nurses. Challenges regarding facilitation appeared as the primary theme from the collected data and subthemes were also identified. Many student nurses stressed how challenging it was to transition from one teaching strategy to another. As a result, students worry excessively about their success with PBL as the newly introduced teaching strategy [13]. The same author further reported that student nurses who adapt to the PBL process experience anxiety and fear of the unknown [13]. Taken together, these findings suggest that transitioning from one teaching strategy to another requires the necessary support for student nurses.

The issue of working in groups was also reported to be a serious challenge mainly because of poor participation by most of the group members. In this context, working in groups refers to a teaching–learning method consisting of both collaborative and cooperative learning launched to achieve a common goal [14]. Pahomov (2018) stated that working in groups requires students to not just work with group members, but truly collaborate with peers to respond to a given assignment and reach a common objective [15]. However, this cannot be achieved if there is poor participation from students. Ideally, when all group members participate in group work, this leads to a product that reflects the full integration of participants' diverse skill sets [15].

Despite PBL promoting the notion that students should conduct independent information searches, the difficulty in searching for and finding relevant information on accessible databases was reported by the student nurses, particularly when one is unfamiliar with searching methods. This discrepancy could be attributed to students having difficulty in transitioning to PBL. According to Spry and Mierzwinski-Urban (2018), successful electronic information searches involve a variety of steps, including selecting the right databases for the search, relevant keywords, acceptable headings as key features, and correct spelling [16]. Finding the appropriate information will be challenging if these factors are not considered [16]. However, Scells et al. (2020) holds the view that the process that mostly influences bias is the creation of search strategies [17]. If the findings of [16,17] Spry and Mierzwinski-Urban (2018) and Scells et al. (2020) are accurate, student nurses must keep both findings in mind.

The fact that there is more work given to complete using PBL, and within a short time, was another significant challenge raised by student nurses. Abdelkarim et al. (2018) acknowledge that PBL has a variety of drawbacks, which include but are not limited to, students' preparation which somehow increases their workload and time constrains [8]. In addition, Ghufron and Ermawati's study (2018) established that it is challenging to implement PBL since it requires a lot of time, planning, and work [7]. It may be argued that it is obvious that transitioning from CBL to PBL does in fact raise challenge and time demands on student nurses. Therefore, one possible implication of this is that while using PBL to approach the curriculum, student nurses should be given adequate time.

A further challenge which emerged was lack of proper guidance from lecturers during the transition from CBL to PBL. Bouwmeester et al. (2019) added that well-informed lecturers are essential for fostering critical thinking and guiding student nurses in problem-solving techniques [18]. Salari et al. (2018) further stated that in PBL, lecturers must strive to guide students as their immediate facilitators and must be considered as a coaches who provide guidance to keep students on track [19]. These literature suggests that [18,19] have similar views. In conclusion, in order to transit properly from CBL to PBL, student nurses should be cautiously guided.

Another significant challenge brought by the student nurses was the constant ongoing learning issues with the PBL curriculum. If a group of student nurses cannot agree on a particular aspect of knowledge presented, it is a "learning issue" and homework is assigned to the students. In this context, a "learning issue" is the homework given to studenst. Consequently, the findings of the study suggest that transitioning from CBL to PBL becomes even more challenging because there are more "learning issues", which in turn result in a greater burden for students. In this regard, students are not corrected or provided with the correct answers and they even go to the examination or test without knowing the appropriate knowledge, which is a challenge because it may lead to poor performances.

A study conducted by Songsirisak and Jitpranee (2019) explains the fundamental objectives of homework, which is to evaluate students' understanding and learning progress [20]. Furthermore, it also gives students the chance to enhance their study habits, academic performance, and academic achievements. However, students' perspectives on homework vary depending on their educational backgrounds, worldviews, attitudes, and cultures [20]. Despite the purported objectives and benefits of homework, the study's finding suggests that student nurses are not content with receiving homework and have negative attitudes towards it. As a result, it can be suggested that to balance workload and ensure that students are acquiring enough knowledge at the same time, student nurses should only be assigned a reasonable workload of homework.

The study's findings also revealed that facilitating online problem-based learning was another significant challenge. This means that the student nurses attended their classes online, utilizing a problem-based learning approach. In the study conducted by García-Morales et al. (2021), students who took classes online experienced difficulties with connectivity issues caused by unexpected network outages [21]. Daugvilaite (2021) further added that disruptions to the connection or freezing of the screen during an online lesson caused students to lose focus and interrupted learning [22]. García-Morales et al. (2021) noted additional significant disadvantages of online learning, which include boredom, a feeling of isolation, a lack of time to study various subjects, and a lack of self-organizational skills [21]. The findings of this study support García-Morales's study in a sense that participants in this study also reported the same challenges.

A lack of student instructors was identified by student nurses as another critical challenge. In the context of this study, senior students in their final year who help junior students with a specific module or offer supplementary classes are known as student instructors. The lack of student instructors in third year has caused a major worry among student nurses, who feel that it disadvantages them. Peer facilitation complements adult learning theories as it unifies cognitive, social, and constructivist theories [23]. Additionally, according to Oh et al. (2018), student nurses reported feeling more comfortable sharing their own thoughts in a peer-facilitation situation and the students preferred discussion that is facilitated by their peers [24]. Moreover, students tended to contribute more original ideas and show a more engaged level of participation when peers facilitated dialogues [24]. In view of the above conversation, a similar recommendation to that made by Davis and Richardson (2017), for universities to empower second- and third-year students to peer facilitate learning sessions for first-year students, can be implemented for the third years [23].

4.2. Challenges Regarding Assessment

The challenges regarding the assessment of student nurses emerged as a second theme of the study. This entails a lack of feedback and lack of revision. The first subtheme to emerge from this theme was the lack of feedback. Seibert (2021) asserts that lecturers must be aware that student nurses require more encouragement, support, and feedback when participating in PBL for the first time to simplify their transition process [13]. On the other hand, the student nurses expressed their gratitude for the lecturers who provided feedback and support and encouragement [13]. Therefore, students should be motivated, supported, and provided with feedback to reduce any anxiety they may be experiencing as a result of taking part in PBL for the first time, thus simplifying their transitioning process.

The lack of revision by student nurses became the second subtheme for this theme. Students stated that while they struggle to transition entirely to PBL, they finish module content late, which leaves them with less time to revise for tests and examinations causing them to panic. According to Cottrell's study (2017), simply having extra time available for studying and revision can be beneficial in a sense that it somehow allays their anxiety relating to tests and examination [25]. Duret et al. (2018) noted that some students cram in the day or even hours prior to a test or examination [26]. It is clear from the literature and study findings that students require ample time for study and revision, to avoid stress and cramming during tests and examinations, because they are not really learning the relevant knowledge, skills, and attitudes inherent to the nursing profession.

4.3. Strategies to Overcome Challenges

The last theme that emerged from the findings of this study was strategies used by the student nurses to overcome the challenges faced during the transition from CBL to PBL. There were four subthemes that emerged from the main theme. The first subtheme to emerge was peer-assisted learning. According to student nurses, transitioning from CBL to PBL brought many challenges as highlighted in the study's findings. However, students developed certain strategies to overcome those challenges, such as learning from what other students do to deal with those challenges and assisting one another.

The evidence from the study findings suggests that this strategy is corroborated by the study of Abdullah and Chan (2018), which states that learning with and from peers enables one to gain learning outcomes, including teamwork, critical thinking, communication, and other skills such as coping mechanisms [27]. Similar to this, Johnson and Johnson's study (2018) established that peer-assisted learning involves classmates of equal status actively helping one another with learning-related issues [28]. Additionally, peer-assisted learning is built on collaboration because support and motivation rarely include competitive engagement [28].

Another of the subthemes that emerged was the usage of pertinent study materials, such as peer-reviewed articles, prescribed books, and past question papers. The utilization of such materials was reported by student nurses as one of the strategies to the overcome challenges they encountered during the transition from CBL to PBL. Most institutions and individuals share their learning resources on the Internet in an open and cost-free manner as open educational resources (OER), even though they are frequently regarded as important intellectual property in the competitive higher education industry [29]. According to Hylén (2021), OER are broadly characterized as digital materials that are freely and openly made available for teachers, students, and self-learners to use and re-use for teaching, learning, and research [29].

Within the higher education context, Colvard et al., (2018) state that OER normally include free, online learning content, software tools, and accumulated digital curricula that are not restricted by copyright licenses and are available to retain, reuse, revise, remix, and redistribute (5Rs). From the literature, it is clear that the usage of pertinent study material is beneficial to the students [30].

Planning study time emerged as another crucial subtheme. One of the strategies used by student nurses to overcome challenges experienced during the transition from CBL to PBL was proper time management. However, Adams and Blair (2019) state that many students struggle to strike a balance between their daily activities and their studies [31]. Effective time management is linked to better academic achievement and decreased levels of anxiety in students, as students learn coping strategies that allow them to negotiate competing demands [31,32]. Additionally, students today frequently complain that they do not have enough time to finish all the duties that have been given to them [32]. The literature supports the concept that suggest that students who plan their study time prosper academically.

Another important subtheme that emerged from the main theme was consultation with lecturers. Student nurses mentioned consultation with lecturers as a strategy for overcoming challenges during the transition from CBL to PBL. According to Agustin et al. (2020), the challenge could be students who are failing academically, which can affect other aspects of the students' lives [33]. One of the strategies to address this is to consult with lecturers who can provide counselling and guidance services, with a primary focus on academic and personal social guidance for students [33].

Furthermore, the knowledgeable lecturers can advise students to direct their explorations to accelerate learning [34]. However, the recommendations of other studies suggest that lecturer must be an expert in the subject being learned to advise students accordingly [34]. Therefore, the literature supports the student nurses' route of consulting with lecturers to assist them with the challenge they experience during the transition period.

5. Conclusions

The study explored and described challenges faced by student nurses during the transition from case-based learning to problem-based learning at one higher institution of learning in the North West Province of South Africa. The study has identified that student nurses were faced with different challenges during the transition from CBL to PBL teaching strategies. Therefore, necessary support should be given to students in order for them to cope with these challenges. However, student nurses suggested strategies that could also be used to overcome such challenges. Furthermore, the findings reported here provided new light that student nurses who are accustomed to CBL may resist taking more responsibility for their own learning when they transition to PBL. This might happen even though there is evidence in the literature which indicates that PBL adds value to the educational experience.

Author Contributions: This manuscript is based on RJP's partial fulfilment of the requirements for a Master of Nursing Science (MNSc) in Community Nursing under the supervision of B.J.M. and M.J.M. at the NWU. The draft of the manuscript was written by R.J.P. and its finalization was equally completed by B.J.M. and M.J.M. All authors have read and agreed to the published version of the manuscript.

Funding: The author(s) received no financial support for the research, however the publication fee of this article will be paid by the North West University (NWU).

Institutional Review Board Statement: The study was conducted in accordance with the Declaration of Helsinki and approved by Health Research Ethics Committee (HREC) of the North West University (Ethics reference number: NWU-00218-21-s1 on 21 January 2022).

Informed Consent Statement: Written informed consent was obtained from all participants involved in the study.

Data Availability Statement: The authors confirm that the data are available. However, it cannot be shared with anyone as per agreement established with participants according to research regulations and Protection of Personal Information Act (POPIA), protected by HREC. However, the data that support the findings of this study are available within the article.

Acknowledgments: We acknowledge the authors of sources cited in this study.

Conflicts of Interest: The authors declare no conflict of interest and have no financial nor personal relationship that could have unduly influenced the writing of this article.

References

1. Günter, T.; Alpat, S.K. The effects of problem-based learning (PBL) on the academic achievement of students studying 'Electrochemistry'. *Chem. Educ. Res. Pract.* **2017**, *18*, 78–98. [CrossRef]
2. Liu, L.; Du, X.; Zhang, Z.; Zhou, J. Effect of problem-based learning in pharmacology education: A meta-analysis. *Stud. Educ. Eval.* **2019**, *60*, 43–58. [CrossRef]
3. Bi, M.; Zhao, Z.; Yang, J.; Wang, Y. Comparison of case-based learning and traditional method in teaching postgraduate students of medical oncology. *Med. Teach.* **2019**, *41*, 1124–1128. [CrossRef]
4. Hassoulas, A.; Forty, E.; Hoskins, M.; Walters, J.; Riley, S. A case-based medical curriculum for the 21st century: The use of innovative approaches in designing and developing a case on mental health. *Med. Teach.* **2017**, *39*, 505–511. [CrossRef] [PubMed]
5. Ali, M.; Han, S.C.; Bilal, H.S.; Lee, S.; Kang, M.J.; Kang, B.H.; Razzaq, M.A.; Amin, M.B. iCBLS: An interactive case-based learning system for medical education. *Int. J. Med. Inform.* **2018**, *109*, 55–69. [CrossRef]
6. Servant-Miklos, V.F. The Harvard connection: How the case method spawned problem-based learning at McMaster University. *Health Professions Education.* **2019**, *5*, 163–171. [CrossRef]
7. Ghufron, M.A.; Ermawati, S. The strengths and weaknesses of cooperative learning and problem-based learning in EFL writing class: Teachers' and students' perspectives. *Int. J. Instr.* **2018**, *11*, 657–672. [CrossRef]
8. Abdelkarim, A.; Schween, D.; Ford, T.G. Advantages and disadvantages of problem-based learning from the professional perspective of medical and dental faculty. *EC Dent. Sci.* **2018**, *17*, 1073–1079.
9. Rakhudu, M.A.; Davhana-Maselesele, M.; Useh, U. Concept analysis of collaboration in implementing problem-based learning in nursing education. *Curationis* **2016**, *39*, 1–3. [CrossRef]

10. Deane, W.H. Transitioning to concept-based teaching: A qualitative descriptive study from the nurse educator's perspective. *Teach. Learn. Nurs.* **2017**, *12*, 237–241. [CrossRef]
11. Jindal-Snape, D.; Cantali, D.; MacGillivray, S.; Hannah, E. Primary-secondary transitions: A systematic literature review. *Soc. Res.* **2019**.
12. Krishnasamy, M.; Hassan, H.; Jewell, C.; Moravski, I.; Lewin, T. Perspectives on Emotional Care: A Qualitative Study with Cancer Patients, Carers, and Health Professionals. *Healthcare* **2023**, *11*, 452. [CrossRef]
13. Seibert, S.A. Problem-based learning: A strategy to foster generation Z's critical thinking and perseverance. *Teach. Learn. Nurs.* **2021**, *16*, 85–88. [CrossRef]
14. Wong, F.M. A phenomenological research study: Perspectives of student learning through small group work between undergraduate nursing students and educators. *Nurse Educ. Today* **2018**, *68*, 153–158. [CrossRef]
15. Pahomov, L. Inventories, Confessionals, and Contracts: Strategies for Effective Group Work. *Educ. Leadersh.* **2018**, *76*, 34–38.
16. Spry, C.; Mierzwinski-Urban, M. The impact of the peer review of literature search strategies in support of rapid review reports. *Res. Synth. Methods* **2018**, *9*, 521–526. [CrossRef]
17. Scells, H.; Zuccon, G.; Koopman, B.; Clark, J. A computational approach for objectively derived systematic review search strategies. In Proceedings of the European Conference on Information Retrieval 2020, Lisbon, Portugal, 14–17 April 2020; Springer: Cham, Switzerland, 2020; pp. 385–398.
18. Bouwmeester, R.A.; de Kleijn, R.A.; van den Berg, I.E.; ten Cate, O.T.; van Rijen, H.V.; Westerveld, H.E. Flipping the medical classroom: Effect on workload, interactivity, motivation and retention of knowledge. *Comput. Educ.* **2019**, *139*, 118–128. [CrossRef]
19. Salari, M.; Roozbehi, A.; Zarifi, A.; Tarmizi, R.A. Pure PBL, Hybrid PBL and Lecturing: Which one is more effective in developing cognitive skills of undergraduate students in pediatric nursing course? *BMC Med. Educ.* **2018**, *18*, 195. [CrossRef] [PubMed]
20. Songsirisak, P.; Jitpranee, J. Impact of homework assignment on students' learning. *J. Educ. Naresuan Univ.* **2019**, *21*, 1–19.
21. García-Morales, V.J.; Garrido-Moreno, A.; Martín-Rojas, R. The transformation of higher education after the COVID disruption: Emerging challenges in an online learning scenario. *Front. Psychol.* **2021**, *12*, 616059. [CrossRef] [PubMed]
22. Daugvilaite, D. Exploring perceptions and experiences of students, parents and teachers on their online instrumental lessons. *Music Educ. Res.* **2021**, *23*, 179–193. [CrossRef]
23. Davis, E.; Richardson, S. How peer facilitation can help nursing students develop their skills. *Br. J. Nurs.* **2017**, *26*, 1187–1191. [CrossRef] [PubMed]
24. Oh, E.G.; Huang, W.H.; Mehdiabadi, A.H.; Ju, B. Facilitating critical thinking in asynchronous online discussion: Comparison between peer-and instructor-redirection. *J. Comput. High. Educ.* **2018**, *30*, 489–509. [CrossRef]
25. Cottrell, S. *The Exam Skills Handbook: Achieving Peak Performance*; Bloomsbury Publishing: London, UK, 2017.
26. Duret, D.; Christley, R.; Denny, P.; Senior, A. Collaborative learning with PeerWise. *Res. Learn. Technol.* **2018**, *26*, 1–3. [CrossRef]
27. Abdullah, K.L.; Chan, C.M. A systematic review of qualitative studies exploring peer learning experiences of undergraduate nursing students. *Nurse Educ. Today* **2018**, *71*, 185–192.
28. Johnson, D.W.; Johnson, R.T. Cooperative learning: The foundation for active learning. In *Active Learning—Beyond the Future*; IntechOpen: London, UK, 2018.
29. Hylén, J. Open educational resources: Opportunities and challenges. *Proc. Open Educ.* **2006**, 4963.
30. Colvard, N.B.; Watson, C.E.; Park, H. The impact of open educational resources on various student success metrics. *Int. J. Teach. Learn. High. Educ.* **2018**, *30*, 262–276.
31. Adams, R.V.; Blair, E. Impact of time management behaviors on undergraduate engineering students' performance. *Sage Open* **2019**, *9*, 2158244018824506. [CrossRef]
32. Razali, S.N.A.M.; Rusiman, M.S.; Gan, W.S.; Arbin, N. The impact of time management on students' academic achievement. *J. Phys. Conf. Ser.* **2018**, *995*, 012042. [CrossRef]
33. Agustin, M.; Setiyadi, R.; Puspita, R.D. Burnout profile of elementary school teacher education students (ESTES): Factors and implication of guidance and counseling services. *Primary Edu. J. Prim. Educ.* **2020**, *4*, 38–47. [CrossRef]
34. Supriyanto, A.; Hartini, S.; Irdasari, W.N.; Miftahul, A.; Oktapiana, S.; Mumpuni, S.D. Teacher professional quality: Counselling services with technology in Pandemic COVID-19. *Couns. J. Bimbing. Dan Konseling* **2020**, *10*, 176–189. [CrossRef]

Disclaimer/Publisher's Note: The statements, opinions and data contained in all publications are solely those of the individual author(s) and contributor(s) and not of MDPI and/or the editor(s). MDPI and/or the editor(s) disclaim responsibility for any injury to people or property resulting from any ideas, methods, instructions or products referred to in the content.

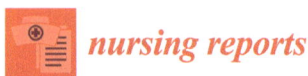

Study Protocol

Nurses' Motivations, Barriers, and Facilitators to Engage in a Peer Review Process: A Qualitative Study Protocol

Júlio Belo Fernandes [1,2,3,*], Josefa Domingos [1,2], John Dean [4], Sónia Fernandes [2,3], Rogério Ferreira [5,6], Cristina Lavareda Baixinho [7,8], Cidália Castro [1,2,3], Aida Simões [1,2,3], Catarina Bernardes [1,2,3], Ana Silva Almeida [9], Sónia Loureiro [10], Noélia Ferreira [1,9], Isabel Santos [11] and Catarina Godinho [1,2,3]

1. Grupo de Patologia Médica, Nutrição e Exercício Clínico (PaMNEC), 2829-511 Almada, Portugal
2. Centro de Investigação Interdisciplinar Egas Moniz (CiiEM), 2829-511 Almada, Portugal
3. Escola Superior de Saúde Egas Moniz, 2829-511 Almada, Portugal
4. Triad Solutions, Aurora, CO 80012, USA
5. Instituto Politécnico de Beja, Escola Superior de Saúde, Departamento de Saúde, 7800-111 Beja, Portugal
6. Comprehensive Health Research Center, 7004-516 Évora, Portugal
7. Nursing School of Lisbon, 1900-160 Lisbon, Portugal
8. Nursing Research, Innovation and Development Centre of Lisbon (CIDNUR), 1900-160 Lisbon, Portugal
9. Department of Nursing, Centro Hospitalar de Setúbal E.P.E., 2910-446 Setúbal, Portugal
10. Department of Nursing, Hospital Garcia de Orta E.P.E., 2805-267 Almada, Portugal
11. Department of Nursing, Unidade de Cuidados na Comunidade de Palmela, 2950-483 Palmela, Portugal

* Correspondence: juliobelo01@gmail.com

Abstract: Peer review supports the integrity and quality of scientific publishing. However, although it is a fundamental part of the publishing process, peer review can also be challenging for reviewers, editors, and other stakeholders. The present study aims to explore the nurses' motivations, barriers, and facilitators in engaging in a peer review process. This qualitative, descriptive exploratory study will be developed in partnerships with three research centers. Researchers followed the consolidated criteria for reporting qualitative research (COREQ) checklist to ensure the quality of this study protocol. According to the selection criteria, the purposive sampling will be used to recruit nurse researchers that act as peer reviewers for several scientific journals in various fields of knowledge. Interviews will be conducted until data have been sufficiently consistent with meeting the initial objectives. Researchers will develop a guide comprising a set of open-ended questions to collect participants' characteristics, descriptive review behavior, and perceptions regarding their motivations, barriers, and facilitators. Researchers will analyze data using an inductive process of content analysis with the help of the QDA Miner Lite database. Findings from this study will generate knowledge that may help stakeholders identify facilitating factors and barriers and guide the development of strategies to remove or minimize these barriers.

Keywords: nurses; peer review; motivation; challenges; difficulties; facilitators

Citation: Belo Fernandes, J.; Domingos, J.; Dean, J.; Fernandes, S.; Ferreira, R.; Baixinho, C.L.; Castro, C.; Simões, A.; Bernardes, C.; Almeida, A.S.; et al. Nurses' Motivations, Barriers, and Facilitators to Engage in a Peer Review Process: A Qualitative Study Protocol. *Nurs. Rep.* **2023**, *13*, 307–314. https://doi.org/10.3390/nursrep13010029

Academic Editors: Antonio Martínez-Sabater, Elena Chover-Sierra and Carles Saus-Ortega

Received: 30 December 2022
Revised: 18 February 2023
Accepted: 20 February 2023
Published: 22 February 2023

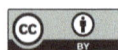

Copyright: © 2023 by the authors. Licensee MDPI, Basel, Switzerland. This article is an open access article distributed under the terms and conditions of the Creative Commons Attribution (CC BY) license (https://creativecommons.org/licenses/by/4.0/).

1. Introduction

Since the 17th century, peer review has been vital in scientific communication in journals [1]. The process of peer review advanced more systematically as a result of the measurable development of research output and expanded fields of specialization [2,3]. Although the concept of peer review is ordinarily used, we can identify different definitions of the term in various scientific journals [3]. Regardless of the several kinds of peer review, the focal aim is to guarantee the integrity and quality of research by evaluating the articles' quality, validity, and originality [4]. The peer reviewer role implies assessing the submitted manuscripts and providing truthful and unbiased feedback to both the authors and editors. To act as peer reviewers, nurses, along with being fair, unbiased, and professional, must be experts in the research being reviewed [5]. By assuming the reviewer role, nurses agree to protect the vital principles of scientific research and to safeguard that research in a practiced manner that is best and safest for the study participants. Peer review is at the heart of the practices of not just scientific journals but of all of science [6]. It supports the integrity and quality of all scientific publishing processes [5]. When employed correctly, peer review has the potential to move science forward [7].

Although it is a crucial part of the scientific publishing process, peer review can also be a largely unrecognized and unacknowledged role. The peer review process can be unquestionably challenging from different perspectives. Authors must face criticism and respond by defending or changing their points of view. Editors sometimes must make tough decisions on their fellow scientists' work, and peer reviewers spend their time uncompensated [8]. Publons estimated that in 2018–2019 the prime 1% of peer reviewers of scientific papers had invested more than 1.3 million hours reviewing [5].

Peer reviewing should be a rewarding task that not only enhances the trust and understanding in research but also has the potential to hasten the nurse's research and academic career [5,9].

The peer review process is one of the most authentic cases of how fellow nurse scientists support one another in shaping a field. All processes of peer review, including the editors' guidance, reviewers' comments, and the authors' responses to debating or acknowledging the expert opinions can give rise to insights of all kinds and inspiration [8].

One major step of the peer review process is choosing adequate peer reviewers. This step is a gatekeeper to the entire peer review process, and although this might appear to be an easy task, this step can be very challenging and rate-limiting for editors. Unfortunately, it is common for a manuscript's assigned editor to obtain recurrent peer rejections to review an article. Even though nurses might have legitimate reasons for refusal, this decision makes the peer review process challenging and time-consuming [10].

As the role of peer reviewer receives more recognition, we expect it will encourage more fellow nurse researchers to accept this role. However, at present, the quest to find committed, high-quality, experienced nurse reviewers available to invest their time in the review process is the core challenge for scientific journals worldwide [5]. This quest becomes even more challenging in nursing because there are various fields in which a nurse may decide to specialize. The guide to nursing specializations and concentrations lists more than 100 nursing specialties [11]. This varied offer allows nurses to advance towards acquiring knowledge and skills in different fields, becoming experts in that area. However, this high level of specialization may limit their participation in peer review processes related to topics outside their specific area of expertise. In addition, we should consider the worldwide shortage of nurses [12], and the results of several studies demonstrating the burden felt by these professionals [13–15].

There is an unmet need to understand these challenges and how to overcome them and facilitate the review process, and to offer more support to reviewers. There is limited knowledge about the reviewers' perspective on participating in the peer review process; therefore, this research explores the nurses' motivations, barriers, and facilitators to engaging in a peer review process.

2. Methods

2.1. Study Design

This is a qualitative study that will use a descriptive exploratory design to explore the nurses' motivations, barriers, and facilitators to engaging in a peer review process. Descriptive exploratory designs are used to investigate a research phenomenon that has not been studied in depth and gather a deeper understanding of a specific phenomenon and its context [16,17].

To ensure the quality of this study protocol, researchers followed the consolidated criteria for reporting qualitative research (COREQ) checklist [18].

2.2. Time Period

The study will be developed from January 2023 to December 2023 (Gantt Chart, Table 1).

Table 1. Project schedule.

Months	1	2	3	4	5	6	7	8	9	10	11	12
Planning	x	x	-	-	-	-	-	-	-	-	-	-
Ethical approval	-	-	x	x	-	-	-	-	-	-	-	-
Participant recruitment	-	-	-	-	x	x	-	-	-	-	-	-
Data collection	-	-	-	-	x	x	x	-	-	-	-	-
Data analysis	-	-	-	-	-	x	x	x	x	x	-	-
Reporting	-	-	-	-	-	-	-	-	-	x	x	x

x: Execution time.

2.3. Setting and Participants

The research sample of this study will include scientific journal reviewers holding academic titles in nursing sciences from three research centers in Portugal. We will focus more on the richness of the cases selected than on the sample size [19,20].

We will reach out to the following:

- The Nursing Research, Innovation, and Development Centre of Lisbon (CIDNUR) is a differentiated unit of the School of Nursing in Lisbon dedicated to developing research. The CIDNUR's mission is to develop fundamental, applied, and experimental research in nursing in line with the Sustainable Development Goals and the principles of Open Science.
- The Research Centre of Egas Moniz—Cooperativa de Ensino Superior CRL (CiiEM) represents a nucleus of innovation and knowledge creation. It fosters a paradigm of translational research and teaching in collaboration with other functional structures of Egas Moniz. It also focuses strongly on community interactions in different contexts, including health, health-related sciences, and social services.
- The Comprehensive Health Research Center is a center of excellence for research, training, and innovation in health promotion, prevention, rehabilitation, and healthcare services. This consortium comprises healthcare professionals, researchers, academics, patients, and entrepreneurs who work together toward a common goal. This research center provides a unifying environment for health research, innovation, and education in public health, lifestyle, nursing, rehabilitation, and clinical research.

In 2022, these research centers aggregated 590 researchers that act as peer reviewers for several scientific journals in various fields of knowledge.

The inclusion and exclusion criteria were as follows.

Inclusion criteria:

- Be a member of one of the research centers;
- Hold an academic title in nursing sciences;
- Had performed at least one peer review for a scientific journal;
- Willingness to participate in the study.

Exclusion criteria:

- Target population unwillingness to participate or comply with all the proceedings.

Researchers will use purposive sampling, widely used in qualitative research, to identify and explore data related to the object of interest. This sampling method will allow the researcher to collect data from the best-fit participants and ensure that the results are relevant to the research context [21,22].

For the first phase of the sample selection, researchers will ask the research centers to provide an initial list of nurse professors/researchers who comply with the study inclusion/exclusion criteria. To obtain sample variation, in the second phase, we will use three criteria: academic title (Assistant Professor, Associate Professor, and Full Professor), time of experience, and time between participation in peer review processes. A previous study revealed differences between tenured and non-tenured referees in the time taken to review [23].

For this study, researchers will consider saturation, as proposed by Glaser and Strauss [24], where researchers will continue to interview new participants until data have reached sufficient consistency to meet the initial objectives. The criteria to decide when to stop sampling the different groups pertinent to a category is when data about a construct reveal no new properties nor yield any further theoretical insights regarding the phenomenon of study whereby researchers can develop properties of each category.

2.4. Data Collection Procedures

The leading researcher will be responsible for recruiting eligible participants and collecting their written informed consent. Participants will be contacted via telephone or email, presenting the research project, its aims, and the importance of the participant's collaboration.

Researchers will safeguard that the chosen location will be free of noise in an environment that ensures the participants' privacy and comfort. Therefore, interviews will be conducted in the office of the leading researcher or the participant's office. No one else will be present during the interviews besides the participant and the interviewer. Every interview will be audio-recorded.

The interviews will be conducted by an experienced researcher: a skilled interviewer [25–27] with a Ph.D. in Nursing Sciences who has no prior relationship with the participants.

The semi-structured interview will follow an interview guide to ensure that central issues are addressed. Reviewers will develop a guide comprising a set of open-ended questions to collect participants' characteristics and descriptive review behavior, covering the following:

- the reviewers' characteristics (sex, age, time of professional experience, time of experience as reviewer), and academic title;
- the characteristics of the participant's behavior (research productivity—measured by the number of articles in Scopus or Web of Science; the quantity of declined reviews; the average number of manuscripts reviewed per year; and the average time invested in each review).

A second set of questions will be developed to gather participants' perceptions regarding the following:

- the motivation for conducting reviews and the outcomes perceived;
- the reasons for declining to review;
- the barriers for review;
- the costs associated with conducting reviews;
- the reasons for accepting reviews;
- the facilitators for review;
- the incentives for the review;
- the relation between the review and the job description.

The guide will be pilot tested among colleagues to assess its suitability for this study. Colleagues will be questioned to know their perceptions regarding the interview guide and determine if they consider it to be sufficiently clear, objective, comprehensive, and to not present questions that could be ambiguous or equivocal.

Based on previous experience, researchers estimate that each interview will take approximately 40 min.

2.5. Data Analysis

We will transcribe verbatim the audio-recorded interviews into a Word file. The final version of the interview transcripts will be returned to participants to assess any discrepancies and provide additional elucidation that may improve data accuracy.

To guarantee the participants' anonymity, in the verbatim transcription, the participants' identification will be replaced by a unique code number (for example, P1, P2, P3, etc.).

Descriptive statistic measures of count, mean (variables sex and academic title), standard deviation, median, minimum, maximum, and range (variables age, time of professional experience, and time of experience as reviewer) will be computed for sample characterization, using the IBM Statistic Package for the Social Sciences software (IBM Corp. Released 2020. IBM SPSS Statistics for Windows, Version 27.0. Armonk, NY, USA: IBM Corp.).

The data analysis of open-ended questions will be conducted by two researchers independently. Textual data from open-ended questions will be exported to the QDA Miner Lite database and analyzed using an inductive process of content analysis as described by Braun, Clarke, Hayfield, and Terry [28]. This process will involve comprehensive readings of the interview transcripts to derive concepts and categories, which allow findings to arise straight from the data analysis rather than from a priori expectations or models.

Therefore, researchers will start with reading the interviews in detail several times. This process will identify differences and similarities between the participants' speech, allowing researchers to see patterns and create initial categories.

The text will be separated into different meaning units of words, phrases, and passages that focus on the same topic. Then, researchers will assign codes to the meaning units and categories using the participants' own words. The codes will reflect the differences and similarities in the participants' perceptions regarding the phenomenon in the study.

Any differences identified during the analysis will be resolved by discussion between the two researchers. If a consensus is not reached, a third researcher will analyze the discrepancy.

Afterward, the research team will review the analysis of data made by the first two researchers and match each quote to one of the identified themes. Finally, the categories and organizing framework will be shared with other researchers external to the study to ratify the final results.

2.6. Trustworthiness

We will implement practices recommended by Nowell, Norris, White, and Moules [29] to ensure the study's trustworthiness. To guarantee credibility, researchers will discuss and detail every decision until consensus during the analysis process and return the initial themes and organizing framework to participants to ratify the researchers' interpretations. In addition, the information on the participants' characteristics and study context will be provided in detail, and participant quotations will be provided through the study report to ensure that readers who sought to transfer the findings to another context could judge transferability. Regarding the study's dependability, researchers will detail every step of the decision-making process to ensure readers can follow the research. Finally, to safeguard confirmability, researchers will request a team of external investigators experienced in qualitative research to search for inconsistencies by comparing their perceptions with those of the researchers.

2.7. Ethics and Procedures

Researchers will conduct this research following the Helsinki Declaration (as revised in 2013) and seek approval from the research center's ethics committee.

In addition, all the participants must sign the informed consent form. The informed consent form will state that participation in this study is entirely voluntary. Therefore, participants are free to not reply to some questions, change or review their responses, or voluntarily quit at any time.

All data will be conducted in compliance with ethical principles guaranteeing the participants' anonymity and confidentiality. Consequently, no individual data will be accessible, a unique code number will replace participants' identification, and only the leading researcher and the interviewer will have access to the identification sheet.

The leading researcher will archive vital documents in a way that ensures that they are readily available, upon request, to the competent authorities. All paper documents will be stored in a locked file. Digital data will be coded and stored on a password-protected computer. After the verbatim transcription, all the audio-recorded data will be destroyed. All data will remain locked in a file cabinet at Egas Moniz University for five years. The leading researcher will destroy all data when this retention period is complete.

3. Discussion

Little is known about the factors that influence the review process. We will study the nurses' motivations, barriers, and facilitators to engage in a peer review process using qualitative research. This study will improve our knowledge regarding the challenges reviewers face in participating in a peer review process and what motivates them to continue to perform peer reviews. Identifying these factors may allow the development of strategies to support nurses' participation in a peer review.

Through peer review, scientific journals validate the published research manuscript and automatically receive credibility [1,5]. High-quality peer review is significant to legitimize the science we publish [5]. A fair, unbiased, and quality review can be challenging to achieve [6]. Although peer review is considered vital to academic quality [4,5] and has the potential to move nursing science forward [7], it is challenging for editors for several reasons, such as difficulty in recruiting expert reviewers with a variety of areas of knowledge and bias in choosing from a list of reviewers who might not be willing or have time available to review the article over the established period [4,6,30].

Even in the case of rejection, when peer preview is performed correctly, it can have positive results for nursing science, as editors will communicate that decision followed by an explanation of the manuscript limitations that led to its rejection and the reviewers' constructive suggestions on how the research could be improved [5].

After completing this study, the team of researchers will work with the research centers to address the barriers to engaging in a peer review process. The peer review process is at the heart of the practices of all science [6]. It is imperative that research centers, in addition to scientific journals, develop strategies that support the participation of nurse researchers in peer review processes.

We draw attention to the fact that peer review needs to be a highly acknowledged and recognized role by the scientific community. The discussion concerning the consequences of external incentives for peer reviewers remains open. Previous studies analyzing the effects of the external review incentives given by the journal or affiliated institution were not enlightening, as Zaharie and Osoian's [3] study identified that the reviewers' internal motivation diminishes in the presence of external rewards. Unlike these results, Chetty, Emmanuel, and Laszlo´s study [23] revealed that cash incentives significantly improve the speed of the reviews. Social incentives have smaller but significant effects on review times and are especially effective among tenured professors, who are less sensitive to deadlines and cash incentives. However, the incentives provided have little or no effect on engagement rates in peer review, quality of reports, or review times at other journals.

We also draw attention to the fact that the publication of study protocols can enhance research transparency, decrease publication bias, prevent duplication of research, and alert the scientific community to know what trials are planned or ongoing, enabling other researchers to adapt and build upon previous researchers' accomplishments [31]. In addition, expert peer review feedback has the potential to help to refine and shape the submitted protocol [32]. Therefore, the publication of study protocols can help improve the medical research standard. We can identify many published study protocols in the literature, from quantitative [33–35] to qualitative [36–38] investigations to literature review protocols [39–41]. As in previously published study protocols, with the writing of this study protocol, we intend to present the aims, methodological approach, and plan to operationalize the research. The results are expected to have straight relevance to the scientific community.

We recognize that the study has limitations. First, researchers and scholars with strong views toward peer review may be unwilling to participate in this study due to perceptions related to social desirability resulting in a possible bias in participant recruitment. Alternatively, if participants perceive it to be socially desirable, they might overstate the frequency of their behavior, increasing the frequency of the positive items. Second, as in preceding studies that rely on data collected from interviews, the participants' perceptions and feelings might deviate from what they expose due to biases such as a lack of confidence in guaranteeing anonymity or protecting identity, values, or beliefs. To overcome these possible limitations, we rely on the research team's skills and experience to ensure that participants trust that their personal information, values, and beliefs will be kept anonymous and confidential while providing rich and detailed accounts of their perceptions regarding the motivations, barriers, and facilitators to engaging in peer review.

4. Conclusions

This study will be the first to explore the nurses' motivations, barriers, and facilitators to engaging in peer review. The study findings can have practical implications for stakeholders to enable improvements in the peer review process. By developing strategies to remove or minimize the influence of the identified barriers and focus on the factor that facilitates the engagement in the peer review process, stakeholders can enable fellow nurse scientists to engage in high-quality peer reviews.

Author Contributions: Conceptualization, J.B.F., J.D. (Josefa Domingos), J.D. (John Dean), S.F., R.F., C.L.B., C.C., A.S., C.B., A.S.A., I.S. and C.G.; methodology, all authors; writing—original draft preparation, all authors; writing—review and editing, all authors; supervision, J.B.F. and C.G.; project administration, J.B.F. and C.G. All authors have read and agreed to the published version of the manuscript.

Funding: This research received no external funding.

Institutional Review Board Statement: Not applicable.

Informed Consent Statement: Not applicable.

Data Availability Statement: Not applicable.

Acknowledgments: The researchers would like to thank the Centro de Investigação Interdisciplinar Egas Moniz (CiiEM) for the support provided for the publication of this article.

Conflicts of Interest: The authors have no relevant financial or non-financial competing interests to report.

References

1. Jacalyn, K.; Sadeghieh, T.; Khosrow, A. Peer Review in Scientific Publications: Benefits, Critiques, & A Survival Guide. *EJIFCC* **2014**, *25*, 227–243.
2. Ross-Hellauer, T. What is open peer review? A systematic review. *F1000Research* **2017**, *6*, 588. [CrossRef]
3. Zaharie, M.A.; Osoian, C. Peer review motivation frames: A qualitative approach. *Eur. Manag. J.* **2016**, *34*, 69–79. [CrossRef]
4. Chien, W.T. Process and quality of peer review in scientific Nursing journals. *Nurs. Rep.* **2011**, *1*, 5. [CrossRef]
5. Hillard, T.; Baber, R. Peer review: The cornerstone of scientific publishing integrity. *Climacteric* **2021**, *24*, 107–108. [CrossRef]
6. Smith, R. Peer review: A flawed process at the heart of science and journals. *J. R. Soc. Med.* **2006**, *99*, 178–182. [CrossRef]
7. Quality in peer review. *Commun. Biol.* **2019**, *2*, 352. [CrossRef]
8. DePellegrin, T.A.; Johnston, M. Opening up Peer Review. *Genetics* **2020**, *216*, 619–620. [CrossRef]
9. Warne, V. Rewarding reviewers—Sense or sensibility? A Wiley study explained. *Learn. Publ.* **2016**, *29*, 41–50. [CrossRef]
10. Medina, M.S.; Draugalis, J. "What if We All Said No?": Removing Barriers to Peer Review. *Am. J. Pharm. Educ.* **2022**, *86*, 8746. [CrossRef]
11. Staff, N. Guide to Nursing Specializations and Concentrations. 2022. Available online: https://nursejournal.org/resources/nursing-specialties-guide/ (accessed on 11 August 2022).
12. Drennan, V.M.; Ross, F. Global nurse shortages-the facts, the impact and action for change. *Br. Med. Bull.* **2019**, *130*, 25–37. [CrossRef]
13. Galanis, P.; Vraka, I.; Fragkou, D.; Bilali, A.; Kaitelidou, D. Nurses' burnout and associated risk factors during the COVID-19 pandemic: A systematic review and meta-analysis. *J. Adv. Nurs.* **2021**, *77*, 3286–3302. [CrossRef]

14. Chen, R.; Sun, C.; Chen, J.-J.; Jen, H.-J.; Kang, X.L.; Kao, C.-C.; Chou, K.-R. A Large-Scale Survey on Trauma, Burnout, and Posttraumatic Growth among Nurses during the COVID-19 Pandemic. *Int. J. Ment. Health Nurs.* **2021**, *30*, 102–116. [CrossRef]
15. Chen, C.; Meier, S. Burnout and depression in nurses: A systematic review and meta-analysis. *Int. J. Nurs. Stud.* **2021**, *124*, 104099. [CrossRef]
16. Doyle, L.; McCabe, C.; Keogh, B.; Brady, A.; McCann, M. An overview of the qualitative descriptive design within nursing research. *J. Res. Nurs.* **2019**, *25*, 443–455. [CrossRef]
17. Hunter, D.J.; McCallum, J.; Howes, D. Defining Exploratory-Descriptive Qualitative (EDQ) research and considering its application to healthcare. *J. Nurs. Health Care* **2019**, *4*, 7.
18. Tong, A.; Sainsbury, P.; Craig, J. Consolidated criteria for reporting qualitative research (COREQ): A 32-item checklist for interviews and focus groups. *Int. J. Qual. Health Care* **2007**, *19*, 349–357. [CrossRef]
19. Gupta, M.; Shaheen, M.; Reddy, K. *Qualitative Techniques for Workplace Data Analysis*; IGI Global: Hershey, PA, USA, 2018.
20. Vasileiou, K.; Barnett, J.; Thorpe, S.; Young, T. Characterising and justifying sample size sufficiency in interview-based studies: Systematic analysis of qualitative health research over a 15-year period. *BMC Med. Res. Methodol.* **2018**, *18*, 148. [CrossRef]
21. Luciani, M.; Campbell, K.; Tschirhart, H.; Ausili, D.; Jack, S.M. How to Design a Qualitative Health Research Study. Part 1: Design and Purposeful Sampling Considerations. *Prof. Inferm.* **2019**, *72*, 152–161.
22. Campbell, S.; Greenwood, M.; Prior, S.; Shearer, T.; Walkem, K.; Young, S.; Bywaters, D.; Walker, K. Purposive sampling: Complex or simple? Research case examples. *J. Res. Nurs.* **2020**, *25*, 652–661. [CrossRef]
23. Chetty, R.; Saez, E.; Sandor, L. What Policies Increase Prosocial Behavior? An Experiment with Referees at the Journal of Public Economics. *J. Econ. Perspect.* **2014**, *28*, 169–188. [CrossRef]
24. Glaser, B.G.; Strauss, A. The Discovery of Grounded Theory. In *Strategies for Qualitative Research*; Taylor & Francis Group: New York, NY, USA, 2017; p. 282.
25. Fernandes, J.B.; Fernandes, S.B.; Almeida, A.S.; Vareta, D.A.; Miller, C.A. Older Adults' Perceived Barriers to Participation in a Falls Prevention Strategy. *J. Pers. Med.* **2021**, *11*, 450. [CrossRef]
26. Fernandes, J.B.; Fernandes, S.B.; Almeida, A.S.; Cunningham, R.C. Barriers to Family Resilience in Caregivers of People Who Have Schizophrenia. *J. Nurs. Scholarsh.* **2021**, *53*, 393–399. [CrossRef]
27. Fernandes, J.B.; Vareta, D.; Fernandes, S.; Almeida, A.S.; Peças, D.; Ferreira, N.; Roldão, L. Rehabilitation Workforce Challenges to Implement Person-Centered Care. *Int. J. Environ. Res. Public Health* **2022**, *19*, 3199. [CrossRef]
28. Braun, V.; Clarke, V.; Hayfield, N.; Terry, G. *Handbook of Research Methods in Health Social Sciences*; Liamputtong, P., Ed.; Springer: Singapore, 2019.
29. Nowell, L.S.; Norris, J.M.; White, D.E.; Moules, N.J. Thematic Analysis. *Int. J. Qual. Methods* **2017**, *16*, 160940691773384. [CrossRef]
30. Gallo, S.A.; Thompson, L.A.; Schmaling, K.B.; Glisson, S.R. The Participation and Motivations of Grant Peer Reviewers: A Comprehensive Survey. *Sci. Eng. Ethics* **2020**, *26*, 761–782. [CrossRef]
31. Gray, R. Nursing Reports: Annual Report Card 2021. *Nurs. Rep.* **2022**, *12*, 397–402. [CrossRef]
32. Sorge, J. Publication of study protocols in the CJRT. *Can. J. Respir. Ther.* **2020**, *56*, v. [CrossRef]
33. Apadula, L.; Capurso, G.; Ambrosi, A.; Arcidiacono, P.G. Patient Reported Experience Measure in Endoscopic Ultrasonography: The PREUS Study Protocol. *Nurs. Rep.* **2022**, *12*, 59–64. [CrossRef]
34. Fernandes, J.B.; Ramos, C.; Domingos, J.; Castro, C.; Simões, A.; Bernardes, C.; Fonseca, J.; Proença, L.; Grunho, M.; Moleirinho-Alves, P.; et al. Addressing Ageism—Be Active in Aging: Study Protocol. *J. Pers. Med.* **2022**, *12*, 354. [CrossRef]
35. Pereira, M.G.; Vilaça, M.; Carvalho, E. Effectiveness of Two Stress Reduction Interventions in Patients with Chronic Diabetic Foot Ulcers (PSY-DFU): Protocol for a Longitudinal RCT with a Nested Qualitative Study Involving Family Caregivers. *Int. J. Environ. Res. Public Health* **2022**, *19*, 8556. [CrossRef]
36. Chen, X.; Su, J.; Bressington, D.T.; Li, Y.; Leung, S.F. Perspectives of Nursing Students towards Schizophrenia Stigma: A Qualitative Study Protocol. *Int. J. Environ. Res. Public Health* **2022**, *19*, 9574. [CrossRef]
37. Laker, C.; Knight-Davidson, P.; Hawkes, D.; Driver, P.; Nightingale, M.; Winter, A.; McVicar, A. The Use of 360-Degree Video in Developing Emotional Coping Skills (Reduced Anxiety and Increased Confidence) in Mental Health Nursing Students: A Protocol Paper. *Nurs. Rep.* **2022**, *12*, 536–544. [CrossRef]
38. Schulz, I.L.; Stegmann, R.; Wegewitz, U.; Bethge, M. The Current Practice of Gradual Return to Work in Germany: A Qualitative Study Protocol. *Int. J. Environ. Res. Public Health* **2022**, *19*, 3740. [CrossRef]
39. Morgado, T.; Lopes, V.; Carvalho, D.; Santos, E. The Effectiveness of Psychoeducational Interventions in Adolescents' Anxiety: A Systematic Review Protocol. *Nurs. Rep.* **2022**, *12*, 217–225. [CrossRef]
40. Ventura, F.; Costeira, C.R.B.; Silva, R.; Cardoso, D.; Oliveira, C. Person-Centered Practice in the Portuguese Healthcare Services: A Scoping Review Protocol. *Nurs. Rep.* **2022**, *12*, 235–244. [CrossRef]
41. Tanner, L.; Sowden, S.; Still, M.; Thomson, K.; Bambra, C.; Wildman, J. Which Non-Pharmaceutical Primary Care Interventions Reduce Inequalities in Common Mental Health Disorders? A Protocol for a Systematic Review of Quantitative and Qualitative Studies. *Int. J. Environ. Res. Public Health* **2021**, *18*, 12978. [CrossRef]

Disclaimer/Publisher's Note: The statements, opinions and data contained in all publications are solely those of the individual author(s) and contributor(s) and not of MDPI and/or the editor(s). MDPI and/or the editor(s) disclaim responsibility for any injury to people or property resulting from any ideas, methods, instructions or products referred to in the content.

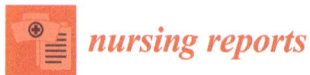

Article

The Effectiveness of NIV and CPAP Training on the Job in COVID-19 Acute Care Wards: A Nurses' Self-Assessment of Skills

Stefano Bambi [1], Eustachio Parente [2], Yari Bardacci [3], Samuele Baldassini Rodriguez [3], Carolina Forciniti [4], Lorenzo Ballerini [5], Christian Caruso [6], Khadija El Aoufy [7], Marta Poggianti [8], Antonio Bonacaro [9], Roberto Rona [10], Laura Rasero [1] and Alberto Lucchini [10],*

1. Department of Health Sciences, University of Florence, 50134 Florence, Italy
2. Neuroscience—Neurosurgery, Meyer Children's Hospital, 50139 Florence, Italy
3. Emergency and Trauma Intensive Care Unit, Careggi University Hospital, 50134 Florence, Italy
4. Medical and Surgical Intensive Care Unit, Careggi University Hospital, 50134 Florence, Italy
5. Emergency Department, Careggi University Hospital, 50134 Florence, Italy
6. Emergency Medical System—AUSL Toscana Centro, 50122 Florence, Italy
7. Department of Experimental and Clinical Medicine, University of Florence, 50121 Florence, Italy
8. Hospital Healthcare Management, Careggi University Hospital, 50134 Florence, Italy
9. School of Health and Sports Sciences, University of Suffolk, Ipswich IP4 1QJ, UK
10. General Intensive Care Unit, San Gerardo Hospital—ASST Monza, Milano Bicocca University, 20900 Monza, Italy
* Correspondence: alberto.lucchini@unimib.it or a.lucchini@asst-monza.it

Abstract: Background: Noninvasive ventilation (NIV) in COVID-19 patients outside of intensive care unit (ICU) settings was a feasible support during the pandemic outbreak. The aim of this study was to assess the effectiveness of an "on the job" NIV training program provided to 66 nurses working in 3 COVID-19 wards in an Italian university hospital. Methods: A quasi-experimental longitudinal before–after study was designed. The NIV Team education program, provided by expert ICU nurses, included: 3 h sessions of training on the job during work-shifts about the management of helmet-continuous positive airway pressure (CPAP) Venturi systems, and NIV with oronasal and full-face masks. An eleven-item "brief skills self-report tool" was administered before and after the program to explore the perception of NIV education program attendees about their level of skills. Results: In total, 59 nurses responded to the questionnaire. There was an improvement in the skill levels of the management of Helmet-CPAP (median before training 2, inter-quartile range (IQR) 0–6; median after training 8, IQR 3–9; $p < 0.0001$), and mask-NIV (median before training 2, IQR 0–6; median after training 8, IQR 3–9; $p < 0.0001$). Conclusions: Training on the job performed by expert ICU nurses can be a valuable and fast means to implement new Helmet-CPAP and mask-NIV skills outside of ICUs.

Keywords: CPAP; noninvasive ventilation; education; COVID-19; general ward; nurses

1. Introduction

In the last 15–20 years, NIV support for acute patients has been "exported" outside the intensive care unit (ICU) "walls", across high dependency units (HDUs) into general wards and finally outside the pre-hospital emergency settings [1,2]. The application of NIV on ARF patients in general medical wards is associated to high success rates, up to 80.9% [3]. During the COVID-19 pandemic BiPAP and CPAP supports have been largely employed to prevent intubation [4], reducing mortality rates, and decreasing the admission rates in ICU [5,6]. A recent systematic review showed that delivering NIV support in COVID-19 patients outside intensive care settings was a feasible strategy during the high demand of ventilatory support provided in pandemic outbreak [7]. The rate of NIV failure

Citation: Bambi, S.; Parente, E.; Bardacci, Y.; Baldassini Rodriguez, S.; Forciniti, C.; Ballerini, L.; Caruso, C.; El Aoufy, K.; Poggianti, M.; Bonacaro, A.; et al. The Effectiveness of NIV and CPAP Training on the Job in COVID-19 Acute Care Wards: A Nurses' Self-Assessment of Skills. *Nurs. Rep.* **2023**, *13*, 17–28. https://doi.org/10.3390/nursrep13010002

Academic Editors: Antonio Martínez-Sabater, Elena Chover-Sierra and Carles Saus-Ortega

Received: 2 December 2022
Revised: 19 December 2022
Accepted: 23 December 2022
Published: 27 December 2022

Copyright: © 2022 by the authors. Licensee MDPI, Basel, Switzerland. This article is an open access article distributed under the terms and conditions of the Creative Commons Attribution (CC BY) license (https://creativecommons.org/licenses/by/4.0/).

was 26% (CI 95%: 21–30%) [7]. The use of NIV or CPAP supports in COVID-19 general ward patients not appropriate for admission to intensive care unit was retrospectively associated to a survival rate of 50% [8]. Behind these data, there were some challenging issues that nurses had to deal with. On one hand there was the transformation of medical general wards in acute COVID-19 wards, by the introduction of new ventilators and CPAP systems. On the other hand, these "new" wards were filled with many newly hired nurses without skills to manage NIV technologies and the patients–interfaces–NIV system interactions [9–11]. In fact, the application of NIV requires special skills and competencies related to set-up and management of ventilators and high-flow devices, achieving adequate levels of patients' compliance to the ventilation, complication's prevention (such as discomfort, pain and interface-related pressure injuries), and optimal troubleshooting about patient–ventilator interaction. Moreover, nurses should be aware of the physical and communication needs of patients during NIV support, and especially the potential condition of anxiety, loss of control feeling and panic that the diverse typologies of interfaces could generate [12,13].

Twenty-four-seven availability of healthcare personnel with adequate skills to manage NIV patient is the clinical key to reach positive outcomes in general wards [14]. Scientific literature frequently showed the lack of doctors' and nurses' knowledge and competence about NIV [15] is the reason behind its scarce application in clinical settings [16–18]. Data from Brazil reported that only 30% of nurses have a know-how to initiate NIV support [19] and that 77% of medical personnel did not know the NIV initiation criteria [20]. The 88% of the surveyed personnel declared not to know how to set ventilator's alarms and identify patient–ventilator dissynchronies [20]. Furthermore, a European survey published in 2014 showed that in 41% of enrolled wards there were less than five nurses with adequate skills for NIV application in acute respiratory failure patients [21]. Nurses seem to have low levels of knowledge and confidence in NIV support [19]. Few nurses know how to choose the right size of NIV facial masks (35%), to identify patient–ventilator dissynchronies, and to change the ventilator's setting parameters (38%) [22]. A Delphi study published in 2012 identified nine core objectives for NIV education programs focusing on modes of ventilation, interfaces, indications and contraindications, evidence for application in various clinical conditions, set-up and initiation of NIV, troubleshooting, monitoring, failure and success indicators, and complications [23]. An adequate NIV educational program should be based on the educational needs assessment, the availability of updated guidelines, clinical procedures, and equipment. The NIV educational program should also be flexible and adaptable to the different needs of multidisciplinary team members and their individual experience levels [24]. NIV requires an education and training time directly proportional to the complex technologies used for delivering [14]. In fact, NIV failure rates are closely related to the levels of training and experience of the healthcare personnel (e.g., the application of an adequate size interface and an appropriate management can reduce air-leaks and risk of unsuccessful outcomes) [25].

Theoretical knowledge is crucial for education for every kind of issue. However, NIV education always requires a clinical practice integration to be really effective. Simulation is a promising educational and training method to acquire adequate competencies for managing NIV patients. Some studies showed that low fi manikin or off-screen feedback sessions can be helpful to reduce the time needed for becoming confident with NIV and patients' management [26,27]. Currently, NIV education performed through high-fidelity simulation is still not largely widespread [28]. An optimal NIV educational program should be composed of theoretical lectures for a third, learner–teacher interaction for a fifth, and the remaining half of time spent for training on the job. Beyond the basis of NIV management, the educational program should focus on critical issues such as nasogastric tube insertion indication, active humidification settings, intra-hospital transport, the use of high-flow oxygen therapy during the breaks from NIV treatment cycles, and the management of patients "NIV-dependent", which are patients with a very low respiratory reserve, that need to be maintained for long period under NIV support. As a general principle, one useful experience during the training course, is to don a helmet or a mask and experience NIV support and feel all the sensations and discomfort suffered by their future patients [29].

Beyond the experiences of educational programs reported by some authors and the experts' recommendations, evidence about the effectiveness of different methods in teaching the management of patients undergoing NIV is still lacking [29]. Moreover, no data about teaching and learning NIV skills in general wards during COVID-19 pandemics were still published in scientific literature.

Based on the above-mentioned issues, this study aimed to demonstrate the effectiveness of an "on the job" NIV training program provided to nurses working in COVID-19 medical wards during the second wave of the COVID-19 pandemic in an Italian university hospital.

2. Materials and Methods

2.1. Design

A quasi-experimental longitudinal single cohort before and after study was designed.

2.2. Sample and Setting

The study involved all the 66 nurses working in three acute medical wards of Careggi University Hospital converted to COVID-19 general wards at the beginning of the second wave of pandemic in October 2020.

The teams of these wards (anonymously called "1", "2", "3") were numerically enhanced with nurses coming from other hospital clinical settings temporarily in stand-by, and many newly hired nurses to consent adequate times of break during the work-shifts with personal protective equipment (PPE). Moreover, these 3 wards were equipped with new ventilators and systems to deliver NIV and CPAP to COVID-19 patients. Therefore, a large educational need emerged by nurses, to manage patients undergoing to these respiratory supports.

2.3. Procedure

The director of healthcare professions department of Careggi university hospital formed a group of four intensive care unit nurses with high skills in noninvasive ventilation and CPAP. This group, called "NIV Team", had the task to plan an on-the-job training program on NIV and CPAP for nurses.

The educational program was based on the hospital official procedure for noninvasive ventilation for patients in general ward, which was specifically updated for the safety issues related to the caring of COVID-19 patients.

The NIV Team education program included: 3 h sessions of training on the job during morning and afternoon work-shifts; the production of simple charts and videos containing the setting-up of the different Helmet-CPAP Venturi systems; and the breathing circuit of NIV performed with oronasal and full-face mask on various mechanical ventilators. Furthermore, a reserved email address was provided to collect and answer the requests of advice by nurses and other healthcare professionals in need.

Lastly, two brief checklists for NIV and CPAP management were drafted and diffused among all the nurses involved in the training program and the physicians working in the three wards.

The NIV Team training on the job program (composed of 2 training sessions) was provided between November 2020 and January 2021, during the morning and afternoon shifts. The aim of NIV Team was to guarantee the presence of at least one expert nurse to perform training-on-the-job session, until every nurse working in the ward had attended the 2 training sessions, giving immediate practical feedback to the trainer about the level of learning obtained.

The educational and training contents of the program were: "refreshing about the use of oxygen therapy, especially through high flow nasal cannula"; "principles of CPAP and NIV supports"; "set-up of Helmet-CPAP through Venturi systems and patients' management"; "set-up of NIV (Spontaneous-Time Mode; Pressure Support Ventilation) with oronasal and full-face masks, and patients' management".

The training was fitted on the educational needs of every single nurse at the bedside following these steps: (1) basic principles of oxygen-therapy and NIV were refreshed and explained; (2) demonstration of NIV and CPAP systems were performed; (3) training of the attendee was carried on until a positive feedback about the acquired skill was obtained; (4) adequate time for answers and questions was provided; (5) training on NIV and CPAP system troubleshooting was performed at the bedside.

Many models of intentional leak NIV ventilators and ICU ventilators were employed in the COVID-19 general wards, increasing the need for focused training sessions as well as for medical personnel. However, the consultations offered to physicians were performed occasionally and were not included in a structured educational program.

2.4. Data Collection and Instrument

An essential "brief skills self-report tool" was designed by the members of NIV Team to explore the perception of NIV education program attendees about their level of skills on the set-up and management of patient undergoing to Helmet-CPAP and NIV. The tool was composed of 11 items investigating the rate of some "core" learned interventions, and 2 items requiring the self-perception of the NIV and CPAP overall management skills levels, before and after the education program. The Items included in the before and after "brief skills self-report tool" with their abbreviations are listed below:

- Maintenance frequency of patients with CPAP-helmet or NIV in Fowler position (Frequency Fowler position).
- Check frequency of the Helmet-CPAP system and/or NIV, and surveillance of patients during the treatment (NIV patients check frequency).
- Frequency of respiratory rate measurement in patients with COVID-19 (RR assessment frequency).
- Frequency of application of 24 h expiring HEPA filters on the exit port of the CPAP-Helmet (HEPA 24-h application frequency).
- Check frequency of pulse-oximetry during helmet CPAP removal pauses or NIV mask breaks (Check SpO_2 frequency).
- Frequency of setting up of the Helmet-CPAP to the patients by 2 healthcare professionals (Frequency of helmet set-up by 2 nurses).
- Frequency of assessment of the Helmet-CPAP system effective performance by appreciating with gloved hands the presence of continuous gas flow leaving the PEEP valve during inspiration and exhalation (CPAP system working check frequency).
- Frequency of use of the Helmet armpits outside the arms of the patient, placing weights (sandbags) to maintain the system in place and limit air leaks [10] (Helmets armpits outside frequency).
- Frequency of use the "off" function instead of "standby" to pause the NIV mask session delivered with a single tube intentional leaks NIV ventilator (Off ventilator frequency).
- Frequency of use of traditional oxygen therapy systems (reservoir masks, standard masks, Venturi masks, nasal cannula) during breaks from Helmet-CPAP and/or NIV mask (O_2 therapy for NIV breaks frequency).
- Frequency of autonomously setting up of a single tube intentional leaks NIV ventilator (Autonomous set-up of NIV circuit frequency).
- Self-perception of skills levels in patient management with Helmet-CPAP (Helmet-CPAP skill levels).
- Self-perception of skills levels in patient management with NIV mask through single tube intentional leaks NIV ventilator (NIV skills levels).

The choice to ask the "frequency" of practicing the learned core intervention was made with the aim of obtaining an indicator of skills acquired as "less subjective" as possible. All the items were evaluated by an eleven-point numerical scale (from 0—"never" or "absent", to 10—"always" or "total").

The brief skills report tool showed high internal consistency (Cronbach Alpha values: 0.977 for all the tool items; 0.930 for the before training tool items; 0.982 for the after-training tool items).

Demographical data were also collected, such as age, gender, ward, total length of service as nurse, current ward length of service, and previously NIV courses attendance.

The before and after "brief skills self-report tool" was transferred on a Google Form sheet and administered to the attendants after a week after the end of the education program. Data were collected on an xls sheet and were stored in personal computer accessible only through a password known by the researchers.

2.5. Statistical Analysis

The collected data underwent a preprocessing (recoding) phase, and after the assessment of the not-normality of distribution through the Shapiro–Wilk test, a descriptive analysis was performed using median and quartile values. Inferential and explorative statistics were performed by non-parametrical statistics using the Wilcoxon Signed Ranks Test for paired groups to highlight the differences between the perception of skills levels before and after the training on the job, while the analysis of the skills levels inter-groups was performed through the Kruskal–Wallis Test. Categorical and binomial data were explored using Chi Square test. IBM SPSS 22 and GraphPad Prism 5 were used for statistical analysis.

2.6. Ethical Issues

The electronic form containing the NIV "brief skills self-report tool" was administered maintaining the anonymity, via the informal WhatsApp chat of the three medical wards involved by the NIV Team training program. The questionnaire did not contain any item requiring data that could identify either the single respondents or the ward of affiliation. Moreover, the data set was stored and protected following the local institutional procedures, and the data analysis was performed in an aggregate way according to the national privacy regulation.

The study was conducted as a part of the outcome evaluation of the training on the job program, after having obtained the consent of the healthcare professions direction office of the hospital.

According to local ethical committee (EC) guidelines, the administration of questionnaires to healthcare workers did not require EC formal approval.

3. Results

3.1. Characteristics of Participants

In total, 59 of the 66 nurses that attended the NIV education program (89.4%) responded to the "brief skills self-report tool" (ward 1: N.16, 27.1%; ward 2: N.23, 39%; ward 3: 20, 33.9%); 48 (81.4%) were female. The median age of respondents was 41 years (IQR 34.5–49; range 22–52). The median total length of service as staff nurse and length of service in the ward of current assignment were 15 years (IQR 10–23; range 2–38) and 6 years (IQR 4–16.5; range 1–20), respectively. None of the respondents had any post-graduate critical care or emergency courses certifications.

The respondents' characteristics, distributed by the three wards of assignment, are shown in Table 1. Although ward 3 accounted for a median age and length of service slightly lower than wards 1 and 2, the differences were not statically significant.

Table 1. Demographical characteristic of the respondents by the ward of current assignation.

Variable	Ward 1	Ward 2	Ward 3	p
Gender Female—n. (%)	14 (87.5)	20 (87)	14 (70)	0.276 [a]
Age—Median (IQR; range)	45 (38.5–49.75; 26–52)	42 (33–50.25; 24–51)	36 (29–48; 22–50)	0.113 [b]
Total length of service as staff nurse—Median (IQR; range)	19.5 (10–21.25; 6–28)	16.5 (9.5–26.5; 2–30)	13 (10–22; 4–38)	0.819 [b]
Length of service in the ward of current assignment—Median (IQR; range)	9 (4.5–17.25; 2–19)	12 (4.5–20; 1–20)	6 (1.5–8; 1–20)	0.137 [b]
NIV/CPAP education courses in the last 5 years	7 (41.2)	11 (45.8)	15 (60)	0.428 [a]

Legend: [a]—Chi square test; [b]—Kruskall–Wallis test.

3.2. Results of the "Brief Skills Self-Report Tool"

After the training on the job, the totality of nurses who filled the questionnaire showed a statistically significant increase in their perception about skill level in management patients undergoing Helmet-CPAP (median before training 2, IQR 0–6, range 0–9; versus median after training 8, IQR 3–9, range 1–10; Wilcoxon Signed Ranks Test $p < 0.0001$) and mask-NIV with single tube ventilator (median before training 2, IQR 0–6, range 0–9; versus median after training 8, IQR 3–9, range 1–10; Wilcoxon Signed Ranks Test $p < 0.0001$) (Figure 1).

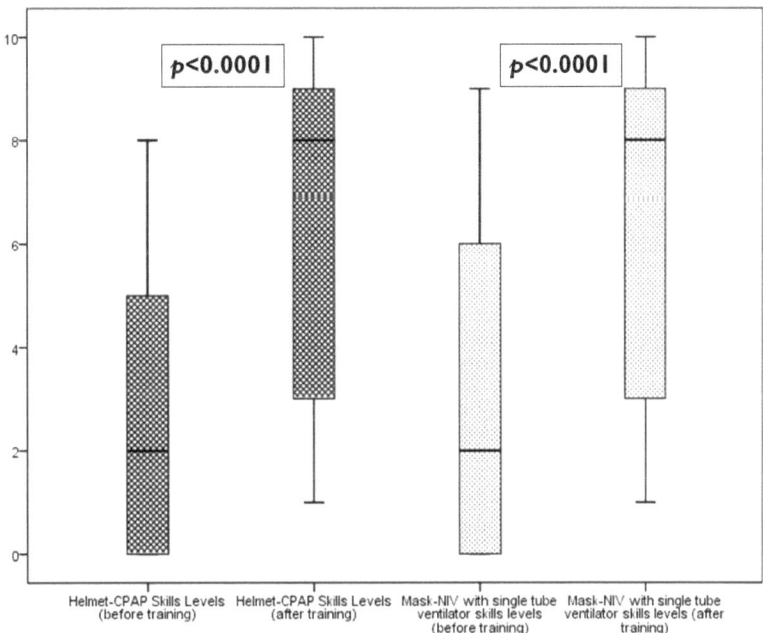

Figure 1. Comparison of Helmet-CPAP and NIV skill levels before and after the training (total sample—59 nurses).

The results of the items related to the frequency of practicing the CPAP and NIV skills before and after the education program in the total sample of nurses are shown in Table 2. The largest differences in the median values before and after the training were recorded in the items related to: (1) the application of HEPA filters at the expiratory port of the

CPAP-Helmet, (2) the control of the CPAP systems effective performance, (3) the use of sandbag weights to maintain the helmet armpits outside the arms of the patient, the set-up of a NIV ventilator breathing circuit, and (4) the use of the ventilators' off function instead of the stand-by to avoid aerosolization exposure during the removal of patients' mask for NIV-breaks. There were no statistically significant differences among the median values of the tool after the training by the three COVID-19 wards, indicating that the aims of the educational programs were homogeneously reached (Table 3). All the COVID-19 wards recorded large differences between the skills levels perceptions of nurses related to CPAP and NIV management before and after the training (Figure 2).

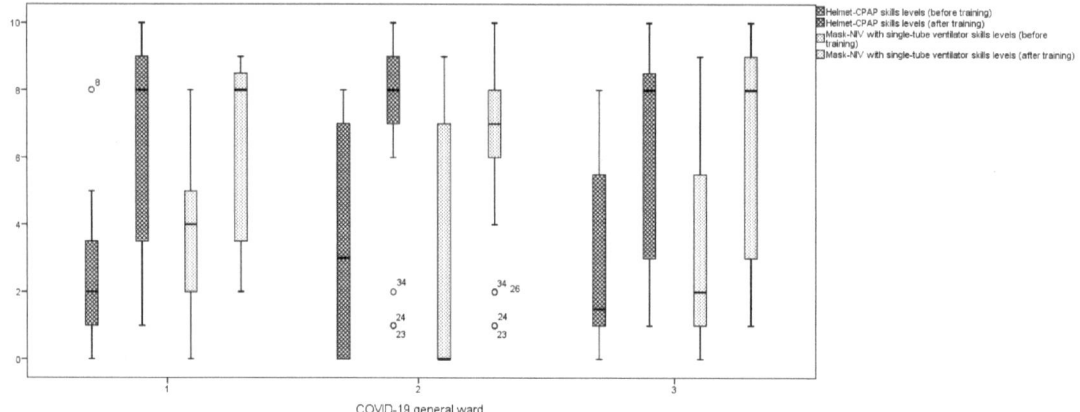

Figure 2. Comparison of Helmet-CPAP and NIV skill levels before and after the training by wards 1, 2, and 3.

Table 2. Frequency of practicing the skills before and after the training on the job in the total sample (59 nurses).

Item (Abbreviated)	Before Training Median (IQR; Range)	After Training Median (IQR; Range)	Wilcoxon SIGNED Rank Test p
Frequency Fowler position	6 (2–9; 0–10)	9 (3–10; 2–10)	<0.0001
NIV patients check frequency	5 (2–8; 0–10)	9 (3–10; 2–10)	<0.0001
RR assessment frequency	5 (2–7; 0–10)	7 (3–10; 0–10)	<0.0001
HEPA 24-h application frequency	3 (0–7; 0–10)	9 (3–10; 1–10)	<0.0001
Check SpO$_2$ frequency	5 (3–9; 0–10)	9 (3–10; 2–10)	<0.0001
Frequency of helmet set-up by 2 nurses	5 (2–8; 0–10)	8 (3–10; 1–10)	<0.0001
CPAP system working check frequency	1 (0–3.25; 0–10)	7 (3–10; 0–10)	<0.0001
Helmets armpits outside frequency	0 (0–0; 0–6)	7 (2–9; 0–10)	<0.0001
Off ventilator frequency	2 (0–6; 0–10)	8 (3–10; 0–10)	<0.0001
O$_2$ therapy for NIV breaks frequency	8.5 (3–10; 0–10)	9 (3–10; 2–10)	<0.0001
Autonomous set-up of NIV circuit frequency	2 (0–6.25; 0–10)	6 (2.5–9; 0–10)	<0.0001

Table 3. Frequency of practicing the acquired skills after the training on the job by wards 1, 2, and 3 (59 nurses).

Item (Abbreviated)	Ward 1 Median (IQR; Range)	Ward 2 Median (IQR; Range)	Ward 3 Median (IQR; Range)	Kruskall Wallis Test p
Frequency Fowler position	9 (3.5–10; 2–10)	9 (8–10; 2–10)	7.5 (2.25–10; 2–10)	0.270
NIV patients check frequency	8.5 (3.5–10; 2–10)	9 (8–10; 2–10)	7.5 (3–10; 2–10)	0.509
RR assessment frequency	6.5 (3–9.75; 1–10)	8 (3–10; 0–10)	8 (2.25–10; 2–10)	0.970
HEPA 24-h application frequency	9 (3.75–10; 2–10)	9 (8–10; 2–10)	8.5 (3–10; 1–10)	0.476
Check SpO_2 frequency	8 (3.5–9.75; 2–10)	9.5 (7.25–10; 2–10)	8 (3–10; 2–10)	0.414
Frequency of helmet set-up by 2 nurses	8.5 (3.75–10; 2–10)	8 (6–9; 2–10)	7.5 (3–10; 1–10)	0.641
CPAP system working check frequency	8 (3.25–9.75; 1–10)	7 (2–10; 0–10)	7 (3–10; 2–10)	0.755
Helmets armpits outside frequency	7.5 (4–8.75; 2–10)	7 (2–9; 0–10)	7 (2–10; 0–10)	0.764
Off ventilator frequency	9 (3–10; 1–10)	8 (2–10; 0–10)	8 (3–10; 2–10)	0.674
O_2 therapy for NIV breaks frequency	9 (4–10; 2–10)	9 (8–10; 2–10)	7 (3–10; 2–10)	0.562
Autonomous set-up of NIV circuit frequency	7.5 (3–9.25; 2–10)	6 (1–8; 0–10)	3 (2.25–9; 0–10)	0.492
Helmet-CPAP skill levels	8 (3.25–9; 1–10)	8 (7–9; 1–10)	8 (3–8.75; 1–10)	0.466
NIV skills levels	8 (3–9; 2–9)	7 (5.5–8.25; 1–10)	8 (3–9; 1–10)	0.977

Concerning risk control, periodical contacts and visits by the NIV Team members were performed across the three wards, and up until now, no adverse events related to the introduction of CPAP and NIV technologies were detected after the education program.

4. Discussion

According to a recent expert consensus, NIV and CPAP should be considered in the support of COVID-19 patients with hypoxemic and hypercapnic respiratory failure showing an increased work of breathing [30]. The benefit of NIV was largely shown in a recent review reporting that in 5120 COVID-19 patients with noninvasive respiratory support (High Flow Nasal Cannula, CPAP, or NIV), the intubation rate was 37% (1880) and survival was 78% (4669) [31].

In a survey among respiratory therapists in Saudi Arabia, the lack of training was one of the main barriers (43%) to ventilatory support management of COVID-19 patients, behind staff shortage, PPE shortage and high workload [32]. As a recent consensus paper stated, healthcare professionals with high expertise in management NIV equipment and patient–ventilator interaction are a key factor to achieve patients' positive outcomes [33] especially in long periods of NIV support application [34]. However, evidence on the best modalities to accomplish educational programs is still lacking [33]. The standards for education in NIV published in 2019 recommended the use of "simulation-based teaching" in NIV, and the need to provide "repetitive sessions depending on the degree of expertise" of the trainees [33]. The training program reported in this paper has moved one step ahead of these recommendations, because the training was provided directly in the clinical setting of the trainees and the duration of the sessions were variable on the single learned feedback.

Authors state that a reasonable NIV educational program time should be made of lectures for 30%, question time for 20%, and training for 50% [33]. The present paper reported on an experience during an emergency, with the aim of providing, in the fastest way possible, a core set of skills and competencies to be immediately applied at patients' bedsides. Therefore, about 80% of the time was spent on the hands-on training, while an essential theoretical refreshing was being provided. In fact, all the education sessions were performed inside the COVID-19 wards, and the speaking for long time could be exhausting for the trainers, due to the presence of personal protective equipment (PPE).

Ramirez et al. (2020) reported that the 58% of patients with CPAP support in COVID-19 internal medicine wards underwent at least a session of prone positioning [35]. The NIV Team training on the job program did not include any specific issue related to the nursing during NIV or CPAP patients undergoing prone position, even if the contents of this educational program covered all the aspects related to the monitoring and management of patients' interactions with the noninvasive respiratory supports, fitting also prone-positioned patients.

Recent research performed on CPAP support applied in COVID-19 wards found high discontinuation rates of CPAP among patients, probably due to an increasing burden of treatment that deserves to be investigated [36]. This potential element should also be taken into account in designing educational programs for nurses because the endurance of patients undergoing to CPAP and NIV support is one of the keys for the treatment success.

Robinson et al. (2021) reported the implementation of CPAP delivered using domiciliary ventilators in an Infectious Disease unit in a UK NHS hospital during the first wave of the COVID-19 pandemic [37]. The ward staff were adequately trained for the use of CPAP home ventilators and supported by the local critical care team. The authors reported a median CPAP length of treatment of 4 days (range 2–5), and 65% of patients (17/26) that avoided the endotracheal intubation were treated [37]. Even if the experience of NIV Team training on the job program lacked in the measures of similar hard outcomes, the reported results show that the aim of education was fully reached because all of the expected behaviors were improved.

Limitations

This study was affected by some limitations due to the "hard time" when it was conducted. The COVID-19 pandemic "healthcare emergency" required a rapid and effective response to new needs coming from the lack of skills and knowledge about new technologies introduced in "usual" low-complexity care settings. Therefore, the choice of the study design was inevitably a quasi-experimental research, with a higher exposure to unobservable sources of bias and confounding (e.g., self-selection bias, differential motivation, previous work experience in critical care settings) than an experimental design, thus limiting the evidence emerging from this study

The evaluation of acquired skills of the nurses attending to the educational program was performed through a self-report tool. Moreover, this tool, even if very simple, did not undergo any validity tests. Finally, we cannot exclude a recall bias (especially for the pre-training item responses) due to the fact that the administration of the tool occurred only after the educational program was termed. Moreover, we could not prevent the possibility of some contaminations among the samples during the filling of the questionnaires; however, this potential bias could have occurred only inside the single wards, not between a ward and another. Thus, the lack of adoption of a validated tool for competency assessment remains probably the main limitation of this study.

The only other mean of skills assessment used by NIV Team was the feedback provided by the trainees during the educational sessions.

No other objective outcomes of this education program could be collected and measured due to the wards' difficulties

5. Conclusions

Educational programs based on training on the job performed by expert professionals can be a valuable and fast means of implementing or updating new Helmet-CPAP and mask-NIV patients' management skills among nurses outside of intensive care settings.

Objective quality indicators as an observational performance checklist or ex post exams to evaluate the maintaining of acquired skills should be implemented.

Since the reconversions of some wards to no-COVID-19 wards, the maintenance of CPAP and NIV competencies and skills should be conducted through refreshing sessions in a high-fidelity-simulation environment and evaluated by study designs with robust internal validity.

Author Contributions: Conceptualization, S.B., Y.B., L.B., C.C., M.P. and L.R.; methodology, S.B., L.R., A.L. and K.E.A.; software, E.P. and S.B.; validation, E.P., S.B.R. and A.L.; formal analysis, S.B. and E.P.; investigation, S.B., Y.B., L.B., C.C., M.P. and L.R.; resources, C.F. and S.B.; data curation, E.P.; writing—original draft preparation, S.B., E.P. and C.F.; writing—review and editing, R.R., A.L. and A.B.; visualization, R.R. and A.B.; supervision, L.R.; project administration, S.B., Y.B. and S.B.R.; funding acquisition, none. All authors have read and agreed to the published version of the manuscript.

Funding: This study was not supported by any external funding.

Institutional Review Board Statement: According to local ethical committee policies, no authorization was needed for this study since patients were not involved in this research.

Informed Consent Statement: Informed consent to participate in this study was required before administering the anonymous "brief skills assessment tool".

Data Availability Statement: Data of this study are available on request to the corresponding author.

Acknowledgments: The authors wish to express their gratitude to all the nurses of medical wards in Careggi University Hospital who cared for COVID-19 patients and faced with enthusiasm and courage the challenge of learning NIV skills in a short time and in the most difficult moment of their professional lives.

Conflicts of Interest: The authors state that they have no conflict of interest in the drafting of this paper.

References

1. Crimi, C.; Noto, A.; Princi, P.; Esquinas, A.; Nava, S. A European survey of noninvasive ventilation practices. *Eur. Respir. J.* **2010**, *36*, 362–369. [CrossRef] [PubMed]
2. Crimi, C.; Noto, A.; Princi, P.; Nava, S. Survey of non-invasive ventilation practices: A snapshot of Italian practice. *Minerva Anestesiol.* **2011**, *77*, 971–978. [PubMed]
3. Ventrella, F.; Giancola, A.; Cappello, S.; Pipino, M.; Minafra, G.; Carbone, M.; Caccetta, L.; Insalata, M.; Iamele, L. Use and performance of non-invasive ventilation in Internal Medicine ward: A real-life study. *Ital. J. Med.* **2015**, *9*, 260–267. [CrossRef]
4. Oranger, M.; Gonzalez-Bermejo, J.; Dacosta-Noble, P.; Llontop, C.; Guerder, A.; Trosini-Desert, V.; Faure, M.; Raux, M.; Decavele, M.; Demoule, A.; et al. Continuous positive airway pressure to avoid intubation in SARS-CoV-2 pneumonia: A two-period retrospective case-control study. *Eur. Respir. J.* **2020**, *56*, 2001692. [CrossRef] [PubMed]
5. Franco, C.; Facciolongo, N.; Tonelli, R.; Dongilli, R.; Vianello, A.; Pisani, L.; Scala, R.; Malerba, M.; Carlucci, A.; Negri, E.A.; et al. Feasibility and clinical impact of out-of-ICU noninvasive respiratory support in patients with COVID-19-related pneumonia. *Eur. Respir. J.* **2020**, *56*, 2002130. [CrossRef]
6. Coppadoro, A.; Zago, E.; Pavan, F.; Foti, G.; Bellani, G. The use of head helmets to deliver noninvasive ventilatory support: A comprehensive review of technical aspects and clinical findings. *Crit. Care* **2021**, *25*, 327. [CrossRef]
7. Cammarota, G.; Esposito, T.; Azzolina, D.; Cosentini, R.; Menzella, F.; Aliberti, S.; Coppadoro, A.; Bellani, G.; Foti, G.; Grasselli, G.; et al. Noninvasive respiratory support outside the intensive care unit for acute respiratory failure related to coronavirus-19 disease: A systematic review and meta-analysis. *Crit. Care* **2021**, *25*, 268. [CrossRef]
8. Burns, G.P.; Lane, N.D.; Tedd, H.M.; Deutsch, E.; Douglas, F.; West, S.D.; Macfarlane, J.G.; Wiscombe, S.; Funston, W. Improved survival following ward-based non-invasive pressure support for severe hypoxia in a cohort of frail patients with COVID-19: Retrospective analysis from a UK teaching hospital. *BMJ Open Respir. Res.* **2020**, *7*, e000621. [CrossRef]
9. Lucchini, A.; Giani, M.; Elli, S.; Villa, S.; Rona, R.; Foti, G. Nursing Activities Score is increased in COVID-19 patients. *Intensive Crit. Care Nurs.* **2020**, *59*, 102876. [CrossRef]
10. Lucchini, A.; Giani, M.; Isgrò, S.; Rona, R.; Foti, G. The "helmet bundle" in COVID-19 patients undergoing non invasive ventilation. *Intensive Crit. Care Nurs.* **2020**, *58*, 102859. [CrossRef]
11. Jackson, D.; Bradbury-Jones, C.; Baptiste, D.; Gelling, L.; Morin, K.; Neville, S.; Smith, G.D. Life in the pandemic: Some reflections on nursing in the context of COVID-19. *J. Clin. Nurs.* **2020**, *29*, 2041–2043. [CrossRef] [PubMed]

12. Sørensen, D.; Frederiksen, K.; Grøfte, T.; Lomborg, K. Practical wisdom: A qualitative study of the care and management of non-invasive ventilation patients by experienced intensive care nurses. *Intensive Crit. Care Nurs.* **2013**, *29*, 174–181. [CrossRef] [PubMed]
13. Torheim, H.; Gjengedal, E. How to cope with the mask? Experiences of mask treatment in patients with acute chronic obstructive pulmonary disease-exacerbations. *Scand J. Caring Sci.* **2010**, *24*, 499–506. [CrossRef] [PubMed]
14. Elliott, M.W.; Confalonieri, M.; Nava, S. Where to perform noninvasive ventilation? *Eur. Respir. J.* **2002**, *19*, 1159–1166. [CrossRef] [PubMed]
15. Rose, L. Management of critically ill patients receiving noninvasive and invasive mechanical ventilation in the emergency department. *Open Access Emerg. Med.* **2012**, *4*, 5–15. [CrossRef]
16. Cox, C.E.; Carson, S.S.; Ely, E.W.; Govert, J.A.; Garrett, J.M.; Brower, R.G.; Morris, D.G.; Abraham, E.; Donnabella, V.; Spevetz, A.; et al. Effectiveness of medical resident education in mechanical ventilation. *Am. J. Respir. Crit. Care Med.* **2003**, *167*, 32–38. [CrossRef]
17. Bierer, G.B.; Soo Hoo, G.W. Noninvasive ventilation for acute respiratory failure: A national survey of Veterans Affairs hospitals. *Respir. Care* **2009**, *54*, 1313–1320.
18. Cabrini, L.; Esquinas, A.; Pasin, L.; Nardelli, P.; Frati, E.; Pintaudi, M.; Matos, P.; Landoni, G.; Zangrillo, A. An international survey on noninvasive ventilation use for acute respiratory failure in general non-monitored wards. *Respir. Care* **2015**, *60*, 586–592. [CrossRef]
19. Nápolis, L.M.; Jeronimo, L.M.; Baldini, D.V.; Machado, M.P.; de Souza, V.A.; Caruso, P. Availability and use of noninvasive ventilation in the intensive care units of public, private and teaching hospitals in the greater metropolitan area of São Paulo, Brazil. *J. Bras Pneumol.* **2006**, *32*, 29. [CrossRef]
20. Tallo, F.S.; de Campos Vieira Abib, S.; de Andrade Negri, F.P.C.; Delascio Lopes, R.; Lopes, A.C. Evaluation of Self-perception of Mechanical Ventilation Knowledge among Brazilian Final-year Medical Students, Residents and Emergency Physicians. *Clinics (Sao Paulo)* **2017**, *72*, 65–70. [CrossRef]
21. Scala, R.; Windisch, W.; Köhnlein, T.; Cuvelier, A.; Navalesi, P.; Pelosi, P.; European Respiratory Society Respiratory Intensive Care Assembly. Targeting European Respiratory Society Group activities: A survey of the Noninvasive Ventilatory Support Group. *Eur. Respir. Rev.* **2014**, *23*, 258–260. [CrossRef]
22. Raurell-Torredà, M.; Argilaga-Molero, E.; Colomer-Plana, M.; Ruiz-García, T.; Galvany-Ferrer, A.; González-Pujol, A. Análisis comparativo de los conocimientos en ventilación mecánica no invasiva de profesionales de cuidados intensivos. *Intensive Care Unit Prof. Knowl. About Non Invasive Vent. Comp. Anal. Enferm Intensiva* **2015**, *26*, 46–53. [CrossRef] [PubMed]
23. Goligher, E.C.; Ferguson, N.D.; Kenny, L.P. Core competency in mechanical ventilation: Development of educational objectives using the Delphi technique. *Crit. Care Med.* **2012**, *40*, 2828–2832. [CrossRef] [PubMed]
24. Davies, J.D.; Gentile, M.A. What does it take to have a successful noninvasive ventilation program? *Respir. Care* **2009**, *54*, 53–61. [PubMed]
25. Nava, S.; Ceriana, P. Causes of failure of noninvasive mechanical ventilation. *Respir. Care* **2004**, *49*, 295–303.
26. McQueen, S.; Dickinson, M.; Pimblett, M. Human patient simulation can aid staff training in non-invasive ventilation. *Nurs. Times* **2010**, *106*, 20.
27. Brill, A.K.; Moghal, M.; Morrell, M.J.; Simonds, A.K. Randomized crossover trial of a pressure sensing visual feedback system to improve mask fitting in noninvasive ventilation. *Respirology* **2017**, *22*, 1343–1349. [CrossRef]
28. Hare, A.; Simonds, A. Simulation-based education for non-invasive ventilation. *Breathe* **2013**, *9*, 366–374. [CrossRef]
29. Bambi, S.; Giani, M.; Lucchini, A. Noninvasive ventilation: Skills, education and training. In *Non-Invasive Ventilation. A Practical Handbook for Understanding the Causes of Treatment and Success*; Esquinas, A., Ed.; Nova Medicine & Health Inc.: New York, NY, USA, 2019; Chapter 40; ISBN 978-1-53615-200-5.
30. Nasa, P.; Azoulay, E.; Khanna, A.K.; Jain, R.; Gupta, S.; Javeri, Y.; Juneja, D.; Rangappa, P.; Sundararajan, K.; Alhazzani, W.; et al. Expert consensus statements for the management of COVID-19-related acute respiratory failure using a Delphi method. *Crit. Care* **2021**, *25*, 106. [CrossRef]
31. Weerakkody, S.; Arina, P.; Glenister, J.; Cotterell, S.; Boscaini-Gilroy, G.; Singer, M.; Montgomery, H.E. Non-invasive respiratory support in the management of acute COVID-19 pneumonia: Considerations for clinical practice and priorities for research. *Lancet Respir. Med.* **2022**, *10*, 199–213, Erratum in *Lancet Respir. Med.* **2021**, *9*, e114. [CrossRef]
32. Alqahtani, J.S.; Aldabayan, Y.S.; AlAhmari, M.D.; AlRabeeah, S.M.; Aldhahir, A.M.; Alghamdi, S.M.; Oyelade, T.; Althobiani, M.; Alrajeh, A.M. Clinical Practice and Barriers of Ventilatory Support Management in COVID-19 Patients in Saudi Arabia: A Survey of Respiratory Therapists. *Saudi. J. Med. Med. Sci.* **2021**, *9*, 223–229. [CrossRef]
33. Karim, H.M.R.; Burns, K.E.A.; Ciobanu, L.D.; El-Khatib, M.; Nicolini, A.; Vargas, N.; Hernández-Gilsoul, T.; Skoczyński, S.; Falcone, V.A.; Arnal, J.M.; et al. Noninvasive ventilation: Education and training. A narrative analysis and an international consensus document. *Adv. Respir. Med.* **2019**, *87*, 36–45. [CrossRef] [PubMed]
34. Lanza, A.; Sommariva, M.; Mariani, S.; Ferreyra, G.; Stagni, G.E.; Tombini, V.; Oppizzi, A.; Pontiggia, C.; Bellone, A. Prolonged non-invasive respiratory support in a COVID-19 patient with severe acute hypoxemic respiratory failure. *Monaldi. Arch. Chest. Dis.* **2021**, *92*. [CrossRef] [PubMed]

35. Ramirez, G.A.; Bozzolo, E.P.; Castelli, E.; Marinosci, A.; Angelillo, P.; Damanti, S.; Scotti, R.; Gobbi, A.; Centurioni, C.; Di Scala, F.; et al. Continuous positive airway pressure and pronation outside the intensive care unit in COVID 19 ARDS. *Minerva Med.* **2020**, *113*, 281–290. [CrossRef] [PubMed]
36. Bradley, P.; Wilson, J.; Taylor, R.; Nixon, J.; Redfern, J.; Whittemore, P.; Gaddah, M.; Kavuri, K.; Haley, A.; Denny, P.; et al. Conventional oxygen therapy versus CPAP as a ceiling of care in ward-based patients with COVID-19: A multi-centre cohort evaluation. *EClinicalMedicine* **2021**, *40*, 101122. [CrossRef]
37. Robinson, R.E.; Nightingale, R.; Frost, F.; Green, T.; Jones, G.; Nwosu, N.; Hampshire, P.; Brown, D.; Beadsworth, M.; Aston, S.; et al. The rapid development and deployment of a new multidisciplinary CPAP service outside of a critical care environment during the early stages of the COVID-19 pandemic. *Future Health J.* **2021**, *8*, e156–e159. [CrossRef]

Disclaimer/Publisher's Note: The statements, opinions and data contained in all publications are solely those of the individual author(s) and contributor(s) and not of MDPI and/or the editor(s). MDPI and/or the editor(s) disclaim responsibility for any injury to people or property resulting from any ideas, methods, instructions or products referred to in the content.

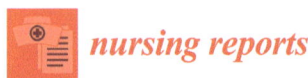 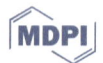

Article

Properties of Polyunsaturated Fatty Acids in Primary and Secondary Prevention of Cardiovascular Diseases in the View of Patients (Silesia, Poland)

Karolina Krupa-Kotara [1,*], Mateusz Grajek [2], Agata Wypych-Ślusarska [1], Sandra Martynus-Depta [1], Klaudia Oleksiuk [1], Joanna Głogowska-Ligus [1], Elżbieta Szczepańska [3] and Jerzy Słowiński [1]

1. Department of Epidemiology, Faculty of Health Sciences in Bytom, Medical University of Silesia in Katowice, 40-055 Katowice, Poland
2. Department of Public Health, Faculty of Health Sciences in Bytom, Medical University of Silesia in Katowice, 40-055 Katowice, Poland
3. Department of Human Nutrition, Faculty of Health Sciences in Bytom, Medical University of Silesia in Katowice, 40-055 Katowice, Poland
* Correspondence: kkrupa@sum.edu.pl

Abstract: Background: Cardiovascular diseases are a major cause of morbidity and mortality in Europe. Lifestyle plays an important role in the primary and secondary prevention of cardiovascular diseases, apart from pharmacotherapy and diagnostics. Numerous studies confirm that the type and quality of fat consumed in the diet have a huge impact on the risk of cardiovascular diseases. Reducing the risk of cardiovascular disease can be helped by minimizing the proportion of saturated fatty acids in the diet and replacing them with polyunsaturated fatty acids. These acids and, above all, their long-chain forms have a positive effect on health. Aim: This study aims to assess the awareness of the properties of polyunsaturated fatty acids in the primary and secondary prevention of cardiovascular diseases in the opinions of patients of the Cardiology Department of the Racibórz Medical Center. Material and Methods: The analysis included 302 patients (113 women and 189 men) hospitalized in the Cardiology Department. The research method was the authors' questionnaire consisting of the patients' record and thirty closed questions. To answer the research questions posed and test the hypotheses, statistical analyses were carried out using the IBM SPSS Statistics version 25 package. Results: Among the respondents, the least frequently used healthy eating habit was the infrequent eating of fried foods. A total of 18.2% of respondents had such a habit. The most commonly used healthy eating habit was checking the fat content in products, which was performed by 67.2% of respondents. Among the respondents, 58.3% said that butter and margarine increase serum cholesterol. Conclusions: The analysis of the data shows that the place of residence, education, sex, and reason for hospitalization of the respondents did not affect the frequency of healthy eating habits. In addition, the subjects had a low amount of healthy eating habits.

Keywords: cardiovascular disease; polyunsaturated fatty acids; eating habits

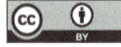

1. Introduction

The main cause of increased morbidity and mortality in Europe is cardiovascular disease. For this reason and due to acute cardiovascular complications, about 45.8% of the country's population dies annually in Poland [1–3]. In addition to pharmacotherapy and diagnostics, lifestyle is an important role in the primary and secondary prevention of cardiovascular diseases. The most important risk factor for the development of cardiovascular disease is inadequate diet. This is mainly related to the excessive consumption of fats and their inadequate composition. The diet of adults in Poland is based primarily on excessive consumption of highly processed products rich in saturated fatty acids. However, due to the functions performed by fats, they should not be completely excluded from the diet, but attention should be paid to the quantity and quality of fats consumed [4,5]. According to the Institute of Food and Nutrition (IŻŻ), the daily intake of fats should be 20–35% [6].

Numerous studies confirm that the type and quality of fat consumed in the diet have a huge impact on the risk of cardiovascular disease [1–5]. Consumption of saturated fatty acids can harm the lipid profile and increase the risk of developing cardiovascular disease. Even though they are the main source of energy in the body, excessive consumption of them raises the concentration of LDL cholesterol, increasing blood clotting, among other things. This, in turn, leads to the development of atherosclerosis and can cause ischemic heart disease. For this reason, their intake should be limited to 10% of daily energy requirements [6]. Reducing the risk of the onset and development of cardiovascular disease can be contributed to reducing the proportion of saturated fatty acids in the diet and replacing them with polyunsaturated fatty acids. These acids, and especially their long-chain forms, have been shown to have positive health effects. Consumption of fish and, therefore, omega-3 polyunsaturated fatty acids reduces the incidence of cardiovascular disease [7,8].

The ratio of fatty acids of the omega-3 to the omega-6 family is also extremely important; it is a determinant of the health-promoting properties of the diet. According to the recommendations for proper nutrition, it should be (4–5):1. An excessive supply of omega-6 fatty acids can lead to a reduction in the beneficial biological effects of omega-3 fatty acids. However, the current, common diet is characterized by an imbalance in the ratio of fatty acids consumed and excessive consumption of saturated fatty acids as well as too little intake of omega-3 fatty acids while consuming too much omega-6 fatty acids [9].

Prevention of cardiovascular disease is defined as activities aimed at both the general population, people with an increased risk of atherosclerosis and its complications, and those with symptoms of atherosclerosis. These activities are aimed at eliminating or minimizing the development of cardiovascular disease and the disability associated with it [10–12]. A properly balanced diet plays an overriding role in the prevention of atherosclerosis and its complications. Of greatest importance is replacing the energy provided by the consumption of saturated fatty acids with energy derived from unsaturated fatty acids and diversifying the daily diet with fish. The main goal of eating a properly fat-balanced diet is to lower serum LDL cholesterol levels and reduce the risk of cardiovascular incidents [12,13]. Secondary prevention applies to those with established coronary artery disease to reduce the risk of subsequent disease [14]. The mortality rate among post-MI patients is twice as high for about 10 years compared to the rest of the population. Having survived a myocardial infarction should mobilize the patient to make lifestyle changes, especially dietary changes. Studies of people after myocardial infarction have proven the benefits of polyunsaturated fatty acids [15]. A study showed that the use of supplementation with DHA and EPA acids reduced the overall mortality by 20% with cardiovascular-related mortality reduced by 30%, which is closely related to the antiarrhythmic properties of omega-3 fatty acids [16,17].

Lipids are the dominant factor in the development of atherosclerotic lesions. Omega-3 fatty acids, through their effect on lipid metabolism, are an important factor in the antiatherosclerotic effect. When used daily, doses of 2–5 g can reduce serum triglyceride concentrations by up to about 30%. Such effects are responsible for increased catabolism and reduced low-density lipoproteins (VLDL) production. Acids from this family minimally raise the concentration of LDL cholesterol and may also raise the concentration of the HDL fraction. Omega-3 PACs contribute to the reduction of postprandial lipemia by activating lipoprotein lipase, the enzyme responsible for the catabolism of very low-density lipoproteins (VLDL) and chylomicrons. The antiarrhythmic effect of omega-3 fatty acids has been widely reported. According to many studies, omega-3 fatty acids directly affect the electrophysiological processes of cardiomyocytes. The action on sodium channels shifts the state of dynamic equilibrium inactivation towards hyperpolarized potentials. The consequence of this action is that cardiomyocytes are less susceptible to excitation. In turn, the anticoagulant effect of omega-3 fatty acids is related to their antiplatelet properties. The mechanism involves inhibiting the formation of prothrombotic factors such as TXA2, interleukin 1 (IL-1), lipoprotein (a), and platelet-activating factor. Omega-3 fatty acid supplementation has been proven to increase the levels of prostacyclins that inhibit platelet aggregation [18–21].

Natural sources of EPA and DHA are algae, phytoplankton, fish fat, and also other marine organisms that feed on plankton and fish. The most important sources of omega-3 fatty acids are oily marine fish and seafood. Fish oils, compared to vegetable oils, are characterized by a lower content of omega-6 fatty acids, which is beneficial for maintaining a normal omega-6/omega-3 ratio [22]. An excess supply of omega-6 acids relative to omega-3 can reduce the beneficial effects of EPA and DHA [16]. The highest levels of omega-3 fatty acids distinguish mackerel fish (tuna, mackerel), herring fish (herring, sardines), salmon fish (trout, salmon), and anchovy fish (anchovies). The species of fish, physiological state, fishing period, and also nature of existence determine the content of omega-3 acids. In addition, rapeseed oil is a valuable source of acids from the omega-3 family [6]. Rich sources of a-linolenic acid (ALA) are vegetable oils (flaxseed, safflower), nuts (walnut, hazelnut, Brazilian), and pumpkin seeds. The main sources of linoleic acid (CLA), which belongs to the omega-6 family, are vegetable oils. The content in grape seed oil ranges from 58–78%, in soybean oil 48–59%, and in safflower oil 68–83% while in canola oil, it accounts for 15–30%. Egg yolk and also meat and meat products are a source of arachidonic acid (ARA). Another source of EPA and DHA supplements in the form of fish oil or capsules. Supplementation is aimed at people whose concentration of omega-3 fatty acids in the body is too low. Sources of omega-3 fatty acids for vegetarians and people allergic to fish protein can be algae, vegetable oils, or nuts [23–27].

Based on the standards of the Institute of Food and Nutrition, the adequate intake (AI) of linoleic acid (LA) is 4% of dietary energy; for a-linolenic acid (AL), the standard was set at 0.5%. The standards for LA and ALA were set based on the lowest average intake of these acids in various population groups of European countries for which no symptoms of deficiency of these acids were found [6]. Numerous studies have shown that regular consumption of fish or supplementation with omega-3 fatty acids contribute to a reduction in mortality from cardiovascular disease. Because of this, the standard AI (adequate intake) level for the intake of EPA and DHA acids in adults is 250 mg [6]. According to the American Heart Association (AHA), patients suffering from ischemic heart disease should consume about 1 g of EPA and DHA each day. As part of the prevention of cardiovascular disease, healthy people are advised to consume oily marine fish about twice a week and eat products that are sources of a-linolenic acid in the amount of 1.5–3 g. The best solution is to provide these acids in the form of fish. Supplementation of these acids in the form of capsules is also acceptable but under the constant supervision of a doctor. Supplementation of DHA and EPA acids in the form of capsules is necessary for patients who need to lower triglycerides [28]. According to the recommendations of the International Society for Study of Fatty Acids and Lipids, the energy from LA intake is 2% while ALA was 0.7%. According to the recommendations, the amount of eicosapentaenoic acid and docosahexaenoic acid in the diet should be 0.65 g and 0.5 g per day, respectively [6]. Current standards in Poland have set the daily energy requirements of omega-6 acids at 5–8%, and the level of omega-3 acids has been set at 1–2% [6].

An extremely important element in the primary and secondary prevention of cardiovascular disease is the use of a well-balanced diet. Numerous observational and experimental studies have shown that the type of fat provided by a diet plays a significant role in the prevention of cardiovascular disease. A diet high in saturated fatty acids significantly affects the lipid profile, thus contributing to the development of cardiovascular disease. For this reason, an appropriately balanced diet should be based on limiting the supply of saturated fatty acids while increasing the supply of acids from the omega-3 and omega-6 families. To achieve a cardioprotective effect, an appropriate quantitative composition and proper proportions of the fatty acids consumed are necessary [6,22–28]. Therefore, the main objective of this study is to evaluate the awareness of the properties of polyunsaturated fatty acids in the primary and secondary prevention of cardiovascular diseases of patients of the Cardiology Department of the Racibórz Medical Center.

Specific objectives of the study:
1. Evaluate the dietary habits of patients hospitalized in a cardiac unit.
2. Evaluate the relationship between place of residence, education, gender, diet and reason for hospitalization, and patients' eating habits.

2. Materials and Methods

2.1. Study Design and Eligibility Criteria

During the study period from 25 November 2019 to 31 January 2020, 302 patients (including 113 females and 189 males) were hospitalized in the Cardiology Department of the Racibórz Medical Center. Written permission from the facility and authorization to process personal data were obtained. The mean age was 50 ± 11.3 (21–71) years. The respondents were informed about the purpose of the study, the use of the obtained results for scientific purposes only, and their anonymity. The characteristics of the study group are shown in Table 1.

The selection of the sample was purposive. The following inclusion criteria were considered: undergoing hospitalization in a cardiology department, age ≥ 18 years, health condition that allows you to take part in the study, and giving written consent to participate in the study.

Patients received the questionnaire in paper form upon admission to the ward, provided that their health condition allowed them to complete it, and they gave informed written consent to complete it, which resulted in such a distribution of age and other variables in the study population.

Table 1. Characteristics of the study group ($n = 302$).

Variable	n (%)
Sex	
Female	113 (37.4)
Male	189 (62.6)
Age	
21–28	1 (0.3)
29–38	15 (4.9)
39–49	46 (15.3)
50–71	240 (79.5)
BMI	
Obesity	85 (28.1)
Overweight	112 (37.1)
Normal weight	105 (34.8)
Underweight	-
Reason for hospitalization	
Shortness of breath	48 (15.9)
Chest pain	39 (12.9)
Myocardial infarction	164 (54.3)
Heart failure	11 (3.6)
Heart rhythm disturbances	27 (8.9)
Uncontrolled hypertension	13 (4.4)
Comorbidities	
Type 2 diabetes	178 (58.9)
Hypertension	267 (88.4)
Atherosclerosis	223 (73.8)
Chronic kidney disease	103 (34.1)
Chronic obstructive pulmonary disease (COPD)	86 (28.8)
Heart failure	167 (55.3)

Table 1. Cont.

Variable	n (%)
Education	
Primary	17 (5.6)
Vocational	176 (58.3)
Secondary	49 (16.2)
Higher	60 (19.9)
Place of residence	
Village or city of up to 20 thousand residents	128 (42.4)
City of 20 thousand–100 thousand residents	118 (39.1)
City of more than 100 thousand residents	56 (18.5)

The survey was conducted using a direct survey method with confidentiality maintained. All data were coded with appropriate symbols to prevent patient identification by the law of 29 August 1997 on the Protection of Personal Data (Journal of Laws 1997 No. 133 item 883).

The study design, in light of the act of 5 December 1996 on the professions of physicians and dentists (Journal of Laws of 2011, No. 277. item 1634, as amended), is not a medical experiment and does not require evaluation by the Bioethics Committee of the Silesian Medical University in Katowice, as it is based on the patient's own experience. In addition, the data collected was based on an anonymous questionnaire to which patients gave written, voluntary consent. The questionnaires were distributed directly to the patients, so the absence of a completed questionnaire also meant that the patients did not agree to participate in the study. The study was conducted according to the principles of clinical research based on the Declaration of Helsinki, as amended.

2.2. Study Procedure and Research Tool

A proprietary questionnaire was prepared to conduct the study (See in Supplementary Materials). The questionnaire consisted of metrics including questions about the year of birth, weight, height, gender, education, social status, and the reason for hospitalization in a cardiac unit. In addition, the questionnaire included thirty closed-ended questions on the properties of polyunsaturated fatty acids in the primary and secondary prevention of cardiovascular disease. Subjects were instructed in detail on how to complete the survey. The questionnaires were reviewed for correct completion and carefully analyzed. Based on the completed metric (weight and height), body mass index (BMI) was calculated. Interpretation of the results obtained was based on the WHO classification of BMI values.

The survey was conducted in three stages. The first stage was a pilot study, during which 20 respondents were asked to fill out a questionnaire to check for understanding of all questions. Most of the questions were found to be clear and understandable to the respondents while questions that were indicated by at least 2 respondents as incomprehensible or unclear were removed or corrected. Stage two was the validation of the questionnaires by distributing them twice to a group of 50 respondents. An interval of 2 weeks was maintained between colocations of the questionnaires. The consistency of answers to the same questions was checked. For the reproducibility of the results obtained by the questionnaire used, the value of the κ (kappa) parameter was calculated for each question in the questionnaire—for 73.8% of the questions, very good ($\kappa \geq 0.80$) method consistency was obtained while for 26.2% of the questions, good ($0.79 \geq \kappa \geq 0.60$) method consistency was obtained. The final stage of the study was to conduct the actual survey.

2.3. Statistical Analyses

Statistical analyses were carried out using the IBM SPSS Statistics version 25 package, with which an analysis of basic descriptive statistics and a series of univariate analyses of variance were performed. The classical threshold of $\alpha = 0.05$ was considered the level of significance; however, the results of probability test statistics at the level of $0.05 < \alpha < 0.1$ were interpreted as significant at the level of the statistical trend.

3. Results

In the first step, the healthy eating habits of the subjects were checked, assuming that more healthy habits would correlate with higher awareness. One point was awarded for each answer indicating healthy habits while zero points were awarded for the others. Thus, respondents could receive a minimum of zero points (no healthy eating habits at all) and a maximum of seven points (completely healthy eating habits). The most common score in the sample was two points, which indicates a very low amount of healthy eating habits. Next, it was checked in which questions the respondents most often showed healthy eating habits and in which the fewest responses indicated adequate habits. As can be seen in Table 2, the least frequent healthy habits included the question about the frequency of eating fried foods, where only 18.2% of respondents answered that they do not eat such dishes. Moreover, only 19.2% consumed fish twice a week, and 19.5% of respondents chose lean cottage cheese. On the other hand, the most common healthy habits included checking the fat content of products, which was done by as many as 67.2% of people, and recognizing that butter and margarine raise cholesterol, which was marked by 58.3% of people.

Table 2. Share of responses indicating healthy eating habits and lack thereof.

Variable	Lack of Healthy Eating Habits		Healthy Eating Habit	
	n	%	n	%
Paying attention to the fat content of products	99	32.8	203	67.2
Recognition that butter and margarine raise cholesterol	126	41.7	176	58.3
Type of fat dominant in the diet	199	65.9	103	34.1
Reaching for lean cottage cheese	243	80.5	59	19.5
Used fat for frying food	213	70.5	89	29.5
Frequency of consumption of fried foods	247	81.8	55	18.2
Frequency of fish consumption	244	80.8	58	19.2

Based on BMI, 34.8% of patients were normal weight (BMI 18.5–24.9 kg/m^2), 37.1% were overweight (BMI 25.0–29.9 kg/m^2), and 28.1% were obese (BMI > 30.0 kg/m^2). There were no underweight patients in the group. About 67% of the overweight and obese patients were male and 33% female (Table 3).

Table 3. WHO classification of patients' BMI values.

BMI (kg/m^2)	WHO Classification	BMI of Patients n (%)
<18.5	Underweight	-
18.5–24.9	Standard	105 (34.8)
25.0–29.9	Overweight	112 (37.1)
30.0–34.9	first-degree obesity	78 (25.8)
35.0–39.9	secondary obesity	4 (1.3)
≥40	tertiary obesity	3 (1.0)

Whether the place of residence is related to healthy eating habits was tested. One-way analysis of variance with the calculation of the omega2 measure was used for calculations. Table 4 shows the results on the healthy eating scale by place of residence.

The results indicated that place of residence was not significant ($p = 0.928$) for the occurrence of healthy eating habits. Respondents obtained similar results regardless of their place of residence.

After verifying the association of healthy eating with education, a one-way analysis of variance was used to see if education correlates with the number of healthy eating habits. Table 5 shows the results of the calculations.

Table 4. Relationship of healthy eating to a place of residence.

Variable: A Place of Residence	Healthy Eating		
	M	SD	n
Village	2.4	1.19	128
City of 50,000 to 100,000 inhabitants	2.44	1.2	118
A city with more than 100,000 inhabitants	2.46	1.09	56
	F	p	ω^2
The relationship between healthy eating and where you live	0.07	0.928	0

Table 5. Relationship of healthy eating with education.

Variable: Education	Healthy Eating		
	M	SD	n
Primary	3	0.94	17
Professional	2.47	1.17	176
Medium	2.33	1.23	49
Higher	2.33	1.16	60
	F	p	ω^2
The link between education and healthy eating	2.12	0.098	0.01

It turned out that the relationship between education and healthy eating was at the level of statistical trend and had weak strength. Post hoc tests comparing the number of healthy eating habits were then performed. However, the analyses showed no statistically significant differences between the pairs ($p = 0.098$).

A t-test for independent samples was used to test the gender difference in healthy eating. The strength of the difference was determined using Cohen's d measure. The results are shown in Table 6.

Table 6. Relationship of gender to healthy eating.

Variable: Gender	Women (n = 113)		Men (n = 189)				95% CI		d Cohen's
	M	SD	M	SD	t	p	LL	UL	
Healthy eating	2.51	1.28	2.38	1.10	0.99	0.323	–0.14	0.41	0.12

The results indicated that there was no statistically significant difference in healthy eating between men and women ($p = 0.323$). Respondents, regardless of gender, had a similar number of healthy eating habits.

Finally, calculations were performed to determine whether the association between the reason for hospitalization and healthy eating habits was statistically significant. A one-way analysis of variance was again used to verify the association. Table 7 presents the results obtained.

Moreover, the reason for hospitalization was not statistically significant for the number of healthy habits ($p = 0.810$). Patients with different reasons for hospitalization scored similarly on the healthy eating scale.

Table 7. Association of healthy eating with the reason for hospitalization.

Variable: The Reason for Hospitalization	Healthy Eating		
	M	SD	n
Shortness of breath	2.54	1.17	48
Chest pains	2.23	1.04	39
Myocardial infarction	2.41	1.26	164
Heart failure	2.63	1.03	11
Heart rhythm disturbance	2.56	0.89	27
Uncontrolled hypertension	2.38	1.12	13
	F	p	ω^2
Relationship between healthy eating and reason for hospitalization	0.46	0.810	0

4. Discussion

The beneficial effects of polyunsaturated fatty acids on the cardiovascular system have been confirmed by numerous observational and experimental studies [29]. The results of these studies confirm the protective properties of polyunsaturated fatty acids on the cardiovascular system. Dietary habits play a significant role in the primary and secondary prevention of cardiovascular diseases [30]. Therefore, it is important to pay attention to the quality and type of fats supplied with the diet. In both the prevention and treatment of cardiovascular disease, it is necessary to follow an appropriate diet. The diet used should contribute to normalizing body weight. An indispensable element in the prevention of cardiovascular disease is to maintain body weight with a BMI in the range of 20–25. In addition, recent studies have shown that following a diet as close as possible to the Mediterranean diet reduces the risk of a cardiovascular incident [31]. A study by Schroeder et al. found that following a Mediterranean diet or habits similar to the principles of the Mediterranean diet negatively correlates with the occurrence of obesity [32].

According to the Position Statement of the Polish Dietetic Association, a controlled fatty acid diet is recommended for primary and secondary prevention and treatment of cardiovascular disease. Dietary fat supply should be limited to below 30% of total energy. Saturated fatty acids should not exceed 7% of dietary energy while cholesterol supply should not exceed 300 mg/d. The recommended supply of EPA and DHA acids is 250–500 mg/d. The source of these acids in the diet should be regularly consumed fish. According to PTD recommendations for cardiovascular prevention, two servings of fish should be consumed per week; each serving should weigh 140 g. At least one of the servings should be of an oily marine fish species [33].

For people postmyocardial infarction, the National Institute for Health and Care Excellence (NICE) recommends a supply of at least 7 g of omega-3 fatty acids per week. The source of these acids should be fatty fish in the amount of two to four servings per week. For those who do not consume the recommended amounts of fish, a supply of 1 g of omega-3 fatty acids in supplement form is recommended [34]. According to the Food Standard Agency's recommendations, the maximum consumption of oily fish per week is four servings (excluding pregnant and lactating women, for whom two servings are recommended). Other recommended sources of omega-3 fatty acids include plant-based products such as soybean oil, canola oil, flaxseed oil, and also walnuts [35].

Unambiguous research results confirm a negative correlation between nut consumption and the risk of cardiovascular disease. Nuts are a highly nutritious source of unsaturated fatty acids. The PREDIMED study showed that a Mediterranean diet enriched each day with a serving of 30 g of nuts plays a beneficial role in the prevention of cardiovascular disease [36].

This survey conducted with patients hospitalized in the Cardiology Department shows that the respondents were characterized by a low number of healthy eating habits. The analysis of the data shows that the most common bad eating habit among the respondents was the consumption of fried foods. This habit affects 81.8% of the respondents. The method of thermal processing of prepared foods is extremely important in the prevention of cardiovascular diseases. The process of frying contributes to the fat content of a given dish or product. The proper technique for preparing meals and dishes is boiling water and steaming or braising food without adding fat using Teflon pans. To ensure that the food being prepared does not absorb extra fat, it can also be prepared on ceramic cookware, combi-brewers, on a grill, and also using an oven sleeve or transparent foil. Another bad habit relates to the frequency of eating fish. Among the respondents, 80.8% admit that they eat fish much less frequently than recommended. A sizable percentage of respondents (80.5%) answered that they choose semiskim or fatty cottage cheese instead of lean cottage cheese, which does not follow the principles of proper nutrition. Choosing cottage cheese with a higher fat content makes it difficult to reduce the amount of fat in the dietary ratio. Among respondents, 70.5% admitted that they do not use the recommended canola oil for frying. Respondents were more likely to use margarine and butter. For short frying, oils high in monounsaturated fatty acids and low in polyunsaturated fatty acids are suitable. The recommended oil for frying is canola oil. In its composition, it contains 61% monounsaturated fatty acids while the content of polyunsaturated acids is 29% [37,38]. The diet of 65.9% of respondents was dominated by animal fats. Only 58.3% of the respondents thought that consuming butter and margarine in excessive amounts can cause elevated serum cholesterol levels. The remaining 41.7% of respondents took the opposite view. In the prevention of cardiovascular disease, products that are a source of saturated fatty acids, which contribute to an increase in the concentration of atherosclerotic cholesterol, should be limited. Such products include butter, margarine, cream, lard, fatty cheeses, and fatty meats. As many as 32.8% of respondents do not pay attention to the fat content of the product they choose. Because of the need to make changes in their current diet, it is necessary to check the fat content on product labels and carefully analyze them. A study by Wegrowski et al. [39] confirms that most patients with cardiovascular diseases are characterized by inappropriate eating habits.

In the study, the relationship between place of residence and eating habits was analyzed. The data showed that the place of residence did not affect the eating habits of the respondents. Analysis of the study conducted by Babiarczyk [40] also did not confirm a statistically significant relationship between place of residence and the eating habits of respondents. In contrast, a study by Bieniasz et al. [41] found statistically significant differences between eating habits and place of residence. Respondents living in cities were more likely to have normal eating habits.

The study analyzed the relationship between education and the eating habits of the respondents. None of the analyses conducted confirmed the relationship studied. A study by Wegrowski et al. [39] found that people with primary, vocational, secondary, and higher education have comparable eating habits. A study by Babiarczyk and Dudek [40] also failed to confirm the relationship between the subjects' education and eating habits.

Another relationship analyzed in the self-reported study concerned gender and eating habits. The results of the analyses do not confirm a gender difference on the subject of eating habits. Respondents, regardless of gender, were characterized by similar eating habits. Different results were obtained in a study conducted by Babiarczyk and Dudek [40]. The results of that study confirmed the relationship between gender and the eating habits of the respondents. In addition, women showed significantly more correct eating habits than men [40]. Women were characterized by higher scores in the category of correct eating habits compared to men [40].

The last relationship analyzed was between the reason for hospitalization and the eating habits of the respondents. This relationship was also not confirmed. Patients hospitalized for different reasons were characterized by similar eating habits.

In conclusion, the survey shows that patient awareness of the properties of polyunsaturated fatty acids in the primary and secondary prevention of cardiovascular diseases is too low. Therefore, it is necessary to conduct health education so that patients acquire the right information and skills to make the right health decisions. This is related to the inseparable making of informed decisions that concern health based on scientifically proven knowledge [42]

Health education methods focus on the patient and his or her coping skills, understanding shared responsibility for health and the impact of health behaviors, and the need to modify them. Health education in which various methods and didactic forms are used contributes to improving the level of patients with cardiovascular diseases [42]. An important role in the formation of proper eating habits among patients with cardiovascular diseases is played by medical personnel. His role should include planning and implementing individual nutrition. A multidisciplinary team including a doctor, nurse, and dietician can develop diet and nutrition recommendations and then supervise the implementation of the nutrition plan. In addition, they shape correct eating behavior among patients by selecting appropriate products and foods and using appropriate thermal processing methods. Health promotion and health education carried out by medical personnel is the most effective way to increase patient knowledge and reduce mortality from cardiovascular diseases [43].

5. Strengths and Limitations

The results of the present study have important utilitarian significance. Pointing out the decidedly inappropriate dietary habits of the patients surveyed, they underscore the need for extensive programs and public campaigns that take dietoprophylaxis into account. The importance of balanced nutrition in diseases of civilization is an indisputable fact. In Poland, however, it seems that nutrition education programs need broader outreach, as they are directed primarily to children and adolescents, young people, and to a lesser extent to the elderly. It is also not out of the question that this group is less receptive to nutrition education due to their previous, often incorrect, dietary habits and patterns. Therefore, the results of the present study make us reflect on the condition, reach, and addressees of dietoprophylaxis.

This study focused on examining awareness of the properties of polyunsaturated fatty acids in the primary and secondary prevention of cardiovascular disease. Other dietary behaviors were not analyzed. On the one hand, this may seem to be a certain limitation of the study but only in appearance. This was a deliberate intention of the authors for reasons regarding the dietary traditions in Poland where, for a long time, mainly fats of animal origin (mainly lard, butter, cream) were consumed, and frying was the basic technique of processing products. Thus, the results of the present analysis identify an area that requires nutrition education or re-education.

Limiting the study to patients with a specific disease entity may not allow for a random sample, so it is difficult to get a representative group, which may lead to bias in the study in some cases, but the authors have made every effort to reduce the risk of error. In addition, the inclusion criteria used did not allow for the inclusion of all people in the study due to health status or age.

The subject under consideration is in line with the strategic and operational objective of the National Health Program for 2021–2025, which is an implementing act of the law of 11 September 2015 on public health, as a strategic response to the need to counteract negative epidemiological trends and the increasing burden of chronic noncommunicable diseases on the population, among which cardiovascular diseases are classified.

This study on the awareness of primary and secondary prevention of cardiovascular diseases in populations already burdened will allow a better definition of the health needs of patients and proper targeting of activities regarding prevention, jurisprudence, social support groups, and thus more effective assistance and reduction of social and economic costs of cardiovascular diseases.

The timing of the study is an undoubted advantage. It was a period before the announcement of the pandemic, so the influence of the SARS-CoV-2 virus on possible cardiovascular complications can be excluded, and thus these circumstances can be ruled out as a cause of hospitalization.

The limitations indicated, however, do not diminish the importance of this study. Indeed, it reveals a significant problem associated with poor eating habits and points to the need for in-depth and nationwide nutrition prevention programs.

6. Conclusions

Based on the study, it was concluded that the awareness of the properties of polyunsaturated fatty acids in the primary and secondary prevention of cardiovascular diseases among patients of the Cardiology Department of the Racibórz Medical Center was insufficient. In addition, the study concluded that:

1. Patients hospitalized in the cardiac unit were characterized by low levels of healthy eating habits.
2. There was no relationship between place of residence, education, gender, or reason for hospitalization and patients' eating habits.

Supplementary Materials: The following supporting information can be downloaded at: https://www.mdpi.com/article/10.3390/nursrep12040094/s1, Questionnaire.

Author Contributions: Conceptualization, K.K.-K.; methodology, M.G.; software, K.K.-K.; validation, M.G.; formal analysis, M.G. and K.K.-K. investigation, S.M.-D.; resources, K.K.-K.; data curation, S.M.-D.; writing—original draft preparation, K.K.-K. and S.M.-D. writing—review and editing, K.K.-K., A.W.-Ś., M.G. and K.O.; visualization, K.K.-K.; supervision, J.G.-L., E.S. and J.S.; project administration, K.K.-K. All authors have read and agreed to the published version of the manuscript.

Funding: This research received no external funding.

Institutional Review Board Statement: This research complies with the provisions of the Helsinki Declaration and local regulations of the Bioethical Commission of the Silesian Medical University in Katowice; the Committee on Publication Ethics (COPE) regulations were followed in this study.

Informed Consent Statement: Informed consent was obtained from all subjects involved in the study.

Data Availability Statement: Not applicable.

Conflicts of Interest: The authors declare no conflict of interest.

References

1. Di Raimondo, D.; Musiari, G.; Rizzo, G.; Pirera, E.; Signorelli, S.S. New Insights in Prevention and Treatment of Cardiovascular Disease. *Int. J. Environ. Res. Public Health* **2022**, *19*, 2475. [CrossRef] [PubMed]
2. Wong, C.X.; Brown, A.; Lau, D.H.; Chugh, S.S.; Albert, C.M.; Kalman, J.M.; Sanders, P. Epidemiology of Sudden Cardiac Death: Global and Regional Perspectives. *Heart Lung Circ.* **2019**, *28*, 6–14. [CrossRef]
3. Eriksson, H.P.; Forsell, K.; Andersson, E. Mortality from cardiovascular disease in a cohort of Swedish seafarers. *Int. Arch. Occup. Environ. Health* **2020**, *93*, 345–353. [CrossRef] [PubMed]
4. Pluta, A.; Sulikowska, B.; Manitius, J.; Posieczek, Z.; Marzec, A.; Morisky, D.E. Acceptance of Illness and Compliance with Therapeutic Recommendations in Patients with Hypertension. *Int. J. Environ. Res. Public Health* **2020**, *17*, 6789. [CrossRef] [PubMed]
5. Kotlęga, D.; Peda, B.; Palma, J.; Zembroń-Łacny, A.; Gołąb-Janowska, M.; Masztalewicz, M.; Nowacki, P.; Szczuko, M. Free Fatty Acids Are Associated with the Cognitive Functions in Stroke Survivors. *Int. J. Environ. Res. Public Health* **2021**, *18*, 6500. [CrossRef]
6. Jarosz, M.; Rychlk, E.; Stoś, K.; Charzewska, J. *Norms of Human Nutrition and Their Application for the Polish Population*; National Institute of Public Health National Institute of Hygiene: Warsaw, Poland, 2020.
7. Santos, H.O.; Price, J.C.; Bueno, A.A. Beyond Fish Oil Supplementation: The Effects of Alternative Plant Sources of Omega-3 Polyunsaturated Fatty Acids upon Lipid Indexes and Cardiometabolic Biomarkers—An Overview. *Nutrients* **2020**, *12*, 3159. [CrossRef]
8. Jain, A.P.; Aggarwal, K.K.; Zhang, P.Y. Omega-3 fatty acids and cardiovascular disease. *Eur. Rev. Med. Pharmacol. Sci.* **2015**, *19*, 441–445.
9. Veselinovic, M.; Vasiljevic, D.; Vucic, V.; Arsic, A.; Petrovic, S.; Tomic-Lucic, A.; Savic, M.; Zivanovic, S.; Stojic, V.; Jakovljevic, V. Clinical Benefits of n-3 PUFA and ɤ-Linolenic Acid in Patients with Rheumatoid Arthritis. *Nutrients* **2017**, *9*, 325. [CrossRef]
10. Ge, L.; Sadeghirad, B.; Ball, G.D.C.; Da Costa, B.R.; Hitchcock, C.L.; Svendrovski, A.; Kiflen, R.; Quadri, K.; Kwon, H.Y.; Karamouzian, M.; et al. Comparison of dietary macronutrient patterns of 14 popular named dietary programmes for weight and cardiovascular risk factor reduction in adults: Systematic review and network meta-analysis of randomised trials. *BMJ* **2020**, *369*, m696. [CrossRef]

11. Ditano-Vázquez, P.; Torres-Peña, J.D.; Galeano-Valle, F.; Pérez-Caballero, A.I.; Demelo-Rodríguez, P.; Lopez-Miranda, J.; Katsiki, N.; Delgado-Lista, J.; Alvarez-Sala-Walther, L.A. The Fluid Aspect of the Mediterranean Diet in the Prevention and Management of Cardiovascular Disease and Diabetes: The Role of Polyphenol Content in Moderate Consumption of Wine and Olive Oil. *Nutrients* **2019**, *11*, 2833. [CrossRef]
12. Trautwein, E.A.; McKay, S. The Role of Specific Components of a Plant-Based Diet in Management of Dyslipidemia and the Impact on Cardiovascular Risk. *Nutrients* **2020**, *12*, 2671. [CrossRef] [PubMed]
13. Siri-Tarino, P.W.; Krauss, R.M. Diet, lipids, and cardiovascular disease. *Curr. Opin. Infect. Dis.* **2016**, *27*, 323–328. [CrossRef] [PubMed]
14. Riegel, B.; Moser, D.K.; Buck, H.G.; Dickson, V.V.; Dunbar, S.B.; Lee, C.S.; Lennie, T.A.; Lindenfeld, J.; Mitchell, J.E.; Treat-Jacobson, D.J.; et al. Self-care for the prevention and management of cardiovascular disease and stroke: A scientific statement for healthcare professionals from the American Heart Association. *J. Am. Heart Assoc.* **2017**, *6*, e006997. [CrossRef] [PubMed]
15. Neto-Neves, E.M.; da Silva Maia Bezerra Filho, C.; Dejani, N.N.; de Sousa, D.P. Ferulic Acid and Cardiovascular Health: Therapeutic and Preventive Potential. *Mini-Rev. Med. Chem.* **2021**, *21*, 1625–1637. [CrossRef] [PubMed]
16. Oppedisano, F.; Mollace, R.; Tavernese, A.; Gliozzi, M.; Musolino, V.; Macrì, R.; Carresi, C.; Maiuolo, J.; Serra, M.; Cardamone, A.; et al. PUFA Supplementation and Heart Failure: Effects on Fibrosis and Cardiac Remodeling. *Nutrients* **2021**, *13*, 2965. [CrossRef]
17. Innes, J.K.; Calder, P.C. Marine Omega-3 (N-3) Fatty Acids for Cardiovascular Health: An Update for 2020. *Int. J. Mol. Sci.* **2020**, *21*, 1362. [CrossRef]
18. Russo, G.L. Dietary n−6 and n−3 polyunsaturated fatty acids: From biochemistry to clinical implications in cardiovascular prevention. *Biochem. Pharmacol.* **2009**, *77*, 937–946. [CrossRef]
19. Sunagawa, Y.; Katayama, A.; Funamoto, M.; Shimizu, K.; Shimizu, S.; Sari, N.; Katanasaka, Y.; Miyazaki, Y.; Hosomi, R.; Hasegawa, K.; et al. The polyunsaturated fatty acids, EPA and DHA, ameliorate myocardial infarction-induced heart failure by inhibiting p300-HAT activity in rats. *J. Nutr. Biochem.* **2022**, *106*, 109031. [CrossRef]
20. Anil, E. The impact of EPA and DHA on blood lipids and lipoprotein metabolism: Influence of apoE genotype. *Proc. Nutr. Soc.* **2007**, *66*, 60–68. [CrossRef]
21. Harris, W.S.; Jackson, K.H.; Brenna, J.T.; Rodriguez, J.C.; Tintle, N.L.; Cornish, L. Survey of the erythrocyte EPA+DHA levels in the heart attack/stroke belt. *Prostaglandins Leukot. Essent. Fat. Acids* **2019**, *148*, 30–34. [CrossRef]
22. Yin, F.; Sun, X.; Zheng, W.; Luo, X.; Zhang, Y.; Yin, L.; Jia, Q.; Fu, Y. Screening of highly effective mixed natural antioxidants to improve the oxidative stability of microalgal DHA-rich oil. *RSC Adv.* **2021**, *11*, 4991–4999. [CrossRef] [PubMed]
23. Saini, R.K.; Prasad, P.; Sreedhar, R.V.; Naidu, K.A.; Shang, X.; Keum, Y.-S. Omega−3 Polyunsaturated Fatty Acids (PUFAs): Emerging Plant and Microbial Sources, Oxidative Stability, Bioavailability, and Health Benefits—A Review. *Antioxidants* **2021**, *10*, 1627. [CrossRef] [PubMed]
24. Kocot, J.; Kiełczykowska, M.; Luchowska-Kocot, D.; Kurzepa, J.; Musik, I. Antioxidant Potential of Propolis, Bee Pollen, and Royal Jelly: Possible Medical Application. *Oxid. Med. Cell. Longev.* **2018**, *2018*, 7074209. [CrossRef] [PubMed]
25. Rodríguez, M.; Rebollar, P.G.; Mattioli, S.; Castellini, C. n-3 PUFA Sources (Precursor/Products): A Review of Current Knowledge on Rabbit. *Animals* **2019**, *9*, 806. [CrossRef] [PubMed]
26. Rogerson, D. Vegan diets: Practical advice for athletes and exercisers. *J. Int. Soc. Sports Nutr.* **2017**, *14*, 36. [CrossRef] [PubMed]
27. Alsenani, F.; Tupally, K.R.; Chua, E.T.; Eltanahy, E.; Alsufyani, H.; Parekh, H.S.; Schenk, P.M. Evaluation of microalgae and cyanobacteria as potential sources of antimicrobial compounds. *Saudi Pharm. J.* **2020**, *28*, 1834–1841. [CrossRef]
28. Skulas-Ray, A.C.; Wilson, P.; Harris, W.S.; Brinton, E.A.; Kris-Etherton, P.M.; Richter, C.K.; Jacobson, T.A.; Engler, M.B.; Miller, M.; Robinson, J.G.; et al. Omega-3 Fatty Acids for the Management of Hypertriglyceridemia: A Science Advisory from the American Heart Association. *Circulation* **2019**, *140*, e673–e691. [CrossRef]
29. Lee, J.H.; O-Keefe, J.H.; Lavie, C.J.; Marchioli, R.; Harris, W.S. Omega-3 Fatty Acids for Cardioprotection. *Mayo Clin. Proc.* **2008**, *83*, 324–332. [CrossRef]
30. van der Meer, P.; Gaggin, H.K.; Dec, G.W. ACC/AHA Versus ESC Guidelines on Heart Failure: A JACC Guideline Comparison. *J. Am. Coll. Cardiol.* **2019**, *73*, 2756–2768. [CrossRef]
31. Visseren, F.; Mach, F.; Smulders, Y.M.; Carballo, D.; Koskinas, K.C.; Bäck, M.; Benetos, A.; Biffi, A.; Boavida, J.-M.; Capodanno, D.; et al. ESC Guidelines on cardiovascular disease prevention in clinical practice. *Eur. Heart J.* **2021**, *42*, 3227–3337. [CrossRef]
32. Schröder, H.; Marrugat, J.; Vila, J.; Covas, M.I.; Elosua, R. Adherence to the Traditional Mediterranean Diet Is Inversely Associated with Body Mass Index and Obesity in a Spanish Population. *J. Nutr.* **2004**, *134*, 3355–3361. [CrossRef] [PubMed]
33. Gajewska, D.; Pałkowska-Goździk, E.; Lange, E.; Niegowska, J.; Paśko, P.; Kościołek, A.; Fibich, K.; Gudej, S. Standardy postępowania dietetycznego w kardiologii u osób dorosłych. Stanowisko Polskiego Towarzystwa Dietetyki 2016. *Dietetyka* **2016**, *9*.
34. Timmis, A.; Roobottom, C.A. National Institute for Health and Care Excellence updates the stable chest pain guideline with radical changes to the diagnostic paradigm. *Heart* **2017**, *103*, 982–986. [CrossRef] [PubMed]
35. Colson, C.; Ghandour, R.A.; Dufies, O.; Rekima, S.; Loubat, A.; Munro, P.; Boyer, L.; Pisani, D.F. Diet Supplementation in ω3 Polyunsaturated Fatty Acid Favors an Anti-Inflammatory Basal Environment in Mouse Adipose Tissue. *Nutrients* **2019**, *11*, 438. [CrossRef]
36. Ros, E. The PREDIMED study. *Endocrinol. Diabetes Nutr.* **2017**, *64*, 63–66. [CrossRef]

37. Amiri, M.; Raeisi-Dehkordi, H.; Sarrafzadegan, N.; Forbes, S.C.; Salehi-Abargouei, A. The effects of Canola oil on cardiovascular risk factors: A systematic review and meta-analysis with dose-response analysis of controlled clinical trials. *Nutr. Metab. Cardiovasc. Dis. NMCD* **2020**, *30*, 2133–2145. [CrossRef]
38. Feingold, K.R. The Effect of Diet on Cardiovascular Disease and Lipid and Lipoprotein Levels. In *Endotext [Internet]*; Feingold, K.R., Anawalt, B., Boyce, A., Eds.; MDText.com, Inc.: South Dartmouth, MA, USA, 2021. Available online: https://www.ncbi.nlm.nih.gov/books/NBK570127/ (accessed on 25 October 2022).
39. Węgorowski, P.; Michalik, J.; Zarzeczny, R.; Domżał-Drzewiecka, R.; Nowicki, G. Health behavior of patients with ischemic heart disease. *J. Educ. Health Sport* **2017**, *7*, 660–670.
40. Babiarczyk, B.; Małutowska-Dudek, B. Assessment of health behaviors undertaken by inpatients and outpatients with hypertension. *Pol. Rev. Health Sci.* **2016**, *1*, 29–35.
41. Schneider-Matyka, D.; Szkup, M.; Owczarek, A.J.; Stanisławska, M.; Knyszyńska, A.; Lubkowska, A.; Grochans, E.; Jurczak, A. The Relationship between the IFNG (rs2430561) Polymorphism and Metabolic Syndrome in Perimenopausal Women. *Medicina* **2020**, *56*, 384. [CrossRef]
42. Michalski, P.; Kosobucka, A.; Nowik, M.; Pietrzykowski, Ł.; Andruszkiewicz, A.; Kubica, A. Health education of patients with cardiovascular diseases. *Folia Cardiol.* **2016**, *11*, 519–524. [CrossRef]
43. Kubica, A.; Kochman, W.; Bogdan, M. Impact of history of coronary angioplasty and hospitalization for myocardial in-farction on knowledge and effectiveness of health education in patients with acute myocardial infarction. *Adv. Interv. Cardiol.* **2009**, *5*, 25–30.

MDPI AG
Grosspeteranlage 5
4052 Basel
Switzerland
Tel.: +41 61 683 77 34

Nursing Reports Editorial Office
E-mail: nursrep@mdpi.com
www.mdpi.com/journal/nursrep

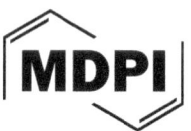

Disclaimer/Publisher's Note: The title and front matter of this reprint are at the discretion of the Guest Editors. The publisher is not responsible for their content or any associated concerns. The statements, opinions and data contained in all individual articles are solely those of the individual Editors and contributors and not of MDPI. MDPI disclaims responsibility for any injury to people or property resulting from any ideas, methods, instructions or products referred to in the content.